The Year in Cognitive Neuroscience 2008

EDITORIAL ADVISORY BOARD

Ralph Adolphs
Pasadena, California

Michael C. Corballis
Auckland, New Zealand

Michael Gazzaniga
Santa Barbara, California

Mel Goodale
London, Ontario, Canada

Scott T. Grafton
Santa Barbara, California

Glyn Humphreys
Birmingham, United Kingdom

Elisabetta Làdavas
Emilia-Romagna, Italy

Adrian M. Owen
Cambridge, United Kingdom

Elizabeth Phelps
New York, New York

Daniel Schachter
Cambridge, Massachusetts

ANNALS OF THE NEW YORK ACADEMY OF SCIENCES
Volume 1124

The Year in Cognitive Neuroscience 2008

Edited by
ALAN KINGSTONE AND MICHAEL B. MILLER

Published by Blackwell Publishing on behalf of the New York Academy of Sciences
Boston, Massachusetts
2008

Library of Congress Cataloging-in-Publication Data

The year in cognitive neuroscience 2008/[edited by] Alan Kingstone and Michael Miller.
    p. cm. – (Annals of the New York Academy of Sciences, ISSN 0077-8923)
   ISBN-13: 978-1-57331-726-9
   ISBN-10: 1-57331-726-8
   1. Cognitive neuroscience. I. Kingstone, Alan. II. Miller, Michael B. III. New York Academy of Sciences.

QP360.5.Y43 2008
612.8'233–dc22

2007051876

The *Annals of the New York Academy of Sciences* (ISSN: 0077-8923 [print]; ISSN: 1749-6632 [online]) is published 28 times a year on behalf of the New York Academy of Sciences by Blackwell Publishing with offices at (US) 350 Main St., Malden, MA 02148-5020, (UK) 9600 Garsington Road, Oxford, OX4 2ZG, and (Asia) 165 Cremorne St., Richmond VIC 3121, Australia. Blackwell Publishing was acquired by John Wiley & Sons in February 2007. Blackwell's program has been merged with Wiley's global Scientific, Technical, and Medical business to form Wiley-Blackwell.

MAILING: *Annals* is mailed Standard Rate. Mailing to rest of world by IMEX (International Mail Express). Canadian mail is sent by Canadian publications mail agreement number 40573520. POSTMASTER: Send all address changes to *Annals of the New York Academy of Sciences*, Blackwell Publishing Inc., Journals Subscription Department, 350 Main St., Malden, MA 02148-5020.

Disclaimer: The Publisher, the New York Academy of Sciences and Editors cannot be held responsible for errors or any consequences arising from the use of information contained in this publication; the views and opinions expressed do not necessarily reflect those of the Publisher, the New York Academy of Sciences and Editors.

Copyright and Photocopying: © 2008 New York Academy of Sciences. All rights reserved. No part of this publication may be reproduced, stored or transmitted in any form or by any means without the prior permission in writing from the copyright holder. Authorization to photocopy items for internal and personal use is granted by the copyright holder for libraries and other users registered with their local Reproduction Rights Organization (RRO), e.g. Copyright Clearance Center (CCC), 222 Rosewood Drive, Danvers, MA 01923, USA (www.copyright.com), provided the appropriate fee is paid directly to the RRO. This consent does not extend to other kinds of copying such as copying for general distribution, for advertising or promotional purposes, for creating new collective works or for resale. Special requests should be addressed to: journalsrights@oxon.blackwellpublishing.com

Blackwell Publishing is now part of Wiley-Blackwell.

Information for subscribers: For ordering information, claims, and any inquiry concerning your subscription please contact your nearest office:

UK: Tel: +44 (0)1865 778315; Fax: +44 (0) 1865 471775
USA: Tel: +1 781 388 8599 or 1 800 835 6770 (toll free in the USA & Canada); Fax: +1 781 388 8232 or Fax: +44 (0) 1865 471775
Asia: Tel: +65 6511 8000; Fax: +44 (0)1865 471775,
Email: customerservices@blackwellpublishing.com

Subscription prices for 2008 are: Premium Institutional: US$4265 (The Americas), £2370 (Rest of World). Customers in the UK should add VAT at 7%; customers in the EU should also add VAT at 7%, or provide a VAT registration number or evidence of entitlement to exemption. Customers in Canada should add 5% GST or provide evidence of entitlement to exemption. The Premium institutional price also includes online access to the current and all online back files to January 1, 1997, where available. For other pricing options, including access information and terms and conditions, please visit www.blackwellpublishing.com/nyas.

Delivery Terms and Legal Title: Prices include delivery of print publications to the recipient's address. Delivery terms are Delivered Duty Unpaid (DDU); the recipient is responsible for paying any import duty or taxes. Legal title passes to the customer on despatch by our distributors.

Membership information: Members may order copies of *Annals* volumes directly from the Academy by visiting www.nyas.org/annals, emailing membership@nyas.org, faxing +1 212 298 3650, or calling 1 800 843 6927 (toll free in the USA), or +1 212 298 8640. For more information on becoming a member of the New York Academy of Sciences, please visit www.nyas.org/membership. Claims and inquiries on member orders should be directed to the Academy at email: membership@nyas.org or Tel: 1 800 843 6927 (toll free in the USA) or +1 212 298 8640.

Printed in the USA. Printed on acid-free paper.

Annals is available to subscribers online at Blackwell Synergy and the New York Academy of Sciences Web site. Visit www.blackwell-synergy.com or www.annalsnyas.org to search the articles and register for table of contents e-mail alerts.

The paper used in this publication meets the minimum requirements of the National Standard for Information Sciences Permanence of Paper for Printed Library Materials, ANSI Z39.48 1984.

ISSN: 0077-8923 (print); 1749-6632 (online)
ISBN-10: 1-57331-726-8 (paper); ISBN-13: 978-1-57331-726-9 (paper)

A catalogue record for this title is available from the British Library.

ANNALS OF THE NEW YORK ACADEMY OF SCIENCES

Volume 1124
March 2008

The Year in Cognitive Neuroscience 2008

Editors
ALAN KINGSTONE AND MICHAEL B. MILLER

CONTENTS

Preface. *By* Alan Kingstone and Michael B. Miller	ix
The Brain's Default Network: Anatomy, Function, and Relevance to Disease. *By* Randy L. Buckner, Jessica R. Andrews-Hanna, and Daniel L. Schacter	1
Episodic Simulation of Future Events: Concepts, Data, and Applications. *By* Daniel L. Schacter, Donna Rose Addis, and Randy L. Buckner	39
Generalization and Differentiation in Semantic Memory: Insights from Semantic Dementia. *By* Matthew A. Lambon Ralph and Karalyn Patterson	61
Spatial Cognition and the Brain. *By* Neil Burgess	77
Multisensory-based Approach to the Recovery of Unisensory Deficit. *By* Elisabetta Làdavas	98
The Adolescent Brain. *By* B.J. Casey, Rebecca M. Jones, and Todd A. Hare	111
Cognitive Neuroscience of Aging. *By* Cheryl L. Grady	127
Can Neurological Evidence Help Courts Assess Criminal Responsibility? Lessons from Law and Neuroscience. *By* Eyal Aharoni, Chadd Funk, Walter Sinnott-Armstrong, and Michael Gazzaniga	145
The Neural Basis of Moral Cognition: Sentiments, Concepts, and Values. *By* Jorge Moll, Ricardo de Oliveira-Souza, and Roland Zahn	161
Intention, Choice, and the Medial Frontal Cortex. *By* Matthew F.S. Rushworth	181
Evaluating Faces on Trustworthiness: An Extension of Systems for Recognition of Emotions Signaling Approach/Avoidance Behaviors. *By* Alexander Todorov	208
Disorders of Consciousness. *By* Adrian M. Owen	225
The Neural Correlates of Consciousness: An Update. *By* Giulio Tononi and Christof Koch	239

Index of Contributors 263

> The New York Academy of Sciences believes it has a responsibility to provide an open forum for discussion of scientific questions. The positions taken by the participants in the reported conferences are their own and not necessarily those of the Academy. The Academy has no intent to influence legislation by providing such forums.

Preface

Welcome to the inaugural volume of *The Year in Cognitive Neuroscience!* It was in March 2007 that we first discussed the idea of editing this peer-reviewed annual review series. Our goal was simple and straightforward—to bring together each year the very best minds in cognitive neuroscience so that they could put forward and review the cutting-edge ideas and issues in the field. A new peer-reviewed volume will be published this time each year, and we expect that it will be a must-read annual review for new and established scientists in the field alike.

The birth of cognitive neuroscience has enabled scientists to come together in their shared enterprise to study the neural basis of cognition across a broad range of traditional domains of research, such as memory, attention, and executive control. As our field has grown, we have moved from studying issues that are specific to cognitive domains to investigating complex issues that cut across traditional domains and that are foundational to science and society. This new annual review, *The Year in Cognitive Neuroscience*, reflects this development within our exciting field. Each of the reviews in this first volume exemplifies an issue-based approach that now defines and fuels cognitive neuroscience, ranging from studies of the brain's default network (Randy Buckner), to investigations of the adolescent brain (B.J. Casey), to matters regarding awareness in the vegetative state (Adrian Owen).

As is always the case with any substantial enterprise, there are many people who have played critical roles in its success. Michael Gazzaniga strongly encouraged us to edit *The Year in Cognitive Neuroscience*. He and our editorial advisory board have contributed greatly to our vision for this series. Kirk Jensen, executive editor of the *Annals of the New York Academy of Sciences*, deserves our most sincere appreciation for his support of our venture. The willingness of these individuals to commit to this initiative is a great testimony to the fact that the time was right for an annual review in cognitive neuroscience. We are also grateful to the referees, who are listed in this publication, for providing their well-considered suggestions and peer commentaries. Finally, and most importantly, we would like to acknowledge the world-class authors who invested a great deal of time and effort to make this annual review an outstanding success.

The Year in Cognitive Neuroscience is published as part of the *Annals of the New York Academy of Sciences*, which is one of the oldest scientific series in the United States and among the most cited of multidisciplinary scientific serials. We are proud and excited to be editors of this new publication and trust that you will find its stimulating articles to be essential reading now and in the years to come.

ALAN KINGSTONE
Department of Psychology
University of British Columbia
Vancouver, British Columbia, Canada

MICHAEL B. MILLER
Department of Psychology
University of California
Santa Barbara, California

List of Reviewers

Jason Barton, University of British Columbia
Kathy Baynes, University of California, Davis
James Bjork, National Institutes of Health
Sarah-Jayne Blakemore, University College London
Kalina Christoff, University of British Columbia
Michael C. Corballis, University of Auckland
Paul Corballis, Georgia Institute of Technology
Mike Dodd, University of Nebraska
Stan Floresco, University of British Columbia
Bill Gehring, University of Michigan
Scott T. Grafton, University of California, Santa Barbara
Scott Guerin, University of California, Santa Barbara
Todd Handy, University of British Columbia
Mary Hegarty, University of California, Santa Barbara
Kent A. Kiehl, University of New Mexico
Stan B. Klein, University of California, Santa Barbara
Neil Macrae, University of Aberdeen
Jason P. Mitchell, Harvard University
Paul Nestor, University of Massachusetts Boston
Lars Nyberg, Umeå University
Lynn Robertson, University of California, Berkeley
Serge Rombouts, Leiden University
Scott Sinnett, University of British Columbia
Walter Sinnott-Armstrong, Dartmouth College
Jonathan Smallwood, University of Aberdeen
Salva Soto, University of Barcelona
Thomas Wolbers, University of California, Santa Barbara

The Brain's Default Network
Anatomy, Function, and Relevance to Disease

RANDY L. BUCKNER,[a,b,c,d,e] JESSICA R. ANDREWS-HANNA,[a,b,c] AND DANIEL L. SCHACTER[a]

[a]*Department of Psychology, Harvard University, Cambridge, Massachusetts, USA*

[b]*Center for Brain Science, Harvard University, Cambridge, Massachusetts, USA*

[c]*Athinoula A. Martinos Center for Biomedical Imaging, Massachusetts General Hospital, Boston, Massachusetts, USA*

[d]*Department of Radiology, Harvard Medical School, Boston, Massachusetts, USA*

[e]*Howard Hughes Medical Institute, Chevy Chase, Maryland 20815, USA*

Thirty years of brain imaging research has converged to define the brain's default network—a novel and only recently appreciated brain system that participates in internal modes of cognition. Here we synthesize past observations to provide strong evidence that the default network is a specific, anatomically defined brain system preferentially active when individuals are not focused on the external environment. Analysis of connectional anatomy in the monkey supports the presence of an interconnected brain system. Providing insight into function, the default network is active when individuals are engaged in internally focused tasks including autobiographical memory retrieval, envisioning the future, and conceiving the perspectives of others. Probing the functional anatomy of the network in detail reveals that it is best understood as multiple interacting subsystems. The medial temporal lobe subsystem provides information from prior experiences in the form of memories and associations that are the building blocks of mental simulation. The medial prefrontal subsystem facilitates the flexible use of this information during the construction of self-relevant mental simulations. These two subsystems converge on important nodes of integration including the posterior cingulate cortex. The implications of these functional and anatomical observations are discussed in relation to possible adaptive roles of the default network for using past experiences to plan for the future, navigate social interactions, and maximize the utility of moments when we are not otherwise engaged by the external world. We conclude by discussing the relevance of the default network for understanding mental disorders including autism, schizophrenia, and Alzheimer's disease.

Key words: default mode; default system; default network; fMRI; PET; hippocampus; memory; schizophrenia; Alzheimer

Introduction

A common observation in brain imaging research is that a specific set of brain regions—referred to as the default network—is engaged when individuals are left to think to themselves undisturbed (Shulman et al. 1997, Mazoyer et al. 2001, Raichle et al. 2001). Probing this phenomenon further reveals that other kinds of situations, beyond freethinking, engage the default network. For example, remembering the past, envisioning future events, and considering the thoughts and perspectives of other people all activate multiple regions within the default network (Buckner & Carroll 2007). These observations prompt one to ask such questions as: What do these tasks and spontaneous cognition share in common? and what is the significance of this network to adaptive function? The default network is also disrupted in autism, schizophrenia, and Alzheimer's disease, further encouraging one to consider how the functions of the default network might be important to understanding diseases of the mind (e.g., Lustig et al. 2003, Greicius et al. 2004, Kennedy et al. 2006, Bluhm et al. 2007).

Motivated by these questions, we provide a comprehensive review and synthesis of findings about the

Address for correspondence: Dr. Randy Buckner, Harvard University, William James Hall, 33 Kirkland Drive, Cambridge, MA 02148. rbuckner@wjh.harvard.edu brain's default network. This review covers both basic science and clinical observations, with its content organized across five sections. We begin with a brief history of our understanding of the default network (section I). Next, a detailed analysis of the anatomy of the default network is provided including evidence from humans and monkeys (section II). The following sections concern the role of the default network in spontaneous cognition, as commonly occurs in passive task settings (section III), as well as its functions in active task settings (section IV). While recognizing alternative possibilities, we hypothesize that the fundamental function of the default network is to facilitate flexible self-relevant mental explorations—simulations—that provide a means to anticipate and evaluate upcoming events before they happen. The final section of the review discusses emerging evidence that relates the default network to cognitive disorders, including the possibility that activity in the default network augments a metabolic cascade that is conducive to the development of Alzheimer's disease (section V).

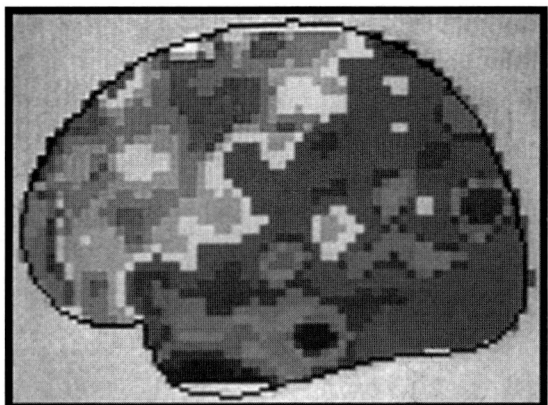

FIGURE 1. An early image of regional cerebral blood flow (rCBF) at rest made by David Ingvar and colleagues using the nitrous oxide technique. The image shows data averaged over eight individuals to reveal a "hyperfrontal" activity pattern that Ingvar proposed reflected "spontaneous, conscious mentation" (Ingvar 1979). Ingvar's ideas anticipate many of the themes discussed in this review (see Ingvar 1974, 1979, 1985).

I. A Brief History

The discovery of the brain's default network was entirely accidental. Evidence for the default network began accumulating when researchers first measured brain activity in humans during undirected mental states. Even though no early studies were explicitly designed to explore such unconstrained states, relevant data were nonetheless acquired because of the common practice of using rest or other types of passive conditions as an experimental control. These studies revealed that activity in specific brain regions increased during passive control states as compared to most goal-directed tasks. In almost all cases, the exploration of activity during the control states occurred as an afterthought—as part of reviews and meta-analyses performed subsequent to the original reports, which focused on the goal-directed tasks.

Early Observations

A clue that brain activity persists during undirected mentation emerged from early studies of cerebral metabolism. It was already known by the late 19th century that mental activity modulated local blood flow (James 1890). Louis Sokoloff and colleagues (1955) used the Kety-Schmidt nitrous oxide technique (Kety & Schmidt 1948) to ask whether cerebral metabolism changes globally when one goes from a quiet rest state to performing a challenging arithmetic problem—a task that demands focused cognitive effort. To their surprise, metabolism remained constant. While not their initial conclusion, the unchanged global rate of metabolism suggests that the rest state contains persistent brain activity that is as vigorous as that when individuals solve externally administered math problems.

The Swedish brain physiologist David Ingvar was the first to aggregate imaging findings from rest task states and note the importance of consistent, regionally specific activity patterns (Ingvar 1974, 1979, 1985). Using the xenon 133 inhalation technique to measure regional cerebral blood flow (rCBF), Ingvar and his colleagues observed that frontal activity reached high levels during rest states (FIG. 1). To explain this unexpected phenomenon, Ingvar proposed that the "hyperfrontal" pattern of activity corresponded "to undirected, spontaneous, conscious mentation, the 'brain work,' which we carry out when left alone undisturbed" (Ingvar 1974). Two lasting insights emerged from Ingvar's work. First, echoing ideas of Hans Berger (1931), his work established that the brain is not idle when left undirected. Rather, brain activity persists in the absence of external task direction. Second, Ingvar's observations suggested that increased activity during rest is localized to specific brain regions that prominently include prefrontal cortex.

The Era of Task-Induced Deactivation

Ingvar's ideas about resting brain activity remained largely unexplored for the next decade until positron emission tomography (PET) methods for brain imaging gained prominence. PET had finer resolution and sensitivity to deep-brain structures than earlier methods and, owing to the development of isotopes with short half-lives (Raichle 1987), typical PET studies included many task and control conditions for comparison. By the mid-1990s several dozen imaging studies were completed that examined perception, language, attention, and memory. Scans of rest-state brain activity[a] were often acquired across these studies for a control comparison, and researchers began routinely noticing brain regions more active in the passive control conditions than the active target tasks—what at the time was referred to as "deactivation."

The term "deactivation" was used because analyses and image visualization were referenced to the target, experimental task. Within this nomenclature, regions *relatively* more active in the target condition (e.g., reading, classifying pictures) compared to the control task (e.g., passive fixation, rest) were labeled "activations"; regions less active in the target condition than the control were labeled "deactivations." Deactivations were present and often the most robust effect in many early PET studies. One form of deactivation for which early interest emerged was activity reductions in unattended sensory modalities because of its theoretical relevance to mechanisms of attention (e.g., Haxby et al. 1994, Kawashima et al. 1994, Buckner et al. 1996). A second form of commonly observed deactivation was along the frontal and posterior midline during active, as compared to passive, task conditions. There was no initial explanation for these mysterious midline deactivations (e.g., Ghatan et al. 1995, Baker et al. 1996).

A particularly informative early study was conducted while exploring brain regions supporting episodic memory. Confronted with the difficult issue of defining a baseline state for an autobiographical memory task, Andreasen and colleagues (1995) explored the possibility that spontaneous cognition makes an important contribution to rest states. Much like other studies at the time, the researchers included a rest condition as a baseline for comparison to their target conditions. However, unlike other contemporary studies, they hypothesized that autobiographical memory (the experimental target of the study) inherently involves internally directed cognition, much like the spontaneous cognition that occurs during "rest" states. For this reason, Andreasen and colleagues explored both the rest and memory tasks referenced to a third control condition that involved neither rest nor episodic memory. Their results showed that similar brain regions were engaged during rest and memory as compared to the nonmemory control. In addition, to better understand the cognitive processes associated with the rest state, they informally asked their participants to subjectively describe their mental experiences.

Two insights originated from this work that foreshadow much of the present review's content. First, Andreasen et al. (1995) noted that the resting state "is in fact quite vigorous and consists of a mixture of freely wandering past recollection, future plans, and other personal thoughts and experiences." Second, the analysis of brain activity during the rest state revealed prefrontal midline regions as well as a distinct posterior pattern that included the posterior cingulate and retrosplenial cortex. As later studies would confirm, these regions are central components of the core brain system that is consistently activated in humans during undirected mental states.

Broad awareness of the common regions that become active during passive task states emerged with a pair of meta-analyses that pooled extensive data to reveal the functional anatomy of unconstrained cognition. In the first study, Shulman and colleagues (1997) conducted meta-analysis of task-induced deactivations to explicitly determine if there were common brain regions active during undirected (passive) mental states. They pooled data from 132 normal adults for which an active task (word reading, active stimulus classification, etc.) could be directly compared to a passive task that presented the same visual words or pictures but contained no directed task goals. Using a similar approach, Mazoyer et al. (2001) aggregated data across 63 normal adults that included both visually and aurally cued active tasks as compared to passive rest conditions.

These two analyses revealed a remarkably consistent set of brain regions that were more active during passive task conditions than during numerous goal-directed task conditions (spanning both verbal and nonverbal domains and visual and auditory conditions). The results of the Shulman et al. (1997) meta-analysis are shown in FIGURE 2. This image displays the full cortical extent of the brain's default network. The broad generality of the rest activity pattern across so many diverse studies reinforced the intriguing possibility that a common set of cognitive processes was used spontaneously during the passive-task states. Motivated by this idea, Mazoyer et al. (2001) explored the content of spontaneous thought by asking participants to describe their musings following the scanned rest periods. Paralleling the informal observations by

---

[a]PET and functional MRI (fMRI) both measure neural activity indirectly through local vascular (blood flow) changes that accompany neuronal activity. PET is sensitive to changes in blood flow directly (Raichle 1987). fMRI is sensitive to changes in oxygen concentration in the blood which tracks blood flow (Heeger and Ress 2002). For simplicity, we refer to these methods as measuring brain activity in this review.

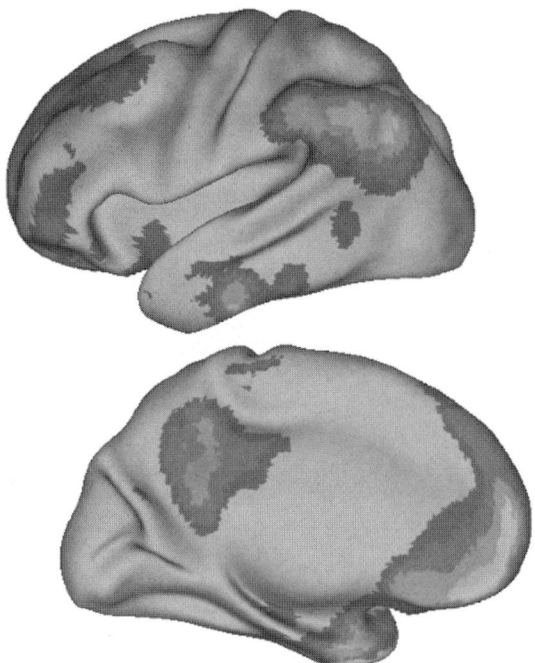

FIGURE 2. The brain's default network was originally identified in a meta-analysis that mapped brain regions more active in passive as compared to active tasks (often referred to as task-induced deactivation). The displayed positron emission tomography (PET) data include nine studies (132 participants) from Shulman et al. (1997; reanalyzed in Buckner et al. 2005). Images show the medial and lateral surface of the left hemisphere using a population-averaged surface representation to take into account between-subject variability in sulcal anatomy (Van Essen 2005). Blue represents regions most active in passive task settings.

Ingvar and Andreasen et al., they noted that the imaged rest state is associated with lively mental activity that includes "generation and manipulation of mental images, reminiscence of past experiences based on episodic memory, and making plans" and further noted that the subjects of their study "preferentially reported autobiographical episodes."

Emergence of the Default Network as Its Own Research Area

The definitive recent event in the explication of the default network came with the a series of publications by Raichle, Gusnard, and colleagues (Raichle et al. 2001, Gusnard & Raichle 2001, Gusnard et al. 2001). A dominant theme in the field during the previous decade concerned how to define an appropriate baseline condition for neuroimaging studies. This focus on the baseline state was central to the evolving concept of a default network. Many argued that passive conditions were simply too unconstrained to be useful as control states. Richard Frackowiak summarized this widely held concern: "To call a 'free-wheeling' state, or even a state where you are fixating on a cross and dreaming about anything you like, a 'control' state, is to my mind quite wrong" (Frackowiak 1991). (For recent discussion of this ongoing debate see Morcom and Fletcher 2007, Buckner & Vincent 2007, Raichle & Snyder 2007). As a result of this uneasiness in interpreting passive task conditions, beyond the few earlier studies mentioned, there was a general trend not to thoroughly report or discuss the meaning of rest state activity.

Raichle, Gusnard, and colleagues reversed this trend dramatically with three papers in 2001 (Raichle et al. 2001, Gusnard & Raichle 2001, Gusnard et al. 2001). Their papers directly considered the empirical and theoretical implications of defining baseline states and what the specific pattern of activity in the default network might represent. Several lasting consequences on the study of the default network emerged. First, they distinguished between various forms of task-induced deactivation and separated deactivations defining the default network from other forms of deactivation (including attenuation of activity in unattended sensory areas). Second, they compiled a considerable array of findings that drew attention to the specific anatomic regions linked to the default network and what their presence might suggest about its function. A key insight was that the medial prefrontal regions consistently identified as part of the default network are associated with self-referential processing (Gusnard et al. 2001, Gusnard & Raichle 2001). Most importantly, the papers brought to the forefront the exploration of the default network as its own area of study (including providing its name, which, as of late 2007, has appeared as a keyword in 237 articles). Our use of the label "default network" in this review stems directly from their labeling the baseline rest condition as the "default mode."[b] Their reviews made clear that the default network is to be studied as a fundamental neurobiological system with physiological and cognitive properties that distinguish it from other systems.

The default network is a brain system much like the motor system or the visual system. It contains a set of interacting brain areas that are tightly functionally

---

[b]References to the default mode appear in the literature on cognition prior to the introduction of the concept as an explanation for neural and metabolic phenomena. Giambra (1995), for example, noted that "Task-unrelated images and thoughts may represent the normal default mode of operation of the self-aware." Thus, the concept of a default mode is converged upon from both cognitive and neurobiological perspectives.

TABLE 1. Core regions associated with the brain's default network

REGION	ABREV	INCLUDED BRAIN AREAS
Ventral medial prefrontal cortex	vMPFC	24, 10m/10r/10p, 32ac
Posterior cingulate/retosplenial cortex	PCC/Rsp	29/30, 23/31
Inferior parietal lobule	IPL	39, 40
Lateral temporal cortex†	LTC	21
Dorsal medial prefrontal cortex	dMPFC	24, 32ac, 10p, 9
Hippocampal formation††	HF+	Hippocampus proper, EC, PH

Notes: Region, abbreviation, and approximate area labels for the core regions associated with the default network in humans. Labels correspond to those originally used by Brodmann for humans with updates by Petrides and Pandya (1994), Vogt et al. (1995), Morris et al. (2000), and Öngür et al. (2003). Labels should be considered approximate because of the uncertain boundaries of the areas and the activation patterns. †LTC is particularly poorly characterized in humans and is therefore the most tentative estimate. ††HF+ includes entorhinal cortex (EC) and surrounding cortex (e.g., parahippocampal cortex; PH).

connected and distinct from other systems within the brain. In the remainder of this review, we define the default network in more detail, speculate on its function both during passive and active cognitive states, and evaluate accumulating data that suggest that understanding the default network has important clinical implications for brain disease.

II. Anatomy of the Default Network

The anatomy of the brain's default network has been characterized using multiple approaches. The default network was originally identified by its consistent activity increases during passive task states as compared to a wide range of active tasks (e.g., Shulman et al. 1997, Mazoyer et al. 2001, FIG. 2). A more recent approach that identifies brain systems via intrinsic activity correlations (e.g., Biswal et al. 1995) has also revealed a similar estimate of the anatomy of the default network (Greicius et al. 2003, 2004). More broadly, the default network is hypothesized to represent a brain system (or closely interacting subsystems) involving anatomically connected and interacting brain areas. Thus, its architecture should be critically informed by studies of connectional anatomy from nonhuman primates and other relevant sources of neurobiological data.

In this section, we review the multiple approaches to defining the default network and consider the specific anatomy that arises from these approaches in the context of architectonic and connectional anatomy in the monkey. We highlight two observations. First, all neuroimaging approaches converge on a similar estimate of the anatomy of the default network that is largely consistent with available information about connectional anatomy (TABLE 1). Second, the intrinsic architecture of the default network suggests that it comprises multiple interacting hubs and subsystems. These anatomic observations provide the foundation on which the upcoming sections explore the functions of the default network.

Blocked Task-Induced Deactivation

Because PET imaging requires about a minute of data accumulation to construct a stable image, the brain's default network was initially characterized using blocked task paradigms. Within these paradigms, extended epochs of active and passive tasks were compared to one another. During these epochs brain activity was averaged over blocks of multiple sequential task trials—hence the label "blocked." Shulman et al. (1997) and Mazoyer et al. (2001) published two seminal meta-analyses based on blocked PET methods to identify brain regions consistently more active during passive tasks as compared to a wide range of active tasks. Tasks spanned verbal and nonverbal domains (Shulman et al. 1997) and auditory and visual modalities (Mazoyer et al. 2001). In total, data from 195 subjects were aggregated across 18 studies in the two meta-analyses.

FIGURE 2 displays the original data of Shulman et al. visualized on the cortical surface to illustrate the topography of the default network; the data from Mazoyer et al. (not shown) are highly similar. FIGURE 3 shows a third meta-analysis of blocked task data from a series of 4 fMRI data sets from 92 young-adult subjects (Shannon 2006). In this meta-analysis of fMRI data, the passive tasks were all visual fixation and the active tasks involved making semantic decisions on visually presented words (data from Gold & Buckner 2002, Lustig & Buckner 2004). Across all the variations, a consistent set of regions increases activity during passive tasks when individuals are left undirected to think to themselves.

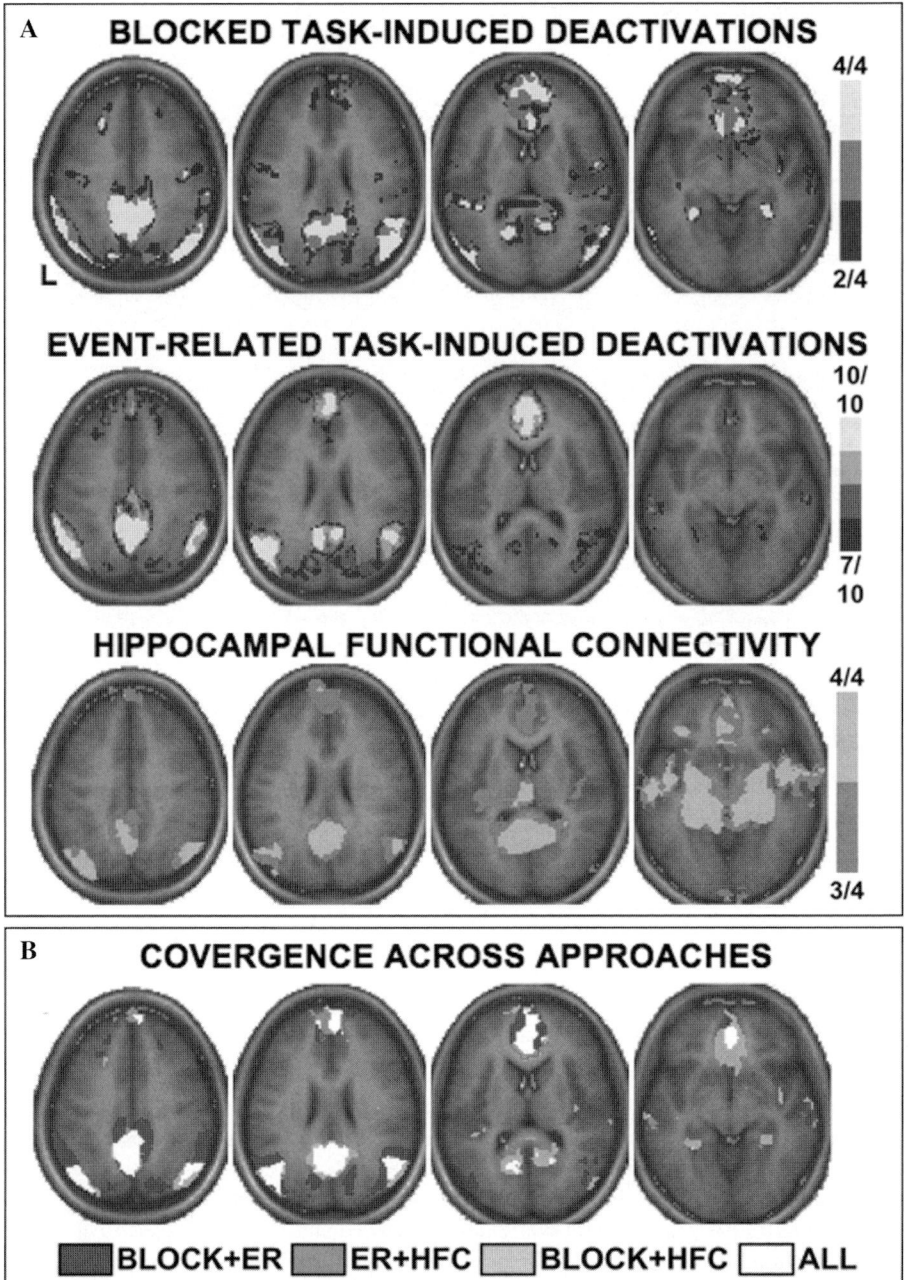

FIGURE 3. The brain's default network is converged upon by multiple, distinct fMRI approaches. **(A)** Each row of images shows a different fMRI approach for defining the default network: blocked task-induced deactivation (top row), event-related task-induced deactivation (middle row), and functional connectivity with the hippocampal formation (bottom row). Within each approach, the maps represent a meta-analysis of multiple data sets thereby providing a conservative estimate of the default network (see text). Colors reflect the number of data sets showing a significant effect within each image (color scales to the right). **(B)** The convergence across approaches reveals the core regions within the default network (legend at the bottom). Z labels correspond to the transverse level in the atlas of Talairach and Tournoux (1988). Left is plotted on the left. Adapted from Shannon (2006).

Event-Related, Task-Induced Deactivation

An alternative to defining the anatomy of the default network based on blocked tasks is to perform a similar analysis on individual task events. Rapid event-related fMRI makes possible such an analysis by presenting task trials at randomly jittered time intervals, typically 2 to 10 seconds apart. The reason to perform such an analysis is the possibility that extended epochs are required to elicit activity during passive epochs, as might be the case if blocked task-induced deactivations arise from slowly evolving signals or sustained task sets that are not modulated on a rapid time frame (e.g., Dosenbach et al. 2006).

FIGURE 3 illustrates the results of a meta-analysis of studies from Shannon (2006) that uses event-related fMRI data to define the default network. In total, data from 49 subjects were pooled for this analysis. The data are based on semantic and phonological classification tasks from Kirchhoff et al. (2005; n = 28) as well as a second sample of event-related data that also involved semantic classification (Shannon 2006; n = 21). As can be appreciated visually, the default network defined based on event-related data is highly similar to that previously reported using blocked data. Thus, the differential activity in the default network between passive and active task states can emerge rapidly, on the order of seconds or less.

Functional Connectivity Analysis

A final approach to defining the functional anatomy of the default network is based on the measurement of the brain's intrinsic activity. At all levels of the nervous system from individual neurons (Tsodyks et al. 1999) and cortical columns (Arieli et al. 1995) to whole-brain systems (Biswal et al. 1995, De Luca et al. 2006), there exists spontaneous activity that tracks the functional and anatomic organization of the brain. The patterns of spontaneous activity are believed to reflect direct and indirect anatomic connectivity (Vincent et al. 2007a) although additional contributions may arise from spontaneous cognitive processes (as will be described in a later section). In humans, low-frequency, spontaneous correlations are detectable across the brain with fMRI and can be used to characterize the intrinsic architecture of large-scale brain systems, an approach often referred to as functional connectivity MRI (Biswal et al. 1995, Haughton & Biswal 1998; see Fox & Raichle 2007 for a recent review). Motor (Biswal et al. 1995), visual (Nir et al. 2006), auditory (Hunter et al. 2006), and attention (Fox et al. 2006) systems have been characterized using functional connectivity analysis (see also De Luca et al. 2006).

Greicius and colleagues (2003, 2004) used such an analysis to map the brain's default network (see also Fox et al. 2005, Fransson 2005, Damoiseaux et al. 2006, Vincent et al. 2006). Functional connectivity analysis is particularly informative because it provides a means to assess locations of interacting brain regions within the default network in a manner that is independent of task-induced deactivation. In their initial studies, Greicius et al. measured spontaneous activity from the posterior cingulate cortex, a core region in the default network, and showed that activity levels in the remaining distributed regions of the system are all correlated together. Their map of the default network, based on intrinsic functional correlations, is remarkably similar to that originally generated by Shulman et al. (1997) based on PET deactivations.

An important further observation from analyses of intrinsic activity is that the default network includes the hippocampus and adjacent areas in the medial temporal lobe that are associated with episodic memory function (Greicius et al. 2004). In fact, many of the major neocortical regions constituting the default network can be revealed by placing a seed region in the hippocampal formation and mapping those cortical regions that show spontaneous correlation (Vincent et al. 2006). FIGURE 3 shows a map of the default network as generated from intrinsic functional correlations with the hippocampal formation in four independent data sets.

Convergence across Approaches for Defining the Default Network

Is there convergence between the three distinct approaches for defining the anatomy of the default network described above? To answer this question, the overlap among the multiple methods for defining default network anatomy is displayed on the bottom panel of FIGURE 3. The convergence reveals that the default network comprises a distributed set of regions that includes association cortex and spares sensory and motor cortex. In particular, medial prefrontal cortex (MPFC), posterior cingulate cortex/retrosplenial cortex (PCC/Rsp), and the inferior parietal lobule (IPL) show nearly complete convergence across the 18 data sets.

Several more specific observations are apparent from this analysis of overlap. First, the hippocampal formation (HF) is shown to be involved in the default network regardless of which approach is used (task-induced deactivation or functional connectivity analysis) but, relative to the robust posterior midline and prefrontal regions, the HF is less prominent using the approach of task-induced deactivations.

MONKEY DEFAULT NETWORK

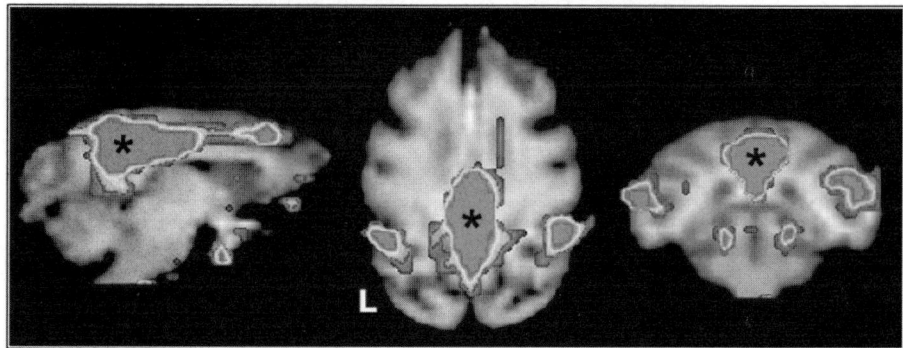

FIGURE 4. The default network in the monkey defined using functional connectivity analysis. A seed was placed in the posterior midline (indicated by asterisk) and the regions showing correlated activity were mapped. The left image shows the medial surface, the middle image a transverse section through parietal cortex, and the right image a coronal section through the hippocampal formation. Left is plotted on the left. Adapted from Vincent et al. (2007a).

Second, multiple default network regions are functionally correlated with the HF, reinforcing the notion that the medial temporal lobe is included in the network. Overlap is not perfect, however, with some indications of more extensive recruitment during passive cognitive states, including both in posterior parietal cortex and in prefrontal cortex. These details will be shown to be informative when subsystems within the default network are discussed. Third, lateral temporal cortex (LTC) extending into the temporal pole is consistently observed across approaches but, like the HF, is less robust. Together these observations tentatively define the core anatomical components of the default network (TABLE 1).

Insights from Comparative Anatomy

Important insights into the organization of human brain systems have been provided by comparative studies in the monkey. Vincent et al. (2007a) recently used functional connectivity analysis to show that the major default network regions in posterior cortex have putative monkey homologues including PCC/Rsp, IPL, and the HF (FIG. 4, see also Rilling et al. 2007). In addition, architectonic maps reveal many similarities between human and monkey anatomy in the vicinity of the default network (e.g., Petrides & Pandya 1994, Morris et al. 2000, Öngür & Price 2000, Vogt et al. 2001). Motivated by these recent observations, we provide here a detailed analysis of the architectonics and connectional anatomy of the default network, while recognizing that there may be fundamental differences in humans. As a means to simplify our analysis, we focus on areas that fall within PCC/Rsp and MPFC and their anatomic relationships with other cortical regions and the HF. Potentially important subcortical connections, such as to the striatal reward pathway and the amygdala, are not covered. Even with this simplification, the details of the anatomy are complex and one is immediately confronted with the observation that each of the activated regions, as defined based on human functional neuroimaging data, extends across multiple brain areas that have distinct architecture and connectivity. Progress will require significantly more detailed analysis of the anatomic extent and locations of default network regions in humans. Nonetheless, using available data we provide an initial analysis of the anatomy recognizing that it is provisional and incomplete.

Posterior cingulate cortex (PCC) and restrosplenial cortex (Rsp) have been extensively studied in the macaque monkey and recently so with focus on direct comparison to human anatomy (e.g., Morris et al. 2000, Vogt et al. 2001). The PCC and Rsp fall along the posterior midline and exist within a region that contains at least three contiguous, but distinct, sets of areas: Rsp (areas 29/30), PCC (areas 23/31), and precuneus (area 7m). Rsp is just posterior to the corpus callosum and, in humans, extends along the ventral bank of the cingulate gyrus (Morris et al. 2000, Vogt et al. 2001). In macaques, Rsp is much smaller and does not encroach onto the cingulate gyrus (Morris et al. 1999, Kobayashi & Amaral 2000). Just posterior to Rsp, along the main portion of the cingulate gyrus, is PCC. The precuneus, a region often cited as being involved in the default network, comprises the posterior and dorsal portion of the medial parietal lobe and includes area 7m (Cavanna & Trimble 2006, Parvizi et al. 2006). As an ensemble, these three structures are sometimes referred to as "posteriomedial cortex," and each structure is interconnected with the others (e.g., Parvizi et al. 2006, Kobayashi & Amaral 2003).

The predominant extrinsic connections to and from the posteriomedial cortex differ by area. Collectively, the connections are widespread and, much like other association areas, are consistent with a role in information integration. Specifically, Rsp is heavily interconnected with the HF and parahippocampal cortex, receiving nearly 40% of its extrinsic input from the medial temporal lobe (Kobayashi & Amaral 2003, see also Suzuki & Amaral 1994, Morris et al. 1999). Rsp also projects back to the medial temporal lobe as well as prominently to multiple prefrontal regions (Kobayashi & Amaral 2007, FIG. 5). PCC area 23 has reciprocal connections with the medial temporal lobe and robust connections with prefrontal cortex and parietal cortex area 7a—an area at or near the putative homologue of the human default network region IPL (Kobayashi & Amaral 2003, 2007, FIG. 5). The medial temporal lobe also has modest, but consistent, connections with area 7a (Suzuki & Amaral 1994, Clower et al. 2001, Lavenex et al. 2002). Thus, PCC/Rsp provides a key hub for overlapping connections between themselves, the medial temporal lobe, and IPL—three of the distributed regions that constitute the major posterior extent of the default network.

An unresolved issue is whether the lateral projection zone of PCC/Rsp is restricted to area 7a in humans or extends to areas 39/40. Macaque PCC has reciprocal projections to superior temporal sulcus (STS) and the superior temporal gyrus (STG; see also Kobayashi & Amaral 2003). Analysis of the default network in macaques provides indication that the network's lateral extent includes STG (Vincent et al. 2007a). Complicating the picture, IPL is greatly expanded in humans, including areas 39/40 (Culham & Kanwisher 2001, Simon et al. 2002, Orban et al. 2006) that are closely localized to the lateral parietal region identified by human neuroimaging as being within the default network (see Caspers et al. 2006). A recent analysis of cortical expansion between the macaque and human brain based on mapping of 23 presumed homologies revealed that IPL is among the regions of greatest increase (Van Essen & Dieker 2007). Thus, these lateral parietal and temporo-parietal areas, which are not as well characterized as PCC/Rsp, are extremely interesting in light of their anatomic connections, involvement in the default network, and potential evolutionary expansion in humans.

The connectional anatomy of area 7m in the precuneus is difficult to understand in relation to the default network even though it is often included in the default network. One possibility is that area 7m is simply not a component of the default network. References to precuneus in the neuroimaging literature are often used loosely to label the general region that includes PCC area 29/30. Precuneus area 7m predominantly connects with occipital and parietal areas linked to visual processing and frontal areas associated with motor planning (Cavada & Goldman-Rakic 1989, Leichnetz 2001). Moreover, medial temporal lobe regions that have extensive projections to PCC and Rsp show minimal connections to area 7m. Connections do exist between area 7m and the PCC, which may be the basis for the extensive activation patterns sometimes observed along the posterior midline, but we suspect that area 7m is not a core component of the network.

Reinforcing this impression, close examination of the many maps that define the human default network in this review shows that the posterior medial extent of the network usually does not encroach on the edge of the parietal midline (where area 7m is located, Scheperjans et al. 2007). This boundary is labeled explicitly in FIGURE 7 by an asterisk. The middle panel of FIGURE 18 shows a particularly clear example of the separation between task-induced deactivation of PCC and its dissociation from the region at or near area 7m. Another example of dissociation between the default network and area 7m can be found in Vogeley et al. (2004; their Figure 2A versus 2B). For all these reasons, we provisionally conclude that area 7m in precuneus is not part of the default network.

The second hub of the default network, MPFC, encompasses a set of areas that lie along the frontal midline (Petrides & Pandya 1994, Öngür & Price 2000). Human MPFC is greatly expanded relative to the monkey (Öngür et al. 2003, FIG. 6). Two differences are notable. First, macaque area 32 is pushed ventrally and rostrally in humans to below the corpus callosum (labeled by Öngür et al. as area 32pl in the human based on Brodmann's original labeling of this area in monkey as the "prelimbic area"). Human area 32ac corresponds to Brodmann's dorsal "anterior cingulate" area. Second, human area 10 is quite large and follows the rostral path of anterior cingulate areas 24 and 32ac much like typical activation of MPFC in the default network. This is relevant because commonly referenced maps based on classic architectonic analyses restrict this area to frontalpolar cortex (e.g., Petrides & Pandya 1994). Some evidence suggests that area 10 is disproportionately expanded in humans even when contrasted to great apes, suggesting specialization during recent hominid evolution (Semendeferi et al. 2001).

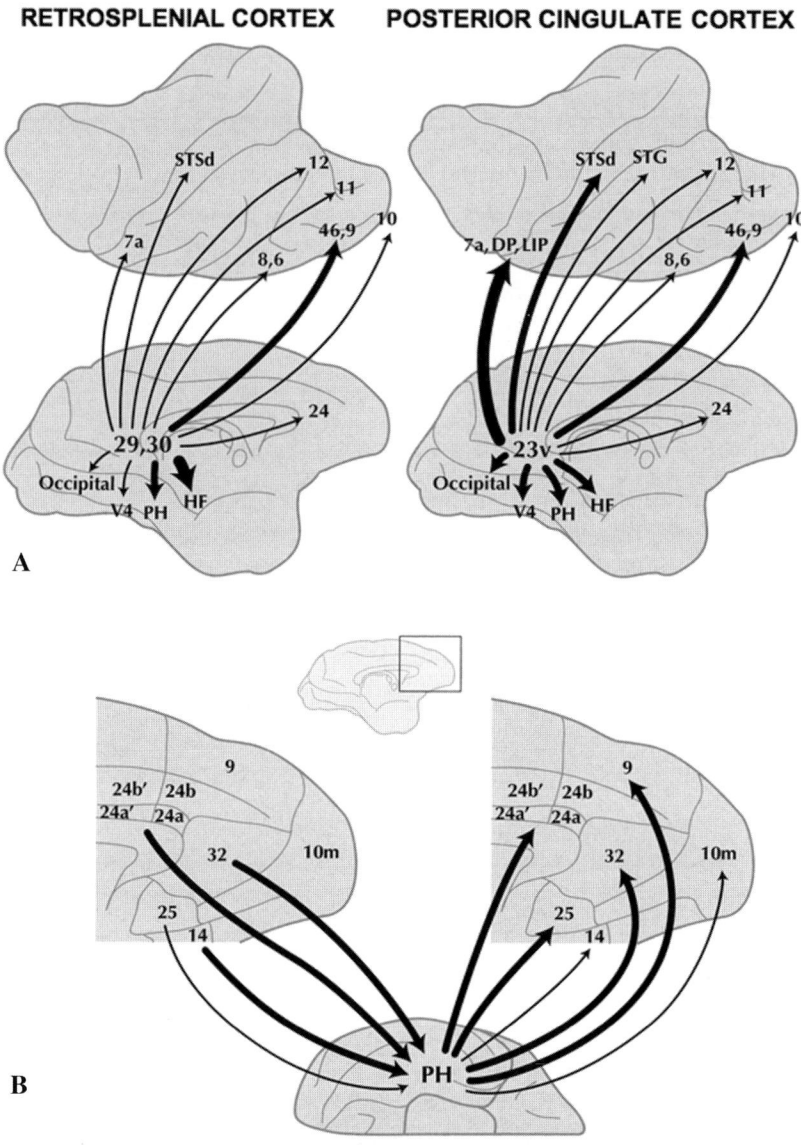

FIGURE 5. Monkey anatomy suggests that the default network includes multiple, distinct association areas, each of which is connected to other areas within the network. Illustrated are two examples of output (efferent) and input (afferent) connections for posterior cingulate/retrosplenial cortex (PCC/Rsp) and parahippocampal cortex (PH). **(A)** Output connections from Rsp (areas 29 and 30) and PCC (area 23) are displayed. Lines show connections to distributed areas; thickness represents the connection strength. Rsp and PCC are heavily connected with the medial temporal lobe (HF, hippocampal formation; PH, parahippocampal cortex), the inferior parietal lobule (IPL) extending into superior temporal gyrus (STG), and prefrontal cortex (PFC). Numbers in the diagram indicate brain areas. Adapted from Kobayashi and Amaral (2007). **(B)** Input and output connections to and from PH to medial prefrontal cortex (MPFC) are displayed. Adapted from Kondo et al. (2005).

Given these details, MPFC activation within the default network is estimated to encompass human areas 10 (10m, 10r, and 10p), anterior cingulate (area 24/32ac), and area 9 in prefrontal cortex. The closest homologues to these areas in the monkey—the medial prefrontal network—show reciprocal connections with the PCC, Rsp, STG, HF, and the perirhinal/parahippocampal cortex; sensory inputs are nearly absent (Barbas et al. 1999, Price 2007). These connectivity patterns closely

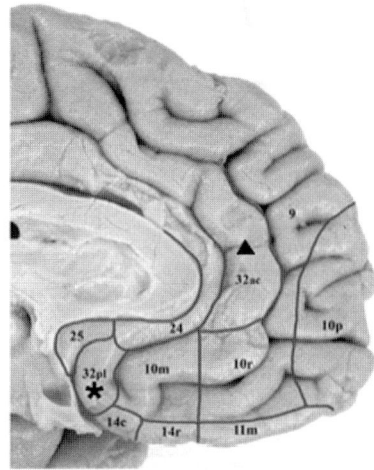

FIGURE 6. Architectonic areas within medial prefrontal cortex (MPFC) are illustrated for the monkey and human. The human MPFC is greatly expanded relative to the macaque monkey. This expansion is depicted by the triangle and asterisk that plot putative homologous areas between species based on Öngür et al. (2003). Area 32 in the macaque is homologous with area 32pl in the human. Area 24c is expanded and homologous to the caudal part of area 32ac in human. The MPFC region activated within the human default network likely corresponds to frontalpolar cortex and its rostral expansion (areas 10m, 10r, and 10p), anterior cingulate (areas 24 and 32ac), and the rostral portion of prefrontal area 9. Because of differences in functional properties, we sometimes differentiate in this review between dorsal and ventral portions of MPFC (dMPFC and vMPFC). Adapted with permission from Öngür et al. (2003).

parallel areas implicated as components of the default network.

At the broadest level, an important principle emerges from considering these anatomic details: the default network is not made up of a single monosynaptically connected brain system. Rather, the architecture reveals a series of interconnected subsystems that converge on key "hubs," in particular the PCC, that are connected with the medial temporal lobe memory system. In the next section, we explore evidence for these subsystems from functional connectivity analysis in humans.

The Default Network Comprises Interacting Subsystems

The default network comprises a set of brain regions that are coactivated during passive task states, show intrinsic functional correlation with one another, and are connected via direct and indirect anatomic projections as estimated from comparison to monkey anatomy. However, there is also clear evidence that the brain regions within the default network contribute specialized functions that are organized into subsystems that converge on hubs.

One way to gain further insight into the organization of the default network is through detailed analysis of the functional correlations between regions. FIGURE 7 plots maps of the intrinsic correlations associated with three separate seed regions within the default network in humans: the hippocampal formation including a portion of parahippocampal cortex (HF+), dMPFC, and vMPFC. The hubs—PCC/Rsp, vMPFC, and IPL—are revealed as the regions showing complete overlap across the maps. HF+ forms a subsystem that is distinct from other major components of default network including the dMPFC: both are strongly linked to the core hubs of the default network but not to each other. We suspect further analyses will reveal more subtle organizational properties. Of note, the map of the default network's hubs and subsystems shown in FIGURE 7 bears a striking resemblance to the original map of Shulman et al. (1997, FIG. 2) and updates the description of the network to show that it comprises at least two interacting subsystems.

Normative estimates of the correlation strengths between regions within the default network are provided in FIGURE 8. The bottom panel of FIGURE 8 is a graph analytic visualization of the correlation strengths using a spring-embedding algorithm to cluster strongly correlated regions near each other and position weakly correlated regions away from each other. This graphical representation illustrates the separation

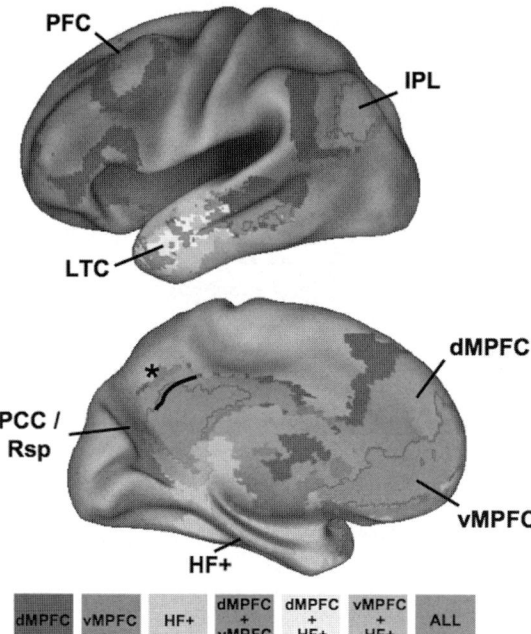

FIGURE 7. Hubs and subsystems within the default network are mapped using functional connectivity analysis. This map was produced by seeding three separate regions (dMPFC, vMPFC, HF+) and plotting the overlap of the functional correlations across the three regions (legend is at bottom; threshold for each map is r = .07). Data are high-resolution rest data (2mm voxels) from 40 participants (mean age = 22 years; 16 male) collected at 3-Tesla using a 12-channel head coil (data from Andrews-Hanna et al. 2007b). Three observations are notable. First, the combined map is remarkably similar to the original estimate of the default network from PET task-induced deactivation (see FIG. 2). Second, PCC/Rsp, IPL, and vMPFC represent anatomic hubs in the default network to which all other regions are correlated. Third, dMPFC and HF+, which are both strongly correlated with the hub regions, are not correlated with each other, indicating that they are part of distinct subsystems. A further interesting feature is that area 7m within the precuneus (indicated by asterisk) is not part of the default network. The black line near the asterisk represents the approximate boundary between areas 7m and 23/31 (estimated boundary based on Vogt & Laureys 2005).

of the medial temporal lobe subsystem. The analysis also reveals that the medial temporal subsystem is less strongly associated with the core of the default network that is centered on MPFC and PCC. However, it is important to note that the correlational strengths associated with the medial temporal lobe are generally weaker than those observed for the distributed neocortical regions. As shown in FIGURE 3, the most robust correlations linked to the medial temporal lobe overlap the default network. It is presently unclear how to interpret the quantitatively lower overall levels of correlations associated with the medial temporal lobe. Functional understanding of the default network should seek to explain both the distinct contributions of the interacting subsystems and the role of their close interaction. Of interest, infants do not show the structured interactions between the default network regions, suggesting that the network develops in toddlers or children (Fransson et al. 2007). At the other end of the age spectrum, it has recently been shown that advanced aging is associated with disrupted correlations across large-scale brain networks including the default network (Andrews-Hanna et al. 2007a, Damoiseaux et al. in press). Thus, the correlation strengths presented in FIGURE 8 are only representative of normal young adults. An interesting topic for future research will be to understand the developmental course of the default network as well as the functional implications of its late life disruption.

Vascular and Other Alternative Explanations for the Anatomy of the Default Network

Given the reproducibility of the specific anatomy of the default network, an important question to ask is whether the pattern can be accounted for by some alternative explanation that is not linked to neural architecture. One possibility is that the observed anatomy reflects a vascular pattern—either draining veins, a global form of "blood stealing" whereby active regions achieve blood flow increases at the expense of nearby regions, or some other poorly understood mechanism of vascular regulation. The methods that have revealed the default network are based on hemodynamic measures of blood flow that are indirectly linked to neural activity (Raichle 1987, Heeger & Ress 2002). This issue is particularly relevant for analyses based on intrinsic correlations because slow fluctuations in vascular properties track breathing as well as oscillations in intracranial pressure. Wise et al. (2004) recently measured fMRI correlations with the slow fluctuations in the partial pressure of end-tidal carbon dioxide that accompany breathing. Their results convincingly demonstrate correlated, spatially specific fMRI responses suggesting that fMRI patterns can reflect vascular responses to breathing (see also Birn et al. 2006). While the spatial patterns associated with respiration do not closely resemble the default network, the results of Wise and colleagues are a reminder that a vascular account should be explored further.

One reason to be skeptical of a vascular account is that the default network is also identified using measures of resting glucose metabolism. In a

INTRINSIC CORRELATIONS WITHIN THE DEFAULT NETWORK

	L LTC	R LTC	dMPFC	vMPFC	L IPL	R IPL	PCC/Rsp	L PHC	R PHC	L HF	R HF
L LTC	1.00	0.41	0.16	0.12	0.14	0.12	0.12	0.11	0.06	0.18	0.14
R LTC		1.00	0.16	0.18	0.07	0.20	0.19	0.08	0.10	0.15	0.17
dMPFC			1.00	0.47	0.22	0.31	0.34	-0.06	-0.10	-0.01	-0.04
vMPFC				1.00	0.27	0.31	0.52	0.11	0.06	0.20	0.16
L IPL					1.00	0.47	0.49	0.25	0.10	0.11	0.06
R IPL						1.00	0.42	0.12	0.05	0.09	0.07
pCC/Rsp							1.00	0.23	0.16	0.26	0.21
L PHC								1.00	0.57	0.31	0.28
R PHC									1.00	0.28	0.28
L HF										1.00	0.61
R HF											1.00

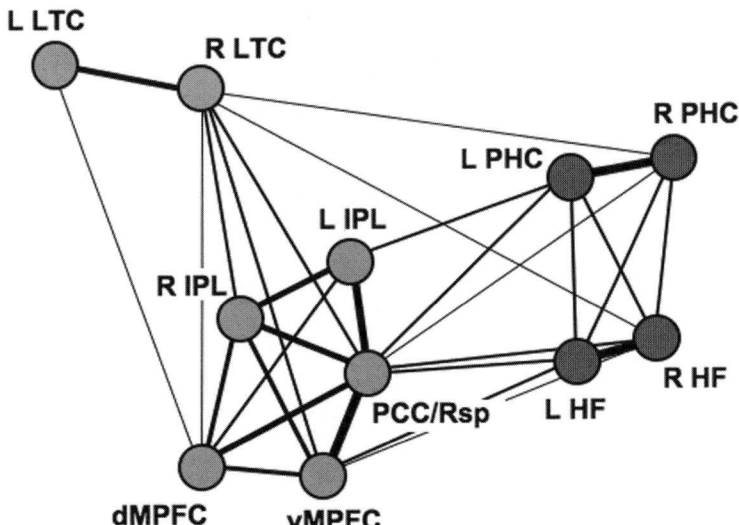

FIGURE 8. (top) Functional correlation strengths are listed for multiple regions within the default network. Each of the regions is displayed on top with the strengths of the region-to-region correlations indicated below (r-values were computed using procedures identical to Vincent et al. 2006). Regions are plotted on the averaged anatomy of the participant group (MNI/ICBM152 atlas with Z coordinates displayed). (bottom) The regions of the default network are graphically represented with lines depicting correlation strengths. The positioning of nodes is based on a spring-embedding algorithm that positions correlated nodes near each other. The structure of the default network has a core set of regions (red) that are all correlated with each other. LTC is distant because of its weaker correlation with the other structures. The medial temporal lobe subsystem (blue) includes both the hippocampal formation (HF) and parahippocampal cortex (PHC). This subsystem is correlated with key hubs of the default network including PCC/Rsp, vMPFC, and IPL. The dMPFC is negatively correlated with the medial temporal lobe subsystem suggesting functional dissociation. Graph analytic visualization provided by Alexander Cohen and Steven Petersen.

particularly informative study, Vogt and colleagues (2006) used [^{18}F]flourodeoxyglucose (FDG) PET to explore anatomy associated with the default network. Critically, FDG-PET measures neuronal activity through glucose metabolism independent of vascular coupling. Vogt et al. first defined regions within the PCC (ventral PCC and dorsal PCC) and Rsp in postmortem human tissue samples. They then measured resting state glucose metabolism in each of these regions across 163 healthy adults and correlated the obtained values across the brain to yield metabolism-based maps of functional correlation. A quite remarkable pattern emerged: ventral PCC showed correlation with the main components of the default network including vMPFC and IPL (see their Figure 7, panel B). Moreover, this pattern was preferential to ventral PCC, suggesting that the posterior hub of the default network may be even more circumscribed than the fMRI data suggest, which have implicated the broader region including dorsal PCC and Rsp. Directly relevant to the question of whether a vascular explanation can account for the default network's anatomy, these results were obtained without relying on vascular coupling.

Glucose Metabolism and the Oxygen Extraction Fraction

Metabolic properties of the default network also set the network apart from other brain systems (Raichle et al. 2001). In particular, regions within the default network show disproportionately high resting glucose metabolism relative to other brain regions as measured using FDG-PET (e.g., Minoshima et al. 1997, Gusnard & Raichle 2001, see FIG. 17) as well as high regional blood flow (Raichle et al. 2001). For example, Minoshima et al. (1997, see their Figure 1) mapped resting glucose metabolism in healthy older adults referenced to the pons, allowing visualization of regional variation across the cortex. Along the midline, normalized glucose metabolism in PCC was about 20% higher than in most other brain regions. However, high glucose metabolism was not selective only to the default network—a region at or near primary visual cortex also showed high resting metabolism. To our knowledge, there has been no systematic investigation of resting glucose metabolism within default network regions as contrasted to regions outside the network; however, all reported exploratory maps of glucose metabolism converge on the observation that the posterior midline near PCC is a region of disproportionately high metabolism (e.g., Minoshima et al. 1997, Figure 1, Gusnard & Raichle 2001, Figure 1). Intriguingly, the regions within the default network that show high resting metabolism are also those affected in Alzheimer's disease, something that will be discussed extensively in the final section of this review. To foreshadow this final discussion, the possibility will be raised that high levels of baseline activity and metabolism (glycolysis) in the default network are conducive to the formation of pathology associated with Alzheimer's disease (Buckner et al. 2005).

A second metabolic property that has been explored in connection with the default network is regional oxygen utilization. In their seminal paper that drew attention to the default network, Raichle et al. (2001) mapped the ratio of oxygen used locally to oxygen delivered by blood flow. This ratio, referred to as the oxygen extraction fraction (OEF), decreases during heightened neural activity because the increased flow of blood into a region exceeds oxygen use (see Raichle & Mintun 2006). Raichle and colleagues (2001) hypothesized that an absolute physiological baseline could be shown to exist if OEF remained constant during passive (rest) task states, suggesting that task-induced deactivations within the default network are physiologically dissimilar from other forms of transient neuronal activity increase. While an intriguing possibility, there are several observations that suggest OEF within the default network does change at rest. First, OEF decreases were noted by Raichle et al. (2001) in several default network regions at rest when each was tested individually at the $p < 0.05$ level of statistical significance. Second, regional variation in OEF across the default network was correlated from one data set to the next (r = .89) indicating systematic modulation; a constant OEF across regions would show zero correlation from one data set to the next. The modulation was quantitatively small, however, with OEF values of most regions falling within 5 to 10% of the other regions. Further exploration will be required to determine if there is an absolute metabolic state that defines a baseline within the default network or whether there are meaningful variations across regions. In the next section, we will specifically explore the possibility that the special properties that arise in the default network associate with its role in spontaneous cognition during freethinking.

III. Spontaneous Cognition

> Human beings spend nearly all of their time in some kind of mental activity, and much of the time their activity consists not of ordered thought but of bits and snatches of inner experience: daydreams, reveries, wandering interior monologues, vivid imagery, and dreams. These desultory concoctions, sometimes unobtrusive but often moving, contribute a great deal to the style and flavor of being human. Their very humanness lends them great intrinsic interest; but beyond that, surely so prominent a set of activities cannot be functionless. (Klinger 1971 p. 347)

A shared human experience is our active internal mental life. Left without an immediate task that demands full attention, our minds wander jumping from one passing thought to next—what William James (1890) called the "stream of consciousness." We muse about past happenings, envision possible future events, and lapse into ideations about worlds that are far from our immediate surroundings. In lay terms, these are the mental processes that make up fantasy, imagination, daydreams, and thought. A central issue for our present purposes is to understand to what degree, if any, the default network mediates these forms of spontaneous cognition. The observation that the default network is most active during passive cognitive states, when thought is directed toward internal channels, encourages serious consideration of the possibility that the default network *is* the core brain system associated with spontaneous cognition, and further that people have a strong tendency to engage the default network during moments when they are not otherwise occupied by external tasks. In considering the relationship between the default network and spontaneous cognition, it is worth beginning with a short review of spontaneous cognition itself.

Descriptions of human nature have alluded to the prominence of private mental experience since the classical period. In a whimsical description, Plato portrayed Socrates as "capable of standing all day in the market place lost in thought and oblivious of the external world," leading Aristophanes to coin the phrase "his head is in the clouds" (Singer 1966). Experimental study of internal mental life originated within the psychological movement of introspection in the late 19th century. Developed by Wilhelm Wundt and continued by the American psychologist Edward Titchener, introspective methods required participants to describe the contents of their internal mental experience. The premise of introspection was that conscious elements and attributes are sufficient to describe the mind. The focus on behaviorism during much of the 20th century, which emphasized measurement of the external factors that control behavior, caused a marked decline in the study of thought in mainstream science. The behaviorists rejected the methods of introspection because they relied on subjective report leading to a global "moratorium on the study of inner experience" (Klinger 1971).

The dark ages of spontaneous cognition ended in 1966 with a seminal publication by Jerome Singer that described an extensive empirical research program on the topic of daydreaming (see also Antrobus et al. 1970, Klinger 1971, Singer 1974). Several important advances emerged from this work. First, behavioral instruments were developed for the measurement of spontaneous cognition that correlated with such factors as individual differences in cognition, physiological measures and eye movements, and were also predictive of response patterns on varied tasks (e.g., Singer & Schonbar 1961, Singer et al. 1963, Antrobus et al. 1966, Antrobus 1968, Antrobus et al. 1970). Second, spontaneous cognition was observed to be quite common: 96% of individuals report daydreaming daily. Moreover, the contents of daydreams were found to include everything from mundane recounts of recent happenings to plans and expectations about the future. Finally, this work emphasized that spontaneous cognition is healthy and adaptive, and not simply a set of distracting processes or fantasies. Singer (1966), Antrobus et al. (1966) and later Klinger (1971) specifically suggested that internal mental activity is important for anticipating and planning the future. We will return to this important idea later.

In the past decade, the study of spontaneous cognition has built upon these foundations and introduced novel experimental approaches to explore the content of people's internal mental states (see Smallwood & Schooler 2006 for review). Critical to understanding the relationship between the default network and spontaneous cognition, measures of sampled thoughts track default network activity. Moreover, individual differences in tendencies to engage spontaneous cognitive processes parallel differences in default network activity. In the following section, we review these findings and discuss their implications.

Stimulus-Independent Thoughts

A number of brain imaging studies have explored stimulus-independent thoughts (SITs).[c] SITs are operationally defined as thoughts about something other than events originating from the environment; they are covert and not directed toward performance of the task at hand. The most common method for measuring SITs involves periodically probing trained participants to indicate whether they are experiencing a SIT. Care is taken to minimize the intrusiveness of the probe, although a limitation of this approach is that the probe nonetheless does interfere with the SIT, most typically to terminate its occurrence (Giambra 1995). Antrobus and colleagues (1966, 1968, 1970) showed that SITs occur quite pervasively—during both resting epochs and also during the performance of concurrent tasks. Even under heavy loads of external information, most individuals still report the presence of some SITs although the number of SITs correlates inversely with the demands of the external task.

---

[c]Various labels have been used in the reviewed papers to describe self-reported thought content including task-irrelevant thoughts (Antrobus et al. 1966), stimulus-independent thoughts (SITs, Antrobus et al. 1970, Teasdale et al. 1995), task-unrelated thoughts (TUTs, Giambra 1989), and task-unrelated images and thoughts (TUITs, Giambra 1995). For simplicity, we use the term "stimulus-independent thoughts" or SITs throughout the text.

Extending from these behavioral observations, several imaging studies have correlated the number of reported SITs with brain activity. In an early study, McGuire et al. (1996) demonstrated that the frequency of SITs estimated following various PET scans correlated with MPFC activity. Following a similar approach, Binder and colleagues (Binder et al. 1999, McKiernan et al. 2003, 2006) conducted two fMRI studies that explored the relationship between SITs and brain activity. In both studies they measured brain activity during rest and various tasks using typical fMRI procedures. Then, within a mock scanning environment, they had participants perform the same tasks while periodically probing for the presence of SITs. This procedure allowed them to sort the fMRI tasks based on their propensity to elicit SITs. The first study (Binder et al. 1999) revealed that rest, as compared to an externally oriented tone detection task, was associated with both increased default network activity, and nearly six times more SITs. The second study parametrically varied task difficulty across six separate tasks such that the easiest task (easy to detect target, slow presentation rate) produced about twice as many SITs as the most difficult task (McKiernan et al. 2003, 2006). Referenced to rest, there was a strong correlation between SITs and activity within the default network.

Mason et al. (2007) recently extended these approaches to study individual differences. Like the earlier work, they measured the propensity of rest and task states to elicit SITs. Task demands were manipulated using practice: a practiced variant of the task (low demands, many SITs) was compared with a novel variant (high demands, few SITs). The researchers replicated the work of Binder and colleagues by showing that default network regions, including MPFC and PCC/Rsp, tracked the different task states in proportion to the numbers of produced SITs. To ascertain who among their group was more likely to produce SITs, they administered a daydreaming questionnaire adopted from Singer and Antrobus (1972) that assessed general tendencies to engage in internal cognition (e.g., Do you daydream at work? When you have time on your hands do you daydream?). There was a strong correlation in regional default network activity with the participant's daydreaming tendencies (FIG. 9). Those individuals who showed the greatest default network activity during the practiced task condition were self-described daydreamers.

Taken collectively, these findings converge to suggest that task contexts that encourage SIT production show the greatest default network activity; furthermore, individuals who daydream most show increased default

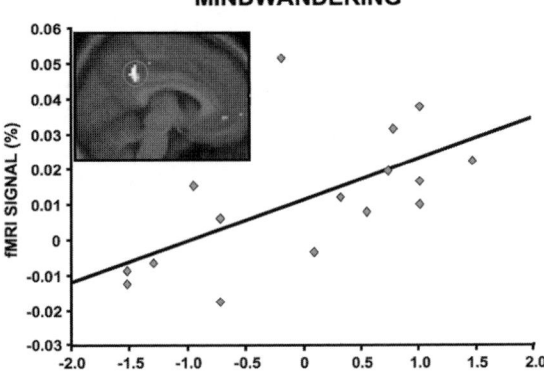

FIGURE 9. The default network is most active in individuals who report frequent mindwandering, suggesting a functional role in spontaneous cognition. Activity estimates are plotted for 16 subjects from PCC/Rsp (region shown in insert) from a task contrast conducive to encouraging mindwandering. The activity within this region is significantly correlated with individual self-reports of daydreaming obtained outside the scanner. Adapted from data published in Mason et al. (2007).

network activity, at least when placed in a conducive experimental setting.

Momentary Lapses in Attention

An idea that emerges repeatedly in the study of internal mental activity is that there is competition between resources for internal modes of cognition and focus on the external world (Antrobus et al. 1966, 1970, Teasdale et al. 1995). In discussing forms of attention, William James (1890) wrote "When absorbed in intellectual attention we become so inattentive to outer things as to be 'absent-minded,' 'abstracted,' or 'distraits.' All revery or concentrated meditation is apt to throw us into this state" (pp. 418–419). In any given task context, there must be assignment of priorities for attending to external or internal channels of information, which in turn will have consequences for task performance (Singer 1966, Smallwood & Schooler 2006). When an external task is performed, focus on internal mental content will likely lead to mistakes or slowed performance on the immediate task at hand. Several studies have explored interactions between external attention and activity within the default network.

In one investigation, Greicius and Menon (2004) studied the dynamics of activity within the default network while people were presented blocks of external visual and auditory stimuli. They first showed that spontaneous activity correlations across regions within the default network continued during the stimulus blocks. The implication of this observation is that spontaneous activity within the default network persists through both experimental and rest epochs. They further observed evidence for competition between sensory processing and spontaneous default network fluctuations: sensory-evoked responses were attenuated in those individuals who showed the strongest spontaneous activity correlations within the default network.

Momentary lapses in external attention were explored directly by Weissman and colleagues (2006) during a demanding perceptual task. Lapses in attention were defined as occurring when participants were slow to respond. Two observations were made. First, just prior to a lapse in attention, activity within brain regions associated with control of attention was diminished, including dorsal anterior cingulate and prefrontal cortex. Second, during the lapse of attention itself, activity within the default network was increased prominently in the PCC/Rsp. These findings suggest that transient lapses in the control of attention may lead to a shift in attention from the external world to internal mentation.

A related observation was made in the context of memory encoding by Otten and Rugg (2001). Brain activity was measured in two studies during the incidental encoding of words. The researchers found that increased activity in the posterior midline near PCC/Rsp and lateral parietal regions near IPL, among other regions, predicted which words would be later forgotten. This observation is consistent with the possibility that transient activity increases in the default network mark those trials on which the memorizers were distracted from their primary task, perhaps lapsing into private channels of thought.

Recently Li et al. (2007) tackled this possibility across two studies using a go/no-go paradigm. In their task, cues signaling participants to make speeded responses were intermixed with infrequent stop signals that mandated the responses should be withheld. Errors occurred when participants responded to stop signals. Exploring brain activity on the trials that preceded errors revealed that regions within the default network (MPFC and PCC/Rsp, but not IPL) augmented activity just prior to errors, an effect replicated in a second study. While again correlational, these data suggest that when the default network is active, lapses in focused external attention occur in ways that affect task performance.

However not all studies have found such relationships. Hahn et al. (2007), for example, noted that fast responses in a target-detection task were associated with increased default network activity (see Figure 3 in Hahn et al. 2007). Gilbert et al. (2006, 2007) hypothesized that the default network is associated with a broadly tuned form of outward attention ("watchfulness"). This idea, as will be discussed more extensively in the upcoming section, is reminiscent of Shulman and colleagues' (1997) suggestion that the default network participates in monitoring the external environment. While difficult to reconcile with the studies discussed earlier, the hypothesis put forward by Gilbert and colleagues is a reminder that evidence to date is limited and correlational, and further that opposing possibilities should be carefully explored. Thus, while an accumulating set of observations suggest that mindwandering is linked to increased activity in regions within the default network, further exploration is warranted to determine if the system is directly supporting the processes underlying the stimulus-independent thoughts that accompany mindwandering.

Spontaneous Activity Dynamics

The default network spontaneously exhibits slow waxing and waning of activity during rest that is correlated across its distributed regions (Greicius et al. 2003, Fox et al. 2005, Fransson 2005, Damoiseaux et al. 2006, Vincent et al. 2006). FIGURE 10 illustrates this robust phenomenon for a 5-minute epoch during which a young adult passively viewed a small fixation crosshair. As can be seen, activity within MPFC and PCC/Rsp—two of the most prominent components of the default network—spontaneously modulates over time. Critically, these two regions, which are anatomically distant from one another and supplied by separate vascular territories, show strong correlation, thereby indicating that the fMRI-measured activity swings arise from coordinated neural activity and not from measurement noise. The presence of fluctuations at rest—when SITs are at their peak—raises the question of whether these unprompted modulations reflect individual thoughts and musings (e.g., Greicius & Menon 2004, Fox et al. 2005, Fransson 2006). In a particularly thoughtful approach to this question, Fransson (2006) showed that correlated spontaneous activity within the default network attenuates when people perform a concurrent demanding cognitive task (see also Shannon et al. 2006). Such forms of tasks are known to reduce the frequency of SITs as discussed above (Antrobus et al. 1966, 1970).

While these observations are intriguing, there are several reasons to be cautious of presuming a simple relationship between spontaneous low-frequency activity modulations and cognitive processes (see Vincent et al. 2006, Fox & Raichle 2007). First,

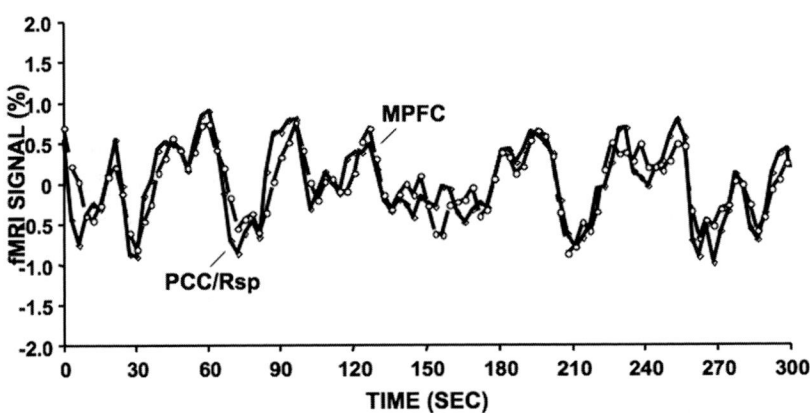

FIGURE 10. Regions within the default network spontaneously increase and decrease activity in a correlated manner. This is illustrated by plotting fMRI signal for two of the regions within the default network (PCC/Rsp and MPFC) as an individual rests in an awake state. Note that the activity slowly drifts about 2% and also that these intrinsic fluctuations are strongly correlated between the two regions. However, similar spontaneous correlations are observed between regions in other brain systems bringing into question whether this particular phenomenon is linked selectively to functional properties of the default network, such as spontaneous cognition. Adapted from data published in Fox et al. (2005).

spontaneous activity simultaneously exists in numerous brain systems including primary sensory and motor systems. It is not selectively observed in higher-order brain systems. Rather, spontaneous activity is pervasive (e.g., see De Luca et al. 2006). Second, spontaneous activity persists during sleep (Fukunaga et al. 2006, Horovitz et al. 2007) and under deep anesthesia verified by concurrently acquired burst-suppression electroencephalographic (EEG) patterns (Vincent et al. 2007a). Third, spontaneous activity is associated with extremely slow fluctuations that are slower than would be expected for cognitive events—less than one cycle every 10 seconds (Cordes et al. 2001, De Luca et al. 2006). Thus, while a considerable amount of data converges on the possibility that default network activity is associated with various forms of thought, the specific phenomenon of intrinsic low-frequency fluctuations may be incidentally related to immediate spontaneous thoughts (Vincent et al. 2006, Raichle 2006, Buckner & Vincent 2007). An intermediate possibility is that spontaneous activity fluctuations measured during rest may reflect *both* intrinsic low-level physiological processes that persist unrelated to conscious mental activity and also spontaneous cognitive events that come to dominate mental content when people are awake and disengaged from their external environments. An interesting future pursuit will be to disentangle these phenomena that are typically concurrent in awake states.

IV. Functions of the Default Network

A unique challenge for understanding the functions of the brain's default network is that the system is most active in passive settings and during tasks that direct attention away from external stimuli. This property informs us that contributions of the default network are suspended or reduced during commonly used active tasks but, unfortunately, tells us little about what the system does do. Two sources of data currently provide information about function. First, while most directed tasks cause task-induced deactivation within the network, there are an accumulating number of tasks that have been shown to elicit increased activity within the default network relative to other tasks. The properties that are common across these tasks provide some insight into function. Second, the specific anatomy of the default network constrains functional possibilities. For example, the default network does not include primary sensory or motor areas but does include areas associated with the medial temporal lobe memory system.

In this section, we explore two possible functions of the network, while recognizing that it is too soon to rule out various alternatives. One possibility is that the default network directly supports internal mentation that is largely detached from the external world. Within this possibility, the default network plays a role in constructing dynamic mental simulations based on personal past experiences such as used during remembering,

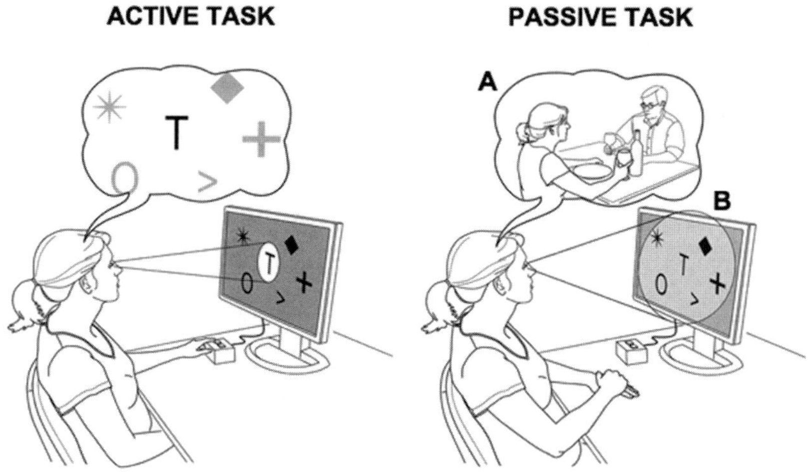

FIGURE 11. The functions of the default network have been difficult to unravel because passive tasks, which engage the default network, differ from active tasks on multiple dimensions. As one goes from an active task demanding focused attention (left panel) to a passive task (right panel), there is both a change in mental content **(A)** and level of attention to the external world **(B)**. Spontaneous thoughts unrelated to the external world increase **(A)**. There is also a shift from focused attention to a diffuse low-level of attention **(B)**. Hypotheses about the functions of the default network have variably focused on one or the other of these two distinct correlates of internally directed cognition.

thinking about the future, and generally when imagining alternative perspectives and scenarios to the present. This possibility is consistent with a growing number of studies that activate components of the default network during diverse forms of self-relevant mentalizing as well as with the anatomic observation that the default network is coupled to memory systems and not sensory systems. Another possibility is that the default network functions to support exploratory monitoring of the external environment when focused attention is relaxed. This alternative possibility is consistent with more traditional ideas of posterior parietal function but does not explain other aspects of the data such as the default network's association with memory structures. It is important to recognize that the correlational nature of available data makes it difficult to differentiate between possibilities, especially because focus on internal channels of thought is almost always correlated with a change in external attention (FIG. 11). We also explore in this section an intriguing functional property of the default network: the default network operates in opposition to other brain systems that are used for focused external attention and sensory processing. When the default network is most active, the external attention system is attenuated and vice versa.

Monitoring the External Environment: The Sentinel Hypothesis

One possibility is that the default network plays a role in monitoring the external environment (Ghatan et al. 1995, Shulman et al. 1997, Gusnard & Raichle 2001, Gilbert et al. 2007, Hahn et al. 2007). The hypothesis is that the critical difference between directed task conditions, which suspend activity within the default network, and passive conditions, which augment activity, is the form of their attentional focus on the external world. Active tasks typically require focused attention on foveal stimuli or on another type of predictable cue. By contrast, passive conditions release the participant to broadly monitor the external environment—what has been termed variably an "exploratory state" (Shulman et al. 1997) or "watchfulness" (Gilbert et al. 2007). Within this possibility, the default network is hypothesized to support a broad low-level focus of attention when one—like a sentinel—monitors the external world for unexpected events.

Hahn and colleagues (2007) specifically suggest that activity at rest "may reflect, among other functions, the continuous provision of resources for spontaneous, broad, and exogenously driven information gathering." By this view, task states represent the exceptional instances when focused attention is harnessed to respond to a specific, predictable event at the expense of broadly monitoring the environment. A variation of this idea is that external monitoring is more passive: the default network may mark a state of awareness of the external environment but should not be conceived of as supporting an active exploration. Rather, the default network may support low levels of attention that are maintained in an unfocused manner while other, internally directed cognitive acts are engaged.

The sentinel hypothesis is consistent with certain properties of the default network as well as attentional deficits following bilateral posterior lesions. First, preliminary evidence suggests that task-induced deactivation in the default network is most pronounced during tasks that involve foveal as compared to parafoveal or peripheral stimuli (Shulman et al. 1997). Second, under some circumstances, performance on sensory processing tasks correlates positively with default network activity. Hahn et al. (2007), for example, observed that the default network was linked to high levels of performance on a target-detection task but only for a diffuse attention condition where targets appeared randomly at multiple possible locations. By contrast, performance was not associated with default network activity when attention was cued to a specific location. Finally, bilateral lesions that extend across precuneus and cuneus can induce Balint's syndrome (Mesulam 2000a). Balint's syndrome is characterized by a form of tunnel vision. Patients can only perceive a small portion of the visual world at one time and often fail to notice the appearance of objects outside the immediate focus of attention (Mesulam 2000a). This deficit is consistent with what might be expected if a brain system that supported global (as opposed to focused) attention were disrupted.

Constructing Alternative Perspectives: The Internal Mentation Hypothesis

An alternative hypothesis about the function of the default network is that it contributes directly to internal mentation. Self-reflective thought and judgments that depend on inferred social and emotional content robustly activate MPFC regions within the default network (e.g., Gusnard et al. 2001, Kelley et al. 2002, Mitchell et al. 2006). The default network also includes connections with the HF and overlaps with regions active during episodic remembering (e.g., Greicius et al. 2004, Buckner et al. 2005, Vincent et al. 2006). These later observations are particularly intriguing because we rely so heavily on memory when imagining social scenarios and other constructed mental simulations. Schacter and colleagues (2008), in this volume, explore the nature of cognitive processes linked to mental simulation (see also Tulving 2005, Gilbert 2006, Buckner & Carroll 2007, Schacter & Addis 2007, Schacter et al. 2007, Hassabis & Maguire 2007, Bar 2007, Gilbert & Wilson 2007). Here we discuss the possibility that the default network underlies these abilities. By mental simulation we mean here imaginative constructions of hypothetical events or scenarios.

Evidence that the default network participates in self-relevant mental simulation arises from the nature of the paradigms that have consistently activated the network. Particularly informative have been those that target autobiographical remembering, theory-of-mind, and envisioning the future (FIG. 12). During autobiographical memory tasks, individuals are encouraged to vividly recall past episodes from their own experiences. Such personal reminiscences are typically experienced as rich, mental simulations of the past event. Andreasen et al. (1995) were the first to note correspondence between autobiographical memory and the default network. In their study, autobiographical memory retrieval (as compared to a word fluency task) activated the major extent of the default network. Svoboda and colleagues (2006) recently conducted a thorough meta-analysis that included 24 separate PET and fMRI studies of autobiographical memory (see also reviews by Maguire 2001, Cabeza & St. Jacques 2007). In all the included studies, participants recalled experiences from their personal pasts. The aggregated plot across these studies highlights a set of regions remarkably similar to the default network including vMPFC, dMPFC, PCC/Rsp, IPL, LTC, and the HF (FIGS. 12 and 13).

Studies of theory of mind also reliably activate components of the default network. Theory of mind—also sometimes called "mentalizing"—refers to thinking about the beliefs and intentions of other people. In a typical test of theory of mind, a story is presented that requires the understanding of another person's perspective. Amodio and Frith (2006) provide the following example introduced by Wimmer and Perner (1983):

> Max eats half his chocolate bar and puts the rest away in the kitchen cupboard. He then goes out to play in the sun. Meanwhile, Max's mother comes into the kitchen, opens the cupboard and sees the chocolate bar. She puts it in the fridge. When Max comes back into the kitchen, where does he look for his chocolate bar: in the cupboard, or in the fridge?

To answer this question one must infer what Max is thinking—an inference that is adaptive and common to many social settings. Awareness of the mental states of people around us is important for anticipating behaviors and successfully navigating social interactions.

Commencing with the study of Fletcher et al. (1995), neuroimaging studies of theory of mind consistently reveal activity overlapping the default network (see Saxe et al. 2004, Amodio & Frith 2006 for recent reviews). FIGURE 12 shows an example using the task of Saxe and Kanwisher (2003, data from Andrews-Hanna et al. 2007b). In both the target and reference tasks,

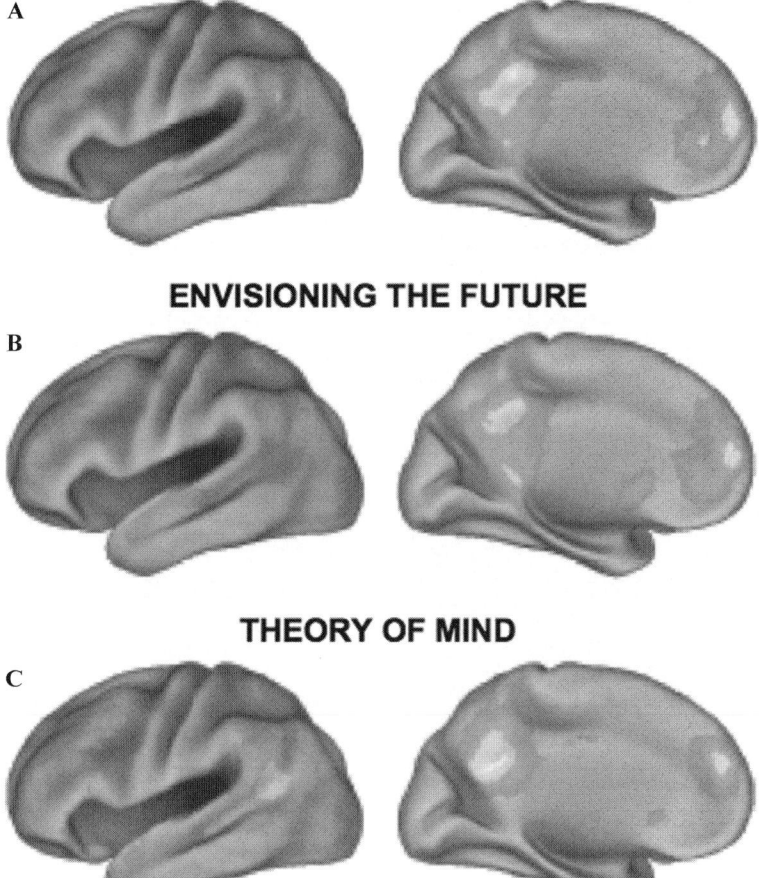

AUTOBIOGRAPHICAL MEMORY

ENVISIONING THE FUTURE

THEORY OF MIND

MORAL DECISION MAKING

FIGURE 12. The default network is activated by diverse forms of tasks that require mental simulation of alternative perspectives or imagined scenes. Four such examples from the literature illustrate the generality. **(A)** Autobiographical memory: subjects recount a specific, past event from memory. **(B)** Envisioning the future: cued with an item (e.g., dress), subjects imagine a specific future event involving that item. **(C)** Theory of mind: subjects answer questions that require them to conceive of the perspective (belief) of another person. **(D)** Moral decision making: subjects decide upon a personal moral dilemma. Data come from prior studies and are here displayed using procedures similar to FIGURE 2. Data in A and B are from Addis et al. (2007). Data in C uses the paradigm of Saxe and Kanwisher (2003). Data in D is from Greene et al. (2001). Note that all the studies activate strongly PCC/Rsp and dMPFC. Active regions also include those close to IPL and LTC, although further research will be required to determine the exact degree of anatomic overlap. It seems likely that these maps represent multiple, interacting subsystems.

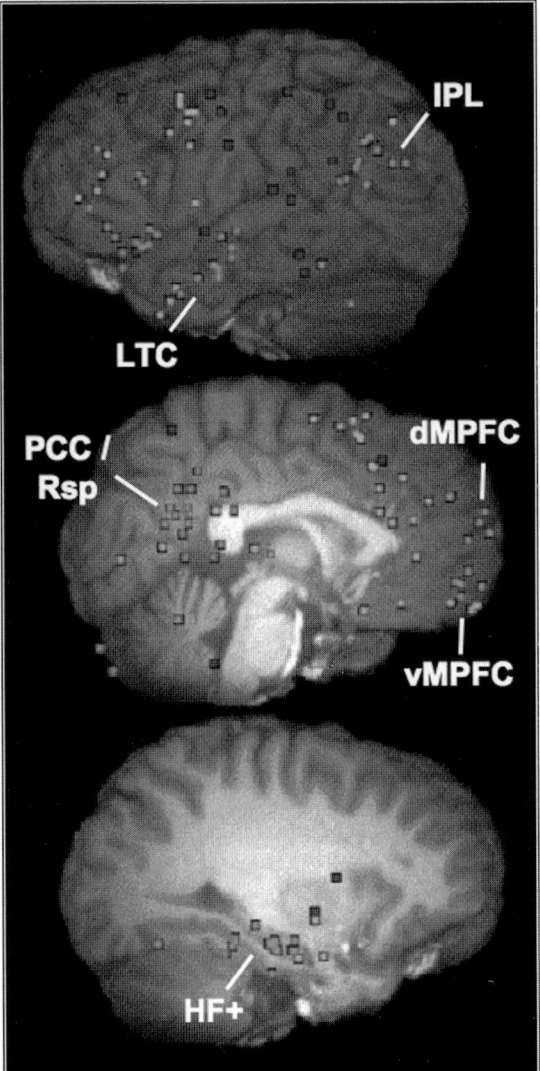

FIGURE 13. Meta-analysis of autobiographical memory tasks. Locations of activation during recall from autobiographical memory are plotted for 24 PET and fMRI studies on the lateral (top) and medial (middle) surfaces. A sagittal cut illustrates the plane of the hippocampal formation (bottom). Colors indicate whether the region contains high (red), medium (green), or low (blue) convergence across studies. Note the clear convergence with the core regions of the default network. Adapted from Svoboda et al. (2006).

subjects read stories that required conceiving a situation like the one above about Max. In one instance, the story was framed in relation to a person's beliefs; in another instance the question was about an inanimate object. For example, a story on what a person believed about an event was compared to a similar story about what a camera captured in a photograph. As can be seen in FIGURE 12, this contrast activates multiple regions within the default network, including prominently dMPFC, PCC/Rsp, and a region near IPL close to the temporo-parietal junction. In a follow-up study, Saxe and Powell (2006) showed that certain regions in the default network, including PCC, did not differentially activate to stories about people's bodily sensations (being hungry, cold) or stories that contained descriptions of people's appearances. PCC was only differentially responsive when stories required conceiving another person's thoughts.

Rilling and colleagues (2004) provide another example of default network activity during interpersonal interactions that depend on inferences about other people's thoughts. In their study, the participants were introduced to 10 living individuals just prior to going into the scanner. While in the scanner, they played a series of game trials where, on each trial, they either chose to cooperate or work against one of the other people. The outcome on each trial was determined both by the participant's decision and also the choice of a putative human playing partner. For example, the playing partner could appear to work against the participant. As a control, the participants performed a rewarded control task that did not involve playing the game. In reality, the participants were always playing a computer but believed fully they were playing real people. Brain activity in the default network differed markedly when the individuals believed they were playing other people as compared to the control task. Moreover, the activity modulation occurred when they received feedback about what the other players chose, suggesting a role in making inferences about other's minds.

The third class of task involves envisioning the future. Schacter et al. (2007, 2008) discuss in detail findings from such paradigms, so we only briefly mention them here. In the prototypical paradigm, participants are given a cue and instructed to imagine a future situation related to that cue. For example, cued with the word "dress," a participant in Addis et al. (2007) reported an imagined scene that included the following: "My sister will be finishing her undergraduate education... And I can see myself sitting in some kind of sundress, like yellow, and under some trees." Behavioral studies show that individuals are quite adept at conceiving plausible future scenarios that contain considerable detail and emotional content (D'Argembeau & Van der Linden 2006). Several such studies have been reported using PET and fMRI (Partiot et al. 1995, Okuda et al. 2003, Szpunar et al. 2007, Addis et al. 2007, Sharot et al. 2007, Botzung et al. 2008, D'Argembeau et al. in press). All these studies activated regions within the default

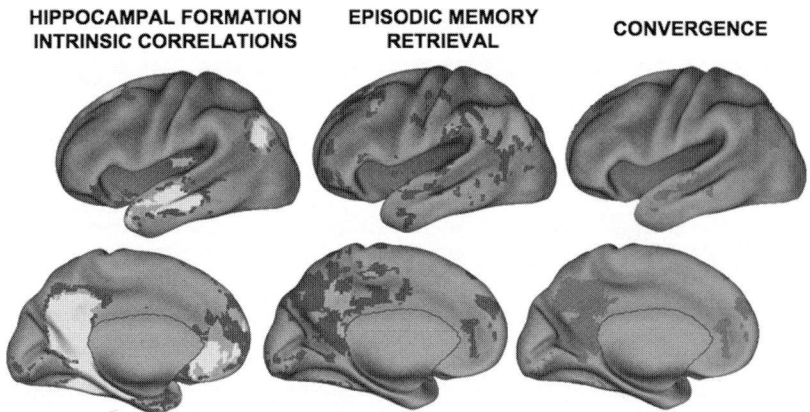

FIGURE 14. Posterior regions within the default network overlap regions that are active during successful episodic memory retrieval. (left) Image of the default network subsystem correlated with the hippocampal formation. These data represent the surface projection of data from FIGURE 3B. Adapted from Vincent et al. (2006). (middle) Image of successful episodic memory retrieval. This image shows regions with high levels of activity during episodic recollection as compared to familiarity-based recognition. Adapted from Wagner et al. (2005). (right) Regions of convergence across the two maps extend to the PCC/Rsp, IPL, and portions of MPFC.

network. Data from Addis et al. (2007) are plotted in FIGURE 12 to illustrate the similarity of the activated region to that of the default network.

An immediate question that arises based on the above observations is: What does this generality mean? While remembering, envisioning the future, and conceiving the mental states of others are different on several dimensions including temporal focus (e.g., past versus present) and personal perspective (e.g., self versus another person), they all converge on similar core processes (Buckner & Carroll 2007, FIGURE 12). In each instance, one is required to simulate an alternative perspective to the present. These abilities, which are most often studied as distinct, rely on a common set of processes by which mental simulations are used adaptively to imagine events beyond those that emerge from the immediate environment.

By this hypothesis, a defining property of the default network is its flexibility. The tasks that activate the default network share core processes in common but differ in terms of the content and goal to which these processes are applied. As a further example that illustrates the breadth of domains that activate the default network, Greene and colleagues (2001) explored brain regions supporting moral decisions. Their paradigms required individuals to evaluate whether a hypothetical action was moral or immoral (Greene & Haidt 2002). They observed that certain forms of moral judgment activated default network regions (Greene et al. 2001, FIG. 12). In particular, the default network was most active when evaluations included personal moral dilemmas (e.g., Consider whether it would be morally acceptable for you to push one person off a sinking boat to save five others). Solving moral dilemmas may be exactly the kind of situation where people simulate alternative events in the service of evaluating them (see Moll et al. 2005 for related discussion). While not explored to date, one wonders whether many reflective cognitive experiences—such as pride, shame, and guilt—are built upon the capacity of the default network to enable contrasts among imagined social scenarios and settings.

The possibility that the default network contributes to internal channels of thought is consistent with the subsystems that comprise its anatomy. The medial temporal lobe subsystem is associated with mnemonic processes and is activated during successful retrieval of old information from memory (see Wagner et al. 2005 for a review). FIGURE 14 illustrates this functional aspect of the medial temporal lobe subsystem by comparing regions intrinsically correlated with the HF to regions responding in traditional memory paradigms. There is considerable overlap between the two approaches, especially for PCC/Rsp and IPL. Furthermore, activity within the medial temporal lobe subsystem increases during retrieval of strong memory traces that include remembered associations and content details (Henson et al. 1999, Eldridge et al. 2000, Wheeler & Buckner 2004, Yonelinas et al. 2005). Taken together, these observations suggest that this subsystem contributes associations and relational information from memory perhaps to provide the critical building blocks of mental exploration (see also Bar 2007, Addis & Schacter 2008).

The second subsystem is linked to the MPFC, specifically dMPFC. dMPFC is activated by many task situations that require participants to make self-referential judgments and engage in other forms of self-relevant mental exploration (e.g., Gusnard et al. 2001, Kelley et al. 2002, Mitchell et al. 2006, see Adolphs 2003, Ramnani & Owen 2004, Amodio & Frith 2006 for relevant reviews). All the task forms noted above that activate the complete, or near complete, default network share in common that the imagined perspectives are self-referenced. Moreover, several findings suggest that reference to the self causes selective and preferential activity within the MPFC subsystem. For example, Szpunar et al. (2007) noted that MPFC was strongly activated by envisioning oneself in the past or future but not so for considering a personally unfamiliar public figure in a future setting. Saxe and Kanwisher (2003) showed greater dMPFC activity for making decisions about conceived perspectives of people as compared to inanimate objects (e.g., a camera). Güroğlu et al. (2008) demonstrated increased activity in the dMPFC and throughout the default network when individuals made judgments about whether to approach familiar peers versus celebrities in an imagined social setting. Mitchell and colleagues (2006) provided a particularly clear example of modulation along the "self" dimension. In their study, individuals made judgments about a fictitious person who was described as being either quite similar in sociopolitical views to the participant or quite different. Judgments made about similar others activated dMPFC to about the same degree as making a judgment about oneself. In contrast, judgments about people perceived as being politically different did not activate dMPFC.[d]

Thus, while it is admittedly difficult to define what is self or self-like, dMPFC is activated when the content of an imagined setting involves social agents that are being considered as such. Note that a subtle distinction is being drawn here: the common element that activates dMPFC does not appear to simply be reference to a person or oneself, which can occur devoid of elaborated context. The common element appears to align more with *thinking* about the complex interactions among people that are conceived of as being social, interactive, and emotive like oneself.

Within this hypothesis, the default network thus comprises at least two distinct interacting subsystems—one subsystem functions to provide information from memory; the second participates to derive self-relevant mental simulations. The adaptive function may be to provide a "life simulator"—a set of interacting subsystems that can use past experiences to explore and anticipate social and event scenarios (Gilbert 2006, Gilbert & Wilson 2007). This idea is similar to a recent hypothesis from Bar (2007) that the HF subsystem serves to supply associations and analogies from past experience to make predictions about upcoming events. An open question is when mental simulation depends on the interactions between both subsystems. As the functional analysis reveals, the dMPFC and medial temporal lobe are not intrinsically correlated with one another, suggesting some level of functional separation (FIG. 8). Certain situations draw heavily on both subsystems such as elicited during autobiographical memory tasks and when thinking about the future. Theory-of-mind tasks, while utilizing the dMPFC subsystem, activate the medial temporal lobe minimally. One possibility is that the dMPFC subsystem interacts with the medial temporal lobe subsystem to the degree that past episodic information is an important constraint on the mental simulation being derived. The convergence of the two subsystems on common hubs, in particular PCC, may serve to prepare the system for these critical interactions.

Competitive Functional Interactions

When initially considering the possibility of a brain system for internal mentation, Ingvar (1979) proposed that such a system might work in opposition to those specialized for sensory processing, which he termed "sensory-gnostic." He noted that

> the low flow/activity in postcentral sensory-gnostic regions appears to agree with a low general awareness of the sensory input from the immediate surroundings, when one is left to oneself, undisturbed, resting awake. Possibly the lower postcentral [flow] signals that the resting consciousness implies an active global inhibition of a sensory input, as if the brain filtered out trivial information in order to let the mind be busy with its own consciousness (p. 20).

The idea that the brain's default network may work in direct opposition to other systems has received recent support from the observation of strong negative activity correlations between the default network and other systems—coined variably "dynamic equilibrium" and "anticorrelations" (Greicius et al. 2003, Fransson 2005, Fox et al. 2005, Golland et al. 2007, Tian et al. 2007). For simplicity, we use the term "anticorrelation" as proposed by Fox et al. (2005).

---

[d] Dorsal and ventral are relative terms and are used variably depending on which regions are being compared. This paper defines dMPFC and vMPFC differently than did Mitchell et al. (2006). The region labeled here as dMPFC is the region Mitchell et al. describe as being ventral.

FIGURE 15 illustrates the phenomenon of anticorrelation. As shown earlier, the distributed regions within the default network show spontaneous correlations with one another (see FIG. 7). These intrinsic correlations also exist in other brain systems including those dedicated to external attention (as described by Corbetta & Shulman 2002). The phenomenon of anticorrelation refers to the additional observation that these distinct brain systems show strong negative correlations with one another: as activity within the default network increases, normalized activity in the external attention system show activity decreases.[e] This finding suggests that the brain may shift between two distinct modes of information processing. One mode, marked by activity within the default network, is detached from focused attention on the external environment and is characterized by mental explorations based on past memories. The second mode is associated with focused information extraction from sensory channels. These systems may be opposed to one another and thus represent functionally competing brain systems.

The possibility of competition raises important questions for future research—how is this competition regulated? Is there a separate control system, perhaps mediated by frontal cortex, that in some manner directs which of these two brain systems is active? Or, are the two systems in direct competition with one another in a way that local competitive interactions between them and input systems define their levels of activity? While minimal data exist to inform this question, Vincent and colleagues (2007b) have recently reported preliminary evidence for a frontal-parietal brain system that is anatomically juxtaposed between the default network and systems associated with external attention, providing a candidate for controlling the functional interactions between the two anticorrelated brain networks.

V. Relevance to Brain Disease

To this point, extensive data have been considered that suggest humans possess a set of closely interacting subsystems known as the default network. One hypoth-

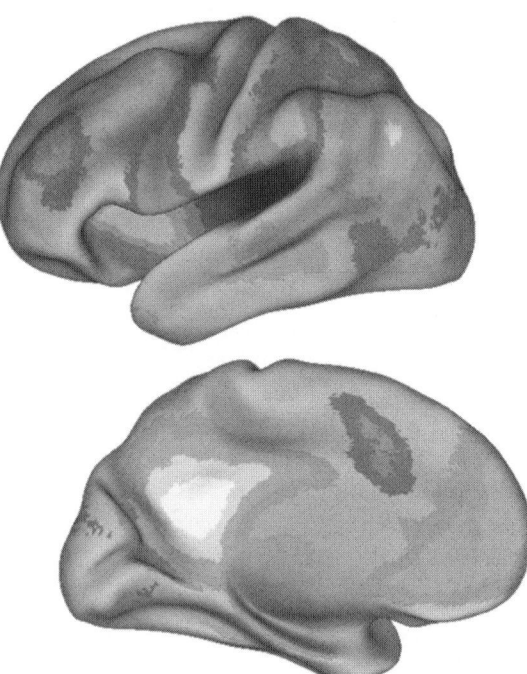

FIGURE 15. Intrinsic activity suggests that the default network is negatively correlated (anticorrelated) with brain systems that are used for focused external visual attention. Anticorrelated networks are displayed by plotting those regions that negatively correlate with the default network (shown in blue) in addition to those that positively correlate (shown in red). These two anticorrrelated networks may participate in distinct functions that compete with one another for control of information processing within the brain. Data are the same as analyzed for FIGURE 7.

esis is that, using memories and associations from past experiences as its building blocks, the default network participates in constructing self-relevant mental simulations that are exploited by a wide range of functions including remembering, thinking about the future, and inferring the perspectives and thoughts of other people. When left undisturbed, this is the network people engage by default. The focus of the present section is to explore the relationship of the default network to mental disorders including autism, schizophrenia, and Alzheimer's disease (TABLE 2). Each of these three clinical conditions is associated with cognitive dysfunction in domains that are linked to the default network. Other disorders for which important links are being made to the default network but are beyond the scope of this review include depression, obsessional disorders, attention-deficit/hyperactivity disorder, and post-traumatic stress disorder.

---

[e]A difficult technical issue associated with spontaneous negative correlations arises because the activity levels are normalized to remove global activity variation. Without such normalization, whole-brain signal fluctuations dominate the local regional correlations. This form of normalization causes the correlation strengths to be distributed around zero (Vincent et al. 2006) forcing negative correlations to emerge. Further research will be required to understand the contributions of normalization to negative correlations in spontaneous activity.

TABLE 2. Selected papers on cognitive disorders associated with the default network

	DATA TYPE
Autism Spectrum Disorders	
Castelli et al. (2002)	Activity–TID
Waiter et al. (2004)	Structure
Kennedy et al. (2006)	Activity–TID
Cherkassky et al. (2006)	Activity–fcMRI
Kennedy & Courchesna (2008)	Activity–fcMRI
Schizophrenia	
Harrison et al. (2007)	Activity–TID
Bluhm et al. (2007)	Activity–fcMRI
Garrity et al. (2007)	Activity–TID/fcMRI
Zhou et al. (2007)	Activity–fcMRI
Alzheimer's Disease	
Reiman et al. (1996)	Metabolism
Minoshima et al. (1997)	Metabolism
Herholtz et al. (2002)	Metabolism
Buckner et al. (2005)	PIB-PET, Structure
Scahill et al. (2002)	Structure
Thompson et al. (2003)	Structure
Lustig et al. (2003)	Activity–TID
Celone et al. (2006)	Activity–TID
Greicius et al. (2004)	Activity–fcMRI
Rombouts et al. (2005)	Activity–fcMRI
Wang et al. (2007)	Activity–fcMRI
Sorg et al. (2007)	Activity–fcMRI, Structure

Notes: Listed are example references that link disruption of the default network with disease. Type refers to the primary form of support in the paper for the association: Activity–TID, Task-induced deactivation data from either PET or fMRI; Activity–fcMRI, functional connectivity analysis from fMRI; Structure, Structural data from MRI; Metabolism, Resting glucose metabolism from PET; PIB-PET, amyloid binding as measured by PET. This list is not comprehensive, especially for metabolism studies that have a long history.

Autism Spectrum Disorders

The autism spectrum disorders (ASD) are developmental disorders characterized by impaired social interactions and communication. Symptoms emerge by early childhood and include stereotyped (repetitive) behaviors. Baron-Cohen and colleagues (1985) proposed that a core deficit in many children with ASD is the failure to represent the mental states of others, as needed to solve theory-of-mind tasks. Based on an extensive review of the functional anatomy that supports theory-of-mind and social interaction skills, Mundy (2003) proposed that the MPFC may be central for understanding the disturbances in ASD. Given the convergent evidence presented here that suggests the default network contributes to such functions, it is natural to explore whether the default network is disrupted in ASD.

Developmental disruption of the default network, in particular disruption linked to the MPFC, might result in a mind that is environmentally focused and absent a conception of other people's thoughts. The inability to interact with others in social contexts would be an expected behavioral consequence. It is important to also note that such disruptions, if identified, may not be linked to the originating developmental events that cause ASD but rather reflect a developmental endpoint. That is, dysfunction of the default network and associated symptoms may emerge as an indirect consequence of early developmental events that begin outside the network.

Many studies have explored whether ASD is associated with morphological differences in brain structure. The general conclusion from this literature is that the brain changes are complex, reflecting differences in growth rates and attenuation of growth (see Brambilla et al. 2003 for review). At certain developmental stages these differences are manifest as overgrowth and at later stages as undergrowth. Early observations have implicated the cerebellum. A further consistent observation has been that the amygdala is increased in volume in children with ASD (e.g., Abell et al. 1999, Schumann et al. 2004), perhaps as a reflection of abnormal regulation of brain growth (Courchesne et al. 2001). While not discussed earlier because of our focus on cortical regions, the amygdala is known to contribute to social cognition (Brothers 1990, Adolphs 2001, Phelps 2006) and interacts with regions within the default network. The amygdala has extensive projections to orbital frontal cortex (OFC) and vMPFC (Carmichael & Price 1995).

Of perhaps more direct relevance to the default network, dMPFC has shown volume reduction in several studies of ASD that used survey methods to explore regional differences in brain volume (Abell et al. 1999, McAlonan et al. 2005). The effects are subtle and will require further exploration, but it is noteworthy that, of those studies that have looked, several have noted dMPFC volume reductions in ASD. Of interest, a study using voxel-based morphometry to investigate grey matter differences in male adolescents with ASD noted that several regions within the default network exhibited a relative increase in grey matter volume compared to the control population (Waiter et al. 2004). Because this observation has generally not been replicated in adult ASD groups, future studies should investigate whether complex patterns of overgrowth and undergrowth of the regions within the default network exist in ASD and, if so, whether they track behavioral improvement on tests of social function (see also Carper & Courchesne 2005).

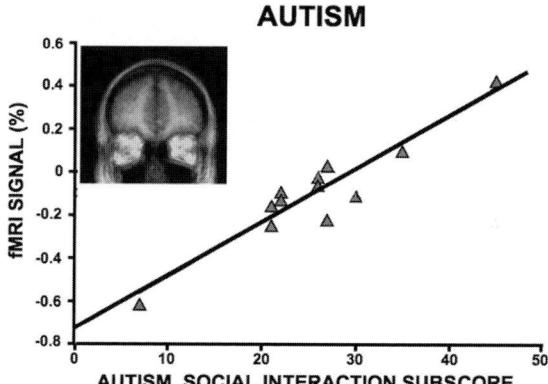

FIGURE 16. Default network activity tracks the severity of social dysfunction in autism. An exploratory correlational analysis by Kennedy et al. (2006) found that activity within MPFC (region shown in inset) was correlated with social impairment as measured by the Autism Diagnostic Interview–Revised. Individuals with autism spectrum disorder who showed less task-induced deactivation had lower social impairment scores. Adapted from Kennedy et al. (2006).

Kennedy and colleagues (2006) recently used fMRI to directly explore the functional integrity of the default network in ASD. In their study, young adults with ASD and age-matched individuals without ASD were imaged during passive tasks and demanding active tasks that elicit strong activity differences in the default network. While the control participants showed the typical pattern of activity in the default network during the passive tasks, such activity was absent in the individuals with ASD. Direct comparison between the groups revealed differences in vMPFC and PCC. Moreover, in an exploratory analysis of individual differences within the ASD group, those individuals with the greatest social impairment (measured using a standardized diagnostic inventory) were those with the most atypical vMPFC activity levels (FIG. 16). An intriguing possibility suggested by the authors of the study and extended by Iacoboni (2006) is that the failure to modulate the default network in ASD is driven by differential cognitive mentation during rest, specifically a lack of self-referential processing.

Another recent study using analysis of intrinsic functional correlations showed that the default network correlations were weaker in ASD (Cherkassky et al. 2006). Of note, the individuals with ASD showed differences in a fronto-parietal network that has been recently hypothesized to control interactions between the default network and brain systems linked to external attention (Vincent et al. 2007b). These data in ASD suggest an interesting possibility: the default network may be largely intact in ASD but under utilized perhaps because of a dysfunction in control systems that regulate its use.

Schizophrenia

Schizophrenia is a mental illness characterized by altered perceptions of reality. Auditory hallucinations, paranoid and bizarre delusions, and disorganized speech are common positive clinical symptoms (Liddle 1987). Cognitive tests also reveal negative symptoms, including impaired memory and attention (Kuperberg & Heckers 2000). These symptoms lead to questions about their relationship to the default network for a few reasons. The first reason surrounds the association of the default network with internal mentation. Many symptoms of schizophrenia stem from misattributions of thought and therefore raise the question of an association with the default network because of its functional connection with mental simulation. A second related reason has to do with the broader context of control of the default network. While still poorly understood, there appears to be dynamic competition between the default network and brain systems supporting focused external attention (Fransson 2005, Fox et al. 2005, Golland et al. 2007, Tian et al. 2007, see also Williamson 2007). Frontal-parietal systems are candidates for controlling these interactions (Vincent et al. 2007b). The complex symptoms of schizophrenia could arise from a disruption in this control system resulting in an overactive (or inappropriately active) default network. The normally strongly defined boundary between perceptions arising from imagined scenarios and those from the external world might become blurry, including the boundary between self and other (similar to that proposed by Frith 1996).

Three studies have provided preliminary data supporting the possibility that the default network is functionally overactive. Garrity and colleagues (2007) recently reported an analysis of correlations among default network regions in patients with schizophrenia. Studying a sizable data sample (21 patients and 22 controls), they explored task-associated activity modulations within the default network and identified largely similar correlations among default network regions in patients and controls. Differences were noted in specific subregions, as were differences in the dynamics of activity as measured from the timecourses of the fMRI signal. Of particular interest, they noted that within the patient group, the positive symptoms of the disease (e.g., hallucinations, delusions, and thought confusions) were correlated with increased default network activity during the passive epochs, including MPFC and PCC/Rsp. In a related analysis, Harrison et al. (2007) noted accentuated default network activity during

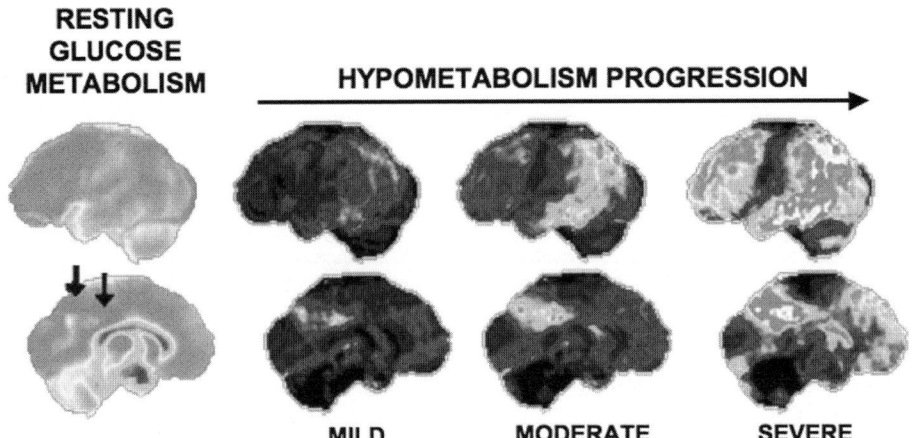

FIGURE 17. Glucose metabolism within the default network is reduced in Alzheimer's disease. Normal resting glucose metabolism shows a disproportionately high level of metabolism in healthy individuals as measured by FDG-PET (left). Arrows indicate high metabolism near PCC/Rsp. Alzheimer's disease is consistently associated with progressive reduction in glucose metabolism (hypometabolism) in specific regions that overlap the default network (right). These data map the glucose metabolism reduction from a cross-sectional sample of older adults across the range of mild (Mini-Mental Status Examination score, MMSE = 30), moderate (MMSE = 20), and severe (MMSE = 0) Alzheimer's disease. Adapted from Minoshima et al. (1997).

passive task epochs in patients with schizophrenia as contrasted to controls, again suggesting an overactive default network. Moreover, within the patient group, poor performance was again correlated with MPFC activation during the passive as compared to the active tasks. Finally, Zhou and colleagues (2007) found that regions constituting the default network were functionally correlated with each other to a significantly higher degree in patients than in control participants. Thus, while the data are limited, these studies converge to suggest that patients with schizophrenia have an overactive default network, as would be expected if the boundary between imagination and reality were disrupted. Overactivity within the network correlates with task performance (Harrison et al. 2007) and clinical symptoms (Garrity et al. 2007).

Alzheimer's Disease

The most compelling link between clinical disease and disruption of the default network occurs in Alzheimer's disease (AD). AD is a progressive dementia typically occurring after the age of 70 and affecting approximately half of older adults above 85. Initial symptoms are memory difficulties, but sensitive tests often reveal disturbances of executive function as well (e.g., Balota & Faust 2001). AD has been extensively studied in living individuals using multiple imaging approaches including measurement of glucose metabolism, measurement of structural atrophy, and measurement of intrinsic and task-evoked brain activity (TABLE 2). All approaches converge to suggest that the default network is disrupted.

The earliest evidence that the default network is disrupted in AD comes from studies of resting glucose metabolism. Patients with AD show a specific anatomic pattern of reduced metabolism relative to age-matched healthy peers (Benson et al. 1983, Kumar et al. 1991, Herholz 1995, Minoshima et al. 1997, de Leon et al. 2001, Alexander et al. 2002, FIG. 17). The pattern of hypometabolism bears a striking resemblance to the regions comprising the posterior components of the default network including PCC/Rsp, IPL, and LTC (Buckner et al. 2005). Hypometabolism in AD progresses with the disease and correlates with mental status (e.g., Minoshima et al. 1997, Herholz et al. 2002). Patients at genetic risk for AD also show similar metabolism differences, implying the disturbances occur early in the course of the disease (Reiman et al. 1996).

Methods that survey atrophy across the brain in AD have also all converged to show disruption in the default network prominently including the medial temporal lobe (Scahill et al. 2002, Thompson et al. 2003, Buckner et al. 2005). Accelerated atrophy is present in PCC/Rsp and the medial temporal lobe at the preclinical stages of the disease, again implying the default network is disrupted early as the disease progresses (Buckner et al. 2005). Recently, functional changes in the default network have been explored in AD using both analysis of task-induced deactivation (Lustig

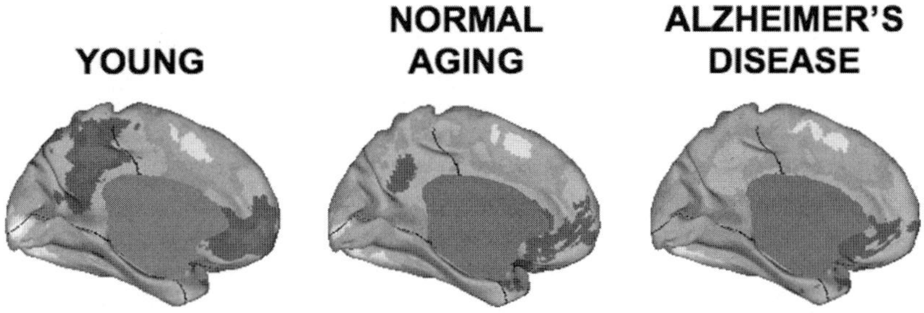

FIGURE 18. Activity within the default network is disrupted in Alzheimer's disease. Task increases (red) and decreases (blue) from a simple word classification task referenced to a passive baseline task are plotted for young adults (left panel), normal older adults (middle panel), and demented older adults with AD (right panel). The young adults show the classic pattern of task-induced deactivation within PCC/Rsp and MPFC. The effect attenuates significantly in AD. Adapted from Lustig et al. (2003, see also Greicius et al. 2004).

et al. 2003, Celone et al. 2006) and analysis of intrinsic activity correlations (Greicius et al. 2004, Rombouts et al. 2005, Celone et al. 2006, Wang et al. 2006). Again, in all instances, disruption has been noted consistent with the metabolic and structural changes. FIGURE 18 shows data from Lustig et al. (2003).

Thus, by all measures the default network appears disrupted in AD, including prominently the medial temporal lobe susbsystem. Recently, molecular imaging methods able to measure AD pathology (Klunk et al. 2004) have revealed an even more surprising link to the default network: pathology preferentially accumulates in the default network even before symptoms emerge. In the next section, we will explore the possibility that metabolic properties or activity patterns within the default network directly relate to— or even cause—the pathology of AD (Buckner et al. 2005).

Default Network Activity May Set the Stage for Alzheimer's Disease: The Metabolism Hypothesis

AD pathology forms preferentially throughout the default network, suggesting the unexpected possibility that activity within the network may facilitate disease processes (Buckner et al. 2005). The leading hypothesis about the cause of AD proposes that toxic forms of the amyloid ß protein (Aß) initiate a cascade of events ending in synaptic dysfunction and cell death (Walsh & Selkoe 2004, Mattson 2004). "Plaques" and "tangles" are the residues of this pathological process. Consistent with the clinical observation that initial symptoms of the disease include memory impairment, the medial temporal lobe and cortical structures linked to memory are affected early in the disease. Several theories have offered explanations for why memory structures are particularly vulnerable to the disease, including ideas based on anatomy (Hyman et al. 1990) and also the possibility that memory structures are sensitive to toxicity because of their role in plasticity (Mesulam 2000b). Early pathological studies also implicated distributed cortical regions as vulnerable to AD (e.g., Brun & Gustafson 1976) leading to a call to explore further systems-level causes of the disease (Saper et al. 1987). The discovery of the default network and the observation that it is active during rest states suggests a novel hypothesis regarding the origins of AD.

The basic idea is that the default network's continuous activity augments an activity-dependent or metabolism-dependent cascade that is conducive to the formation of AD pathology. Buckner and colleagues (2005) referred to this idea as the "metabolism hypothesis." Maps of Aß plaques in living individuals provide the key evidence (Klunk et al. 2004), as images of Aß plaques taken at the earliest stages of AD show a distribution that is remarkably similar to the anatomy of the default network (Buckner et al. 2005, FIG. 19). About 10% of nondemented older individuals also show this pattern, presumably reflecting the preclinical stage of the disease (Buckner et al. 2005, Mintun et al. 2006a). The preferential use of the default network throughout life may be conducive to increased accumulation of Aß and its pathological sequelae. By this view, memory systems may be preferentially affected by the disease because these systems play a central role in resting brain activity as part of the default network.

Several recent observations lend support to the metabolism hypothesis, although it should still be considered highly speculative. Of particular interest is the discovery of a plausible biological link between neural activity and upregulation of Aß. In a technically innovative study, Cirrito and colleagues (2005) showed that Aß levels increased following stimulation of the brain

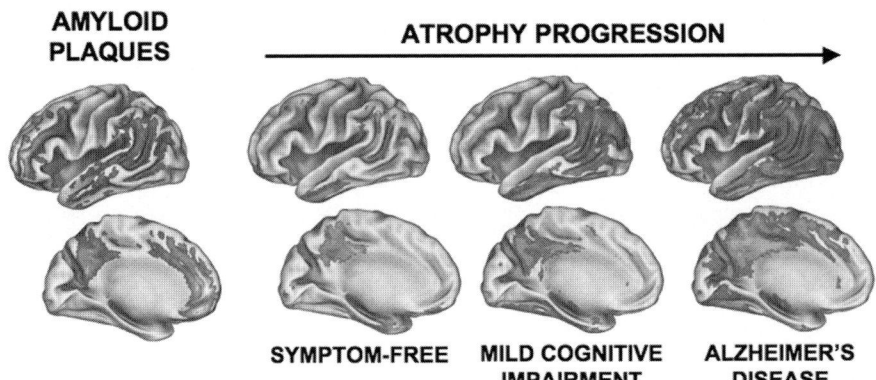

FIGURE 19. Alzheimer's disease may be causally related to default network activity. Regions manifesting default activity in young adults (e.g., FIGS. 2 and 7) are highly similar to those that show pathology in early stages of the disease as measured by molecular imaging of amyloid plaques using PET (left). These regions, in turn, appear affected by structural atrophy as measured by longitudinal MRI (right). One possibility is that activity within the default network augments an activity-dependent or metabolism-dependent cascade that leads to the formation of Alzheimer's disease pathology. Adapted from Buckner et al. (2005).

in living genetically engineered mice expressing human proteins that form the building blocks of Aß. This observation suggests that synaptic activity can increase the presence of extracellular Aß (see also Selkoe 2006). A further supporting observation comes from a new PET method to map glycolysis based on measuring the ratio of oxygen to glucose consumption. Glycolysis is the process by which glucose is metabolized into cellular energy. The map of rest-state glycolysis correlates remarkably well with the distribution of amyloid plaques (Mintun et al. 2006a). The metabolism hypothesis might also explain certain risk factors for AD. Specifically, a genetic risk factor was recently discovered that links to the enzyme GAPDH involved in glycolysis (Li et al. 2004). If AD takes foothold earliest in regions of high glycolytic metabolism within the default network, it is possible that the explanation for this genetic risk factor may lie in differences in metabolic efficiency across individuals (Buckner et al. 2005).

At the most global level, the possibility that brain activity states can influence a disease process has implications for intervention and understanding of disease. We so often think about how aberrant molecular and cellular processes affect brain circuits and cognitive processes. The present hypothesis highlights a potential influence in the opposite direction: brain activity patterns may directly modulate the molecular cascades that are relevant to disease. In the case of AD, rest-state activity may accelerate the formation of pathology. Intervention may take the form of a therapy that modifies glycolysis or other aspect of brain metabolism.

VI. Conclusions

The brain's default network is a recently described brain system that has been identified using neuroimaging methods. The reviewed findings suggest properties of the network that set it apart from other brain systems. In particular, the default network is the most active brain system when individuals are left to think to themselves undisturbed. The default network also increases activity during mental explorations referenced to oneself including remembering, considering hypothetical social interactions, and thinking about one's own future. These properties suggest that the default network functions to allow flexible mental explorations—simulations—that provide a means to prepare for upcoming, self-relevant events before they happen.

Analysis of connectional anatomy in the monkey and intrinsic functional correlations between regions in the human suggest that the default network is organized around a set of interacting subsystems that comprise distributed association areas of the brain (TABLE 2, FIGS. 7 and 8). The main hubs of the default network are within the MPFC cortex and along the posterior midline including PCC. A particularly important direction for future research will involve the study of behavioral deficits following damage to regions within the network and also the study of nonhuman primate models that allow causal inferences about function to be explored.

Characterization of the default network, unlike study of other brain systems, arose almost entirely from correlational imaging approaches. The study of most other brain systems has been initiated by a neurological syndrome and then probed further using animal models and neuroimaging approaches. On the one hand, the discovery of the brain's default network represents a unique contribution of neuroimaging to cognitive neuroscience. On the other hand, there have been no lesion studies that motivate their behavioral probes based on the recent characterization of the network, leaving a large number of questions unanswered. Providing some information, studies of patients with lesions to regions overlapping the default network are noted in the present review and also discussed in the companion paper of Schacter et al. (2008). However, considerably more work needs to be conducted.

A further open issue is how the default network interacts with the distributed brain systems that contribute content to the process of mental exploration. Studies of episodic memory retrieval have shown that visual cortex and auditory cortex are preferentially activated during the recollection of visual objects and sounds (e.g., Nyberg et al. 2000, Wheeler et al. 2000). Imagining the personal future, which activates the default network under many contexts, has also been demonstrated to additionally recruit the anterior temporal cortex (Partiot et al. 1995) and the amygdala (Sharot et al. 2007, see also Güroğlu et al. 2008) when strong emotional context is a component of the upcoming episode. Judgments about inferred emotions have been linked to regions within the default network (e.g., Ochsner et al. 2004, see also Maddock 1999). One possibility is that the regions within the default network transiently interact with sensory, motor, and emotional systems to represent the content of the imagined event.

Germane to this possibility, Hassabis and Maguire (2007) recently proposed that interactions among regions within the default network may "facilitate the retrieval and integration of relevant informational components, stored in their modality-specific cortical areas, the product of which has a coherent spatial context, and can then later be manipulated and visualized." They refer to this process as "scene construction," a term emphasizing that mental simulation often unfolds in one's mind as an imagined scene with rich visual and spatial content (see also Hassabis et al. 2007). Vogeley and colleagues (2004) have also noted that regions within the default network are differentially active depending on the perspective taken when imaging a scene. The default network is most active when one takes a first-person perspective centered upon one's own body as opposed to a third-person perspective.

Perhaps the most intriguing avenue for future exploration surrounds the implication that specific brain systems are devoted to internal modes of cognition. To date, cognitive and systems neuroscience has concerned itself primarily with how information is extracted from sensory inputs and integrated over time to make decisions and plan actions. Knowledge that the default network exists reminds us that there may be specialized brain systems that underlie our abilities to mentally explore and anticipate future situations. Such constructive processes may be adaptive because they allow the brain to preexperience upcoming events and to derive prospectively useful forms of representation that are many steps removed from their originally encoded sources.

Relevant to this possibility, studies of neural activity in the rat hippocampus have recently revealed that future event sequences are the beginnings of journeys (Diba & Buzáki 2007) and choice points (Johhnson & Redish 2007) providing a candidate neural mechanism for evaluating the consequences of upcoming actions before they happen (see also Shapiro et al. 2006, Buckner & Carroll 2007). In a series of recent studies, Johnson and Redish (2007) focused on the behavior of rats at a critical choice point in a maze where they were confronted with a high-cost decision. The rats had to follow a path to the right or left, and the incorrect choice required an extended journey to obtain another chance for reward. By recording from ensembles of cells with place fields in the hippocampus, they were able to visualize the representation of space in the rat brain at these critical decision junctures. What emerged was quite remarkable: when the rats paused before their decision, the neurons fired in patterns that swept ahead of the location, first down one choice and then the other. This prospective coding occurred, on average, for about 10% of the time the rats were at the choice point. Moreover, on some trials where the rats made decision errors, the representations of space swept back toward the choice point and down the path of the correct journey. Although a direct causal link to the decision choice has yet to be uncovered, these findings suggest a candidate neural mechanism by which potential future choices can be simulated in the rat brain in the service of planning.

The default network's prominent use during passive epochs may contribute adaptive function by allowing event scenarios to be constructed, replayed, and explored to enrich the remnants of past events in order to derive expectations about the future. This functional role may explain why the default network increases its activity during passive moments when the demands for processing external information are minimal. Rather than let the moments pass with idle brain activity, we capitalize on them to consolidate past experience in ways that are adaptive for our future needs.

Acknowledgments

We thank Justin Vincent, Avi Snyder, Peter Fransson, Michael Greicius, Daniel Gilbert, Cindy Lustig, Moshe Bar, Daphne Holt, Britta Hahn, Marcus Raichle, Mike Fox, Jason Mitchell, Michael Miller, and two reviewers for valuable discussion and comments on the paper. Avi Snyder and Itamar Kahn provided assistance with computational techniques for constructing the figures. Data for figures were generously provided by Mike Fox, Joshua Greene, Malia Mason, Jason Mitchell, Marcus Raichle, Ben Shannon, Avi Snyder, Satoshi Minoshima, and Justin Vincent. Ben Shannon compiled the data illustrated in FIGURE 3. Steve Petersen and Alex Cohen contributed the graph analytic visualization displayed in FIGURE 8. Katie Powers assisted with manuscript preparation and Haderer & Müller Biomedical Art illustrated FIGURES 5 and 11. Funding was provided by the National Institute on Aging (AG021910, JAG08441), National Institute of Mental Health (MH060941), and the Howard Hughes Medical Institute.

Conflict of Interest

The authors declare no conflicts of interest.

References

Abell, F., Krams, M., Ashburner, J., Passingham, R., Friston, K., et al. (1999). The neuroanatomy of autism: a voxel-based whole brain analysis of structural scans. *Neuroreport, 10*, 1647–51.

Addis, D. R., & Schacter, D. L. (2008). Constructive episodic simulation: Temporal distance and detail of past and future events modulate hippocampal engagement. *Hippocampus, 18*, 227–237.

Addis, D. R., Wong, A. T., & Schacter, D. L. (2007). Remembering the past and imagining the future: common and distinct neural substrates during event construction and elaboration. *Neuropsychologia, 45*, 1363–77.

Adolphs, R. (2001). The neurobiology of social cognition. *Curr. Opin. Neurobiol., 11*, 231–9.

Adolphs, R. (2003). Cognitive neuroscience of human social behaviour. *Nat. Rev. Neurosci., 4*, 165–78.

Amodio, D. M., & Frith, C. D. (2006). Meeting of minds: the medial frontal cortex and social cognition. *Nat. Rev. Neurosci., 7*, 268–77.

Andreasen, N. C., O'Leary, D. S., Cizadlo, T., Arndt, S., Rezai, K., et al. (1995). Remembering the past: two facets of episodic memory explored with positron emission tomography. *Am. J. Psychiatry, 152*, 1576–85.

Andrews-Hanna, J. R., Snyder, A. Z., Vincent, J. L., Lustig, C., Head, D., et al. (2007a). Disruption of large-scale brain systems in advanced aging. *Neuron, 56*, 924–35.

Andrews-Hanna, J. R., Saxe, R., Poulin, R., & Buckner, R. L. (2007b). The default system overlaps activation during theory of mind and episodic memory retrieval tasks. *Soc. Neurosci. Abstr.*

Antrobus, J. S. (1968). Information theory and stimulus-independent thought. *Br. J. Psychol., 59*, 423–30.

Antrobus, J. S., Singer, J. L., & Greenberg, S. (1966). Studies in the stream of consciousness: experimental enhancement and suppression of spontaneous cognitive processes. *Perceptual and Motor Skills, 23*, 399–417.

Antrobus, J. S., Singer, J. L., Goldstein, S., & Fortgang, M. (1970). Mindwandering and cognitive structure. *Trans. N. Y. Acad. Sci., 32*, 242–52.

Alexander, G. E., Chen, K., Pietrini, P., Rapoport, S. I., & Reiman, E. M. (2002). Longitudinal PET evaluation of cerebral metabolic decline in dementia: a potential outcome measure in Alzheimer's disease treatment studies. *Am. J. Psychiatry, 159*, 738–45.

Arieli, A., Shoham, D., Hildesheim, R., & Grinvald, A. (1995). Coherent spatiotemporal patterns of ongoing activity revealed by real-time optical imaging coupled with single-unit recording in the cat visual cortex. *J. Neurophysiol., 73*, 2072–93.

Baker, S. C., Rogers, R. D., Owen, A. M., Frith, C. D., Dolan, R. J., et al. (1996). Neural systems engaged by planning: a PET study of the Tower of London task. *Neuropsychologia, 34*, 515–26.

Balota, D. A., & Faust, M. E. (2001). Attention in dementia of the Alzheimer's type. In F. Boller & S. Cappa (Eds.) Handbook of Neuropsychology VI: Aging and Dementia (pp. 51–80). Amsterdam: Elsevier Science B.V.

Bar, M. (2007). The proactive brain: using analogies and associations to generate predictions. *Trends Cogn. Sci., 11*, 280–9.

Barbas, H., Ghashghaei, H., Dombrowski, S. M., & Rempel-Clower, N. L. (1999). Medial prefrontal cortices are unified by common connections with superior temporal cortices and distinguished by input from memory-related areas in the rhesus monkey. *J. Comp. Neurol., 410*, 343–67.

Baron-Cohen, S., Leslie, A. M., & Frith, U. (1985). Does the autistic child have a "theory of mind"? *Cognition, 21*, 37–46.

Benson, D. F., Kuhl, D. E., Hawkins, R. A., Phelps, M. E., Cummings, J. L., & Tsai, S. Y. (1983). The fluorodeoxyglucose ^{18}F scan in Alzheimer's disease and multi-infarct dementia. *Arch. Neurol., 40*, 711–4.

Berger, H. (1931/1969). On the electroencephalogram of man: third report. *Electroenceph. Clin. Neurophysiol. Supplement No., 28*, 95–132.

Binder, J. R., Frost, J. A., Hammeke, T. A., Bellgowan, P. S., Rao, S. M., & Cox, R. W. (1999). Conceptual processing during the conscious resting state. a functional MRI study. *J. Cogn. Neurosci., 11*, 80–95.

Birn, R. M., Diamond, J. B., Smith, M. A., & Bandettini, P. A. (2006). Separating respiratory-variation-related fluctuations from neuronal-activity-related fluctuations in fMRI. *Neuroimage, 31*, 1536–48.

Biswal, B., Yetkin, F. Z., Haughton, V. M., & Hyde, J. S. (1995). Functional connectivity in the motor cortex of resting human brain using echo-planar MRI. *Magn. Reson. Med., 34*, 537–41.

Bluhm, R. L., Miller, J., Lanius, R. A., Osuch, E. A., Boksman, K., et al. (2007). Spontaneous low-frequency fluctuations in the BOLD signal in schizophrenic patients:

anomalies in the default network. *Schizophr. Bull.*, *33*, 1004–12.

Botzung, A., Denkova, E., & Manning, L. (2008). Experiencing past and future personal events: functional neuroimaging evidence on the neural bases of mental time travel. *Brain and Cognition*, *66*, 202–12.

Brambilla, P., Hardan, A., di Nemi, S. U., Perez, J., Soares, J. C., & Barale, F. (2003). Brain anatomy and development in autism: review of structural MRI studies. *Brain. Res. Bull.*, *61*, 557–69.

Brothers, L. (1990). The social brain: A project for integrating primate behavior and neurophysiology in a new domain. *Concepts Neurosci.*, *1*, 27–51.

Brun, A., & Gustafson, L. (1976). Distribution of cerebral degeneration in Alzheimer's disease: A clinico-pathological study. *Arch. Psychiat. NervKrankh.*, *223*, 15–33.

Buckner, R. L., Raichle, M. E., Miezin, F. M., & Petersen, S. E. (1996). Functional anatomic studies of memory retrieval for auditory words and visual pictures. *J. Neurosci.*, *16*, 6219–35.

Buckner, R. L., Snyder, A. Z., Shannon, B. J., LaRossa, G., Sachs, R., et al. (2005). Molecular, structural, and functional characterization of Alzheimer's disease: evidence for a relationship between default activity, amyloid, and memory. *J. Neurosci.*, *25*, 7709–17.

Buckner, R. L., & Carroll, D. C. (2007). Self-projection and the brain. *Trends Cogn. Sci.*, *11*, 49–57.

Buckner, R. L., & Vincent, J. L. (2007). Unrest at rest: default activity and spontaneous network correlations. *Neuroimage*, *37*, 1091–6.

Cabeza, R., & St Jacques, P. (2007). Functional neuroimaging of autobiographical memory. *Trends Cogn. Sci.*, *11*, 219–27.

Carmichael, S. T., & Price, J. L. (1995). Limbic connections of the orbital and medial prefrontal cortex in macaque monkeys. *J. Comp. Neurol.*, *363*, 615–41.

Carper, R. A., & Courchesne, E. (2005). Localized enlargement of the frontal cortex in early autism. *Biol. Psychiatry.*, *57*, 126–33.

Caspers, S., Geyer, S., Schleicher, A., Mohlberg, H., Amunts, K., & Zilles, K. (2006). The human inferior parietal cortex: cytoarchitectonic parcellation and interindividual variability. *Neuroimage*, *33*, 430–48.

Castelli, F., Frith, C., Happé, F., & Frith, U. (2002). Autism, Asperger syndrome and brain mechanisms for the attribution of mental states to animated shapes. *Brain*, *125*, 1839–49.

Cavada, C., & Goldman-Rakic, P. S. (1989). Posterior parietal cortex in rhesus monkey: I. parcellation of areas based on distinctive limbic and sensory corticocortical connections. *J. Comp. Neurol.*, *287*, 393–421.

Cavanna, A. E., & Trimble, M. R. (2006). The precuneus: a review of its functional anatomy and behavioural correlates. *Brain*, *129*, 564–83.

Celone, K. A., Calhoun, V. D., Dickerson, B. C., Atri, A., Chua, E. F., et al. (2006). Alterations in memory networks in mild cognitive impairment and Alzheimer's disease: an independent component analysis. *J. Neurosci.*, *26*, 10222–31.

Cherkassky, V. L., Kana, R. K., Keller, T. A., & Just, M. A. (2006). Functional connectivity in a baseline resting-state network in autism. *Neuroreport*, *17*, 1687–90.

Cirrito, J. R., Yamada, K. A., Finn, M. B., Sloviter, R. S., Bales, K. R., et al. (2005). Synaptic activity regulates interstitial fluid amyloid-beta levels in vivo. *Neuron*, *48*, 913–22.

Clower, D. M., West, R. A., Lynch, J. C., & Strick, P. L. (2001). The inferior parietal lobule is the target of output from the superior colliculus, hippocampus, and cerebellum. *J. Neurosci.*, *21*, 6283–91.

Corbetta, M., & Shulman, G. L. (2002). Control of goal-directed and stimulus-driven attention in the brain. *Nat. Rev. Neurosci.*, *3*, 201–15.

Cordes, D., Haughton, V. M., Arfanakis, K., Carew, J. D., Turski, P. A., et al. (2001). Frequencies contributing to functional connectivity in the cerebral cortex in "resting-state" data. *Am. J. Neuroradiol.*, *22*, 1326–33.

Courchesne, E., Karns, C. M., Davis, H. R., Ziccardi, R., Carper, R. A., et al. (2001). Unusual brain growth patterns in early life in patients with autistic disorder: an MRI study. *Neurology*, *57*, 245–54.

Culham, J. C., & Kanwisher, N. G. (2001). Neuroimaging of cognitive functions in human parietal cortex. *Curr. Opin. Neurobiol.*, *11*, 157–63.

D'Argembeau, A., & Van der Linden, M. (2006). Individual differences in the phenomenology of mental time travel: the effect of vivid visual imagery and emotion regulation strategies. *Conscious Cogn.*, *15*, 342–50.

D'Argembeau, A., Xue, G., Lu, Z.-L., Van der Linden, M., & Bechara, A. (In press). Neural correlates of envisioning emotional events in the year and far future. *Neuroimage*.

Damoiseaux, J. S., Beckmann, C. F., Arigita, E. J., Barkhof, F., Scheltens, P., et al. (In press). Reduced resting-state brain activity in the "default network" in normal aging. *Cereb. Cortex*.

Damoiseaux, J. S., Rombouts, S. A., Barkhof, F., Scheltens, P., & Stam, C. J., et al. (2006). Consistent resting-state networks across healthy subjects. *Proc. Natl. Acad. Sci. U.S.A.*, *103*, 13848–53.

de Leon, M. J., Convit, A., Wolf, O. T., Tarshish, C. Y., DeSanti, S., et al. (2001). Prediction of cognitive decline in normal elderly subjects with 2-[(18)F]fluoro-2-deoxy-D-glucose/positron-emission tomography (FDG/PET). *Proc. Natl. Acad. Sci. U.S.A.*, *98*, 10966–71.

De Luca, M., Beckmann, C. F., De Stefano, N., Matthews, P. M., & Smith, S. M. (2006). fMRI resting state networks define distinct modes of long-distance interactions in the human brain. *Neuroimage*, *29*, 1359–67.

Diba, K., & Buzsaki, G. (2007). Forward and reverse hippocampal place-cell sequences during ripples. *Nat. Neurosci.*, *10*, 1241–2.

Dosenbach, N. U., Visscher, K. M., Palmer, E. D., Miezin, F. M., Wenger, K. K., et al. (2006). A core system for the implementation of task sets. *Neuron*, *50*, 799–812.

Eldridge, L. L., Knowlton, B. J., Furmanski, C. S., Bookheimer, S. Y., & Engel, S. A. (2000). Remembering episodes: a selective role for the hippocampus during retrieval. *Nat. Neurosci.*, *3*, 1149–52.

Fletcher, P. C., Happé, F. Frith, U., Baker, S. C., Dolan, R. J., et al. (1995). Other minds in the brain: A functional imaging study of "theory of mind" in story comprehension. *Cognition*, *57*, 109–28.

Fox, M. D., Snyder, A. Z., Vincent, J. L., Corbetta, M., Van Essen, D. C., & Raichle, M. E. (2005). The human brain is intrinsically organized into dynamic, anticorrelated functional networks. *Proc. Natl. Acad. Sci. U.S.A.*, *102*, 9673–8.

Fox, M. D., Corbetta, M., Snyder, A. Z., Vincent, J. L., & Raichle, M. E. (2006). Spontaneous neuronal activity distinguishes human dorsal and ventral attention systems. *Proc. Natl. Acad. Sci. U.S.A.*, *103*, 10046–51.

Fox, M. D., & Raichle, M. E. (2007). Spontaneous fluctuations in brain activity observed with functional magnetic resonance imaging. *Nat. Rev. Neurosci.*, *8*, 700–11.

Frackowiack, R. S. J. (1991). Language activation studies with positron emission tomography. In D. J. Chadwick & J. Whelan (Eds.) *Exploring Brain Functional Anatomy with Positron Emission Tomography* (p. 231). Chichester, UK: John Wiley & Sons Ltd.

Fransson, P. (2005). Spontaneous low-frequency BOLD signal fluctuations: an fMRI investigation of the resting-state default mode of brain function hypothesis. *Hum. Brain Mapp.*, *26*, 15–29.

Fransson, P. (2006). How default is the default mode of brain function? Further evidence from intrinsic BOLD signal fluctuations. *Neuropsychologia*, *44*, 2836–45.

Fransson, P., Skiold, B., Horsch, S., Nordell, A., Blennow, M., et al. (2007). Resting-state networks in the infant brain. *Proc. Natl. Acad. Sci. U.S.A.*, *104*, 15531–6.

Frith, C. (1996). The role of the prefrontal cortex in self-consciousness: the case of auditory hallucinations. *Philos. Trans. R. Soc. Lond. B. Biol. Sci.*, *351*, 1505–12.

Fukunaga, M., Horovitz, S.G., van Gelderen, P., de Zwart, J. A., Jasma, J. M., et al. (2006). Large-amplitude, spatially correlated fluctuations in BOLD fMRI signals during extended rest and early sleep stages. *Magn. Reson. Imaging*, *24*, 979–92.

Garrity, A. G., Pearlson, G. D., McKiernan, K., Lloyd, D., Kiehl, K. A., & Calhoun, V. D. (2007). Aberrant "default mode" functional connectivity in schizophrenia. *Am. J. Psychiatry*, *164*, 450–7.

Ghatan, P. H., Hsieh, J. C., Wirsen-Meurling, A., Wredling, R., Eriksson, L., et al. (1995). Brain activation induced by the perceptual maze test: a PET study of cognitive performance. *Neuroimage*, *2*, 112–24.

Giambra, L. M. (1989). Task-unrelated-thought frequency as a function of age: a laboratory study. *Psychol. Aging*, *4*, 136–43.

Giambra, L. M. (1995). A laboratory method for investigating influences on switching attention to task-unrelated imagery and thought. *Conscious Cogn.*, *4*, 1–21.

Gilbert, D. T. (2006). *Stumbling on Happiness*. New York: Alfred A. Knopf. xvii, 277 pp.

Gilbert, D. T., & Wilson, T. D. (2007). Prospection: experiencing the future. *Science*, *317*, 1351–4.

Gilbert, S. J., Dumontheil, I., Simons, J. S., Frith, C. D., & Burgess, P. W. (2007). Comment on "Wandering minds: the default network and stimulus-independent thought". *Science 317*, 43.

Gilbert, S. J., Simons, J. S., Frith, C. D., & Burgess, P. W. (2006). Performance-related activity in medial rostral prefrontal cortex (area 10) during low-demand tasks. *J. Exp. Psychol. Hum. Percept. Perform.*, *32*, 45–58.

Gold, B. T., & Buckner, R. L. (2002). Common prefrontal regions coactivate with dissociable posterior regions during controlled semantic and phonological tasks. *Neuron*, *35*, 803–12.

Golland, Y., Bentin, S., Gelbard, H., Benjamini, Y., Heller, R., et al. (2007). Extrinsic and intrinsic systems in the posterior cortex of the human brain revealed during natural sensory stimulation. *Cereb. Cortex*, *17*, 766–77.

Greene, J., & Haidt, J. (2002). How (and where) does moral judgment work? *Trends Cogn. Sci.*, *6*, 517–23.

Greene, J. D., Sommerville, R. B., Nystrom, L. E., Darley, J. M., & Cohen, J. D. (2001). An fMRI investigation of emotional engagement in moral judgment. *Science*, *293*, 2105–8.

Greicius, M. D., Krasnow, B., Reiss, A. L., & Menon, V. (2003). Functional connectivity in the resting brain: a network analysis of the default mode hypothesis. *Proc. Natl. Acad. Sci. U.S.A.*, *100*, 253–8.

Greicius, M. D., & Menon, V. (2004). Default-mode activity during a passive sensory task: uncoupled from deactivation but impacting activation. *J. Cogn. Neurosci.*, *16*, 1484–92.

Greicius, M. D., Srivastava, G., Reiss, A. L., & Menon, V. (2004). Default-mode network activity distinguishes Alzheimer's disease from healthy aging: evidence from functional MRI. *Proc. Natl. Acad. Sci. U.S.A.*, *101*, 4637–42.

Güroğlu, B., Haselager, G. J., van Lieshout, C. F., Takashima, A., Rijpkema, M., et al. (2008). Why are friends special? Implementing a social interaction stimulation task to probe the neural correlates of friendship. *Neuroimage*, *39*, 903–910.

Gusnard, D. A., Akbudak, E., Shulman, G. L., & Raichle, M. E. (2001). Medial prefrontal cortex and self-referential mental activity: relation to a default mode of brain function. *Proc. Natl. Acad. Sci. U.S.A.*, *98*, 4259–64.

Gusnard, D. A., & Raichle, M. E. (2001). Searching for a baseline: functional imaging and the resting human brain. *Nat. Rev. Neurosci.*, *2*, 685–94.

Hahn, B., Ross, T. J., & Stein, E. A. (2007). Cingulate activation increases dynamically with response speed under stimulus unpredictability. *Cereb. Cortex*, *17*, 1664–71.

Harrison, B. J., Yücel, M., Pujol, J., & Pantelis, C. (2007). Task-induced deactivation of midline cortical regions in schizophrenia assessed with fMRI. *Schizophr. Res.*, *91*, 82–6.

Hassabis, D., Kumaran, D., & Maguire, E. A. (2007). Using imagination to understand the neural basis of episodic memory. *J. Neurosci.*, *27*, 14365–74.

Hassabis, D., & Maguire, E. A. (2007). Deconstructing episodic memory with construction. *Trends Cogn. Sci.*, *11*, 299–306.

Haughton, V., & Biswal, B. (1998). Clinical application of basal regional cerebral blood flow fluctuation measurements by fMRI. *Adv. Exp. Med. Biol.*, *454*, 583–90.

Haxby, J. V., Horwitz, B., Ungerleider, L. G., Maisog, J. M., Pietrini, P., & Grady, C. L. (1994). The functional organization of human extrastriate cortex: a PET-rCBF study of selective attention to faces and locations. *J. Neurosci.*, *14*, 6336–53.

Heeger, D. J., & Ress, D. (2002). What does fMRI tell us about neuronal activity? *Nat. Rev. Neurosci.*, *3*, 142–51.

Henson, R. N., Rugg, M. D., Shallice, T., Josephs, O., & Dolan, R. J. (1999). Recollection and familiarity in recognition memory: an event-related functional magnetic resonance imaging study. *J. Neurosci.*, *19*, 3962–72.

Herholz, K. (1995). FDG PET and differential diagnosis of dementia. *Alzheimer Dis. Assoc. Disord.*, *9*, 6–16.

Herholz, K., Salmon, E., Perani, D., Baron, J. C., Holthoff, V., et al. (2002). Discrimination between Alzheimer dementia and controls by automated analysis of multicenter FDG PET. *Neuroimage*, *17*, 302–16.

Horovitz, S. G., Fukunaga, M., de Zwart, J. A., van Gelderen, P., Fulton, S. C., et al. (2007). Low frequency BOLD fluctuations during resting wakefulness and light sleep: a simultaneous EEG-fMRI study. *Hum. Brain Mapp.*

Hunter, M. D., Eickhoff, S. B., Miller, T. W., Farrow, T. F., Wilkinson, I. D., & Woodruff, P. W. (2006). Neural activity in speech-sensitive auditory cortex during silence. *Proc. Natl. Acad. Sci U.S.A.*, *103*, 189–94.

Hyman, B. T., Van Hoesen, G. W., & Damasio, A. R. (1990). Memory-related neural systems in Alzheimer's disease: an anatomic study. *Neurology*, *40*, 1721–30.

Iacoboni, M. (2006). Failure to deactivate in autism: the co-constitution of self and other. *Trends Cogn. Sci.*, *10*, 431–3.

Ingvar, D. H. (1974). Patterns of brain activity revealed by measurements of regional cerebral blood flow. *Alfred Benzon Symposium VIII*. Copenhagen.

Ingvar, D. H. (1979). "Hyperfrontal" distribution of the cerebral grey matter flow in resting wakefulness: on the functional anatomy of the conscious state. *Acta Neurol. Scand.*, *60*, 12–25.

Ingvar, D. H. (1985). "Memory of the future": an essay on the temporal organization of conscious awareness. *Hum. Neurobiol.*, *4*, 127–36.

James, W. (1890). *The Principles of Psychology*. New York: Henry Holt and Company.

Johnson, A., & Redish, A. D. (2007). Neural ensembles in CA3 transiently encode paths forward of the animal at a decision point. *J. Neurosci.*, *27*, 12176–89.

Kawashima, R., Roland, P. E., & O'Sullivan, B. T. (1994). Fields in human motor areas involved in preparation for reaching, actual reaching, and visuomotor learning: a positron emission tomography study. *J. Neurosci.*, *14*, 3462–74.

Kelley, W. M., Macrae, C. N., Wyland, C. L., Caglar, S., Inati, S., & Heatherton, T. F. (2002). Finding the self? An event-related fMRI study. *J. Cogn. Neurosci.*, *14*, 785–94.

Kennedy, D. P., & Courchesne, E. (2008). The intrinsic functional organization of the brain is altered in autism. *Neuroimage*, *39*, 1877–85.

Kennedy, D. P., Redcay, E., & Courchesne, E. (2006). Failing to deactivate: resting functional abnormalities in autism. *Proc. Natl. Acad. Sci. U.S.A.*, *103*, 8275–80.

Kety, S. S., & Schmidt, C. F. (1948). The nitrous oxide method for the quantitative determination of cerebral blood flow in man: theory, procedure and normal values. *J. Clin. Invest.*, *27*, 476–83.

Kirchhoff, B. A., Schapiro, M. L., & Buckner, R. L. (2005). Orthographic distinctiveness and semantic elaboration provide separate contributions to memory. *J. Cogn. Neurosci.*, *17*, 1841–54.

Klinger, E. (1971). *Structure and Functions of Fantasy*. New York: John Wiley & Sons, Inc.

Klunk, W. E., Engler, H., Nordberg, A., Wang, Y., Blomqvist, G., et al. (2004). Imaging brain amyloid in Alzheimer's disease with Pittsburgh Compound-B. *Ann. Neurol.*, *55*, 306–19.

Kobayashi, Y., & Amaral, D. G. (2000). Macaque monkey retrosplenial cortex: I. three-dimensional and cytoarchitectonic organization. *J. Comp. Neurol.*, *426*, 339–65.

Kobayashi, Y., & Amaral, D. G. (2003). Macaque monkey retrosplenial cortex: II. cortical afferents. *J. Comp. Neurol.*, *466*, 48–79.

Kobayashi, Y., & Amaral, D. G. (2007). Macaque monkey retrosplenial cortex: III. cortical efferents. *J. Comp. Neurol.*, *502*, 810–33.

Kondo, H. Saleem, K. S., & Price, J. L. (2005). Differential connections of the perirhinal and parahippocampal cortex with the orbital and medial prefrontal networks in macaque monkeys. *J. Comp. Neurol.*, *493*, 479–509.

Kumar, A., Schapiro, M. B., Grady, C., Haxby, J. V., Wagner, E., et al. (1991). High-resolution PET studies in Alzheimer's disease. *Neuropsychopharmacology*, *4*, 35–46.

Kuperberg, G., & Heckers, S. (2000). Schizophrenia and cognitive function. *Curr. Opin. Neurobiol.*, *10*, 205–10.

Lavenex, P., Suzuki, W. A., & Amaral, D. G. (2002). Perirhinal and parahippocampal cortices of the macaque monkey: projections to the neocortex. *J. Comp. Neurol.*, *447*, 394–420.

Leichnetz, G. R. (2001). Connections of the medial posterior parietal cortex (area 7m) in the monkey. *Anat. Rec.*, *263*, 215–36.

Li, C.-S. R., Yan, P., Bergquist, K. L., & Sinha, R. (2007). Greater activation of the "default" brain regions predicts stop signal errors. *NeuroImage*, *38*, 640–8.

Li, Y., Nowotny, P., Holmans, P., Smemo, S., & Kauwe, J. S., et al. (2004). Association of late-onset Alzheimer's disease with genetic variation in multiple members of the GAPD gene family. *Proc. Natl. Acad. Sci. U.S.A.*, *101*, 15688–93.

Liddle, P. F. (1987). Schizophrenic syndromes, cognitive performance and neurological dysfunction. *Psychol. Med.*, *17*, 49–57.

Lustig, C., Snyder, A. Z., Bhakta, M., O'Brien, K. C., McAvoy, M., et al. (2003). Functional deactivations: change with age and dementia of the Alzheimer type. *Proc. Natl. Acad. Sci. U.S.A.*, *100*, 14504–9.

Lustig, C., & Buckner, R. L. (2004). Preserved neural correlates of priming in old age and dementia. *Neuron*, *42*, 865–75.

Maddock, R. J. (1999). The retrosplenial cortex and emotion: new insights from functional neuroimaging of the human brain. *Trends Neurosci*, *22*, 310–6.

Maguire, E. A. (2001). Neuroimaging studies of autobiographical event memory. *Philos. Trans. R. Soc. Lond. B. Biol. Sci.*, *356*, 1441–51.

Mason, M. F., Norton, M. I., Van Horn, J. D., Wegner, D. M., Grafton, S. T., & Macrae, C. N. (2007). Wandering minds: the default network and stimulus-independent thought. *Science*, *315*, 393–5.

Mattson, M. P. (2004). Pathways towards and away from Alzheimer's disease. *Nature*, *430*, 631–9.

Mazoyer, B., Zago, L., Mellet, E., Bricogne, S., Etard, O., et al. (2001). Cortical networks for working memory and executive functions sustain the conscious resting state in man. *Brain Res. Bull.*, *54*, 287–98.

McAlonan, G. M., Cheung, V., Cheung, C., Suckling, J., Lam, G. Y., et al. (2005). Mapping the brain in autism: a voxel-based MRI study of volumetric differences and intercorrelations in autism. *Brain*, *128*, 268–76.

McGuire, P. K., Paulesu, E., Frackowiak, R. S., & Frith, C. D. (1996). Brain activity during stimulus independent thought. *Neuroreport*, *7*, 2095–9.

McKiernan, K. A., D'Angelo, B. R., Kaufman, J. N., & Binder, J. R. (2006). Interrupting the "stream of consciousness": an fMRI investigation. *Neuroimage*, *29*, 1185–91.

McKiernan, K. A., Kaufman, J. N., Kucera-Thompson, J., & Binder, J. R. (2003). A parametric manipulation of factors affecting task-induced deactivation in functional neuroimaging. *J. Cogn. Neurosci.*, *15*, 394–408.

Mesulam, M. M. (2000a). *Principles of Behavioral and Cognitive Neurology*. New York: Oxford University Press.

Mesulam, M. M. (2000b). A plasticity-based theory of the pathogenesis of Alzheimer's disease. *Ann. N.Y. Acad. Sci.*, *924*, 42–52.

Minoshima, S., Giordani, B., Berent, S., Frey, K. A., Foster, N. L., & Kuhl, D. E. (1997). Metabolic reduction in the posterior cingulate cortex in very early Alzheimer's disease. *Ann. Neurol.*, *42*, 85–94.

Mintun, M. A., Sacco, D., Snyder, A. Z., Couture, L., Powers, W. J., Hornbeck, R., et al. (2006a). Distribution of glycolysis in the resting healthy human brain correlates with distribution of beta-amyloid plaques in Alzheimer's disease. *Soc. Neurosci. Abstr.*, 707.6.

Mintun, M. A., Larossa, G. N., Sheline, Y. I., Dence, C. S., Lee, S. Y., et al. (2006b). [^{11}C]PIB in a nondemented population: potential antecedent marker of Alzheimer disease. *Neurology*, *67*, 446–52.

Mitchell, J. P., Macrae, C. N., & Banaji, M. R. (2006). Dissociable medial prefrontal contributions to judgments of similar and dissimilar others. *Neuron*, *50*, 655–63.

Moll, J., Zahn, R., de Oliveira-Souza, R., Krueger, F., & Grafman, J. (2005). Opinion: the neural basis of human moral cognition. *Nat. Rev. Neurosci.*, *6*, 799–809.

Morcom, A. M., & Fletcher, P. C. (2007). Does the brain have a baseline? Why we should be resisting a rest. *Neuroimage*, *37*, 1073–82.

Morris, R., Petrides, M., & Pandya, D. N. (1999). Architecture and connections of retrosplenial area 30 in the rhesus monkey (Macaca mulatta). *Eur. J. Neurosci.*, *11*, 2506–18.

Morris, R., Paxinos, G., & Petrides, M. (2000). Architectonic analysis of the human retrosplenial cortex. *J. Comp. Neurol.*, *421*, 14–28.

Mundy, P. (2003). The neural basis of social impairments in autism: the role of the dorsal medial-frontal cortex and anterior cingulate system. *J. Child. Psychol. Psychiatry*, *44*, 793–809.

Nir, Y., Hasson, U., Levy, I., Yeshurun, Y., & Malach, R. (2006). Widespread functional connectivity and fMRI fluctuations in human visual cortex in the absence of visual stimulation. *Neuroimage*, *30*, 1313–24.

Nyberg, L., Habib, R., McIntosh, A. R., & Tulving, E. (2000). Reactivation of encoding-related brain activity during memory retrieval. *Proc. Natl. Acad. Sci. U.S.A.*, *97*, 11120–4.

Ochsner, K. N., Knierim, K., Ludlow, D. H., Hanelin, J., Ramachandran, T., Glover, G., et al. (2004). Reflecting upon feelings: an fMRI study of neural systems supporting the attribution of emotion to self and other. *J. Cogn. Neurosci.*, *16*, 1746–72.

Okuda, J., Fujii, T., Ohtake, H., Tsukiura, T., Tanji, K., et al. (2003). Thinking of the future and past: the roles of the frontal pole and the medial temporal lobes. *Neuroimage*, *19*, 1369–80.

Öngür, D., & Price, J. L. (2000). The organization of networks within the orbital and medial prefrontal cortex of rats, monkeys and humans. *Cereb. Cortex*, *10*, 206–19.

Öngür, D., Ferry, A. T., & Price, J. L. (2003). Architectonic subdivision of the human orbital and medial prefrontal cortex. *J. Comp. Neurol.*, *460*, 425–49.

Orban, G. A., Claeys, K., Nelissen, K., Smans, R., Sunaert, S., et al. (2006). Mapping the parietal cortex of human and non-human primates. *Neuropsychologia*, *44*, 2647–67.

Otten, L. J., & Rugg, M. D. (2001). When more means less: neural activity related to unsuccessful memory encoding. *Curr. Biol.*, *11*, 1528–30.

Partiot, A., Grafman, J., Sadato, N., Wachs, J., & Hallett, M. (1995). Brain activation during the generation of nonemotional and emotional plans. *Neuroreport*, *6*, 1397–400.

Parvizi, J., Van Hoesen, G. W., Buckwalter, J., & Damasio, A. (2006). Neural connections of the posteromedial cortex in the macaque. *Proc. Natl. Acad. Sci. U.S.A.*, *103*, 1563–8.

Petrides, M., & Pandya, D. N. (1994). Comparative architectonic analysis of the human and the macaque frontal cortex. In F. Boller, & H. Spinnler (Eds.) *Handbook of Neuropsychology* (pp. 17–58). Amsterdam: Elsevier Science B.V.

Phelps, E. A. (2006). Emotion and cognition: insights from studies of the human amygdala. *Annu. Rev. Psychol.*, *57*, 27–53.

Price, J. L. (2007). Definition of the orbital cortex in relation to specific connections with limbic and visceral structures, and other cortical regions. *Ann. N.Y. Acad. Sci.*, *1121*, 54–71.

Raichle, M. E. (1987). Circulatory and metabolic correlates of brain function in normal humans. In V. Mountcastle, & F. Plum (Eds.) *Handbook of Physiology, The Nervous System. V. Higher Functions of the Brain, Part 2* Bethesda: American Psychological Society.

Raichle, M. E. (2006). The brain's dark energy. *Science*, *314*, 1249–50.

Raichle, M. E., MacLeod, A. M., Snyder, A. Z., Powers, W. J., Gusnard, D. A., et al. (2001). A default mode of brain function. *Proc. Natl. Acad. Sci. U.S.A.*, *98*, 676–82.

Raichle, M. E., & Mintun, M. A. (2006). Brain work and brain imaging. *Annu. Rev. Neurosci.*, *29*, 449–76.

Raichle, M. E., & Snyder, A. Z. (2007). A default mode of brain function: a brief history of an evolving idea. *Neuroimage*, *37*, 1083–1090.

Ramnani, N., & Owen, A. M. (2004). Anterior prefrontal cortex: insights into function from anatomy and neuroimaging. *Nat. Rev. Neurosci.*, *5*, 184–94.

Reiman, E. M., Caselli, R. J., Yun, L. S., Chen, K., Bandy, D., et al. (1996). Preclinical evidence of Alzheimer's disease in persons homozygous for the epsilon 4 allele for apolipoprotein E. *N. Engl. J. Med.*, *334*, 752–8.

Rilling, J. K., Sanfey, A. G., Aronson, J. A., Nystrom, L. E., & Cohen, J. D. (2004). The neural correlates of theory of mind within interpersonal interactions. *Neuroimage, 22,* 1694–703.

Rilling, J. K., Barks, S. K., Parr, L. A., Preuss, T. M., Faber, T. L., et al. (2007). A comparison of resting-state brain activity in humans and chimpanzees. *Proc. Natl. Acad. Sci. U.S.A., 104,* 17146–51.

Rombouts, S. A., Barkhof, F., Goekoop, R., Stam, C. J., & Scheltens, P. (2005). Altered resting state networks in mild cognitive impairment and mild Alzheimer's disease: an fMRI study. *Hum. Brain Mapp., 26,* 231–9.

Saper, C. B., Wainer, B. H., & German, D. C. (1987). Axonal and transneuronal transport in the transmission of neurological disease: Potential role of system degenerations, including Alzheimer's disease. *Neuroscience, 23,* 389–98.

Saxe, R., & Kanwisher, N. (2003). People thinking about thinking people: the role of the temporo-parietal junction in "theory of mind". *Neuroimage, 19,* 1835–42.

Saxe, R., Carey, S., & Kanwisher, N. (2004). Understanding other minds: linking developmental psychology and functional neuroimaging. *Annu. Rev. Psychol., 55,* 87–124.

Saxe, R., & Powell, L. J. (2006). It's the thought that counts: specific brain regions for one component of theory of mind. *Psychol. Sci., 17,* 692–9.

Scahill, R. I., Schott, J. M., Stevens, J. M., Rossor, M. N., & Fox, N. C. (2002). Mapping the evolution of regional atrophy in Alzheimer's disease: unbiased analysis of fluid-registered serial MRI. *Proc. Natl. Acad. Sci. U.S.A., 99,* 4703–7.

Schacter, D. L., & Addis, D. R. (2007). The cognitive neuroscience of constructive memory: remembering the past and imagining the future. *Philos. Trans. R. Soc. Lond. B. Biol. Sci., 362,* 773–86.

Schacter, D. L., Addis, D. R., & Buckner, R. L. (2007). Remembering the past to imagine the future: the prospective brain. *Nat. Rev. Neurosci., 8,* 657–61.

Schacter, D. L., Addis, D. R., & Buckner, R. L. (2008). Episodic simulation of future events: concepts, data, and applications. In *The Year in Cognitive Neuroscience 2008, Ann. N.Y. Acad. Sci., 1124,* 39–60.

Scheperjans, F., Hermann, K., Eickhoff, S. B., Amunts, K., Schleicher, A., et al. (2007). Observer-independent cytoarchitectonic mapping of the human superior parietal cortex. *Cereb. Cortex.*

Schumann, C. M., Hamstra, J., Goodlin-Jones, B. L., Lotspeich, L. J., Kwon, H., et al. (2004). The amygdala is enlarged in children but not adolescents with autism; the hippocampus is enlarged at all ages. *J. Neurosci., 24,* 6392–401.

Selkoe, D. J. (2006). The ups and downs of Abeta. *Nat. Med., 12,* 758–9.

Semendeferi, K., Armstrong, E., Schleicher, A., Zilles, K., & Van Hoesen, G. W. (2001). Prefrontal cortex in humans and apes: a comparative study of area 10. *Am. J. Phys. Anthropol., 114,* 224–41.

Shannon, B. J. (2006). *Functional anatomic studies of memory retrieval and the default mode.* Washington University in St. Louis, St. Louis. 184 pp.

Shannon, B. J., Snyder, A. Z., Vincent, J. L., & Buckner, R. L. (2006). Spontaneous correlations and the default network: effects of task performance. *Soc. Neurosci. Abstr.,* 119.5.

Shapiro, M. L., Kennedy, P. J., & Ferbinteanu, J. (2006). Representing episodes in the mammalian brain. *Curr. Opin. Neurobiol., 16,* 701–9.

Sharot, T., Riccardi, A. M., Raio, C. M., & Phelps, E. A. (2007). Neural mechanisms mediating optimism bias. *Nature, 450,* 102–5.

Shulman, G. L., Fiez, J. A., Corbetta, M., Buckner, R. L., Miezin, F. M., et al. (1997). Common blood flow changes across visual tasks: II.: decreases in cerebral cortex. *J. Cogn. Neurosci., 9,* 648–63.

Simon, O., Mangin, J. F., Cohen, L., Le Bihan, D., & Dehaene, S. (2002). Topographical layout of hand, eye, calculation, and language-related areas in the human parietal lobe. *Neuron, 33,* 475–87.

Singer, J. L., & Antrobus, J. S. (1963). A factor-analytic study of daydreaming and conceptually-related cognitive and personality variables. *Perceptual and Motor Skills, 17,* 187–209.

Singer, J. L., & Schonbar, R. A. (1961). Correlates of daydreaming: a dimension of self-awareness. *Journal of Consulting Psychology, 25,* 1–6.

Singer, J. L. (1966). *Daydreaming: An Introduction to the Experimental Study of Inner Experience.* New York: Random House, Inc.

Singer, J. L. (1974). Daydreaming and the stream of thought. *American Scientist, 62,* 417–25.

Singer, J. L., & Antrobus, J. S. (1972). Daydreaming, imaginal processes, and personality: a normative study. In P. W. Sheehan (Ed.) *The Function and Nature of Imagery* (pp. 175–202). New York: Academic Press, Inc.

Smallwood, J., & Schooler, J. W. (2006). The restless mind. *Psychol. Bull., 132,* 946–58.

Sokoloff, L., Mangold, R., Wechsler, R. L., Kenney, C., & Kety, S. S. (1955). The effect of mental arithmetic on cerebral circulation and metabolism. *J. Clin. Invest., 34,* 1101–8.

Sorg, C., Reidl, V., Muhlaü, M., Calhoun, V. D., Eichele, T., et al. (2007). Selective changes of resting-state networks in individuals at risk for Alzheimer's disease. *Proc. Natl. Acad. Sci. U.S.A., 104,* 18760–5.

Suzuki, W. A., & Amaral, D. G. (1994). Perirhinal and parahippocampal cortices of the macaque monkey: cortical afferents. *J. Comp. Neurol., 350,* 497–533.

Svoboda, E., McKinnon, M. C., & Levine, B. (2006). The functional neuroanatomy of autobiographical memory: a meta-analysis. *Neuropsychologia, 44,* 2189–208.

Szpunar, K. K., Watson, J. M., & McDermott, K. B. (2007). Neural substrates of envisioning the future. *Proc. Natl. Acad. Sci. U.S.A., 104,* 642–7.

Talairach, J., & Tournoux, P. (1988). *Co-planar stereotaxic atlas of the human brain.* New York: Thieme.

Teasdale, J. D., Dritschel, B. H., Taylor, M. J., Proctor, L., Lloyd, C. A., et al. (1995). Stimulus-independent thought depends on central executive resources. *Mem. Cognit., 23,* 551–9.

Thompson, P. M., Hayashi, K. M., de Zubicaray, G., Janke, A. L., Rose, S. E., et al. (2003). Dynamics of gray matter loss in Alzheimer's disease. *J. Neurosci., 23,* 994–1005.

Tian, L., Jiang, T., Liu, Y., Yu, C., Wang, K., et al. (2007). The relationship within and between the extrinsic and intrinsic systems indicated by resting state correlational patterns of sensory cortices. *Neuroimage, 36,* 684–90.

Tsodyks, M., Kenet, T., Grinvald, A., & Arieli, A. (1999). Linking spontaneous activity of single cortical neurons and the underlying functional architecture. *Science, 286,* 1943–6.

Tulving, E. (2005). Episodic memory and autonoesis: Uniquely human? In H. Terrance, & J. Metcalfe (Eds.) *The missing link in cognition: Origins of self-reflective consciousness* (pp. 3–56). New York: Oxford University Press.

Van Essen, D. C. (2005). A Population-Average, Landmark- and Surface-based (PALS) atlas of human cerebral cortex. *Neuroimage, 28*, 635–62.

Van Essen, D. C., & Dieker, D. L. (2007). Surface-based and probabilistic atlases of primate cerebral cortex. *Neuron, 56*, 209–25.

Vincent, J. L., Snyder, A. Z., Fox, M. D., Shannon, B. J., Andrews, J. R., et al. (2006). Coherent spontaneous activity identifies a hippocampal-parietal memory network. *J. Neurophysiol., 96*, 3517–31.

Vincent, J. L., Patel, G. H., Fox, M. D., Snyder, A. Z., Baker, J. T., et al. (2007a). Intrinsic functional architecture in the anaesthetized monkey brain. *Nature, 447*, 83–6.

Vincent, J. L., Kahn, I., Snyder, A. Z., Fox, M. D., Raichle, M. E., & Buckner, R. L. (2007b). Evidence for three distinct, bilateral frontoparietal associative brain systems revealed by spontaneous fMRI correlations. *Soc. Neurosci. Abstr.*

Vogeley, K., May, M., Ritzl, A., Falkai, P., Zilles, K., & Fink, G. R. (2004). Neural correlates of first-person perspective as one constituent of human self-consciousness. *J. Cogn. Neurosci., 16*, 817–27.

Vogt, B. A., Vogt, L. J., Perl, D. P., & Hof, P. R. (2001). Cytology of human caudomedial cingulate, retrosplenial, and caudal parahippocampal cortices. *J. Comp. Neurol., 438*, 353–76.

Vogt, B. A., & Laureys, S. (2005). Posterior cingulate, precuneal and retrosplenial cortices: cytology and components of the neural network correlates of consciousness. *Prog. Brain Res., 150*, 205–17.

Vogt, B. A., Nimchinsky, E. A., Vogt, L. J., & Hof, P. R. (1995). Human cingulate cortex: Surface features, flat maps, and cytoarchitecture. *J. Comp. Neurol., 359*, 490–506.

Vogt, B. A., Vogt, L., & Laureys, S. (2006). Cytology and functionally correlated circuits of human posterior cingulate areas. *Neuroimage, 29*, 452–66.

Wagner, A. D., Shannon, B. J., Kahn, I., & Buckner, R. L. (2005). Parietal lobe contributions to episodic memory retrieval. *Trends Cogn. Sci., 9*, 445–53.

Waiter, G. D., Williams, J. H., Murray, A. D., Gilchrist, A., Perrett, D. I., & Whiten, A. (2004). A voxel-based investigation of brain structure in male adolescents with autistic spectrum disorder. *Neuroimage, 22*, 619–25.

Walsh, D. M., & Selkoe, D. J. (2004). Deciphering the molecular basis of memory failure in Alzheimer's disease. *Neuron, 44*, 181–93.

Wang, K., Liang, M., Wang, L., Tian, L., Zhang, X., et al. (2006). Altered functional connectivity in early Alzheimer's disease: a resting-state fMRI study. *Hum. Brain Mapp., 28*, 967–78.

Weissman, D. H., Roberts, K. C., Visscher, K. M., & Woldorff, M. G. (2006). The neural bases of momentary lapses in attention. *Nat. Neurosci., 9*, 971–8.

Wheeler, M. E., Petersen, S. E., & Buckner, R. L. (2000). Memory's echo: vivid remembering reactivates sensory-specific cortex. *Proc. Natl. Acad. Sci. U.S.A., 97*, 11125–9.

Wheeler, M. E., & Buckner, R. L. (2004). Functional-anatomic correlates of remembering and knowing. *Neuroimage, 21*, 1337–49.

Williamson, P. (2007). Are anticorrelated networks in the brain relevant to schizophrenia? *Schizophr. Bull., 33*, 994–1003.

Wimmer, H., & Perner, J. (1983). Beliefs about beliefs: representation and constraining function of wrong beliefs in young children's understanding of deception. *Cognition, 13*, 103–28.

Wise, R. G., Ide, K., Poulin, M. J., & Tracey, I. (2004). Resting fluctuations in arterial carbon dioxide induce significant low frequency variations in BOLD signal. *Neuroimage, 21*, 1652–64.

Yonelinas, A. P., Otten, L. J., Shaw, K. N., & Rugg, M. D. (2005). Separating the brain regions involved in recollection and familiarity in recognition memory. *J. Neurosci., 25*, 3002–8.

Zhou, Y., Liang, M., Tian, L., Wang, K., Hao, Y., et al. (2007). Functional disintegration in paranoid schizophrenia using resting-state fMRI. *Schizophr. Res, 97*, 194–205.

Episodic Simulation of Future Events

Concepts, Data, and Applications

DANIEL L. SCHACTER,[a,c] **DONNA ROSE ADDIS,**[a,c] **AND RANDY L. BUCKNER**[a,b,c,d]

[a]*Department of Psychology, Harvard University, Cambridge, Massachusetts, USA*

[b]*Center for Brain Science, Harvard University, Cambridge, Massachusetts, USA*

[c]*Athinoula A Martinos Center for Biomedical Imaging, Massachusetts General Hospital, Boston, Massachusetts, USA*

[d]*Howard Hughes Medical Institute, Harvard University, Cambridge, Massachusetts, USA*

This article focuses on the neural and cognitive processes that support imagining or simulating future events, a topic that has recently emerged in the forefront of cognitive neuroscience. We begin by considering concepts of simulation from a number of areas of psychology and cognitive neuroscience in order to place our use of the term in a broader context. We then review neuroimaging, neuropsychological, and cognitive studies that have examined future-event simulation and its relation to episodic memory. This research supports the idea that simulating possible future events depends on much of the same neural machinery, referred to here as a core network, as does remembering past events. After discussing several theoretical accounts of the data, we consider applications of work on episodic simulation for research concerning clinical populations suffering from anxiety or depression. Finally, we consider other aspects of future-oriented thinking that we think are related to episodic simulation, including planning, prediction, and remembering intentions. These processes together comprise what we have termed "the prospective brain," whose primary function is to use past experiences to anticipate future events.

Key words: episodic memory; simulation of future events; neuroimaging; constructive memory; episodic future thinking; prospective memory; foresight; hippocampus; prefrontal cortex; mental time travel

The study of episodic memory has constituted one of the most vigorous research areas in all of cognitive neuroscience for more than two decades. Neuroimaging and patient studies have examined a wide variety of topics, including the nature of encoding and retrieval processes, the relation between recollection and familiarity, and the basis of memory accuracy versus distortion, along with many others. During the past year or two, a less familiar topic has burst onto the landscape of memory research: the role of episodic memory in imagining or simulating possible future events. Though seeds of interest in the topic had been sown in earlier years, the simultaneous publication within a brief time span of neuroimaging, neuropsychological, and cognitive studies, as well as the appearance of several theoretically oriented integrative articles, has brought much greater attention to the issue.

The purpose of the present article is to consider this emerging collection of empirical findings and ideas in a broad context of relevant research, concepts, and applications. We will focus on the recent evidence indicating that episodic memory is critically involved in our ability to carry out simulations of future happenings and to imagine novel events, and that brain regions traditionally identified with memory, including the hippocampus, appear to be similarly engaged when people imagine future experiences. Because we have reviewed some of this work elsewhere (Buckner & Carroll 2007; Schacter & Addis 2007a; Schacter et al. 2007), here we will focus on delineating some of the key concepts in this emerging area and discussing research that we have not considered in our previous papers. We will also attempt to link work on episodic simulation to related research that fits under the rubric of an organizing concept that we have termed "the prospective brain," which proposes that a crucial function of the brain is to use stored information to allow us to imagine, plan for, and predict possible future events (Schacter et al. 2007). The recent studies alluded to above have

Address for correspondence: Daniel L. Schacter, Department of Psychology, Harvard University, 33 Kirkland St., Cambridge, MA 02138. dls@wjh.harvard.edu focused on imagining or simulating future events, but these are only a subset of processes that are relevant to the prospective brain.

We will begin by focusing on the concept of *simulating* possible future events, which we believe is central to understanding the prospective brain. The concept of simulation has played an important role in a number of areas of psychology and cognitive neuroscience but has been relatively little used in memory research. We will consider its various uses in order to help sharpen our own conceptualization of the term. Next, we will review neuroimaging, neuropsychological, and cognitive studies that have examined future-event simulation and its relation to episodic memory. A major message of this research is that simulating possible future events depends on much of the same neural machinery—what we will refer to as a core network—as does remembering past events.

We will then consider the applications of this work for research concerning clinical populations suffering from anxiety or depression in which pathological future thinking is a central feature. Finally, we place the process of event simulation into the broader context of the prospective brain by considering briefly research concerning related processes of planning, prediction, and remembering intentions. We offer a few preliminary thoughts concerning how simulation may be related to these other key processes of the prospective brain.

Episodic Simulation: Delineating a Concept

Consider a scenario in which you are preparing a talk that you will give the following week to a small group of experts in your field. You are trying to decide whether to include a particular analysis in your talk: is it necessary to present the analysis to buttress your case, or will it simply complicate and slow down your talk? You imagine yourself giving this talk, standing in front of an audience in the room the conference was held in last year. You consider each of the experts who will likely be in the audience and imagine how they would react to your claims with and without the extra analysis slide. You remember vividly how one of these colleagues objected fiercely to one of your earlier talks when you did not include a similar analysis and try to figure out whether a similar response is likely in this new situation. You also recall hearing from a collaborator that one of the attendees who you do not know well is a stickler for details; you can envisage her questioning why you did not include the extra analysis. Though it will add length to the talk, these imaginary exercises convince you to err on the side of caution and include the extra analysis. When that analysis turns out the following week to be crucial to addressing the concerns of these colleagues, you are quite pleased that you took the time to imagine the possible outcomes before giving the talk.

This fictional (though not unfamiliar) scenario illustrates what we have in mind when we talk about episodic simulation of future events: drawing on elements of past experiences in order to envisage and mentally "try out" one or more versions of what might happen. Though memory researchers have until recently paid scant attention to the nature and implications of such episodic simulations, the general notion of mental simulation has been discussed by investigators in a number of areas of psychology and cognitive neuroscience.

Perhaps the first researcher to invoke the construct of simulation in a cognitive neuroscience context was the Swedish brain physiologist David Ingvar (see also Buckner et al. 2008 and Schacter et al. 2007 for discussion of Ingvar's work). Ingvar (1979) described studies in which he and his colleagues observed high levels of blood flow in prefrontal cortex during a resting awake state in which subjects sat quietly with eyes closed. Observing that the activated prefrontal regions are involved in "programming our behavior in general," Ingvar (1979, p. 21) theorized that the activity observed during resting states reflects an internal connection between the past and the future: "On the basis of previous experiences, represented in memories, the brain—one's mind—is automatically busy with extrapolation of future events and, as it appears, constructing alternative hypothetical behavior patterns in order to be ready for what may happen." Further, claimed Ingvar, "the high frontal cortical flows ... could be ascribed to a '*simulation of behavior*,' i.e., an inner anticipatory programming of several alternative behavioral modes prepared to be used depending upon what will happen" (p. 21).

Ingvar's use of the concept of simulation is quite similar to the one that we will adopt in this article, and his general interpretation of his early data (see also Ingvar 1985; Ingvar & Philipson 1977) receives strong support from recent research that we will consider. Nonetheless, Ingvar's ideas regarding memory-based simulation of future events were largely ignored by memory researchers of the day (an inspection of the Web of Science citation database turns up only a few scattered citations to his work among memory researchers through the late 1980s; cf. Olton 1989; Schacter 1987; Tulving 1985, 1987; Tulving et al. 1988; Wood 1987).

At around the same time as Ingvar discussed simulation of possible future behavior patterns, Amos Tversky and Daniel Kahneman stressed the importance of simulation in their pioneering research concerning the role of heuristics and biases in human decision making. Tversky and Kahneman (1973) reported classic studies showing that subjects' estimates of the likelihood of an event happening in the future were greatly influenced by the ease of retrieving similar examples from memory, a process that they termed "the availability heuristic." In closing their 1973 article, Tversky and Kahneman also briefly discussed a related heuristic that is used when people make judgments about rare or unique events in which similar instances are not available in memory. Here, individuals construct scenarios related to the target events, and the ease of scenario construction influences likelihood estimates, such that more easily constructed scenarios are judged to be more likely to occur in the future. A decade later, Kahneman and Tversky (1982) noted that this latter mechanism had been relatively neglected in prior research and called it the "simulation heuristic." According to Kahneman and Tversky (1982), "There appear to be many situations in which questions about events are answered by an operation that resembles the running of a simulation model" (p. 201). They suggested further that "A simulation does not necessarily produce a single story, which starts at the beginning and ends with a definite outcome." Instead, "we construe the output of simulation as an assessment of the ease with which the model could produce different outcomes" (p. 201). Commenting that contemporary understanding of the simulation heuristic "is still rudimentary," Kahneman and Tversky called for further research "in a domain that appears exceptionally rich and promising" (p. 204). Although there has been relatively little research on the simulation heuristic during the past 25 years, we will discuss later some interesting explorations of this heuristic in the future thinking of psychopathological populations (e.g., Brown et al. 2002; Raune et al. 2005; Vaughn & Weary 2002).

Note that Kahneman and Tversky's ideas about the simulation heuristic were not specifically restricted to future events; they also discussed the role of simulation in reconstructing and revisiting past events (i.e., counterfactual thinking; see also Byrne 2005; Kahneman & Miller 1986). Taylor and Schneider (1989) invoked an even broader notion of simulation in the context of a cognitive theory of coping and emotion regulation. They defined simulation as "the imitative representation of the functioning or process of some event or series of events ... We will use the term to mean the cognitive construction of hypothetical scenarios or the reconstruction of real scenarios" (p. 175). Taylor and Schneider ascribed great functional importance to simulation because it provides a kind of cognitive flexibility that exceeds what can be accomplished by behavior alone: "Unlike actual behavior, the cognitive system is capable of rerunning past events, altering their components or changing their endings, and projecting multiple versions of imaginary or future events with considerable virtuosity" (p. 175). Taylor and Schneider went on to outline and discuss specific functions for simulation of future events, including checking the viability of plans (cf. Miller et al. 1960), regulating emotions, and facilitating links between thought and action. They also discussed how simulation of past events can aid coping with prior stressors (see Taylor et al. 1998 for an update; for related work, see Sanna 2000).

The foregoing uses of the concept of simulation have for the most part focused on simulation of particular episodes or events. An even broader use of the concept can be found in research exploring the hypothesis that thinking and categorizing involve the simulation of perception and action (Barsalou 1999, 2003; Hesslow 2002, for review see Decety & Grezes 2006). Thus, for example, Barsalou (2003, p. 521) argued that "conceptual processing uses reenactments of sensory-motor states—simulations—to represent categories." Hesslow (2002, p. 242) contended that conscious thought reflects the simulation of perception and action. For example, simulation of perception occurs in the sense that "imagining perceiving something is essentially the same as actually perceiving it, only the perceptual activity is generated by the brain itself rather than by external stimuli," whereas simulation of action occurs because "we can activate motor structures of the brain in a way that resembles activity during a normal action but does not cause any overt movement." Interestingly, these broad conceptions of simulation were influenced by early work from David Ingvar that showed similar patterns of cerebral blow flow when subjects carried out a movement and when they only imagined carrying out the movement. Decety and Ingvar (1990) provided a comprehensive review of then-extant studies concerning brain structures that participate in simulation of various kinds of actions. There has been considerable cognitive neuroscience research on the topic since that time (Decety & Grezes 2006) as well as on related topics such as the overlapping brain regions activated during perceiving and imagining (e.g., Kosslyn 1994, 2005).

Finally, the concept of simulation has played an important role in developmental research concerning theory of mind and related work on "mentalizing," or the processes involved in reading the mental states of other individuals (for reviews, see Frith & Frith 2006; Goldman 2006; Oberman & Ramachandran 2007). This approach stems from philosophical analyses that emphasize the critical importance of simulation in mentalizing (Goldman 1989; Gordon 1986; Heal 1986). According to the simulation account, attributions about another individual's mental state involve imaginatively placing oneself in the other's situation and pretending to have the same desires or beliefs as the other individual (Goldman 2006). The results of this mental simulation can then be used to make predictions or inferences about how another individual will behave. The simulation account contrasts with the so-called theory-theory, which holds that folk psychology or commonsense theories about other individuals' minds constitute the basis for mentalizing (e.g., Gopnik & Meltoff 1997; Gopnik & Wellman 1992). Debates about the viability of simulation and theory-theory accounts of mentalizing in both children and adults remain active and unsettled (cf. Davies & Stone 1995; Goldman 2006; Gordon 1992; Heal 1994; Mitchell et al. 2006; Saxe 2005).

It seems clear, then, that the concept of simulation has been used in diverse settings and for a variety of theoretical purposes. In the present article, our use of the term "simulation" most closely resembles that of Taylor and Schneider (1989) in that we use the term to refer to *imaginative constructions of hypothetical events or scenarios*. We note several points about our use of the concept. First, we view simulation as a goal-directed process that involves more than simple imagery. People generate simulations with a view toward addressing a current or future problem. Second, we emphasize that simulation is critical for envisaging possible future events, but we do not restrict our application of simulation to the future. People also engage in simulations of present and past events, a point to which we return later when considering theoretical approaches to recent neuropsychological and neuroimaging data. Given the range of situations in which simulations are used, it would be easy to use the concept of simulation interchangeably with more general notions such as "thought" or "thinking." We view simulation as a particular kind or subset of thinking that involves imaginatively placing oneself in a hypothetical scenario and exploring possible outcomes. Third, we focus our review and theoretical claims on simulation of events or episodes. While acknowledging that others use the concept much more broadly to make claims about the nature and basis of perception, categorization, mentalizing, and the like, our own emphasis on episodic simulation is neutral with respect to the various theoretical debates that exist concerning these related issues. It may turn out that there is a common underlying basis for various kinds of simulation-based processes, and we indeed consider later some data bearing on this point. We are hopeful that by delineating some key features of episodic simulation and suggesting a neural basis for this process that we can help to pave the way for a broader understanding of simulation processes is several domains.

Episodic Simulation of Future Events: The Core Network

The emerging interest in future-event simulation within cognitive neuroscience is no doubt attributable, at least in part, to recent studies that provide converging evidence for shared neural processes underlying remembering past events and imagining future events. These studies show, to varying degrees, that regions previously thought to play a role in episodic remembering, including prefrontal and medial temporal regions, are also implicated in simulation of future events. While a role for prefrontal cortex in future thinking dates to the early work of Ingvar (1979, 1985), observations of medial temporal contributions to future-event simulation are of more recent vintage. Relevant evidence has been provided by behavioral studies of amnesic patients and neuroimaging studies of individuals with intact memory.

The first indications that future-event simulation might rely on the same structures as episodic memory came from observations of amnesic patients. In his famous monograph concerning patients with Korsakoff's amnesia, Talland (1965) observed that many of his patients exhibited deficits in making personal plans. However, it was unclear from these observations whether and how the memory and planning deficits are linked. Patients with Korsakoff's syndrome often exhibit problems not observed in other amnesic patients as a result of their relatively more diffuse pathology (e.g., Schacter 1987; Squire 1982), and it is possible that the planning deficits are incidental or unrelated to the memory deficits. Somewhat more compelling evidence was provided by observations concerning the severely amnesic patient K.C., who fails to remember *any* specific episodes from his past (for a review of K.C., see Rosenbaum et al. 2005). Strikingly, K.C. showed a parallel difficulty envisaging any specific episodes in his future (Tulving 1985; Tulving et al. 1988). However, as with the Korsakoff patients, K.C. is characterized by fairly extensive brain damage, affecting medial temporal, prefrontal, and other regions; though episodic memory loss clearly constitutes his most severe problem, it is not his only deficit (see Rosenbaum et al. 2005).

Klein et al. (2002) reported a more extensive investigation of past and future events in patient D.B., who became amnesic as a result of cardiac arrest and consequent anoxia. They gave D.B. a 10-item questionnaire probing past and future events that were matched for temporal distance from the present (e.g., What did you do yesterday? What are you going to do tomorrow?). Since it is not entirely clear what constitutes a correct answer for questions about the personal future, Klein et al. evaluated D.B.'s responses in light of information provided by his family. For example, D.B. was asked "When will be the next time you see a doctor?" and responded "Sometime in the next week." This response was judged correct because his daughter confirmed that he did have an appointment with the doctor the next week. D.B. was also asked "Who are you going to see this evening?" and said that he was going to visit his mother. This response was judged incorrect (i.e., confabulatory) because D.B.'s mother had died nearly two decades earlier. Consistent with the previous observations, D.B. was highly impaired on the both past and future versions of this task. D.B.'s deficit in simulating future events appeared to be specific to his *personal* future: D.B. showed little difficulty imagining possible future events in the public domain, such as political events and issues. As Schacter and Addis (2007b) have noted, however, many of the items concerning the public domain did not ask about specific events, so the evidence for a personal/public distinction is not clear cut. Furthermore, little information was provided concerning the location of D.B.'s lesion, limiting the inferences that could be made concerning the basis for the future simulation deficit and its relation to his episodic memory problems.

A number of the foregoing limitations were addressed in a more recent study by Hassabis et al. (2007). They examined the ability of five patients with documented bilateral hippocampal amnesia to imagine novel experiences. Amnesic patients and matched controls generated everyday imaginary experiences, such as "Imagine you're lying on a white sandy beach in a beautiful tropical bay." Subjects were specifically instructed to construct something new and not to provide a memory of a past event. Participants described their imaginary scenarios in the presence of a cue card to remind them of the task, and experimenters probed subjects for further details and elaboration. Protocols were scored based on the content, spatial coherence, and subjective qualities of the participants' imagined scenarios.

The imaginary constructions produced by four of the five hippocampal patients were greatly reduced in richness and content compared with those of controls. The impairment was especially pronounced for the measure of spatial coherence, indicating that the constructions of the hippocampal patients tended to consist of isolated fragments of information, rather than connected scenes. Interestingly, the one patient who performed normally on the imaginary scene task exhibited some residual hippocampal tissue, which may have contributed to the intact performance.

Compared with previous studies of amnesic patients, this study provides a tighter link between event simulation and brain function, since the lesions in these cases appear to be restricted to hippocampal formation. However, in contrast to the earlier observations, this study did not specifically require participants to construct scenes pertaining to *future* events, suggesting that the amnesic patients suffer from a more general event simulation deficit that pertains to constructing novel scenes irrespective of time period. Of course, the fact that the instructions for this study failed to specify a time period need not necessarily mean that participants did not imagine the scenes in a temporal frame. For example, when asked to imagine yourself on a white sandy beach, you might envision yourself taking next winter's vacation in a warm climate. We return to this point later when discussing various theoretical interpretations of future-event simulation.

Recent neuroimaging studies converge nicely with the data from amnesic patients in pointing toward regions that are associated with past and future-event simulation. An early neuroimaging study investigating future-event simulation was reported by Okuda et al. (2003). During a PET scan, participants were instructed to talk freely about either the near past or future (i.e., the last or next few days) or the distant past or future (i.e., the last or next few years). There was evidence of shared activity during past and future conditions in several prefrontal regions, as well as in the medial temporal lobe, including right hippocampus and bilateral parahippocampal gyrus. The effect of temporal distance on neural activity in these regions revealed that in eight out of the nine foci the same neural response to temporal distance (i.e., either an increase or decrease with increasing distance) was evident for both past and future events.

Although participants in this study talked about their personal past or future, it is unclear whether these events were episodic (unique events specific in time and place), rather than reflecting general or semantic information about one's past or future. More recent fMRI studies have used event-related designs to yield information regarding the neural bases of specific past and future events.

Szpunar et al. (2007) instructed participants to remember specific past events, imagine specific future events, or imagine specific events involving a familiar individual (Bill Clinton) in response to event cues (e.g., past birthday, retirement party). Again, there was striking overlap in activity associated with past and future events in the bilateral frontopolar and medial temporal lobe regions, as well as posterior cingulate cortex. Importantly, these regions were not activated to the same magnitude when imagining events involving Bill Clinton, seeming to demonstrate a neural signature that is unique to the construction of events in one's *personal* past or future.

A point of general concern in studies that compare the neural correlates of remembering past events and imaging future events is that remembering is typically associated with greater levels of episodic detail than is imagining (e.g., Johnson et al. 1988). If so, then comparisons between past and future events may be partly or entirely confounded by differences in level of detail. To address this issue, Addis et al. (2007) attempted to equate experimentally the level of detail and related phenomenological features of past and future events. Also, taking advantage of the temporal resolution of fMRI, the past and future tasks were divided into two phases: (1) an initial construction phase during which participants generated a past or future event in response to an event cue (e.g., "dress") and made a button-press when they had an event in mind; and (2) an elaboration phase during which participants generated as much detail as possible about the event. The construction phase was associated with some common past–future activity in posterior visual regions and left hippocampus. During the elaboration phase, when participants focused on generating details about the remembered or imagined event, there was even more extensive overlap between the past and future tasks. Both event types were associated with activity in a network of regions including not only medial temporal (hippocampus and parahippocampal gyrus) and prefrontal cortex, but also in posterior cingulate and retrosplenial cortex.

Botzung et al. (in press) have recently reported data from an fMRI study that largely converge with those of the foregoing studies. The day before scanning, subjects initially reported on 20 past events from the previous week and 20 future events planned for the upcoming week. The subjects constructed cue words for these events, which were presented to them the next day during scanning, when they were instructed to think of past or future events related to each cue. Past and future events produced activation in a similar network to that reported by Addis et al. (2007), including precuneus, medial temporal, medial prefrontal, and dorsolateral prefrontal regions.

In light of these recent studies, it is interesting to note partly overlapping findings in an older study by Partiot et al. (1995) concerning what the authors termed "emotional and nonemotional plans." Subjects were asked to imagine a single nonemotional script ("the sequence of events and feelings concerned with preparation and dressing before [their] mother comes over for dinner") or an emotional script ("the sequence of events and feelings concerned with preparation and dressing to go to [their] mother's funeral"). Compared with linguistic and imagery control tasks, a number of regions similar to those documented in recent studies show increased activation, including dorsolateral prefrontal, left frontopolar, left precuneus/posterior cingulate, and right inferior parietal cortex for the nonemotional condition, medial prefrontal and cingulate for the emotional condition, and medial retrosplenial for both conditions. This study used only a single script for each condition, and it is unclear whether or not subjects imagined specific events; thus, the results must be interpreted with some caution. Nonetheless, there are clear points of overlap with more recent work.

Taken together and in relation to previous studies of autobiographical memory (Cabeza & St Jacques 2007; Gilboa 2004; Maguire 2001; Svoboda et al. 2006), these studies support the idea that a specific core network of regions supports both remembering the past and imagining the future (Buckner & Carroll 2007; Schacter et al. 2007; see FIGURE 1). Buckner et al. (2008), in this volume, provide a detailed analysis of the anatomy of this core network, which involves prefrontal and medial temporal lobe regions, as well as posterior regions including the posterior cingulate and retrosplenial cortex that are consistently observed as components of brain networks important to memory retrieval (Wagner et al. 2005).

Furthermore, analyses of the interactions among the brain regions within this core system demonstrate that many of the component regions are selectively correlated with one another within a large-scale brain system that includes the hippocampal formation (Buckner et al., 2008; Greicius et al. 2004; Vincent et al. 2006).

While the data support the idea that a brain system involving direct contributions from the medial temporal lobe supports both remembering the past and imagining the future, it is important to note that direct comparisons also provided some evidence for greater activity during imagining the future than remembering

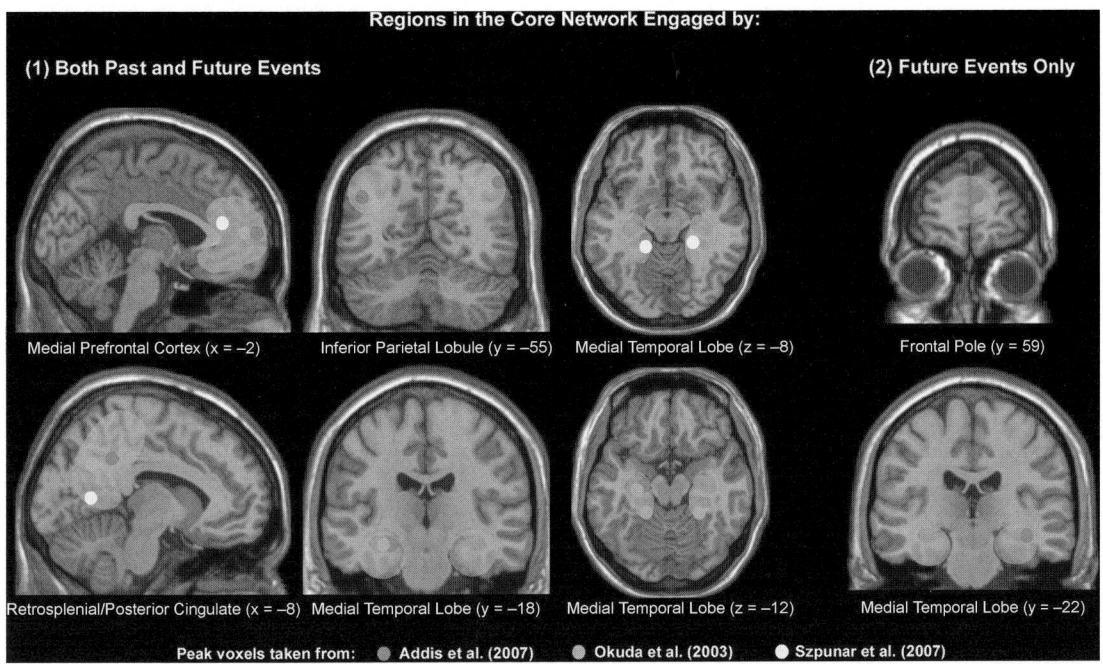

FIGURE 1. Regions making up the core network supporting the simulation of events are highlighted in blue, including medial prefrontal cortex, medial temporal lobe, retrosplenial/posterior cingulate cortex, and inferior parietal lobule. The regions making up this core network have been shown to functionally correlate with each other, and in particular, the hippocampus. Peak voxels from relevant contrasts in neuroimaging studies of past and future events (Addis et al. 2007; Okuda et al. 2003; Szpunar et al. 2007) are overlaid on the schematic of the core network. Included are peak voxels that exhibited (1) common responses to past and future events and (2) differential responses to future events relative to past events.

the past. Okuda et al. (2003) reported greater activity in frontopolar and medial temporal regions during future than past conditions. Szpunar et al. (2007) reported several regions that were significantly more active for future relative to past events, but not vice versa. Addis et al. (2007) found that during the early construction phase of future simulation, several regions showed greater activity for future versus past events (but not the reverse), including frontopolar cortex.

How can we interpret these findings? Szpunar et al. (2007) suggested that this pattern could reflect a more active type of imagery processing required by future than past events. Addis et al. (2007) hypothesized that the pattern reveals the more intensive constructive processes required by imagining future events relative to retrieving past events. While both past and future event tasks require the retrieval of information from memory, thus engaging common memory networks, only the future task requires that event details gleaned from various past events be flexibly recombined into a novel future event, perhaps resulting in increased activity during such tasks.

Note also that Botzung et al. (in press) found no evidence for future greater than past activation in any region; in fact, they found that three regions of interest (right and left hippocampus and anterior medial prefrontal cortex) showed the opposite pattern. However, as noted earlier, in the Botzung et al. study—unlike those of Addis et al., Okuda et al., and Szpunar et al.—subjects initially carried out their simulations of future events in a separate session prior to scanning. During scanning, subjects may have recalled their prior simulation, rather than constructing it for the first time, as subjects did in earlier studies. Botzung et al. attempted to address this issue by asking subjects whether they produced the original past or future event during scanning, or the descriptions of those events from the prescan interview; they excluded those trials where subjects stated that they produced an event from the prescan interview. Nonetheless, since subjects had previously encoded their future-event simulation, rather than constructing it during scanning as in previous studies, there may have been less recruitment of processes involved in recombining details from past experiences. If so, it is perhaps not surprising that they failed to observe the neural correlates of such processes, that is, greater activity for future than past events. Indeed, in an earlier electrophysiological study of memory for previously imagined versus previously experienced events, Conway et al. (2003) reported evidence of greater activity in posterior regions for experienced than imagined events. Additional research is required to compare on-line construction of imagined events and memory for imagined events.

Further evidence concerning differential neural responses to past and future events comes from a study by Addis and Schacter (2008) that examined further the responses of several regions of interest from the Addis et al. (2007) study. While emphasizing the theoretical importance of the overlapping network of regions activated during elaboration of past and future events, Addis and Schacter also noted the possibility that regions within the network respond differently to particular event characteristics, such as temporal distance and the amount of detail generated, depending on whether the event is in the past or future. Addis and Schacter explored the issue by conducting parametric modulation analyses, with temporal distance and detail as covariates, focusing on the medial temporal lobes and the frontopolar cortex. They hypothesized that the integration of increasing amounts of detail for either a past or future event would be associated with increasing levels of hippocampal activity. Moreover, because future events are thought to require more intensive processing to recombine disparate details into a coherent event, the hippocampal response to increasing amounts of future-event detail should be larger than that for past-event detail. In addition, since the right frontal pole is thought to play a role in prospective thinking (e.g., Burgess et al. 2001; Okuda et al. 2003), this region should also exhibit a future–past detail response if it is involved in the generation of future details.

Consistent with predictions, the analysis showed that the left posterior hippocampus was responsive to the amount of detail comprising both past and future events. In contrast, a separate region in the left anterior hippocampus responded differentially to the amount of detail comprising future events, possibly reflecting the recombination of details into a novel future event. Moreover, the right frontal pole responded significantly more to the generation of future relative to past-event details, suggesting that this region might be involved specifically in prospective thinking.

The parametric modulation analysis of temporal distance revealed that the increasing recency of past events was associated with activity in the right parahippocampus gyrus (BA 35/36), while activity in the bilateral hippocampus was associated with the increasing remoteness of future events. Addis and Schacter proposed that the hippocampal response to the distance of future events reflects the increasing disparateness of details likely included in remote future events and the intensive relational processing required for integrating such details into a coherent episodic simulation of the future. More generally, these results suggest that the core network supporting past- and future-event simulation can be recruited in different ways depending on whether the generated event is in the past or future.

This latter observation raises a general point concerning the growing number of studies that have compared remembering the past with imagining the future. When differences between these two conditions are observed, they are typically attributed to differences in the way the brain handles past and future events. However, because in the reviewed studies past events are remembered whereas future events are imagined, the differences could equally well be attributed to differences between remembering and imagining, rather than differences between past and future per se. Of course, the future cannot be remembered because it has not yet happened. However, both the past and the future can be imagined. Therefore, it would be useful for researchers to consider including conditions in their experiments in which participants imagine events as having occurred in the past; any past–future differences observed under these conditions cannot be attributed to differences between remembering and imagining. Such a comparison should allow further refinement of theoretical conclusions concerning how the brain simulates events.

Cognitive Neuroscience of Episodic Simulation: Theoretical Accounts

The foregoing observations have led to several recent hypotheses regarding the nature of episodic simulation and the brain regions that support it. Two different types of theoretical accounts can be distinguished: one type is concerned primarily with understanding the relation between past and future events; the second type is concerned with specifying the critical conditions under which the core network is activated and understanding the functions served by this network. Though the two types of accounts are related, they focus on slightly different questions and different data sets.

Perhaps the best known attempt to link past and future events is Tulving's notion of "mental time travel" (e.g., Tulving 1983, 2002, 2005). From this perspective, remembering past experiences and simulating future events are linked because they both depend on an episodic memory system that allows individuals to detach from the present environment and project themselves into the past or the future. This view accounts naturally for the overlap in brain regions activated during past and future events and for the parallel past–future deficits observed in amnesic patients. The hypothesis is also supported by developmental studies indicating both episodic remembering and future thinking emerge roughly in parallel, between approximately three and five years of age (Atance & O'Neill 2005; Suddendorf & Busby 2005), and by cognitive studies that have shown that remembering past events and imagining future events are affected similarly by a number of experimental manipulations. For example, in a study of college students, D'Armgembeau and van der Linden (2004) found that positive events were associated with increased subjective ratings of reexperiencing for past events and "preexperiencing" for future events and that temporally close events in either the past or future included more sensory and contextual details, and greater feelings of reexperiencing and preexperiencing, than temporally distant events (see also Nussbaum et al. 2006; Trope & Liberman 2003). D'Argembeau and van der Linden (2006) showed that individual differences in imagery ability and emotion-regulation strategies are similarly related to past and future events. Spreng and Levine (2006) reported striking similarities in the shapes of the temporal distributions of past and future autobiographical events provided by college students and older adults.

Much discussion regarding mental time travel has centered on the question of whether nonhuman animals exhibit this ability. Tulving (2005) and others (e.g., Suddendorf & Corballis 1997, 2007) have argued strongly that the capacity for mental time travel is uniquely human. While acknowledging that nonhuman animals can use stored information by relying on semantic or procedural memory systems, they contend that such processes need not involve mental time travel in the sense of detaching oneself from the present moment and either recollectively reexperiencing a past event or simulating and "preexperiencing" a future event. In fact, Tulving (2005) and Suddendorf and Corballis (1997, 2007) argued that animals lack the episodic memory capacities required for time travel into past or future. This strong claim has spurred research examining whether nonhuman animals are capable of mental time travel (for recent reviews, see Clayton et al. 2003; Suddendorf & Corballis 2007), including compelling experimental demonstrations that, at the very least, cast doubt on the strong claim for human uniqueness. For example, Clayton and Dickinson (1998) showed that food-caching scrub jays are able to retrieve detailed information about what food they cached as well as when and where they cached it. More recently, they have devised clever paradigms that establish that jays can cache food in a manner that reflects some form of planning for the future (Raby et al. 2007). Further, they have carried out control tasks indicating that such planning-like behavior is not merely a reflection of the jays' current motivational state (Correia et al. 2007). There is also evidence from rats that suggests some of type of prospective coding. Ferbinteanu and Shapiro (2003) recorded hippocampal activity during a spatial task that required them to find food at the end of a goal arm; multiple trials were performed at each goal arm. The investigators reported evidence that the hippocampal neurons encoded not only current location and recent memory, but also prospective information concerning where the rat needed to go in the immediate future. More recently, Diba and Buzsaki (2007) recorded hippocampal activity while rats ran back and forth on a track to obtain a water reward at each end of the track. At the end of a run, they found that hippocampal neurons exhibited "reverse replay" (Foster & Wilson 2006) of the route, firing in reverse order of activity during the run. In addition, Diba and Buzsaki also found evidence that hippocampal neurons exhibited "forward preplay" in anticipation of an upcoming run, perhaps suggesting the formulation of some type of route planning. Johnson and Redish (in press) reported similar phenomena in a cleverly designed series of experiments that examined place cell activity during choices made by rats in spatial decision tasks. They recorded from ensembles of neurons with place fields in the CA3 region of hippocampus, allowing them to analyze activity at critical decision points. They found that on some trials, the spatial representation reconstructed from the neural ensemble "swept ahead" of the animal, appearing to indicate possible future paths. These observations lead the authors to suggest that the hippocampus may provide prospective memory signals that serve as a basis for making decisions.

Suddendorf and Corballis (2007) provided a conceptual "theater production metaphor" to promote discussion of whether nonhuman animals are capable of mental time travel. They liken the experience of envisioning the future or recollecting the past to a theater production involving several key components: a stage on which the production unfolds (working memory), a playwright who scripts the production (combining and recombining stored information), actors who play characters in the production (knowledge of self and others), a set that reflects aspect or principles of the real world (knowledge of time), a director who tries out different versions of the production (monitoring and metacognition), an executive producer who organizes high-level aspects of the production (executive control), and a broadcaster who communicates the production (language or nonlinguistic communication). Suddendorf and Corballis considered the extent to which nonanimals possess each of these critical components of mental time travel.

We think that this theater production metaphor constitutes a useful approach to addressing issues of mental time travel in animals. As we have argued elsewhere (Schacter et al. 2007), however, it is unclear whether debates about mental time travel in nonhuman animals will ever be settled definitively, given that animals do not possess the linguistic capacity to describe mental contents (or without detailed measurements of neural activity that reflects mental content). From a theoretical perspective, however, this aspect of the mental time travel hypothesis—that is, can nonhuman animals engage in mental time travel—can be treated separately from issues concerning how well the hypothesis handles data from human subjects. For example, Suddendorf and Corballis's theater production metaphor may prove a useful heuristic for thinking about mental time travel independent of how questions concerning mental time travel in animals are ultimately resolved. Similarly, a critical question concerns whether mental time travel specifically or uniquely activates the core network. Although Tulving (2002, 2005) has not made any strong claims on this score, the core network does appear to be involved in functions other than those strictly involving mental time travel.

Several recent proposals have considered the functions of regions within the core network in a range of simulation processes (Buckner & Carroll 2007; Hassabis et al. 2007; Hassabis & Maguire 2007; Schacter & Addis 2007a, 2007b). Schacter and Addis (2007a, 2007b) focused on the constructive processes involved in future-event simulations, suggesting that this property of adaptive simulations could help to explain why memories for the past are subject to errors and misattributions. Buckner and Carroll (2007) focused on the anatomy of the core network and its generality across many tasks that demand mental simulations, including but extending beyond those that are simulations of the past and future. Hassabis and Maguire (2007) explored the degree to which a proposed form of mental imagery—scene construction—is the common process linking together various tasks that depend on the core network. We discuss each of these ideas in more detail below.

The *constructive episodic simulation hypothesis* (Schacter & Addis 2007a, 2007b) maintains that simulation of future events requires a system that can flexibly recombine details from past events. The idea was proposed in the context of attempting to understand why memory involves a constructive process of piecing together bits and pieces of information, rather than a literal replay of the past. The constructive nature of memory can result in various kinds of errors and distortions (e.g., Bartlett 1932; Loftus 2003; Roediger & McDermott 1995; Schacter 1999, 2001). However, it has also been suggested that some of these memory errors serve an adaptive role (cf. Anderson & Schooler 1991; Bjork & Bjork 1988; Schacter 1999, 2001). For example, Anderson and Schooler (1991) argued that memory is adapted to retain information that is most likely to be needed in the environment in which it operates. Because we do not often need to remember all the exact details of our experiences, an adapted system would not automatically preserve all such details. Thus, by producing what we can think of as data compression or economy of storage, a constructive memory system may promote adaptive functions.

Arguing from a different kind of adaptive perspective, Schacter and Addis (2007a, 2007b) suggested that a critical function of a constructive memory is to make information available for simulation of future events (see also relevant discussion by Dudai & Carruthers 2005; Suddendorf & Corballis 1997). By this view, past and future events draw on similar information stored in episodic memory and rely on similar underlying processes; episodic memory supports the construction of future events by extracting and recombining stored information into a simulation of a novel event. The adaptive value of such a system is that it enables past information to be used flexibly in simulating alternative future scenarios without engaging in actual behavior. A potential downside of such a system is that it is vulnerable to memory errors, such as misattribution and false recognition (see, e.g., Schacter & Addis 2007a, 2007b). While focusing on processes that support future-event simulation, the constructive episodic simulation hypothesis does not explicitly embrace or reject the idea that the core network is specifically involved in mental time travel.

The constructive episodic simulation hypothesis receives general support from the previously reviewed findings of neural and cognitive overlap between past and future events. Further support is provided by recent data from Szpunar and McDermott (in press). They reported more vivid and detailed future-event simulations when college students imagined events that might occur within the next week in a familiar context (home, friend's apartment) than in a novel context (jungle, North Pole), and also that future events were more vivid and detailed when imagined in recently experienced contexts (university locations) than in remotely experienced contexts (high school). Familiar and recently experienced contexts are usually represented in greater episodic detail than novel and remote ones. Accordingly, these results support the idea that episodic information is used to construct future-event simulations.

Because the constructive episodic simulation hypothesis specifically emphasizes the importance of flexibly relating and recombining information from past episodes, it is supported by the evidence discussed earlier that links hippocampal function and relational processing with future-event simulation. The hippocampal region is thought to support relational memory processes (e.g., Eichenbaum & Cohen 2001), and these processes are hypothesized to be crucial for recombining stored information into future-event simulations. Further support along these lines comes from a behavioral study of future-event simulation in older adults. Addis et al. (2008) provided younger and older adults with event cues and provided them three minutes to generate, in as much detail as possible, episodes from specified periods in the past or future. Consistent with previous work (Levine et al. 2002), older adults reported less detailed episodic memories of past events than did younger adults. A parallel effect occurred for future events: the episodes imagined by older adults also contained sparser episodic information compared to younger adults. Critically, as predicted by the constructive episodic simulation hypothesis, the ability of older adults to generate episode-specific details of both the past and future events was correlated with a measure of their ability to integrate information and form relations between items—that is, with their relational memory performance.

While the available data are thus consistent with the constructive episodic simulation hypothesis, a number of issues need to be addressed. For example, it remains unclear whether and to what extent future-event simulations are based on retrieval of individual fragments of prior episodes, or whether recombining elements from different episodes, as emphasized by the constructive episodic simulation hypothesis, is a critical process in future-event simulation. Also, the constructive episodic simulation hypothesis is likely incomplete because it emphasizes the contribution of episodic memory to future-event simulation, while remaining mute about possible contributions of semantic memory. Although the distinction between episodic and semantic memory continues to inspire debate and discussion (cf. Foster & Jelicic 1999; Moscovitch et al. 2006; Tulving 1983, 2002), it seems clear that as the source of knowledge about general properties of events, semantic memory presumably is used to guide the construction of future scenarios in line with known event properties. Research that directly compares episodic and semantic contributions to future-event simulations may well require extension or modification of the constructive episodic simulation hypothesis. Finally, while the constructive episodic simulation hypothesis holds that there is a direct link between future-event simulation and memory distortion, no such link has yet been established empirically.

While sharing some of the core assumptions of the constructive episodic simulation hypothesis regarding the use of episodic information to build future-event simulations, other theories have focused on broader issues concerning the conditions under which the core network is engaged. Buckner and Carroll (2007) argued that the core brain system serves a common set of processes by which past experiences are used adaptively to imagine perspectives and events beyond those that emerge from the immediate environment. In addition to the system's role in remembering the past and envisioning the future, they argued, it serves an even more general function, extending to diverse tasks that require mental simulation of alternative perspectives. They observed that regions within the core network, in particular the posterior cingulate/retrospenial region, are engaged during theory-of-mind tasks that require thinking about the perspectives of others (e.g., Saxe & Kanwisher 2003), and also noted that such regions may be engaged in certain kinds of spatial navigation tasks (e.g., Byrne et al. 2007). In light of these results, the mental time travel hypothesis seems too restrictive to accommodate the range of conditions in which the core network is active. Buckner and Carroll suggested that the core brain network is commonly engaged when individuals are simulating alternative perspectives, including alternatives in the present and possibilities in the future—a process they provisionally termed "self-projection." By this view, the core brain system allows one to shift from perceiving the immediate environment as constrained by the external world to an alternative, imagined perspective that is based largely on memories of the past. This view encourages further analysis of the common features of the various tasks subserved by the core network, including to what extent imagined perspectives always include visual imagery and self-referential processes. A clear prediction from this view is that activation of the core network should correspond to the extent that a task encourages simulation of an alternative perspective not required by the immediate environment.

It is interesting to note, however, that even though certain regions within the core network are active during theory-of-mind tasks (Saxe & Kanwisher 2003), Bird et al. (2004) reported that a patient with damage to part of the network (the medial prefrontal region) and who exhibited "severe" memory problems, nonetheless performed normally on theory-of-mind tasks. These observations contrast with those indicating that amnesic patients have difficulty simulating future events and raise questions concerning which regions in the core network (if any) are *necessary* for carrying out the kind of perspective taking involved in theory-of-mind tasks. Furthermore, these findings suggest that imagining the future may depend on remembering the past in a way that adopting the perspective of others does not. Analysis of functional connectivity provisionally suggests that medial prefrontal and medial temporal subsystems within the core network make distinct contributions to simulation (Buckner et al. 2008). Therefore, a full understanding of the roles of these individual regions within the core network is still evolving.

Hassabis and Maguire (2007) advanced a related though distinct view that "scene construction" is the critical process associated with activation of the core network, thereby emphasizing the visual–spatial aspects of the simulation. This view was motivated in part by the finding that amnesic patients showed deficits on a task that required them to imagine novel scenes (Hassabis et al. 2007); the spatial coherence of patients' constructions were particularly impaired. Further, Hassabis and Maguire (2007) refered to a neuroimaging study they conducted using their novel-scenes task that produced activation of the core network, both when subjects constructed novel scenes and when they remembered actual experiences. Critically, the novel-scenes task does not explicitly require mental time travel, thereby leading Hassabis and Maguire to contend that projecting oneself into the past or the future is not the critical process for activating the core network, similar to Buckner and Carroll's proposal. Hassabis and Maguire went on to argue that scene construction, rather than self-projection, can best account for the array of findings noted earlier without postulating that the scenes are referenced to a personal perspective. Further research will be required to determine whether scene construction is sufficient to account for all findings associated with the core network, including observations that the some regions in the network are used during forms of mentalizing, such as theory-of-mind tasks whose underlying processes are presently unclear.

Cognitive Neuroscience of Episodic Simulation: Applications and Extensions

The foregoing findings and ideas have begun to establish a foundation for understanding the brain systems involved in episodic simulation of future events. We now consider some applications and extensions of this work. First, we consider future-event simulation in psychopathological conditions—depression, anxiety, and schizophrenia. This has been an active area of research, including some of the earliest work on simulation of future events; we believe that recent cognitive neuroscience research has some interesting implications for this research. Second, we consider future-event simulation in relation to other processes that comprise the "prospective brain": the formation of plans and intentions, and making predictions about future events.

Simulation of Future Events: Relation to Psychological Well-Being and Psychopathology

Simulations play an important role in psychological well-being. The ability to generate specific and detailed simulations of future events is associated with effective coping; it enables one to engage in emotional regulation and appropriate problem-solving activities (Brown et al. 2002; Taylor et al. 1998; Taylor & Schneider 1989). Simulating future events can regulate emotion by allowing one to envision the feeling of relief associated with a positive outcome. For instance, coherent and detailed simulations of positive future outcomes have been found to correlate with increased subjective probability of a positive outcome and decreased amounts of worry related to the future event (Brown et al. 2002). Simulations can also enable identification of problem-solving activities. For instance, subjects who simulated the details of an ongoing stressful event were found to subsequently increase their use of active coping strategies and seeking social support, compared with participants who simulated the relief of the stressor resolving or with controls who did not engage in future-event simulation (Taylor et al. 1998). Moreover, simulating future stressful situations and mentally rehearsing appropriate actions in these situations can enhance one's ability to cope if and when those situations arise (Taylor & Schneider 1989).

These observations fit well with the results of a recent fMRI study by Sharot et al. (2007), who examined the relation of future-event simulation to optimism—specifically, the pervasive optimistic bias whereby people maintain unrealistically positive expectations of their futures (Weinstein 1980). During scanning, 15 healthy young subjects were given brief descriptions of significant events, such as "the end of a romantic relationship" or "winning an award," and were cued to think about either a past event that had actually occurred or a future event that might occur. Subjects made a button-press response when the memory or simulation began to take shape, and then again when it was fully formed. They also rated each event for its emotional valence (positive, neutral, or negative). After the scanning session, subjects provided additional ratings concerning their memories and simulations: how vivid they were, how strongly they felt they were reliving their pasts or "preexperiencing" their futures, the time of the event, and their subjective sense of how close in time they felt to the event. Finally, subjects also completed a scale that assessed their degree of optimism (Scheier et al. 1994).

Behavioral data showed that a) subjects felt that positive future events were closer in time than negative future events, b) they rated positive events in the future as more positive than positive events from the past, and c) they indicated that positive future events were more intensely "preexperienced" than negative future events. These effects were strongest in the most optimistic subjects. The fMRI results revealed a possible brain basis for these optimistic biases. Several regions in the core network discussed earlier showed similarly increased activity when subjects recalled past events and imagined future events, including rostral anterior cingulate cortex (rACC) extending into ventral medial prefrontal cortex, dorsal medial prefrontal cortex, and posterior cingulate cortex. There was also significant activation in the amygdala. The amygdala as well the rACC showed less activity when people imagined negative future events compared with any of the other conditions (positive future events, positive past events, or negative past events). When people imagined positive future events, the activities of the rACC and the amygdala were more strongly correlated with one another than when the subjects imagined negative future events. Importantly, more optimistic individuals showed relatively greater rACC activation when imagining positive versus negative future events than did less optimistic individuals.

The results thus provide clues concerning the neural underpinnings of optimistic bias by showing that areas involved in emotional processing (amygdala and rACC) selectively decrease their activity when people think about negative future events and co-ordinate activity when people think about positive future events, and that these effects are most pronounced in the most optimistic individuals. Given other behavioral evidence indicating that anticipating both negative and positive future events can be more emotionally intense than remembering negative and positive events (Van Boven & Ashworth 2007), additional studies are needed to delineate the conditions under which future-event simulations are associated with optimistic biases (for more detailed discussion of the Sharot et al. findings and their possible implications for understanding optimism, see Schacter & Addis 2007c).

Given the role of simulations in healthy and effective coping, it is not surprising that maladaptive coping strategies and psychopathological disorders are associated with changes in the ability to generate future simulations. To date, most theories advanced to explain simulation deficits in psychiatric disorders have focused on psychological and cognitive factors. We suggest that emerging knowledge concerning the neural regions supporting the simulation of past and future events provides a basis for formulating hypotheses regarding the mechanisms underlying simulation deficits in some psychiatric populations.

In an early study, Williams et al. (1996) reported that suicidally depressed patients have difficulty recalling specific memories of past events and also in generating specific simulations of future events. The past and future events generated by depressed patients in response to cue words lacked detail and were "overgeneral" relative to those produced by nondepressed controls. Importantly, the reductions in specificity of past and future events were significantly correlated. Numerous studies have since replicated the finding of reduced specificity and increased overgenerality of past and future events, not only in patients with major depressive disorder (Williams et al. 1996), but also those with mild depression (e.g., Dickson & Bates 2005; MacLeod et al. 1993), schizophrenia (D'Argembeau et al. in press), and depressed patients with borderline personality disorder (Kremers et al. 2006). Similarly, the worries of anxious individuals often exhibit reduced concreteness compared with those of healthy individuals (Stöber & Borkovec 2002).

In order to explain decreases in the specificity of simulated events in depression, Williams and colleagues (Williams 1996, 2006; Williams et al. 1996) advanced the *affect regulation hypothesis*. According to this hypothesis, the production of overgeneral events reflects the truncation of the event search as a protective mechanism to prevent retrieval of potentially destabilizing memories. The search for an event may be aborted at various stages of the retrieval process, as reflected by the search output. For example, an omission would result if the search for an event is not initiated at all, whereas a general event would be produced if an initial search is completed but not further refined to locate a specific event. Moreover, ruminating on general events may cause "mnemonic interlock": when an individual cannot inhibit all the generic representations activated so that the search for a specific event can continue (Williams 1996, 2006). The affect regulation hypothesis is supported by studies reporting that specific memories of negative events cause more stress than general memories (Raes et al. 2003), and also by findings of more severe reductions in event specificity in individuals with a history of trauma (Kuyken & Brewin 1995; Raes et al. 2005) and those with a repressive coping style (Dickson & Bates 2005).

The neural mechanisms that might underlie the use of an overgeneral affective regulation have not been identified. However, one electrophysiological study of memory retrieval in healthy adults does lend support to the affect regulation hypothesis. Using event-related potentials, Conway et al. (2001) found that immediately following cue presentation emotional memories were associated with less activity across the prefrontal cortices as well as longer retrieval latencies. These findings were interpreted as reflecting an initial inhibition of the retrieval process due to the potentially destabilizing nature of emotional memories.

Williams et al. (1996) found that past and future events generated by suicidally depressed patients were overgeneral irrespective of the valence of the event. However, others have reported effects of valence, particularly with respect to the ease of access to future events. For instance, MacLeod et al. (1993) found that suicidally depressed patients were less able to envision *positive* future episodes. Similarly, dysphoric individuals took significantly longer to access pleasant past and future events but did not differ from controls with respect to unpleasant events (Dickson & Bates 2006). Moreover, slower and less successful access to positive future events, as well as the belief that positive future events are less likely to happen, has been found to correlate with the severity of hopelessness (MacLeod & Cropley 1995). This observation suggests that simulation deficits may be critical in maintaining the sense of hopelessness often evidence in depression.

Pessimistic views of the future have also been shown to play a role in psychiatric disorders. For instance, the severity of depression correlates with faster and more successful access to negative future events and a belief that negative events will happen in future (MacLeod & Cropley 1995). Moreover, dysphoric individuals have easier access to reasons why negative events will happen in future relative to nondepressed controls (Vaughn & Weary 2002). Similarly, increased access to simulations of negative future events is a characteristic of anxiety disorders (e.g., MacLeod et al. 1997; Ruane et al. 2005), including post-traumatic stress disorder (Lavi & Solomon 2005). In line with our earlier discussion of the simulation heuristic, whereby more easily constructed scenarios are judged to be more likely to occur in the future (Kahneman & Tversky 1982), the ability of anxious patients to gain access to simulations of negative future events, and to form visual images of the event, was found to correlate significantly with their predicted probability that these events would occur in the future (Ruane et al. 2005). Moreover, anxious patients were less able to generate reasons why negative events would *not* happen, relative to nonanxious controls (MacLeod et al. 1997). Pessimism has also been shown to differentiate anxiety from depression. Using a verbal fluency paradigm in which patients were required to generate as many positive and negative, past and future events as possible, MacLeod et al. (1997) found that anxious patients generated significantly more negative events than did controls, but not fewer positive events, while depressed patients generated significantly fewer positive events but not more negative events.

While applicable to mood disorders, the role of maladaptive affect regulation and pessimism is not as easily applicable to other psychiatric populations exhibiting simulation deficits, such as schizophrenia. In a recent study, D'Argembeau et al. (in press) found that schizophrenic patients generated significantly fewer specific past and future events than did healthy controls. Such observations encourage consideration of the possible role of factors other than affect regulation in the simulation deficits that are evident in psychiatric disorders, such as neuropsychological impairments that have been documented in psychiatric populations. While it is highly likely that affect regulation and pessimism influence the valance of future events accessible to patients with mood disorders, understanding the neural regions mediating the simulation of past and future events enables the generation of specific predictions regarding the neuropsychological deficits that may contribute to the reduced specificity of events evident in psychiatric disorders. This approach will hopefully enable development of integrative theories for understanding simulation deficits across various neuropsychological and psychiatric populations.

One such hypothesis is that executive dysfunction plays a critical role in simulation deficits. In this view, the search for a specific past or future event fails, not because it is truncated by affect regulation processes, but because the patient fails to engage effective search processes as a consequence of executive dysfunction (Dalgleish et al. 2007; Hertel 2000). Simulation of an event is a relatively unconstrained task that places many demands on executive functions, including devising strategies to aid specification of effective cues, determining whether the simulated event meets the search criteria (e.g., a specific, plausible event), and inhibiting output which does not meet these criteria. Although reduced specificity of past events has been shown to correlate with reduced performance on executive tasks such as verbal fluency in depressed patients (Dalgleish et al. 2007), neither past nor future simulation deficits in schizophrenic patients correlated with verbal fluency measures (D'Argembeau et al. in press). Further research is needed to clarify the role of executive dysfunction in simulation deficits.

The recent data considered earlier from neuroimaging studies and amnesic patients, implicating the hippocampus as part of the core network subserving event simulation, suggest that hippocampal dysfunction might also contribute to overgeneral simulations of past and future events. Hippocampal atrophy and/or elevated hippocampal glucocorticoid levels are evident in a number of psychiatric conditions in which simulation deficits have been documented, including depression (Bremner et al. 2000; Campbell & Macqueen 2004), post-traumatic stress disorder (Sapolsky 2000), and schizophrenia (Velakoulis et al. 2006). Given that the hippocampus is crucial to the reintegration of details in order to recollect a specific past event and thought to be necessary for the recombination of details into a simulation of a specific future event (Addis et al. 2007, in press; Buckner & Carroll 2007; Hassabis et al. 2007; Schacter & Addis 2007a, 2007b), the various ideas discussed earlier suggest that hippocampal dysfunction is a candidate neural mechanism for simulation deficits observed in psychiatric populations.

A link between hippocampal dysfunction and relational memory deficits has been documented in some psychiatric disorders. For instance, fMRI studies have demonstrated that schizophrenic patients exhibit underrecruitment of the hippocampus during relational memory tasks, including transitive inference tasks that require flexible use of previously learned information (Öngür et al. 2006). However, despite the central role of the hippocampus in the simulation of past and future events, the link between reduced autobiographical event specificity and hippocampal dysfunction has been considered only occasionally in the psychiatric literature (Barnhofer et al. 2005). Further studies are needed to determine whether ability to generate specific simulations of past and future events is correlated with the structural and functional integrity of the hippocampus, as well as other regions comprising the core network that supports future-event simulation.

Finally, the Sharot et al. (2007) experiment concerning neural correlates of optimism, which we discussed earlier, fits nicely with studies indicating that depressed patients show reduced volume and metabolism in the same subregion of the rACC that Sharot et al. found to correlate strongly with optimism. When corrected for volume loss, metabolism in remaining rACC tissue is actually elevated in depressed patients relative to controls, and effective antidepressant treatment reduces rACC metabolism to normal levels (for review, see Drevets 2000).

Plans and Intentions: Links to Episodic Simulation?

We have emphasized that cognitive neuroscience research on episodic simulation of future events, though not without historical precedent, is of relatively recent vintage, with a good deal of focus on the topic emerging in the past couple of years. However, this is not to say that psychologists and cognitive neuroscientists have only recently begun to focus on future-oriented cognitive and memory processes; far from it. For example, cognitive and social psychologists have long been interested in the processes underlying planning (e.g., Miller et al. 1960; Morris & Ward 2005), and neuropsychologists and neurologists have conducted numerous studies of planning deficits in patients with frontal lobe lesions (e.g., Fellows & Farah 2005; Luria 1966; Mesulam 2002; Shallice 1982; Shallice & Burgess 1996; Stuss & Benson 1986). Similarly, for the past 20 years or more, cognitive psychologists and neuropsychologists have been interested in how people formulate and remember intentions to carry out future actions, an area of research that has come to be known as prospective memory (e.g., Brandimonte et al. 1996; Einstein & McDaniel 1990, 2005; Harris 1984).

What is the role of future-event simulation in such prospective processes? For the most part, researchers in the areas of planning and prospective memory have focused on issues other than episodic simulation. For example, planning researchers have examined the role of executive control and working memory processes in complex problem-solving tasks such as the Tower of London (e.g., Owen 2005; Philips et al. 1999; Shallice 1982), the relations among various kinds of planning tasks (e.g., Burgess et al. 2005), and the role of top-down and bottom-up processes in formulating and executing plans (e.g., Hayes-Roth & Hayes-Roth 1979). Prospective memory researchers have spent a good deal of time examining such issues as the properties of cues that trigger recall of intentions, how individuals generate their own cues, the processes involved in monitoring whether an action needs to be performed, and distinctions among different types of prospective memory, such as event-based (remembering to carry out a task when a specific event occurs) versus time based (remembering to carry out an action at a specific time in the future; for review, see Brandimonte et al. 1996; Einstein & McDaniel 2005). Some of the issues have been studied from a cognitive neuroscience perspective with neuroimaging techniques. For example, Simons et al. (2006) asked whether the processes involved in recognizing the appropriate context to act (cue identification) and remembering the action to be performed (intention retrieval) have a common neural basis. They reported evidence that the frontal pole (BA 10) exhibited similar responses to cue identification and intention retrieval: in lateral BA 10, these two tasks resulted in increased activity, while in medial BA 10 decreased activity was evident during both tasks. Moreover, these effects within lateral and medial BA 10 were greater for intention retrieval than cue identification (see also Burgess et al. 2001; Okuda et al. 1998).

It is difficult to find much discussion in the literature on planning and prospective memory concerning the processes of future-event simulation, but we think that there may be points of connection at both the cognitive and neural levels. At the cognitive level, one can ask whether the kinds of episodic simulation processes considered here are relevant or important for understanding how people remember to carry out future actions. For example, when formulating the intention to pick up milk and butter on the way home from work, is it necessary or useful to imagine carrying out the action, or to mentally simulate the context in which the action will occur? Similarly, does the formulation of more complex plans benefit from simulating alternative scenarios? Some evidence suggests affirmative answers to these questions.

Marsh et al. (2006) reported data suggesting that prospective memory may indeed benefit from processes that would appear to involve episodic simulation. They focused on the question of whether holding an intention to perform a future action results in a cost to other activities during the time period over which the intention is held. If holding intentions interferes with other tasks, then the cost of engaging in prospective activities in everyday life could be prohibitively high. In two experiments investigating event-based and time-based prospective memory, Marsh et al. reported that associating an intention with a specific future context significantly reduced interference with carrying out other tasks during the interval when subjects held the intention, prior to executing the target action. The act of associating an intention with a specific future context can be viewed as a type of episodic simulation, perhaps related to the kinds of simulation processes discussed earlier. If so, then the act of associating an intention with a specific future context might well recruit some or all regions in the core network associated with future-event simulation.

These processes bear a close resemblance to what Gollwitzer (1999) has termed "implementation intentions": plans that link an intention with a specific anticipated situation in which the plan is to be executed. Gollwitzer (1999, p. 494) contrasted implementation intentions ("When situation x arises, I will perform response y!") with goal intentions ("I intend to reach x!"). People form implementation intentions by imagining and rehearsing a plan with respect to the specific future context in which they will execute it. Forming implementation intentions can increase significantly the chances of carrying out an intention or plan. For example, Orbell et al. (1997) asked some women who had the goal of performing a breast self-examination within the next month to imagine exactly when and where they would want to perform the exam. All of the women who formed these implementation intentions reported later that they indeed carried out the exam. By contrast, only half the women who had strong intentions to perform the exam, but were not asked to form additional implementation intentions, later performed the exam. More recent research shows that there are conditions in which older adults can benefit from forming implementation intentions (Chasteen et al. 2001). Older adults who envisaged themselves performing a prospective memory task (writing the day of the week on sheets they would be receiving) were twice as likely to do so as older adults who were asked to perform the same task but did not form this implementation intention.

Implementation intentions likely aid performance by linking an intention to a context-specific mental representation of a future situation that can later cue the intention (see also Seifert & Patalano 2001 for related work). Further study of implementation intentions could represent an informative intersection between episodic simulation processes on the one hand and the formation of intentions and plans on the other.

Neuroimaging research on intentional processing and prospective memory can also inform work on future-event simulation given that there are points of overlap among the regions activated during simulation and prospective memory. Notable among these regions is frontopolar region (BA 10), which as reviewed earlier has shown preferential activation when people simulate future events (Addis et al. 2007; Okuda et al. 2003), and also during prospective memory tasks (Burgess et al. 2001; Okuda et al. 2003; Simons et al. 2006). Such findings encourage further research that examines whether and to what extent frontopolar regions are specifically related to the prospective aspects of event simulation.

Prediction and Simulation

Predictions are a key component of many kinds of future-related thinking (Hawkins & Blakesee 2005). Predictions about the future may occur at a variety of different time scales and for different purposes. When entering a novel context, such as an office, park, or museum, people use past experiences and associations to generate predictions about what kinds of objects and events are likely to be encountered next (e.g., Bar 2007). When making major life decisions, such as where to accept a job or whom to marry, or more minor ones such as where to spend a vacation or eat dessert, people try to generate predictions about their likely future happiness (Gilbert 2006). Simulations of the future may serve as the basis for many kinds of predictions, and their properties can help to understand why predictions about the future are often erroneous (Gilbert & Wilson 2007).

As Gilbert and Wilson (2007) noted, a key to understanding prediction errors is that future simulations are often based on memories, which are themselves prone to various kinds of inaccuracies. Supporting this idea, Morewedge et al. (2005) found that people often make predictions of their future happiness based on atypical past experiences that are highly memorable to them. However, these atypical experiences do not accurately predict what is likely to occur in the future, thereby resulting in prediction errors. Another example that frequently impacts everyday behavior concerns the fact that individuals often underestimate how long it will take them to complete a task in the future. Roy et al. (2005) summarized evidence indicating that predictions about future task duration are often based on memories of past event duration, which are themselves underestimates of the actual duration. If one mistakenly remembers, for instance, that serving as a grant reviewer took a few hours rather than an entire day, then one may be unpleasantly surprised to discover that a new review cannot be completed during the hours one predicted would be sufficient to complete the task.

Summarizing a broad range of studies, Gilbert and Wilson (2007) distinguished among four properties of simulations that reflect the influence of memory and are likely to contribute to prediction errors: simulations are 1) *unrepresentative*, often capturing the most salient but not the most likely elements of an experience; 2) *essentialized*, omitting some nonessential details that can impact future happiness; 3) *abbreviated*, often overemphasizing the initial part of an event; and 4) *decontextualized*, ignoring aspects of a future context that affect the experience of an event.

Gilbert and Wilson (2007) summarized research from social and cognitive psychology that provides evidence that each of the four key properties of future-event simulations can impact the predictions individuals make about the future happiness or likelihood of engaging in future behaviors. These findings dovetail nicely with the cognitive neuroscience evidence reviewed here, inasmuch as both point to an intimate link between the processes subserving episodic memory and future-event simulation. Nonetheless, the link between simulation and prediction has not yet been made empirically at a brain-systems level. A number of neuroimaging studies using conditioning procedures or decision-making paradigms have examined the brain systems that are involved in generation of signals related to prediction of future reward or punishment, with several studies highlighting a key role for specific regions within the striatum (e.g., Knutson et al. 2000; Seymour et al. 2007; Yacubian et al. 2006). Such findings, coupled with the previously mentioned findings on simulation-based prediction errors, led Gilbert and Wilson (2007) to conceive of future predictions in terms of an interaction between cortically driven simulations and subcortical affective responses to those simulations. These kinds of ideas suggest that neuroimaging and neuropsychological studies of the link between simulation and prediction constitute a promising area for research.

Concluding Comments

Episodic simulation of future events has emerged only recently as a topic of intense interest in cognitive neuroscience, but we hope that we have shown in this article that the issue fits into a broader landscape of research in multiple disciplines. We view the issue as fundamental with respect to both theoretical and applied concerns. On the theoretical side, the study of future-event simulation represents the intersection of memory processes with those involved in imagination, planning, and prediction. Further study of the issue therefore promises to both broaden and deepen our understanding of the nature and function of memory. As we and others have argued, since planning for the future is a task of paramount adaptive importance, it makes sense to conceive of the brain as a fundamentally prospective organ that is designed to use information from the past and present to generate predictions about the future (e.g., Bar 2007; Buckner & Carroll 2007; Gilbert 2006; Hawkins & Blakesee 2005; Schacter & Addis 2007b; Schacter et al. 2007). Such a perspective encourages us to view memory as a key component of the prospective brain that helps to generate simulations of possible future events that contribute to the formation of plans and predictions. Such a perspective calls for a shift not only in conceptual emphasis, but also a change in methodology. Rather than focusing predominantly on assessing memory with tasks that query the past, greater emphasis should be placed on the development of tasks that capture how memory is used to simulate, plan, and predict the future.

On the applied side, future thinking is crucial to understanding well-being (e.g., Gilbert 2006; Taylor et al. 1998), achievement and goal attainment (e.g., Ajzen 1991; Aspinwall 2005), aging (e.g., Addis et al. in press; Carstensen et al. 1999; Einstein & McDaniel 1990), optimism (Schacter & Addis 2007c; Sharot et al. 2007), and various clinical conditions discussed earlier (e.g., MacLeod et al. 1997; Mesulam 2002). However, despite some progress in the analysis of cognitive and social aspects of these phenomena, our understanding of the neural correlates and basis of the relevant prospective processes is exceedingly modest. Advances in our understanding of the cognitive neuroscience of future-event simulation are thus likely to have implications for addressing a wide array of issues that are essential to everyday life.

Acknowledgments

Preparation of this paper was supported by grants from the National Institute on Aging, National Institute of Mental Health, and Howard Hughes Medical Institute. We thank Adrian Gilmore for invaluable aid with preparation of the manuscript.

Conflict of Interest

The authors declare no conflicts of interest.

References

Addis, D. R., & Schacter, D. L. (2008). Constructive episodic simulation: Temporal distance and detail of past and future events modulate hippocampal engagement. *Hippocampus, 18*, 227–237.

Addis, D. R., Wong, A. T., & Schacter, D. L. (2007). Remembering the past and imagining the future: Common and distinct neural substrates during event construction and elaboration. *Neuropsychologia, 45*, 1363–1377.

Addis, D. R., Wong, A. T., & Schacter, D. L. (2008). Age-related changes in the episodic simulation of future events. *Psychol. Sci., 19*, 33–41.

Ajzen, I. (1991). The theory of planned behavior. *Organ. Behav. Hum. Decis. Process., 50*, 179–211.

Anderson, J. R., & Schooler, L. J. (1991). Reflections of the environment in memory. *Psychol. Sci., 2*, 396–408.

Aspinwall, L. G. (2005). The psychology of future-oriented thinking: From achievement to proactive coping, adaptation, and aging. *Motiv. Emot., 29*, 203–235.

Atance, C. M., & O'Neill, D. K. (2005). The emergence of episodic future thinking in humans. *Learn. Motiv., 36*, 126–144.

Bar, M. (2007). The proactive brain: Using analogies and associations to generate predictions. *Trends Cogn. Sci., 11*, 280–289.

Barnhofer, T., Kuehn, E. M., & de Jong-Meyer, R. (2005). Specificity of autobiographical memories and basal cortisol levels in patients with major depression. *Psychoneuroendocrinology, 30*, 403–411.

Barsalou, L. W. (1999). Perceptual symbol systems. *Behav. Brain Sci., 22*, 577–609.

Barsalou, L. W. (2003). Situated simulation in the human conceptual system. *Lang. Cogn. Process., 18*, 513–562.

Bartlett, F. C. (1932). *Remembering*. Cambridge, UK: Cambridge University Press.

Bird, C. M., Castelli, F., Malik, O., Frith, U., & Husain, M. (2004). The impact of medial frontal lobe damage on "Theory of Mind" and cognition. *Brain, 127*, 914–928.

Bjork, R. A., & Bjork, E. L. (1988). On the adaptive aspects of retrieval failure in autobiographical memory. In M. M. Gruneberg, P. E. Morris, & R. N. Sykes (Eds.), *Practical aspects of memory: Current research and issues* (pp. 283–288). Chichester, UK: Wiley.

Botzung, A., Denkova, E., & Manning, L. (in press). Experiencing past and future personal events: Functional neuroimaging evidence on the neural bases of mental time travel. *Brain Cogn.*

Brandimonte, M., Einstein, G. O., & McDaniel, M. A. (Eds.). (1996). *Prospective memory: Theory and applications*. Mahwah, NJ: Lawrence Erlbaum Associates.

Bremner, J. D., Narayan, M., Anderson, E. R., Staib, L. H., Miller, H. L., & Charney, D. S. (2000). Hippocampal volume reduction in major depression. *Am. J. Psychiatry, 157*, 115–117.

Brown, G. P., MacLeod, A. K., Tata, P., & Goddard, L. (2002). Worry and the simulation of future outcomes. *Anxiety Stress Copin., 15*, 1–17.

Buckner, R. L., Andrews-Hanna, J. R., & Schacter, D. L. (2008). The brain's default system: Anatomy, function, and relevance to disease. In *The Year in Cognitive Neuroscience 2008, Ann. N. Y. Acad. Sci., 1124,* 1–38.

Buckner, R. L., & Carroll, D. C. (2007). Self-projection and the brain. *Trends Cogn. Sci., 11,* 49–57.

Burgess, P., Simons, J. S., Coates, L. M. A., & Channon, S. (2005). The search for specific planning processes. In R. Morris & G. Ward (Eds.), *The cognitive psychology of planning* (pp. 199–227). Hove, UK and New York: Psychology Press.

Burgess, P. W., Quayle, A., & Frith, C. D. (2001). Brain regions involved in prospective memory as determined by positron emission tomography. *Neuropsychologia, 39,* 545–555.

Byrne, P., Becker, S., & Burgess, N. (2007). Remembering the past and imagining the future: A neural model of spatial memory and imagery. *Psychol. Rev., 114,* 340–375.

Byrne, R. M. J. (2005). *The rational imagination: How people create alternatives to reality.* Cambridge, MA: MIT Press.

Cabeza, R., & St Jacques, P. (2007). Functional neuroimaging of autobiographical memory. *Trends Cogn. Sci., 11,* 219–227.

Campbell, S., & Macqueen, G. (2004). The role of the hippocampus in the pathophysiology of major depression. *J. Psychiatry Neurosci., 29,* 417–426.

Carstensen, L. L., Isaacowitz, D., & Charles, S. T. (1999). Taking time seriously: A theory of socioemotional selectivity. *Am. Psychol., 54,* 165–181.

Chasteen, A. L., Park, D. C., & Schwarz, N. (2001). Implementation intentions and facilitation of prospective memory. *Psychol. Sci., 12,* 457–461.

Clayton, N. S., Bussey, T. J., & Dickinson, A. (2003). Can animals recall the past and plan for the future? *Nat. Rev. Neurosci., 4,* 685–691.

Clayton, N. S., & Dickinson, A. (1998). Episodic-like memory during cache recovery by scrub jays. *Nature, 395,* 272–274.

Conway, M. A., Peydell-Pearce, C. W., & Whitecross, S. E. (2001). The neuroanatomy of autobiographical memory: A slow cortical potential study of autobiographical memory retrieval. *J. Mem. Lang., 45,* 493–524.

Conway, M. A., Peydell-Pearce, C. W., Whitecross, S. E., & Sharpe, H. (2003). Neurophysiological correlates of memory for experienced and imagined events. *Neuropsychologia, 41,* 334–340.

Correia, S. P. C., Dickinson, A., & Clayton, N. S. (2007). Western scrub-jays anticipate future needs independently of their current motivational state. *Curr. Biol., 17,* 856–861.

D'Argembeau, A., Raffard, S., & Van Der Linden, M. (in press). Remembering the past and imagining the future in schizophrenia. *J. Abnorm. Psychol.*

D'Argembeau, A., & Van Der Linden, M. (2004). Phenomenal characteristics associated with projecting oneself back into the past and forward into the future: Influence of valence and temporal distance. *Conscious Cogn., 13,* 844–858.

D'Argembeau, A., & Van Der Linden, M. (2006). Individual differences in the phenomenology of mental time travel. *Conscious Cogn., 15,* 342–350.

Dalgleish, T., Williams, J., Golden, A., Perkins, N., Barett, L., et al. (2007). Reduced specificity of autobiographical memory and depression: The role of executive control. *J. Exp. Psychol. Gen., 136,* 23–42.

Davies, M., & Stone, T. (Eds.). (1995). *Mental simulation.* Oxford, UK: Blackwell Publishers.

Decety, J., & Grezes, J. (2006). The power of simulation: Imagining one's own and other's behavior. *Brain Res., 1079,* 4–14.

Decety, J., & Ingvar, D. (1990). Brain structures participating in mental simulation of motor behavior: A neuropsychological interpretation. *Acta. Psychol. (Amst.), 73,* 13–24.

Diba, K., & Buzsaki, G. (2007). Forward and reverse hippocampal place-cell sequences during ripples. *Nature Neurosci., 10,* 1241–1242.

Drevets, W. C. (2000). Neuroimaging studies of mood disorders. *Biol. Psychiatry, 48,* 813–829.

Dickson, J. M., & Bates, G. W. (2005). Influence of repression on autobiographical emories and expectations of the future. *Aust. J. Psychol., 57,* 20–27.

Dickson, J. M., & Bates, G. W. (2006). Autobiographical memories and views of the future: In relation to dysphoria. *Int. J. Psychol., 41,* 107–116.

Dudai, Y., & Carruthers, M. (2005). The Janus face of mnemosyne. *Nature, 434,* 823–824.

Eichenbaum, H., & Cohen, N. J. (2001). *From conditioning to conscious recollection: memory systems of the brain.* New York: Oxford University Press.

Einstein, G. O., & McDaniel, M. A. (1990). Normal aging and prospective memory. *J. Exp. Psychol. Learn. Mem. Cogn., 16,* 717–726.

Einstein, G. O., & McDaniel, M. A. (2005). Prospective memory: Multiple retrieval processes. *Curr. Dir. Psychol. Sci., 14,* 286–290.

Fellows, L. K., & Farah, M. J. (2005). Dissociable element of human foresight: A role for te ventromedial frontal lobes in framing the future, but not in discounting future rewards. *Neuropsychologia, 43,* 1214–1221.

Ferbinteanu, J., & Shapiro, M. L. (2003). Prospective and retrospective memory coding in the hippocampus. *Neuron, 40,* 1227–1239.

Frith, C. D., & Frith, U. (2006). The neural basis of mentalizing. *Neuron, 50,* 531–534.

Gilbert, D. T. (2006). *Stumbling on happiness.* New York: Alfred A. Knopf.

Gilbert, D. T., & Wilson, T. (2007). Prospection: Experiencing the future. *Science, 317,* 1351–1354.

Gilboa, A. (2004). Autobiographical and episodic memory – one and the same? Evidence from prefrontal activation in neuroimaging studies. *Neuropsychologia, 42,* 1336–1349.

Goldman, A. I. (1989). Interpretation psychologized. *Mind Lang., 4,* 161–185.

Goldman, A. I. (2006). *Simulating minds: The philosophy, psychology, and neuroscience of mind reading.* New York: Oxford University Press.

Gollwitzer, P. M. (1999). Implementation intentions: Strong effects of simple plans. *Am. Psychol., 54,* 493–503.

Gopnik, A., & Meltoff, A. (1997). *Words, thoughts, and theories.* Cambridge, MA: MIT Press.

Gopnik, A., & Wellman, H. (1992). Why the child's theory of mind really is just a theory. *Mind Lang., 7,* 145–171.

Gordon, R. M. (1986). Folk psychology as simulation. *Mind Lang., 1,* 158–171.

Gordon, R. M. (1992). The simulation theory: Objects and misconceptions. *Mind Lang., 7,* 11–34.

Greicius, M. D., Srivastava, G., Reiss, A. L., & Menon, V. (2004). Default-mode network activity distinguishes Alzheimer's disease from healthy aging: Evidence from functional MRI. *Proc. Natl. Acad. Sci. U.S.A., 101*, 4637–4642.

Harris, J. E. (1984). Remembering to do things: A forgotten topic. In J. E. Harris & P. E. Morris (Eds.), *Everyday memory, actions, and absent-mindedness* (pp. 71–92). New York: Academic Press.

Hassabis, D., Kumaran, D., Vann, S. D., & Maguire, E. A. (2007). Patients with hippocampal amnesia can not imagine new experiences. *Proc. Natl. Acad. Sci. U.S.A., 104*, 1726–1731.

Hassabis, D., & Maguire, E. A. (2007). Deconstructing episodic memory with construction. *Trends Cogn. Sci., 11*, 299–306.

Hawkins, J., & Blakesee, S. (2005). *On intelligence*. New York: Times Books.

Hayes-Roth, B., & Hayes-Roth, F. (1979). A cognitive model of planning. *Cognit. Sci., 3*, 275–310.

Heal, J. (1986). Replication and functionalism. In J. Butterfield (Ed.), *Language, mind, and logic* (pp. 135–150). Cambridge, UK: Cambridge University Press.

Heal, J. (1994). Simulation vs theory-theory: What's at issue? In C. Peacocke (Ed.), *Objectivity, simulation and the unity of consciousness* (pp. 129–144). Oxford, UK: Oxford University Press.

Hertel, P. T. (2000). The cognitive-initiative account of depression-related impairments in memory. In D. Medin (Ed.), *The psychology of learning and motivation* (pp. 12–25). New York: Academic Press.

Hesslow, G. (2002). Conscious thought as simulation of behavior and perception. *Trends Cogn. Sci., 6*, 242–247.

Ingvar, D. H. (1979). Hyperfrontal distribution of the cerebral grey matter flow in resting wakefulness: On the functional anatomy of the conscious state. *Acta Neurol. Scand., 60*, 12–25.

Ingvar, D. H. (1985). "Memory of the future": An essay on the temporal organization of conscious awareness. *Hum. Neurobiol., 4*, 127–136.

Ingvar, D. H., & Philipson, L. (1977). Distribution of cerebral blood-flow in dominant hemisphere during motor ideation and motor-performance. *Ann. Neurol., 2*, 230–237.

Foster, D. J., & Wilson, M. A. (2006). Reverse replay of behavioural sequences in hippocampal place cells during the awake state. *Nature, 440*, 680–683.

Foster, J. K., & Jelicic, M. (Eds.). (1999). *Memory: Systems, process, or function?* Oxford, UK: Oxford University Press.

Johnson, A., & Redish, A. D. (2007). Neural ensembles in CA3 transiently encode paths forward of the animal at a decision point. *J. Neurosci., 27*, 12176–12189.

Johnson, M. K., Foley, M. A., Suengas, A. G., & Raye, C. L. (1988). Phenomenal characteristics of memories for perceived and imagined autobiographical events. *J. Exp. Psychol. Gen., 117*, 371–376.

Kahneman, D., & Miller, D. T. (1986). Norm theory: Comparing reality to its alternatives. *Psychol. Rev., 93*, 136–153.

Kahneman, D., & Tversky, A. (1982). The simulation heuristic. In D. Kahneman, P. Slovic, & A. Tversky (Eds.), *Judgment under uncertainty* (pp. 201–208). Cambridge, UK: Cambridge University Press.

Klein, S. B., Loftus, J., & Kihlstrom, J. F. (2002). Memory and temporal experience: The effects of episodic memory loss on an amnesic patient's ability to remember the past and imagine the future. *Soc. Cogn., 20*, 353–379.

Knutson, B., Westdorp, A., Kaiser, E., & Hommer, D. (2000). FMRI visualization of brain activity during a monetary incentive delay task. *Neuroimage, 12*, 20–27.

Kosslyn, S. M. (1994). *Image and brain*. Cambridge, MA: MIT Press.

Kosslyn, S. M. (2005). Mental images and the brain. *Cogn. Neuropsychol., 22*, 333–347.

Kremers, I. P., Spinhoven, P., Van Der Does, A. J., & van Dyck, R. (2006). Social problem solving, autobiographical memory and the future specificity in outpatients with borderline personality disorder. *Clin. Psychol. Psychot., 13*, 131–137.

Kuyken, W., & Brewin, C. R. (1995). Autobiographical memory functioning in depression and reports of early abuse. *J. Abnorm. Psychol., 104*, 585–591.

Lavi, T., & Solomon, Z. (2005). Palestinian youth of the Intifada: PTSD and future orientation. *J. Am. Acad. Child Adolesc. Psychiatry, 44*, 1176–1183.

Levine, B., Svoboda, E., Hay, J. F., Winocur, G., & Moscovitch, M. (2002). Aging and autobiographical memory: Dissociating episodic from semantic retrieval. *Psychol. Aging, 17*, 677–689.

Loftus, E. F. (2003). Make-believe memories. *Am. Psychol., 58*, 867–873.

Luria, A. R. (1966). *Human brain and psychological processes*. New York: Harper & Row.

MacLeod, A. K., & Cropley, M. L. (1995). Depressive future-thinking: The role of valence and specificity. *Cognit. Ther. Res., 19*, 35–50.

MacLeod, A. K., Rose, G., & Williams, J. M. (1993). Components of hopelessness about the future in parasuicide. *Cognit. Ther. Res., 17*, 441–455.

MacLeod, A. K., Tata, P., Kentish, J., Carroll, F., & Hunter, E. (1997). Anxiety, depression, and explanation-based pessimism for future positive and negative events. *Clin. Psychol. Psychother., 4*, 15–24.

Maguire, E. A. (2001). Neuroimaging studies of autobiographical event memory. *Philos. Trans. R. Soc. Lond., B, Biol. Sci., 356*, 1441–1451.

Marsh, R. L., Hicks, J. L., & Cook, G. I. (2006). Task interference from prospective memories covaries with contextual associations of fulfilling them. *Mem. Cognit., 34*, 1037–1045.

Mesulam, M. M. (2002). The human frontal lobes: Transcending the default mode through contingent encoding. In D. T. Stuss & R. T. Knight (Eds.), *Principles of frontal lobe function* (pp. 8–30). New York: Oxford University Press.

Miller, G. A., Galanter, E., & Pribram, K. (1960). *Plans and the structure of behavior*. New York: Holt, Rinehart, and Winston.

Mitchell, J. P., Macrae, C. N., & Banaji, M. R. (2006). Dissociable medial prefrontal contributions to judgments of similar and dissimilar others. *Neuron, 50*, 655–663.

Morewedge, C. K., Gilbert, D. T., & Wilson, T. D. (2005). The least likely of times: How remembering the past biases forecasts of the future. *Psychol. Sci., 16*, 626–630.

Moscovitch, M., Nadel, L., Winocur, G., Gilboa, A., & Rosenbaum, R. S. (2006). The cognitive neuroscience of episodic, semantic and spatial remote memory. *Curr. Opin. Neurobiol., 16*, 179–190.

Morris, R., & Ward, G. (Eds.). (2005). *The cognitive psychology of planning*. Hove, UK and New York: Psychology Press.

Nussbaum, S., Liberman, N., & Trope, Y. (2006). Predicting the near and distant future. *J. Exp. Psychol. Gen., 135*, 152–161.

Oberman, L. M., & Ramachandran, V. S. (2007). The simulating social mind: The role of the mirror neuron system and simulation in the social and communicative deficits of autistic spectrum disorder. *Psychol. Bull., 133*, 310–327.

Okuda, J., Fujii, T., Ohtake, H., Tsukiura, T., Tanji, K., et al. (2003). Thinking of the future and the past: The roles of the frontal pole and the medial temporal lobes. *Neuroimage, 19*, 1369–1380.

Okuda, J., Fujii, T., Yamadori, A., Kawashima, R., Tsukiura, T., et al. (1998). Participation of the prefrontal cortices in prospective memory: Evidence from a PET study in humans. *Neurosci. Lett., 253*, 127–130.

Olton, D. S. (1989). Inferring psychological dissociation from experiment dissociations: The temporal context of episodic memory. In H. L. Roediger & F. I. M. Craik (Eds.), *Varieties of memory and consciousness: Essays in honour of Endel Tulving* (pp. 161–177). Hillsdale, NJ: Lawrence Erlbaum.

Öngür, D., Cullen, T. J., Wolf, D. H., Rohan, M., Barreira, P., et al. (2006). The neural basis of relational memory deficits in schizophrenia. *Arch. Gen. Psychiatry, 63*, 356–365.

Orbell, S., Hodgkins, S., & Sheeran, P. (1997). Implementation intentions and the theory of planned behavior. *Pers. Soc. Psychol. Bull., 23*, 945–954.

Owen, A. M. (2005). Cognitive planning in humans: New insights from the tower of london (TOL) task. In R. Morris & G. Ward (Eds.), *The cognitive psychology of planning* (pp. 135–151). Hove, UK and New York: Psychology Press.

Partiot, A., Grafman, J., Sadato, N., Wachs, J., & Hallett, M. (1995). Brain activation during the generation of emotional and non-emotional plans. *Neuroreport, 6*, 1269–1272.

Philips, L. H., Wynn, V. E., Gilhooly, K. J., Della Sala, S., & Logie, R. H. (1999). The role of memory in the Tower of London task. *Memory, 7*, 209–231.

Raby, C. R., Alexis, D. M., Dickinson, A., & Clayton, N. S. (2007). Planning for the future by western scrub-jays. *Nature, 445*, 919–921.

Raes, F., Hermans, D., der Decker, A., Eelen, P., & Wiliams, J. M. (2003). Autobiographical memory specificity and affect regulation: an experimental approach. *Emotion, 3*, 201–206.

Raes, F., Hermans, D., Williams, G. G., & Eelen, P. (2005). Autobiographical memory specificity and emotional abuse. *Br. J. Clin. Psychol., 44*, 133–138.

Raune, D., MacLeod, A., & Holmes, E. A. (2005). The simulation heuristic and visual imagery in pessimism for future negative events in anxiety. *Clin. Psychol. Psychother., 12*, 313–325.

Roediger, H. L., & McDermott, K. B. (1995). Creating false memories: Remembering words not presented in lists. *J. Exp. Psychol. Learn. Mem. Cogn., 21*, 803–814.

Rosenbaum, R. S., Kohler, S., Schacter, D. L., Moscovitch, M., Westmacott, R., et al. (2005). The case of K.C.: Contributions of a memory-impaired person to memory theory. *Neuropsychologia, 43*, 989–1021.

Roy, M. M., Christenfeld, N. J. S., & McKenzie, C. R. M. (2005). Underestimating the duration of future events: Memory incorrectly used or memory bias? *Psychol. Bull., 131*, 738–756.

Ruane, D., MacLeod, A. K., & Holmes, E. A. (2005). The simulation heuristic and visual imagery in pessimism for negative events in anxiety. *Clin. Psychol. Psychother., 12*, 313–325.

Sanna, L. J. (2000). Mental simulation, affect, and personality: A conceptual framework. *Curr. Dir. Psychol. Sci., 9*, 168–173.

Sapolsky, R. M. (2000). Glucocorticoids and hippocampal atrophy in neuropsychiatric disorders. *Arch. Gen. Psychiatry, 57*, 925–935.

Saxe, R. (2005). Against simulation: The argument from error. *Trends Cogn. Sci., 9*, 174–179.

Saxe, R., & Kanwisher, N. (2003). People thinking about thinking people: The role of the temporo-parietal junction in "theory of mind". *Neuroimage, 19*, 1835–1842.

Schacter, D. L. (1987). Memory, amnesia, and frontal lobe dysfunction. *Psychobiology, 15*, 21–36.

Schacter, D. L. (1999). The seven sins of memory: Insights from psychology and cognitive neuroscience. *Am. Psychol., 54*, 182–203.

Schacter, D. L. (2001). *The seven sins of memory: How the mind forgets and remembers*. Boston: Houghton Mifflin.

Schacter, D. L., & Addis, D. R. (2007a). The cognitive neuroscience of constructive memory: Remembering the past and imagining the future. *Philo. Trans. R. Soc. Lond., B, Biol. Sci., 362*, 773–786.

Schacter, D. L., & Addis, D. R. (2007b). The ghosts of past and future. *Nature, 445*, 27.

Schacter, D. L., & Addis, D. R. (2007c). The optimistic brain. *Nat. Neurosci., 10*, 1345–1347.

Schacter, D. L., Addis, D. R., & Buckner, R. L. (2007). Remembering the past to imagine the future: The prospective brain. *Nat. Rev. Neurosci., 8*, 657–661.

Scheier, M. F., Carver, C. S., & Bridges, M. W. (1994). Distinguishing optimism from neuroticism (and trait anxiety, self-mastery, and self-esteem): A reevaluation of the Life Orientation Test. *J. Pers. Soc. Psychol., 67*, 1063–1078.

Seifert, C. M., & Patalano, A. L. (2001). Opportunism in memory: Preparing for chance encounters. *Curr. Dir. Psychol. Sci., 6*, 198–201.

Seymour, R., Daw, N., Dayan, P., Singer, T., & Dolan, R. (2007). Differential encoding of losses and gains in the human striatum. *J. Neurosci., 27*, 4826–4831.

Shallice, T. (1982). Specific impairments of planning. *Philos. Trans. R. Soc. Lond., B, Biol. Sci., 298*, 199–209.

Shallice, T., & Burgess, P. (1996). The domain of supervisory processes and the temporal organization of behaviour. *Philos. Trans. R. Soc. Lond., B, Biol. Sci., 351*, 1405–1411.

Sharot, T., Riccardi, A. M., Raio, C. M., & Phelps, E. A. (2007). Neural mechanisms mediating optimism bias. *Nature, 450*, 102–105.

Simons, J. S., Schölvinck, M. L., Gilbert, S. J., Frith, C. D., & Burgess, P. W. (2006). Differential components of prospective memory? Evidence from fMRI. *Neuropsychologia*, *44*, 1388–1397.

Spreng, R. N., & Levine, B. (2006). The temporal distribution of past and future autobiographical events across the lifespan. *Mem. Cognit.*, *34*, 1644–1651.

Squire, L. R. (1982). Comparisons between forms of amnesia: Some deficits are unique to Korsakoff's syndrome. *J. Exp. Psychol. Learn. Mem. Cogn.*, *8*, 560–571.

Stöber, J., & Borkovec, T. D. (2002). Reduced concreteness of worry in generalized anxiety disorder: Findings from a therapy study. *Cognit. Ther. Res.*, *26*, 89–96.

Stuss, D. T., & Benson, D. F. (1986). *The frontal lobes*. New York: Raven Press.

Suddendorf, T., & Busby, J. (2005). Making decisions with the future in mind: Developmental and comparative identification of mental time travel. *Learn. Motiv.*, *36*, 110–125.

Suddendorf, T., & Corballis, M. C. (1997). Mental time travel and the evolution of the human mind. *Genet. Soc. Gen. Psychol. Monogr.*, *123*, 133–167.

Suddendorf, T., & Corballis, M. C. (2007). The evolution of foresight: What is mental time travel and is it unique to humans? *Behav. Brain Sci.*, *30*, 299–313.

Svoboda, E., McKinnon, M. C., & Levine, B. (2006). The functional neuroanatomy of autobiographical memory: A meta-analysis. *Neuropsychologia*, *44*, 2189–2208.

Szpunar, K. K., & McDermott, K. B. (in press). Episodic future thought and its relation to remembering: Evidence from ratings of subjective experience. *Conscious. Cogn.*

Szpunar, K. K., Watson, J. M., & McDermott, K. B. (2007). Neural substrates of envisioning the future. *Proc. Natl. Acad. Sci. U.S.A.*, *104*, 642–647.

Talland, G. A. (1965). *Deranged memory: A psychonomic study of the amnesic syndrome*. New York and London: Academic Press.

Taylor, S. E., Pham, L. B., Rivkin, I. D., & Armor, D. A. (1998). Harnessing the imagination: Mental simulation, self-regulation, and coping. *Am. Psychol.*, *53*, 429–439.

Taylor, S. E., & Schneider, S. K. (1989). Coping and the simulation of events. *Soc. Cogn.*, *7*, 174–194.

Trope, Y., & Liberman, N. (2003). Temporal construal. *Psychol. Rev.*, *110*, 401–421.

Tulving, E. (1983). *Elements of episodic memory*. Oxford, UK: Clarendon Press.

Tulving, E. (1985). Memory and consciousness. *Can. Psychol.*, *26*, 1–12.

Tulving, E. (1987). Introduction: Multiple memory systems and consciousness. *Hum. Neurobiol.*, *6*, 67–80.

Tulving, E. (2002). Episodic memory: From mind to brain. *Annu. Rev. Psychol.*, *53*, 1–25.

Tulving, E. (2005). Episodic memory and autonoesis. In H. Terrance & J. Metcalfe (Eds.), *The missing link in cognition: Origins of self-reflective consciousness* (pp. 3–56). New York: Oxford University Press.

Tulving, E., Schacter, D. L., McLachlan, D. R., & Moscovitch, M. (1988). Priming of semantic autobiographical knowledge: A case study of retrograde amnesia. *Brain Cogn.*, *8*, 3–20.

Tversky, A., & Kahneman, D. (1973). Availability: A heuristic for judging frequency and probability. *Cognit. Psychol.*, *5*, 207–232.

Van Boven, L., & Ashworth, L. (2007). Looking forward, looking back: Anticipation is more evocative than retrospection. *J. Exp. Psychol. Gen.*, *136*, 289–300.

Vaughn, L. A., & Weary, G. (2002). Roles of the availability of explanations, feelings of ease, and dysphoria in judgements about the future. *J. Soc. Clin. Psychol.*, *21*, 686–704.

Velakoulis, D., Wood, S. J., Wong, M. T., McGorry, P. D., Yung, A., et al. (2006). Hippocampal and amygdala volumes according to psychosis stage and diagnosis: A magnetic resonance imaging study of chronic schizophrenia, first-episode psychosis, and ultra-high-risk individuals. *Arch. Gen. Psychiatry*, *63*, 139–149.

Vincent, J. L., Snyder, A. Z., Fox, M. D., Shannon, B. J., Andrews, J. R., et al. (2006). Coherent spontaneous activity identifies a hippocampal-parietal memory network. *J. Neurophysiol.*, *96*, 3517–3531.

Wagner, A. D., Shannon, B. J., Kahn, I., & Buckner, R. L. (2005). Parietal lobe contributions to episodic memory retrieval. *Trends Cogn. Sci.*, *9*, 445–453.

Weinstein, N. D. (1980). Unrealistic optimism about future life events. *J. Pers. Soc. Psychol.*, *39*, 806–820.

Williams, J. M. (1996). Depression and the specificity of autobiographical memory. In D. C. Rubin (Ed.), *Remembering our past: Studies in autobiographical memory* (pp. 244–267). Cambridge, UK: Cambridge University Press.

Williams, J. M. (2006). Capture and rumination, functional avoidance, and executive control (CaRFAX): Three processes that underlie overgeneral memory. *Cogn. Emot.*, *20*, 139–149.

Williams, J. M., Ellis, N. C., Tylers, C., Healy, H., Rose, G., et al. (1996). The specificity of autobiographical memory and imageability of the future. *Mem. Cognit.*, *24*, 116–125.

Wood, F. (1987). Focal and diffuse memory activation assessed by localized indicators of CNS metabolism: The semantic-episodic memory distinction. *Hum. Neurobiol.*, *6*, 141–151.

Yacubian, J., Gladcher, J., Schroeder, K., Sommer, T., Braus, D. F., et al. (2006). Dissociable systems for gain- and loss-related value predictions and errors of prediction in the human brain. *J. Neurosci.*, *26*, 9530–9537.

Generalization and Differentiation in Semantic Memory

Insights from Semantic Dementia

MATTHEW A. LAMBON RALPH[a] AND KARALYN PATTERSON[b]

[a]*Neuroscience and Aphasia Research Unit, School of Psychological Sciences, University of Manchester, Manchester, United Kingdom*

[b]*MRC Cognition and Brain Sciences Unit, Cambridge, United Kingdom*

According to many theories, semantic representations reflect the parallel activation of information coded across a distributed set of modality-specific association brain cortices. This view is challenged by the neurodegenerative condition known as semantic dementia (SD), in which relatively circumscribed, bilateral atrophy of the anterior temporal lobes results in selective degradation of core semantic knowledge, affecting all types of concept, irrespective of the modality of testing. Research on SD suggests a major revision in our understanding of the neural basis of semantic memory. Specifically, it is proposed that the anterior temporal lobes form amodal semantic representations through the distillation of the multimodal information that is projected to this region from the modality-specific association cortices. Although cross-indexing of modality-specific information could be achieved by a web of direct connections between pairs of these regions, amodal semantic representations enable semantic generalization and inference on the basis of conceptual structure rather than modality-specific features. As expected from this hypothesis, SD is characterized by impaired semantic generalization, both clinically and in formal assessment. The article describes a comprehensive array of under- and overgeneralization errors by patients with SD when engaged in receptive and expressive verbal and nonverbal tasks and everyday behaviors.

Key words: semantic dementia; semantic memory; anterior temporal lobes

Introduction

The British poet Philip Larkin once famously quipped that sexual intercourse began in 1963, between the end of the Lady Chatterley ban and the arrival of the Beatles' first LP. Just as remarkably, though perhaps less sensationally, semantic memory appears to have begun around the same time. The first documented use of the term is probably the title of Quillian's (1966) Ph.D. thesis; it subsequently appeared as part of the title of the well-known article by Collins and Quillian (1969) and, even more famously, in Tulving's (1972) chapter on the distinction between episodic and semantic memory.

Of course, even before the 1960s, everyone really knew that people had semantic memory (as well as sex), but it is perhaps not so surprising that semantic memory has only recently achieved independent status. What we mean by having independent status is the equivalent of what Shallice (1988) refers to as a cognitive subsystem that is isolable or anatomically distinct. Semantic memory is usually assumed not to be localized to one neuroanatomical region but rather to reflect activation of modality-specific information encoded within a widely distributed network of regions. This view is perhaps most often found in the discussion sections of articles on functional imaging of semantic processing in normal individuals (e.g., Thompson-Schill 2003), though it is also sometimes found in studies of neuropsychological disorders. Here is one example. Some objects, such as elephants or spinach, have characteristic colors, and all cognitive scientists would probably agree that people's knowledge of these standard colors is part of semantic memory. But suppose, as some researchers have concluded in their imaging or patient studies, that color knowledge has its own module in the brain, separate from other aspects of knowledge even about the same objects (e.g., what shape elephants are,

Address for correspondence: Prof. Matthew A. Lambon Ralph, Neuroscience and Aphasia Research Unit, School of Psychological Sciences, University of Manchester, Manchester, UK.
matt.lambon-ralph@manchester.ac.uk

what sound they make, and how they move). Then color knowledge would have independent status and a specific neuroanatomical location, and so would each of the other attribute-specific components of semantic memory (Martin 2007); but central conceptual knowledge would not have this characteristic.

In this article we will outline a different hypothesis about semantic memory, in which—in addition to the modality-specific components of the broader semantic network on which essentially all theories agree—the central aspects of conceptual knowledge are and in fact need to be synthesized into a localized subsystem of unified, amodal representations. More specifically, the hypothesis comes in two parts: (a) as conceptual knowledge is acquired, the brain constructs amodal semantic representations that knit together the collection of attribute-specific features about a concept; and (b) neuroanatomically speaking, these amodal representations are supported by anterior regions of the temporal lobes bilaterally. Why do we claim that central semantic memory ought to be localized in this fashion? The argument, developed below, is that amodal conceptual representations support the vital function of semantic generalization. The corollary of this argument is that, when the brain region supporting these representations is damaged, a key consequence will be a failure of appropriate generalization.

Conceptualization without Amodal Representations

Before laying out the theory and evidence for amodal semantic representations, we will first briefly review both historical and contemporary views of semantic memory. Long before the term "semantic memory" was introduced to the world, in fact going back more than a century, Wernicke and Meynert (see Eggert 1977) were interested in how the brain formed and reactivated concepts—a process they referred to as "conceptualization." Unlike the language centers that Wernicke, more famously, described in his work on aphasia, Meynert and Wernicke's model of conceptualization made the following assumptions: (a) that the building blocks of concepts were modality-specific engrams (stores of information) localized to the cortical areas responsible for the corresponding sensory, motor, or verbal domain; (b) that these modality-specific engrams, in widespread brain regions, were fully interconnected; and (c) that this web of connections was the basis of conceptualization—a specific concept being represented by the coactivation of all its associated engrams (FIG. 1A). For example, if you taste an apple (even with your eyes closed), the taste-specific engram will automatically activate all the other associated modality-linked engrams, enabling your brain to retrieve other knowledge concerning the object: its visual form, probable color, name, presence of seeds, how you would peel it, and so on. In this proposal, modality-specific engrams were located in particular brain regions, but conceptualization was not. Indeed, Wernicke and Meynert argued that, unlike forms of agnosia and aphasia, central disorders of conceptualization occurred only as a consequence of global brain damage (dementia) because only such widespread cortical damage would disrupt the engram reactivation process.

Conceptualization Requires Amodal Representations

In this article we advance the hypothesis that semantic memory is, in fact, critically based on the formation of amodal representations, and we attempt to explain why this form of semantic organization might be required for the complexities of conceptual behaviour in which humans specialize. The first significant modern evidence for this hypothesis came in the form of a neuropsychological study by Warrington (1975). She described three patients with progressive brain disease resulting in a range of semantic deficits that cut across different modalities but were nonetheless restricted to the domain of semantics. That is, other aspects of the patients' cognition, including perceptual abilities and even other forms of memory (everyday episodic memory and short-term memory) were well preserved. Referring to Tulving's (1972) then–recently proposed distinction between episodic and semantic memory, Warrington (1975) labeled the disorder one of semantic memory. Snowden et al. (1989) later identified the condition as part of the spectrum of frontotemporal dementia (FTD) and gave it the label that has stuck, semantic dementia (SD).

There was little or no neuroanatomical information about the patients in Warrington's original study, but as further similar cases were published in tandem with advances in structural brain imaging, it became clear that SD was consistently associated with selective atrophy of the anterior temporal lobes bilaterally (Hodges et al. 1992; Snowden et al. 1996). Quantitative structural magnetic resonance imaging (MRI) studies, using both manual methods and automatic voxel–based morphometry, reveal consistent and substantial atrophy (often 50–80% gray matter loss) of the polar and perirhinal cortices and the anterior fusiform gyri (Williams et al. 2005; Brambati et al. 2007). In a neurodegenerative condition, precise boundaries of the pathological process are admittedly not easy to define; but, with the advent of functional brain imaging,

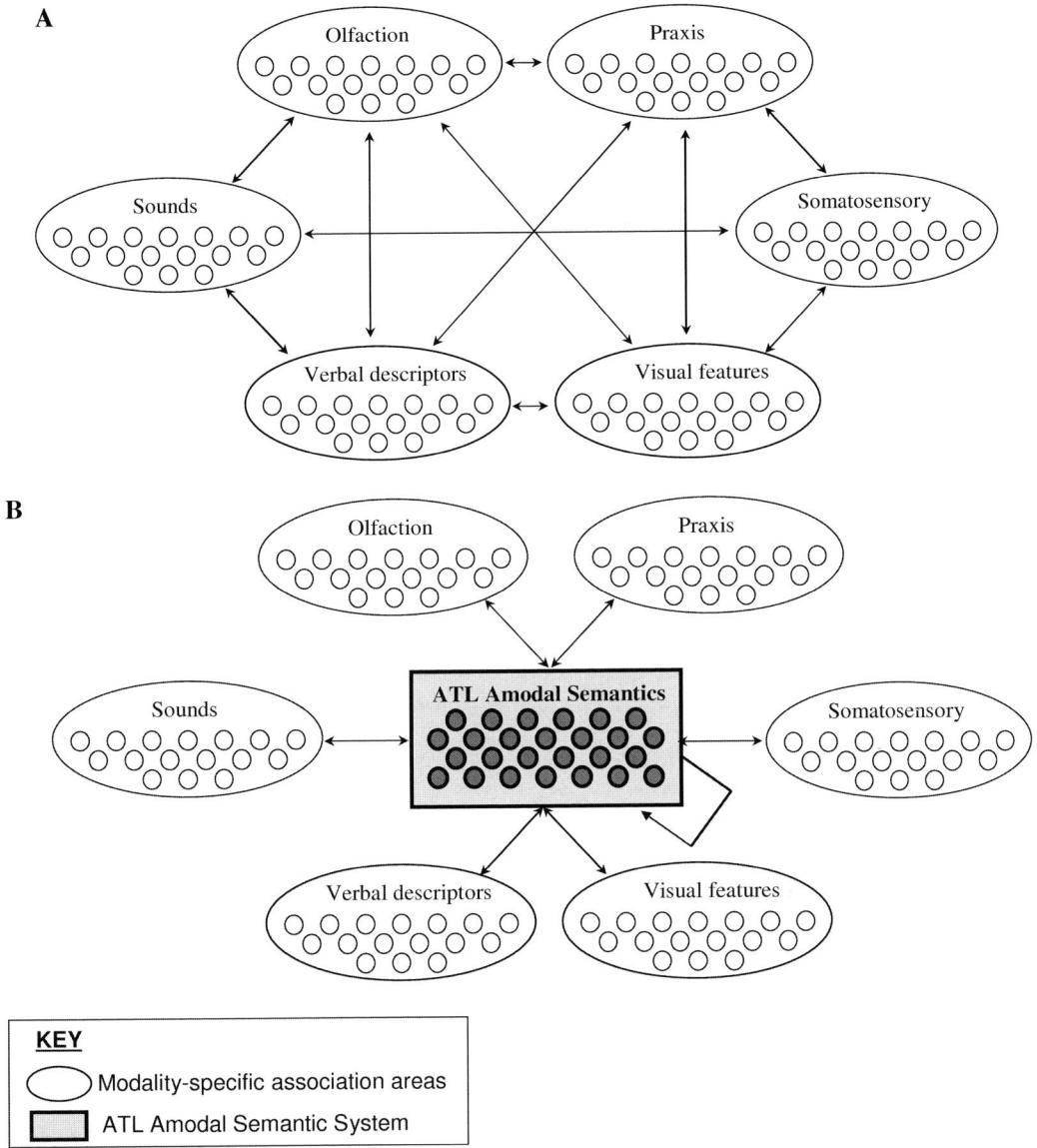

FIGURE 1. (A) Wernicke–Meynert model of conceptualization. **(B)** Model of ATL amodal semantic system (Rogers et al. 2004).

researchers have been able to demonstrate that not only the atrophy but also the hypometabolism in SD is restricted largely to the anterior temporal lobes, suggesting that the associated cognitive disorder is attributable to damage in this region rather than to widespread functional abnormality (Desgranges et al. in press; Diehl et al. 2004; Nestor et al. 2006).

While patients are alive, the nature of the dysfunction in neurodegenerative disease can only be guessed at or predicted, albeit often (and increasingly) with reasonably high confidence. Confirmed pathological diagnosis requires postmortem analysis of brain tissue, and researchers studying FTD in general and SD in particular have only recently begun to accumulate sufficient postmortem samples to be able to offer meaningful summary statistics. In patients coming to postmortem from our Cambridge series, of 20 cases with a clinical diagnosis of SD in life, 14 had ubiquitin-positive neuronal inclusions of the kind associated with motor neuron disease; four had the τ-positive inclusions characteristic of Pick's disease; and two had the plaques and tangles of Alzheimer's disease.

As well as data on the regions of atrophy and underlying dysfunction in SD, there is a considerable wealth of detailed neuropsychological findings about this disorder (Rogers et al. 2004; Patterson et al. 2007; Hodges & Patterson 2007). In short, the patients present with a *progressive* and *selective* deterioration of semantic memory. *Progressive* means that, especially if the patients come to appropriate assessment early enough, their performance on tests requiring conceptual knowledge can be tracked from mildly to moderately to severely abnormal; *selective* means that many other aspects of cognition, memory, and language are relatively well preserved until late in the disorder. This specificity is important for several reasons. Clinically, it is an important aspect for differential diagnosis of SD as opposed to other forms of dementia or conditions in which semantic impairment can be observed (Hodges & Patterson 2007; Kipps et al. 2008). From a research perspective, the specificity of the semantic decline means that SD provides a neurological model of semantic impairment and its effect on cognition without major complications from co-occurring non-semantic deficits. Of course, semantic impairment can be found in several other neurological conditions, including Alzheimer's disease, herpes simplex virus encephalitis, head injury, and stroke. Almost inevitably, however, the semantic impairment in these disorders is (a) less pervasive than that observed in SD and (b) accompanied by other deficits affecting episodic or short-term memory, attention, executive, and/or language processing.

SD challenges the assumption that semantic memory is based on a widely distributed system of modality-specific representations and links between them and does not require amodal representations localized to a specific brain region. For this article two more characteristics of SD are important: (a) semantic impairment is a graded phenomenon in which concepts and the boundaries between concepts gradually "dissolve" or "dim," rather than dropping out abruptly (Lambon Ralph et al. 2007; Patterson & Hodges 2000); (b) the degradation of concepts is amodal, thereby producing poor comprehension and production of information across all verbal and nonverbal domains, including words, objects, pictures, sounds, smells, and touch, etc., in receptive mode, and speech, writing, object use, drawing, etc., in expressive mode (Rogers et al. 2004).

These characteristics of SD can be understood on the hypothesis that the area of focal atrophy in this disorder, the anterior temporal lobe (ATL), supports the formation of amodal semantic representations. Using a computational model, Rogers et al. (2004) demonstrated that a central component of the model's architecture that draws together modality-specific information will behave as an amodal semantic system. The Rogers et al. model is an extension of the Meynert–Wernicke framework (FIG. 1B). Information arising in each specific modality (e.g., the elephant's shape, color, smell, form of movement, name, and verbal descriptors) is coded in the corresponding specific cortical sensory or motor or language region; in this sense, the semantic network as a whole *is* neuroanatomically widespread. The information from the modality-specific regions, however, is fused through amodal representations. We assume these representations to be supported by the bilateral ATL, not only because this is the location of the focal atrophy/hypometabolism in SD but also because this region is highly interconnected with many modality-specific association cortices (Gloor 1997); it thus has the necessary neuroanatomical connectivity to provide the neural substrate for the fusion of multimodal information into amodal representations. The Rogers et al. model was trained to take a piece of modality-specific information (e.g., an outline of the elephant's visual form) as input and to reproduce the correct information across the remaining information layers (e.g., its color or name or various things people might say about it) by propagating activation through the intermediate units. Rogers et al. demonstrated that simulated damage to these intermediate semantic units of the trained model reproduced the core features of SD. That is, increasing degrees of damage produced gradual decline in performance of any task requiring conceptual knowledge and, because of its intermediate location, damage to this central component of semantic memory resulted in deficits across various receptive and productive verbal and nonverbal domains.

At this level of description, the implemented Rogers model provides an alternative to the Wernicke–Meynert solution to the riddle of conceptualization (how to draw together multimodal experience, coded in different brain regions, into a unified concept). The Rogers formulation also resembles the notion of "convergence zones" proposed by Damasio (1989), whereby various brain regions link or index corresponding features and attributes. Logically speaking, conceptualization could be achieved either by the full set of direct connections between individual pairs of modality-specific regions (Wernicke–Meynert) or by a common amodal portal (Rogers/Damasio et al.). Semantic dementia, however, in which a selective but multimodal semantic impairment results from circumscribed ATL damage, argues for the second solution. If this assertion is correct, one might want to inquire why nature has selected against what might seem the simpler brain-engineering solution (a web of direct connections) and instead used a corner of the brain (the ATL) to underpin conceptualization. The answer, or at least one potential answer, lies in generalization. Knowing the range of concepts over which a component of knowledge should be generalized is a multilevel, nonlinear problem; its solution probably requires representations that abstract away from surface similarities.

The Conundrum of Semantic Generalization and Inference

The following example captures critical aspects of the semantic conundrum of generalization and inference. Various exemplars of five different yet related objects are shown in FIGURE 2. The items are grouped horizontally in terms of visual similarity, whereas the vertical structure reflects their most typical function. One can immediately see that superficial, surface similarity is not a reliable guide to other types of information. Thus, to know which subset of objects would be used to make and serve tea (a nonverbal generalization) or be referred to as a "teapot" (a verbal generalization) requires us to step away from visual similarities to select the correct subset. Matters are made more complex because different pieces of verbal or nonverbal knowledge can be generalized at different levels across this set. For example, all the items are used to contain and pour liquids (and we might refer to them verbally as "containers" to denote this level of generality). Consequently, they need to be set down on a level surface, and the liquid level needs to be kept below the tip of the spout to avoid spillage. The exact form of the liquid, however, varies across these objects—one set takes oil, one group takes wine, whereas the others hold water. Then at a more specific level, two of the five are used to hold very hot water (yet we do not use the same name to refer to them), but only one of these is used to generate it. Each of the five main groups of items can be subdivided again in terms of both the verbal and nonverbal features applied to them. For example, some of the kettles are heated by being set on a flame or external electric element, whereas others incorporate an internal electric element and so are plugged in (a distinction that can confuse British and American people when they visit each other's houses). A subset of teapots are made of metal or china (the latter therefore fragile), but the teapots can also be divided along completely different lines in terms of those that would be used to serve "English" versus Chinese or Japanese tea. Finally, we can use our complex semantic knowledge of these items to make new inferences on the basis of their meaning rather than their visual or structural characteristics. For example, if we learn about a new type of tea or learn that the Japanese word for teapot is *kyusu*, we would all pick the same subset of items to infuse the new tea or to apply the new label to—and we would do so on the basis of conceptual rather than visual similarity.

In summary, an amodal semantic system performs five key yet computationally demanding functions: (a) it provides a method to link multimodal experience and information to a core concept; (b) it allows us to step away from surface similarities (e.g., similar-sounding or -looking objects) to generalize on the basis of conceptual similarity; (c) it permits generalization of features simultaneously at different levels of specificity; (d) it allows appropriate generalization to be computed for all types of verbal and nonverbal information; and (e) it provides a sophisticated knowledge base on which to make new inferences when we acquire a new piece of information.

SD: A Disorder of Failing Semantic Generalization?

If the neuroanatomical basis of amodal semantic representations is the ATL, patients with SD—in whom focal brain disease gradually destroys the ATL—should exhibit disorders in all five functions listed above. To date, research on SD has concentrated largely on the first of these—the ability to link verbal and nonverbal information to each concept. As expected, disease progression in SD leads to a striking and eventually profound disruption of semantic knowledge. Thus, the patients have significant deficits in understanding and producing the names of objects (Hodges et al. 1992; Warrington 1975), provide increasingly impoverished definitions and drawings of objects (Lambon Ralph et al. 1999), have a reducing repertoire of everyday behavior such as knowing how to cook or cut the lawn or replace a fuse (Hodges & Patterson 2007), and so on. More recently, however, researchers studying SD have begun to investigate the other four, arguably more complex, aspects of conceptualization (e.g., Patterson 2007). The next section of this article will review and synthesize current evidence for disorders of these functions in SD, drawing upon evidence from both formal neuropsychological assessment and from everyday, real-world examples. Specifically, by assessing the effect of ATL degeneration in SD, we will evaluate the hypothesis that the ATL semantic system provides the mechanism for appropriate generalization on the basis of amodal, conceptual knowledge

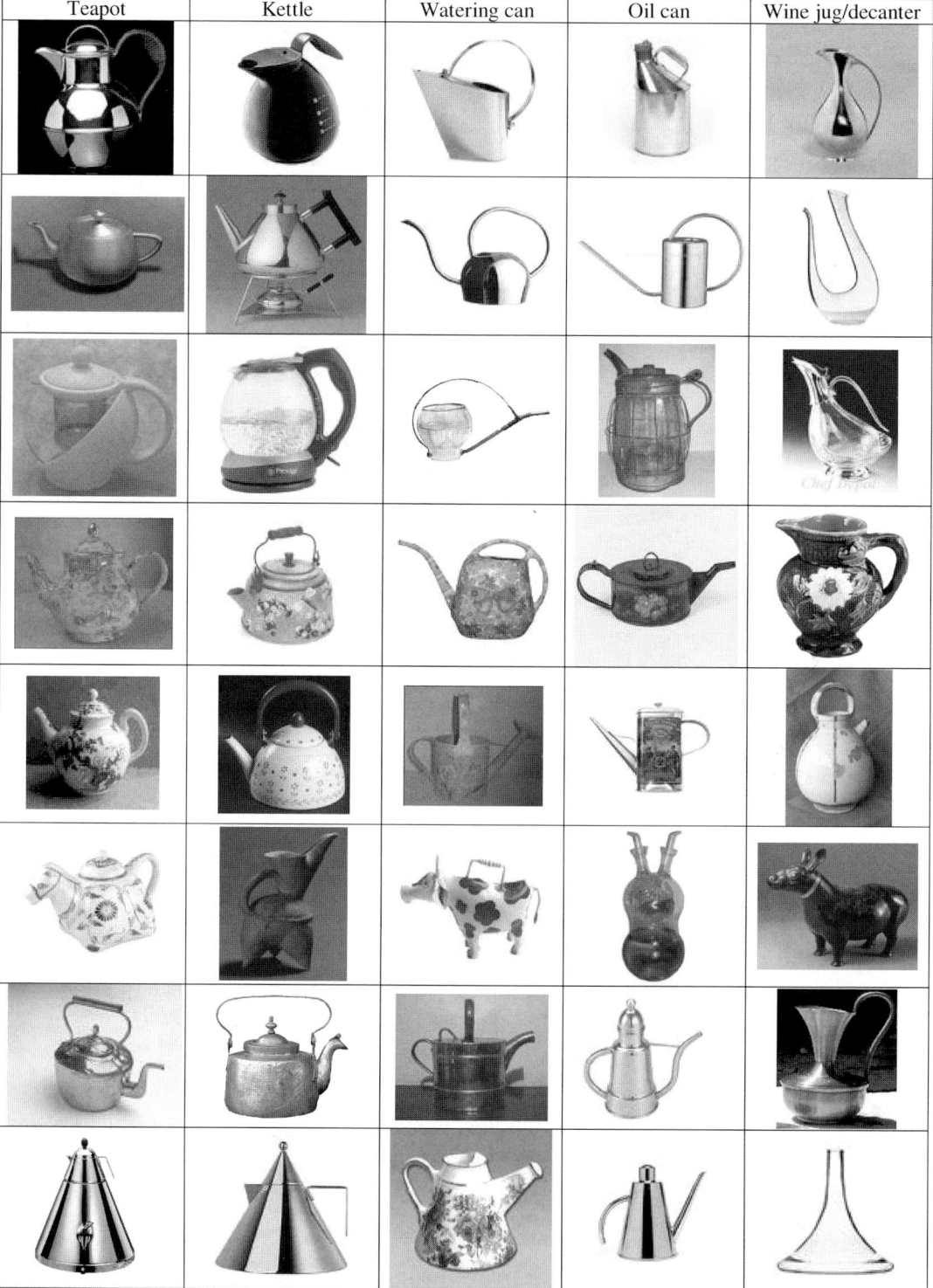

FIGURE 2. Examples of "liquid containers" ordered by visual similarity (rows) and principal function (columns).

(i.e., not on the basis of modality-specific similarities). If this notion is correct, then we should be able to find evidence for the following three predictions:

(a) Patients with SD should both over- and undergeneralize knowledge, being increasingly influenced by information that is general to many items rather than specific to a given concept, and by superficial, nonsemantic similarities.
(b) They should exhibit over- and undergeneralization in both verbal and nonverbal domains.
(c) They should exhibit over- and undergeneralization in both receptive and expressive tasks.

Evidence from SD Regarding the Nature of Under- and Overgeneralization

Word Production and Comprehension

The first—and throughout the course of the disease, perhaps always most obvious—symptom of SD is anomia: inability to retrieve the appropriate word for an object or concept. This anomia should not be thought of as word-finding difficulty in the sense experienced by many patients with aphasia after a stroke, or indeed sometimes momentarily by normal people. In the latter cases, people will often spontaneously retrieve the desired word a few minutes later or on another occasion; and even when in the anomic state they can often be helped to retrieve it by a simple cue such as its initial letter or sound (Jefferies & Lambon Ralph 2006). The anomia in SD is neither temporary nor cueable, and for good reason: The source of SD anomia is not in fact a failure of word retrieval. Its cause is that the patients lack sufficiently precise knowledge of the concept for the semantic system to activate the concept's name. Cueing (e.g., for violin, "it begins with /v/") will help normal speakers and most patients who suffered an aphasic stroke because they have substantial semantic information about the concept; the experimenter's additional bit of phonological information (/v/) can then push the word's phonological representation over the threshold for production. Patients with mild SD, looking at a picture of a violin, know only that it is a musical thing; patients with more severe SD may not know what it is at all. This degraded information is insufficient for them to find the word on another occasion or to benefit from a phonological cue (Graham et al. 1995).

Given that the anomia in SD derives from degraded knowledge, anomia is naturally accompanied by a parallel deficit in word comprehension. Asked "What is a violin?" the patients' responses mimic their attempts to name a picture of it: That is, at a mild stage, the patient may say that "It's for playing music"; at a more severe stage, he or she will just say "I don't know." Indeed, in clinic we often observe something like "word alienation," where a patient responds by repeating "violin, violin, violin" over and over again, with perfect phonological production but no apparent experience of familiarity with the word or its referent (Hodges & Patterson 2007).

How do the phenomena of under- and overgeneralization reveal themselves in the word production and comprehension deficits of patients with SD? For production, there are three sources of evidence: formal object-naming tests, formal analyses of target word production in a task like picture description, and anecdotal observations of the things that patients say in conversation or in clinic interview.

On naming tests, one prominent form of overgeneralization in SD is the production of semantic coordinate errors in which the name produced is a more common, more typical instance of the category to which the target instance belongs. This error occurs most often in the domain of animals because the category structure of animals lends itself most naturally to this kind of error. Hence the most common coordinate errors are the most typical and most familiar animal names ("cat," "dog," and "horse" in Britain). One additional intriguing component of this phenomenon is that, even though the line drawings usually used in these naming tests are all roughly the same size, the patients' semantic errors can indicate some residual knowledge of real-world size, with an elephant named as "horse," a goat named as "dog," and a rabbit named as "cat" (Hodges et al. 1995; Patterson et al. 2007). Another component of interest, and more directly relevant to the nature of overgeneralization, is that semantic coordinate errors (a) occur more often for moderately typical instances of a category than for atypical ones and (b) are more likely to be the prototypical dog–cat–horse responses if the target itself is fairly typical. In a recent large analysis of naming in patients with SD, for example, Woollams et al. (2007) reported on the fate of the tortoise and the hare (or rabbit), the former being an atypical animal and the latter a fairly typical one as indicated by category typicality norms (Morrow & Duffy 2005). Of incorrect responses to these two pictures, a significantly higher proportion were semantic coordinate errors for the rabbit than for the tortoise; and of the semantic coordinate errors, a much higher proportion were "cat" or "dog" for the rabbit than for the tortoise. Our way of thinking about this phenomenon is that the amodal semantic representations for typical instances with many shared features are clustered together at the center of semantic space. When a patient's conceptual representation of rabbit is too degraded to generate the correct name, the brain activation produced by looking at a rabbit can be captured by a more intact and close concept like "cat" or "dog." "Tortoise," on the other hand, is far from the center of this space and so is less prone to being overgeneralized to the prototypical animals (Garrard et al. 2001; Woollams et al. 2007).

The other main form of overgeneralization in naming by patients with SD is production of a superordinate label such as "animal." Again, this type of error is more commonly observed for living things than for synthetic artifacts, though sometimes patients will use an artifact superordinate like "container" for objects that can hold things, such as cups, bowls, dustbins, suitcases, boxes, or bottles.

The results of tests like picture description tell a similar story, indicating that the profound anomia and overgeneralization observed in SD is not related to the perhaps odd and out-of-context experience of being asked to name a series of single, unrelated objects. In the picture-description task most often used in the aphasia literature, the Cookie Theft picture from Goodglass and Kaplan (1983), a woman is washing dishes at an overflowing sink, while behind and unseen by her, her son (presumably) is standing on a tipping stool as he tries to steal cookies from a cupboard. Almost every normal speaker, in describing this picture, uses the terms "stool" for what the boy is standing on and starting to fall off of, "sink" for what the woman is standing at, and "overflowing" for what is happening to the water in the sink. Of 21 patients with SD (whose descriptions of this picture were analyzed by Patterson & MacDonald 2006), none produced the word "stool"; three managed to say "sink"; and two, "overflowing." Most patients, though not all, did produce a verb to describe what was happening to the water, but it was usually a more general term than "overflowing," such as "coming down" or "running out."

In spontaneous conversation, speech of patients with SD is replete with overgeneralizations, though of course they often just say little and so do not give researchers an opportunity to observe their word production failures—which is, of course, partly why we resort to tests like object naming or picture description. Virtually all the patients overuse terms like "thing" and "place" in conversation to substitute for the objects and locations that they cannot name. One patient began to call everyone of relevance in her life (e.g., her sisters, her son) "my person." Individual patients, as their semantic deficit worsens, often seem to alight on particular words to serve as general terms, and these are sometimes terms such as "situation" or "portion" that give the patient's speech an odd and almost formal-sounding quality.

Overgeneralization is somewhat harder to observe in comprehension than production, in part because of the major difference in the nature of the mapping from words versus objects (or pictures of them) to concepts. A simple experiment, or even "thought" experiment, of removing one part of a stimulus easily illustrates this concept. If a picture of a duck is presented minus one component such as its head, feet, or tail, an observer is still likely to be able to identify it as a duck, or at least as a bird. By contrast, if we remove one letter from the written name of this object: _uck could be *duck* or *luck*; d_ck could be *duck* or *dock*; du_k could be *duck* or *dusk*; and duc_ could be *duck* or *duct*. There is no "duckiness" about any of these alternative words. Despite the limited ability to infer anything about a word's meaning from its phonological or orthographic shape, at least early in the semantic deterioration of SD, patients will sometimes, as indicated above, comprehend a spoken word in an overgeneral fashion, as in "What's a violin?" → "A musical thing." One can also observe something akin to overgeneralization in the patients' word comprehension by constructing word-to-picture matching tests in which the semantic proximity of the target to the foils is manipulated. Patients with SD achieve reasonable (though certainly below normal) scores in pointing to a picture of a kingfisher in response to its spoken name when the foils are things like a shoe, a piece of cheese, or a desk; their success in selecting the self-same kingfisher is significantly lower if it occurs among pictures of other small birds (Adlam et al. 2006).

What about undergeneralization in word production and comprehension? One of the most striking instances actually comes from a contrast of these two reflections of word knowledge in a fashion that we have not yet had the opportunity to document or quantify in an experimental context but that we have observed during clinic assessments. Patients will sometimes use a specific term in talking about a particular episode involving that concept and then fail to recognize or comprehend the same term when it is presented to them in a different context. One of the patients with SD in our cohort told us that "Those trees in my garden that usually have something to eat on them didn't have anything this year because we had an early frost" (he was referring to apples). Later in the same session, when we asked him what the word "frost" means, he had no idea. Another patient, in describing his life history, said that he had worked as a petroleum engineer; asked later to define "petroleum," he looked puzzled, hesitated for a long time, and then hesitantly replied, "I'm not sure; is it something that uses petrol?" What is happening when a patient's comprehension fails to generalize appropriately to a term that he himself has spontaneously produced? We assume that the word can be produced when it is part of a specific scenario like apple trees in the garden or a career in petroleum engineering; the same word—when offered at a different time and in a different (or indeed without any) context—fails to make contact with that limited, scenario-specific knowledge.

A version of this undergeneralization phenomenon was documented experimentally in a clever study by Snowden et al. (1995). A patient with SD who could both produce and comprehend the term "driving license" was unable to comprehend either the more general unmodified word "license" or the compound term "dog license," even though she knew what a dog was. Over a set of such terms, the patient scored more than 90% correct in defining the personally familiar compound terms but fewer than 30% of the new compound terms, and she made no attempt to infer or guess the meanings of the latter. Making this kind of appropriate inference, even if one has never heard specifically of a dog license, is precisely the achievement of a functioning semantic memory system.

There are many anecdotal examples of undergeneralization in word production. For example, all Japanese people can tell you the name of the prefecture in which they live. One patient with SD studied by our colleague Dr. Manabu Ikeda could not produce the name of her prefecture; but she had learned, by rote memory, a list of the various prefectures in her area. If asked to name her own prefecture, she would reel off the list in order, like an overlearned poem, and stop when she got to the correct name.

Object Use and Knowledge

SD is an amodal disorder. Productive and expressive tasks involving words may be most sensitive at unveiling the deficits, especially early in the disease progression, but SD is never just a language disorder (Adlam et al. 2006). Therefore, patients with SD not only fail to name objects and people but also gradually, increasingly fail to know what the objects are and what to do with them and to know who the people are. How do these deficits exhibit the over- and undergeneralization that is the core topic of this chapter?

One dramatic form of overgeneralization of object knowledge can be observed in the task of delayed-copy drawing. There is relatively little point in trying to acquire information about the object knowledge of patients with SD by asking them to draw named objects: If a patient is asked, "Please draw a rhinoceros," his or her most likely response will be "What's a rhinoceros?" But patients with SD have no impairment to the visuospatial skills required to produce a drawing of a rhinoceros, as indicated by the task of giving them such a picture and asking them to copy it. The rhino stimulus picture and one direct copy of it of a patient with SD are shown in the left and middle positions in the first row of FIGURE 3, respectively. So far, so fairly normal. On another occasion, however, we showed this patient the same rhino picture and allowed him to look at it for several seconds to extract all the information he wanted from the stimulus; we neither asked him to name it nor offered him its name, thus making this exposure purely nonverbal. We then removed the picture and asked the patient to count from 1 to 15, which patients with SD do without difficulty and about as rapidly as an unimpaired person, taking about 10 seconds. We then said (again without giving the picture a name), "Please draw what you were looking at a minute ago." The result is illustrated at the right-hand side of the top row of FIGURE 3. The rhino now has no horns, no armored skin—indeed, no rhino-specific features. It has become a generalized animal, more like a pig or a dog than a rhinoceros. Another example, this time for a peacock, is in the bottom row of FIGURE 3; in the patient's delayed-copy drawing, the peacock has the four legs typical of most land animals rather than the two legs standard for birds. Many more examples of such overgeneralization in delayed-copy drawing can be found in Bozeat et al. (2003), Caine et al. (in press), Lambon Ralph and Howard (2000), and Patterson and Erzinclioglu (in press).

What is happening here? Human visual memory is not very precise or literal, at least not for more than about a second. When a normal person is asked to produce a delayed-copy drawing of a rhinoceros, the response will contain horns partly because the person remembers seeing them in the stimulus but at least as much because, having identified the picture as a rhino, the person's semantic memory will insist that the response include horns. The patient with SD cannot recognize the stimulus picture as a rhinoceros; he knows only that it is some sort of animal. After a 10-second gap, short-term visual memory—which as far as we know is reasonably normal in SD—has lost substantial detail. The patient's drawing response, just like the normal individual's drawing response, will then

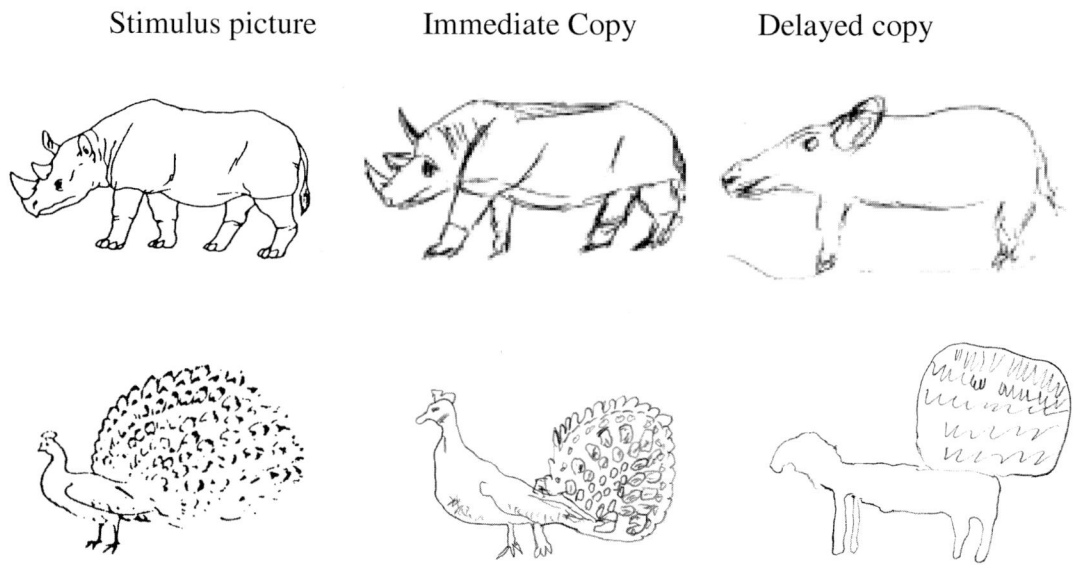

FIGURE 3. Examples of nonverbal overgeneralization: delayed-copy drawing.

be informed by conceptual knowledge of the stimulus. But for the patient, the response is degraded and overgeneralized conceptual knowledge—hence, no horns. The omission of appropriate features and the insertion of inappropriate features are anything but random in these delayed-copy drawings. Atypical features like rhinoceros horns and camel humps get omitted from the concepts where they belong and are never added to ones where they do not. Typical features like tails are rarely omitted from truly tailed animals, are often inserted onto tailless animals (like frogs and seals), and never get added to trees or chairs. As a result, the drawing response is almost invariably more typical of the stimulus class than the real stimulus was.

With respect to the overgeneralization of patients with SD of object/person recognition or object use in the real world, we have mainly anecdotal evidence to offer. For example, during a meal with one of the authors of this chapter, a patient with SD stirred sugar into his glass of wine (presumably generalizing to other drinks like tea or coffee, not to mention feeding the "sweet tooth" that many patients with FTD develop). He also used two spoons, one in each hand, to eat a plate of spaghetti, instead of the fork and knife or fork and large spoon that people who are not semantically impaired would use. With regard to overgeneralized person recognition, we have seen a woman with advanced SD emerge from the clinic room out into the public area where her husband was waiting for her, walk up to a man standing in the waiting room, and say, "I can go now"; but the recipient of this message was a stranger, not her husband. We also have anecdotal evidence of overgeneralization in everyday behavior: The wives of three different male case patients with SD in our patient cohort over the years have reported to us that their husbands continued to shave their faces much as they had done all their adult lives but also began, as the disease progressed, to shave hair on other parts of their bodies.

Undergeneralization in object use is one of the most striking aspects of the SD syndrome and brings us to the topic of how—in the context of degraded conceptual knowledge—everyday behavior comes increasingly to be dominated by current episodic and procedural experience. First documented experimentally by Snowden, Griffiths, and Neary (1994) and subsequently by Bozeat et al. (2002), patients with SD continue until late in the disease to use their own familiar objects at home but often fail to generalize such recognition and use appropriately to other exemplars of the same objects. In one example in the Bozeat et al. study, the patient J.H. could find (in its usual drawer in her kitchen) and correctly use her own cheese grater. When the experimenter offered her another grater that would, to a normal person, be equivalent, J.H. did not know what to do with it. It was furthermore clear that such "knowledge" was being maintained by regular experience. In a subsequent study (Bozeat et al. 2004), J.H.'s husband helped us to select a set of objects that his wife had recently stopped using, including the cheese grater. The experimenter successfully retrained her to use these, but after the training sessions ended, tests designed to probe the persistence of this regained ability demonstrated a gradual but steady decline in J.H.'s success.

We placed "knowledge" in quotation marks in the previous paragraph because there has been some debate about what exactly is maintained by regular experience (Graham et al. 1999a, 1999b; Snowden et al. 1999). Although the issue is not yet resolved, and the answer is probably not "either–or," we are inclined to think that it is more in the line of episodic, autobiographical, and/or procedural memory that is being reinforced and maintained by regular experience than it is true semantic knowledge. This may seem like slightly circular reasoning, but our conclusion is based on the fact that generalization is such a hallmark of semantic memory that, if using one's own familiar cheese grater were boosting semantic knowledge of what cheese graters are for and how they are used, this boost *should* generalize to a different but equally good exemplar of a cheese grater, which it tends not to do.

A similar form of undergeneralization has also been experimentally demonstrated in studies of episodic recognition memory in SD. In two studies, one of recognition memory for objects (Graham et al. 2000) and the other for famous people (Simons et al. 2001), the stimulus items were selected for each patient with SD to be either still relatively "known" or now significantly "degraded" for that patient on the basis of other tests of naming and name–picture matching. Sets of photographs of items from these known and degraded categories were presented to the patients with SD in a study phase. In the subsequent test phase of each experiment, all the studied photos plus an equal number of previously unencountered photos of objects or people were presented for yes–no recognition memory judgments ("Did you see this thing/person before in this experiment?"). In a further experimental manipulation, the photo at test was either identical to the one at study or was a different exemplar of the same concept or person. For famous people, participants might see one photo of Princess Diana at study and a different one at test; for objects, they might see a square stainless-steel toaster at study and a rectangular white plastic-bodied toaster at test. The instructions, of course, included, with many examples, the information that the participant should make "yes" responses in the test when shown different exemplars of the same person or object presented during the study phase. For normal control participants there was no significant advantage for correct "Yes, I saw this before" judgments in the same—as opposed to different—photo conditions; the same was true for the patients with SD, provided that the items came from the "known" set. There was, however, a substantial and significant drop in the number of recognition memory hits for the patients' degraded items in the different-photo condition of both experiments. In other words, generalization between different photos of Princess Diana or different toasters is supported by semantic knowledge and disabled when that knowledge deteriorates.

At least anecdotally, there is evidence that the boundaries of generalization can be shockingly reduced by degraded knowledge. One of the authors of this article when doing some extensive testing with a particular patient with SD, went to test the patient at the patient's home at 2 PM every Tuesday for several weeks. After about five of these visits, during which she always welcomed the author on his arrival at 2 PM, on one Tuesday he was unavoidably detained in arriving at her house. He stopped on the way to telephone her to explain his delay, but it was clear that she did not really understand who he was or what he was telling her. When he arrived at about 3:15, she completely failed to recognize him and, until he pulled out the standard sorts of testing materials, she was reluctant to believe that she knew him and that he was supposed to be there. With a grain of humor (but many more grains of sadness about the fate of such patients), we describe this as the "Mr. Two O'Clock" episode. This patient, like many SD cases, was an avid clockwatcher and associated the researcher's arrival with a specific time; when he arrived at a different time, he was not the same person.

Report of another dramatic occurrence of undergeneralization comes from a neurologist colleague of ours in Barcelona, Dr. Raquel Sanchez-Valle. Several patients with SD develop a passion for puzzles of one kind or another; in our experience in Britain, it is most often jigsaw puzzles, perhaps because these seem to require only elements of cognition that are well preserved in SD until late in the disease, such as good visuospatial function and good color matching. For the particular patient with SD being studied by Sanchez-Valle, however, the puzzle passion was for Sudoku. Each morning, this man would arise, put on some clothes, go out to the local news agent, buy his regular daily newspaper, return home, and complete the Sudoku puzzle; until it was finished, nothing else (such as eating breakfast) held any interest for him. Sanchez-Valle knew of the patient's fascination with Sudoku and wanted to observe him engaging in this activity, so on one of his clinic visits, she gave him a newspaper containing a Sudoku puzzle. He said (in his native Catalan), "I don't know what this is or what I should do with it." The Sudoku instructions were printed beside the puzzle, so

Sanchez-Valle asked him to read them aloud, which he did perfectly but could not understand them and so still claimed to have no idea what to do with the puzzle. Because she had not seen him in several months, and because eventually even such nonsemantic activities and abilities do decline, she assumed that the patient was no longer doing Sudoku. Half an hour later, chatting with the patient's wife, Sanchez-Valle commented that he had apparently given up Sudoku. "What do you mean?" asked the wife in surprise. "He does them every day. In fact, I have this morning's newspaper here in which he completed the Sudoku puzzle." Sudoku exemplars in different newspapers do look slightly different; they may have different sizes or typeface fonts or background color or position on the page. It nevertheless seems almost inconceivable that someone who does Sudoku every day could fail to recognize a new "token" as belonging to that "type." We can assume only that, for this patient who was semantically impaired, Sudoku is not a token of a general type but is rather an event that belongs specifically to his morning routine of fetching the newspaper and doing the puzzle before breakfast. When a similar puzzle is produced by someone else, out of its normal context, he cannot generalize it to his everyday Sudoku experience.

As acknowledged when we first raised the question about the nature of the knowledge or memory that is maintained by everyday experience, this issue is unresolved. It seems clear from the examples given above that the concepts of frost, cheese grater, and Sudoku have severely reduced boundaries for these patients. This could be the result of a diminished semantic representation combined with specific reinforcement from a particular, repeated aspect of the meaning. In other words, just as concepts in a normal individual change and develop over time as a result of continued experience, J.H.'s concept of a grater may be not only diminished in breadth because of her disease but also strengthened in its narrow instantiation because of her regular experience (see Welbourne & Lambon Ralph 2005, in press, for discussion of the interaction of damage with continued learning/plasticity). Alternatively, as suggested earlier, such severely reduced boundaries could reflect the fact that when a semantic concept is sufficiently degraded, the person is forced to rely on one or more different kinds of memory or knowledge that, by their nature, do not support an appropriate level of generalization. Perhaps both explanations are partially correct. It may also be that different kinds of experience lend themselves to different degrees of reliance on these two kinds of knowledge. In the delayed-copy task, for example, we argued that literal visual memory provides a poor basis for performing the task and that therefore both normal individuals and patients with SD must refer to the way in which their semantic memory processed the stimulus. The patient with SD can code the rhinoceros only as an overgeneralized animal, and his or her response will reflect that semantic coding. Regular use of a specific cheese grater, on the other hand, may be capable of producing fairly durable episodic and procedural memories that can stand in for the general concept.

A similar kind of analysis of type of task or experience might apply to the perhaps obvious question: What determines whether the abnormal boundaries for concepts in SD are too wide, hence resulting in overgeneralization, or too narrow, thus yielding undergeneralization? We have already mentioned one general principle that will contribute to this balance: Within the domain of objects or concrete concepts, a real object or picture of it gives more clues to the approximate nature of the object than its name does. Thus, presentation of an object or picture to be named or defined is more likely to result in an overgeneralization response from a patient with SD than presentation of its name, which is likely to produce "I don't know" (Lambon Ralph et al. 1999). In the domain of person recognition, we gave examples above of both over- and undergeneralization in SD behavior. Again, the task or situation may in large part determine which will occur. If a patient genuinely no longer recognizes Princess Diana, then, when presented with a picture of her to name or identify, there is really no level at which overgeneralization can occur: She is just an unknown person. But when the patient with severe SD went out into the waiting room at the hospital to find her husband, she was confronted with several men to whom her profoundly impaired person recognition could overgeneralize. We realize that this is a somewhat post-hoc analysis and that we need to make more precise predictions in advance about the circumstances under which one would expect to obtain these striking phenomena of over- and undergeneralization resulting from degraded semantic memory. We are only just beginning....

Importance of the ATLs in Semantic Memory: What Is the Evidence from Other Sources?

Although the data from SD clearly implicate the bilateral ATL in semantic representation, these areas are often overlooked or even disputed in other research on semantic memory (Hickok & Poeppel 2007; Martin 2007; Wise 2003). It is claimed that semantic tasks rarely activate the ATL in functional MRI (fMRI) but rather, in line with some aphasiological models (see below), implicate left posterior temporal, temporoparietal, and prefrontal regions (Devlin et al. 2000; Garavan et al. 2000; Martin 2007). It is also claimed that, were the ATL to be so vital to semantic memory, resection of the ATL for intractable epilepsy should result in major semantic impairment, which it does not (Hermann et al. 1999).

Recent studies indicate, however, that the results underlying these claims are not as contradictory as they might seem to the results from SD. First, the failure to find ATL activation in semantic tasks reflects, at least in part, technical limitations of fMRI. Field inhomogeneities around air-filled cavities lead to signal dropout and distortions that are particularly pronounced in the orbitofrontal cortex and the inferior and polar aspects of the temporal lobes (Devlin et al. 2000; Wise 2003). Functional neuroimaging that uses positron emission tomography (which does not suffer from the same problems) does detect semantically related activation in the ATL, even when the same experiment conducted in fMRI does not (Devlin et al. 2000). Because of the preeminence of fMRI in cognitive neuroscience, the potentially central importance of the ATL within a network of regions that support semantic cognition can be overlooked (Patterson et al. 2007; Rogers & McClelland 2004; Wise 2003).

Second, interpretation of the cognitive consequences of epilepsy surgery is complicated by two factors: (a) Longstanding epilepsy can lead to changes in neural organization and, indeed, recent imaging studies have shown that white matter connectivity and neurotransmitter function are significantly altered in this condition (Hammers et al. 2003; Powell et al. 2007); and (b) epilepsy surgery is unilateral, whereas patients with SD invariably have bilateral, even if asymmetrical, lesions. In the rare cases where we have been able to assess patients with SD at a sufficiently early stage that there is only minor atrophy on the less affected side, the patients have tended to show rather slight semantic deficits unless taxed with especially difficult tasks. We therefore infer that substantial semantic deficit results only from significant bilateral ATL abnormality. This supposition would account for the fact that semantic deficits observed after temporal lobe resection are mild (Wilkins & Moscovitch 1978), or indeed absent, if the tests are too easy.

Other neurological disorders, such as herpes simplex virus encephalitis, do produce semantic impairment when damage affects the same bilateral temporal lobe regions as SD (Lambon Ralph et al. 2007; Noppeney et al. 2007). Also, we have recently demonstrated that repetitive transcranial magnetic stimulation of the ATL in normal participants produces a selective slowing of semantically related tasks (synonym judgment and naming) but not of equally demanding, nonsemantic tasks—exactly as expected from SD (Pobric et al. in press).

Beyond Semantic Memory and the ATL

The focus of this article has been the role of the ATLs in achieving conceptualization and appropriate levels of semantic generalization. We have, therefore, said nothing thus far about the role of other brain regions or different aspects of semantic cognition. There is no doubt that parts of the brain other than the ATL play critical roles in other aspects of semantically driven behavior, as evidenced by activation of these other regions in functional neuroimaging studies of semantic processing in normal participants and by some varieties of semantic disorders when these other regions are damaged. These other aspects can be divided into two broad types: impairments of semantic access and disorders of semantic control.

Most models of semantic memory assume that semantic activation is initiated by input from one or more modality-specific forms of knowledge/engrams. Sensory input must be processed well enough to enable semantic processing. Failures of comprehension or semantically driven behavior can follow, therefore, from impaired mechanisms of perceptual analysis or from damaged connections between perception and central semantic representations. Classically, these two forms of impairment are labelled "apperceptive" and "associative" agnosia (Brown 1972). The crucial characteristic of these disorders is that comprehension/semantic behavior is impaired only when input arrives in the affected modality (e.g., visual or auditory or tactile or linguistic); comprehension initiated by a stimulus in any other modality should be fairly normal. These modality-specific agnosias, or impairments of semantic access, are unlike the amodal impairment of patients with SD.

What about the other type of problem, a disorder of semantic "control"? There is recent evidence to suggest that patients with damage to non-ATL regions can exhibit multimodal semantic impairment. Some patients classified as aphasic after a left-hemisphere stroke, whose deficits might be expected to affect only language comprehension, in fact perform poorly on purely nonverbal receptive tests, such as matching of different pictures on a semantic basis, and/or on purely nonverbal production tests such as object use (especially in a complex sequence of behavior such

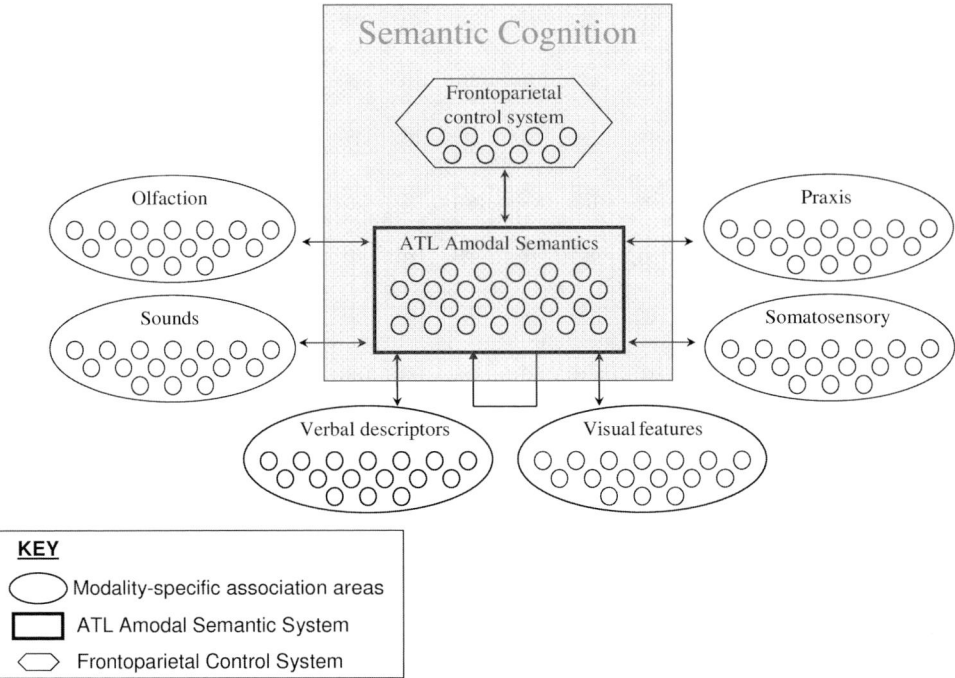

FIGURE 4. Extended theoretical framework for semantic cognition.

as making a cup of tea). These patients, described as having semantic aphasia (SA; Jefferies & Lambon Ralph 2006), have lesions of either the left inferior frontal gyrus and/or the left temporoparietal junction (Berthier 1999). Although their multimodal semantic impairment might prompt one to think that SA is the stroke/aphasic equivalent of SD, direct formal comparisons between the patient groups indicate that the two disorders are qualitatively different (Jefferies & Lambon Ralph 2006). SA seems to arise not from degraded knowledge itself but rather from an impairment of semantic control—that is, difficulty in manipulating and shaping semantic knowledge in a fashion appropriate for the specific task in hand or for the specific moment within a task. SD is a disorder of core conceptual knowledge. Because all semantic tasks (though to different degrees) require executive control as well as conceptual knowledge, both patient groups reveal deficits across both verbal and nonverbal domains. The lesion locations of the patients with SA (inferior frontal gyrus and/or temporoparietal junction) align with results from functional neuroimaging of normal subjects undertaking not only semantic tasks but also other cognitive assessments that require executive processing (Badre et al. 2005; Gold et al. 2006).

These comparative studies generate a more extensive framework (summarized in FIG. 4) about the processes and their associated brain regions that support semantically driven behavior, which we refer to as "semantic cognition" (Rogers & McClelland 2004). We have adopted this broader term to encompass the two major, interactive dimensions that are required for flexible semantic behavior. Semantic control allows task-relevant aspects of meaning to be brought to the fore, whereas other, currently irrelevant pieces of information are inhibited, thus enabling semantic flexibility and novel semantic problem solving. As described more fully in this article semantic memory or conceptual knowledge provides the basis on which semantic information can be retrieved, and generalized at an appropriate level, irrespective of modality or task.

Conflicts of Interest

The authors declare no conflicts of interest.

References

Adlam, A.-L. R., Patterson, K., Rogers, T. T., Nestor, P., Salmond, C. H., Acosta-Cabronero, J., et al. (2006). Semantic dementia and fluent primary progressive aphasia: two sides of the same coin? *Brain, 129*, 3066–3080.

Badre, D., Poldrack, R., Paré-Blagoev, E., Insler, R., & Wagner, A. (2005). Dissociable controlled retrieval and generalized selection mechanisms in ventrolateral prefrontal cortex. *Neuron, 47*, 907–918.

Berthier, M. (1999). *Transcortical Aphasias*. Hove, East Sussex: Psychology Press.

Bozeat, S., Lambon Ralph, M. A., Graham, K. S., Patterson, K., Wilkin, H., Rowland, J., et al. (2003). A duck with four legs: investigating the structure of conceptual knowledge using picture drawing in semantic dementia. *Cognitive Neuropsychology, 20*, 27–47.

Bozeat, S., Lambon Ralph, M. A., Patterson, K., & Hodges, J. R. (2002). The influence of personal familiarity and context on object use in semantic dementia. *Neurocase, 8*, 127–134.

Bozeat, S., Patterson, K., & Hodges, J. R. (2004). Relearning object use in semantic dementia. *Neuropsychological Rehabilitation, 14*, 351–363.

Brambati, S. M., Rankin, K. P., Narvid, J., et al. (in press). 2007. Atrophy progression in semantic dementia with asymmetric temporal involvement: a tensor-based morphometry study. *Neurobiol. Aging.* [Epub ahead of print: doi:10.1016/j.neurobiolaging.2007.05.014]

Brown, J. W. (1972). *Aphasia, Apraxia and Agnosia*. Springfield, IL: Charles C Thomas.

Caine, D., Breen, N., & Patterson, K. (2007). Emergence and progression of "non-semantic" deficits in semantic dementia. *Cortex*, in press.

Collins, A. M., & Quillian, M. R. (1969). Retrieval time from semantic memory. *Journal of Verbal Learning and Verbal Behavior, 8*, 240–247.

Damasio, A. R. (1989). The brain binds entities and events by multiregional activation from convergence zones. *Neural Computation, 1*, 123–132.

Desgranges, B. et al. (2007) Anatomical and functional alterations in semantic dementia: a voxel-based MRI and PET study. *Neurobiology of Aging, 28*, 1904–1913.

Devlin, J. T., Russell, R. P., Davis, M. H., Price, C. J., Wilson, J., Moss, H. E., et al. (2000). Susceptibility-induced loss of signal: comparing PET and fMRI on a semantic task. *Neuroimage, 11*, 589–600.

Diehl, B. et al. (2004). Cerebral metabolic patterns at early stages of frontotemporal dementia and semantic dementia. A PET study. *Neurobiology of Aging, 25*, 1051–1056.

Eggert, G. H. (1977). *Wernicke's Works on Aphasia: A Sourcebook and Review* (Vol.1). The Hague: Mouton.

Garavan, H., Ross, T. J., Li, S. J., & Stein, E. A. (2000). A parametric manipulation of central executive functioning. *Cerebral Cortex, 10*, 585–592.

Garrard, P., Lambon Ralph, M. A., Hodges, J. R., & Patterson, K. (2001). Prototypicality, distinctiveness, and intercorrelation: analyses of the semantic attributes of living and nonliving concepts. *Cognitive Neuropsychology, 18*, 125–174.

Gloor, P. (1997). *The Temporal Lobe and the Limbic System*. Oxford, UK: Oxford University Press.

Gold, B. T. et al. (2006). Dissociation of automatic and strategic lexical-semantics: functional magnetic resonance imaging evidence for differing roles of multiple frontotemporal regions. *Journal of Neuroscience, 26*, 6523–6532.

Goodglass, H., & Kaplan, E. (1983). *The Assessment of Aphasia and Related Disorders*. 2nd ed. Philadelphia: Lea & Febiger.

Graham, K. S., Lambon Ralph, M. A., & Hodges, J. R. (1999a). Determining the impact of autobiographical experience on "meaning": new insights from investigating sports-related vocabulary and knowledge in two cases of semantic dementia. *Cognitive Neuropsychology, 14*, 801–837.

Graham, K. S., Lambon Ralph, M. A., & Hodges, J. R. (1999b). A questionable semantics: the interaction between semantic knowledge and autobiographical experience in semantic dementia. *Cognitive Neuropsychology, 16*, 689–698.

Graham, K. S., Patterson, K., & Hodges, J. R. (1995). Progressive pure anomia: insufficient activation of phonology by meaning. *Neurocase, 1*, 25–38.

Graham, K. S., Simons, J. S., Pratt, K. H., Patterson, K., & Hodges, J. R. (2000). Insights from semantic dementia on the relationship between episodic and semantic memory. *Neuropsychologia, 38*, 313–324.

Hammers, A., Koepp, M. J., Richardson, M. P., Hurlemann, R., Brooks, D. J., & Duncan, J. S. (2003). Grey and white matter flumazenil binding in neocortical epilepsy with normal MRI. A PET study of 44 patients. *Brain, 126*, 1300–1318.

Hermann, B., Davies, K., Foley, K., & Bell, B. (1999). Visual confrontation naming outcome after standard left anterior temporal lobectomy with sparing versus resection of the superior temporal gyrus: a randomized prospective clinical trial. *Epilepsia, 40*, 1070–1076.

Hickok, G., & Poeppel, D. (2007). Opinion—the cortical organization of speech processing. *Nature Reviews Neuroscience, 8*, 393–402.

Hodges, J. R., Graham, N., & Patterson, K. (1995). Charting the progression in semantic dementia: implications for the organisation of semantic memory. *Memory, 3*, 463–495.

Hodges, J. R., & Patterson, K. (2007). The neuropsychology of frontotemporal dementia. In J. R. Hodges (Ed.), *Frontotemporal Dementia Syndromes* (pp. 102–133). Cambridge, UK: Cambridge University Press.

Hodges, J. R., Patterson, K., Oxbury, S., & Funnell, E. (1992). Semantic dementia: progressive fluent aphasia with temporal lobe atrophy. *Brain, 115*, 1783–1806.

Jefferies, E., & Lambon Ralph, M. A. (2006). Semantic impairment in stroke aphasia vs. semantic dementia: a case-series comparison. *Brain, 129*, 2132–2147.

Kipps, C. M., Knibb, J. A., Patterson, K., & Hodges, J. H. (2008). Neuropsychology of frontotemporal dementia. In G. Goldenberg & B. Miller (Eds.), *Handbook of Clinical Neurology*. Amsterdam: Elsevier.

Lambon Ralph, M. A., Graham, K. S., Patterson, K., & Hodges, J. R. (1999). Is a picture worth a thousand words? Evidence from concept definitions by patients with semantic dementia. *Brain & Language, 70*, 309–335.

Lambon Ralph, M. A., & Howard, D. (2000). Gogi aphasia or semantic dementia? Assessing poor verbal comprehension in a case of fluent progressive aphasia. *Cognitive Neuropsychology, 17*, 437–466.

Lambon Ralph, M. A., Lowe, C., & Rogers, T. T. (2007). Both type and distribution of damage are critical for category-specific semantic deficits: evidence from semantic dementia, herpes simplex virus encephalitis and a neural network model of conceptual knowledge. *Brain, 130*, 1127–1137.

Martin, A. (2007). The representation of object concepts in the brain. *Annual Review of Psychology, 58*, 25–45.

Morrow, L. I., & Duffy, F. M. (2005). The representation of ontological category concepts as affected by healthy aging: normative data and theoretical implications. *Behavior Research Methods, 37*, 608–625.

Nestor, P. J., Fryer, T. D., & Hodges, J. R. (2006). Declarative memory impairments in Alzheimer's disease and semantic dementia. *NeuroImage, 30*, 1010–1020.

Noppeney, U., Patterson, K., Tyler, L. K., Moss, H., Stamatakis, E. A., Bright, P., et al. (2007). Temporal lobe lesions and semantic impairment: a comparison of herpes simplex virus encephalitis and semantic dementia. *Brain, 130*, 1138–1147.

Patterson, K. (2007). The reign of typicality in semantic memory. *Philosophical Transactions of the Royal Society B, 362*, 813–821.

Patterson, K., & Erzinçlioğlu, S. (in press). Drawing as a "window" on deteriorating conceptual knowledge in neurodegenerative disease. In C. Lange-Kuettner & A. Vinter (Eds.), *Drawing and the Non-Verbal Mind. A Life-Span Perspective*. Cambridge, UK: Cambridge University Press.

Patterson, K., Graham, N. L., Lambon Ralph, M. A., & Hodges, J. R. (2008). Varieties of silence: the impact of neurodegenerative diseases on language systems in the brain. In J. R. Pomerantz (Ed.), *Topics in Integrative Neuroscience: From Cells to Cognition* (pp. 181–205). Cambridge, UK: Cambridge University Press.

Patterson, K., & Hodges, J. R. (2000). Semantic dementia: one window on the structure and organization of semantic memory. In L. Cermak (Ed.), *Handbook of Neuropsychology, 2nd Edition, Vol. 2: Memory and Its Disorders* (pp. 313–333). Amsterdam/London: Elsevier.

Patterson, K., & MacDonald, M. C. (2006). Sweet nothings: Narrative speech in semantic dementia. In S. Andrews (Ed.), *From Inkmarks to Ideas: Current Issues in Lexical Processing* (pp. 288–317). Hove, UK: Psychology Press.

Patterson, K., Nestor, P. J., & Rogers, T. T. (2007). Where do you know what you know? the representation of semantic knowledge in the human brain. *Nature Reviews Neuroscience, 8*, 976–987.

Pobric, G., Jefferies, E., & Lambon Ralph, M. A. (2007). Anterior temporal lobes mediate semantic representation: mimicking semantic dementia by using rTMS in normal participants. *Proceedings of the National Academy of Sciences USA, 104*, 20137–20141.

Powell, H. W. R., Parker, G. J. M., Alexander, D. C., Symms, M. R., Boulby, P. A., Wheeler-Kingshott, C. A. M., et al. (2007). Abnormalities of language networks in temporal lobe epilepsy. *Neuroimage, 36*, 209–221.

Quillian, M. R. (1966). *Semantic Memory*. Ph.D. thesis, Carnegie Institute of Technology.

Rogers, T. T., Lambon Ralph, M. A., Garrard, P., Bozeat, S., McClelland, J. L., Hodges, J.R., et al. (2004). The structure and deterioration of semantic memory: a neuropsychological and computational investigation. *Psychological Review, 111*, 205–235.

Rogers, T. T., & McClelland, J. L. (2004). *Semantic Cognition: A Parallel Distributed Processing Approach*. Cambridge, MA: MIT Press.

Shallice, T. (1988). *From Neuropsychology to Mental Structure*. Cambridge, UK: Cambridge University Press.

Simons, J. S., Graham, K. S., Galton, C. J., Patterson, K., & Hodges, J. R. (2001). Semantic knowledge and episodic memory for faces in semantic dementia. *Neuropsychology, 15*, 101–114.

Snowden, J. S., Goulding, P. J., & Neary, D. (1989). Semantic dementia: a form of circumscribed cerebral atrophy. *Behavioural Neurology, 2*, 111–138.

Snowden, J. S., Griffiths, H. L., & Neary, D. (1994a). Semantic dementia: autobiographical contribution to preservation of meaning. *Cognitive Neuropsychology, 11*, 265–288.

Snowden, J. S., Griffiths, H. L., & Neary, D. (1995). Autobiographical experience and word meaning. *Memory, 3*, 225–246.

Snowden, J. S., Griffiths, H. L., & Neary, D. (1999). The impact of autobiographical experience on meaning: reply to Graham, Lambon Ralph and Hodges. *Cognitive Neuropsychology, 16*, 673–687.

Snowden, J. S., Neary, D., & Mann, D. M. A. (1996). *Fronto-Temporal Lobar Degeneration*. New York: Churchill Livingstone.

Thompson-Schill, S. L. (2003). Neuroimaging studies of semantic memory: inferring "how" from "where." *Neuropsychologia, 41*(3), 280–292.

Tulving, E. (1972). Episodic and semantic memory. In E. Tulving & W. Donaldson (Eds.), *Organisation of Memory* (pp. 381–403). New York: Academic Press.

Warrington, E. K. (1975). The selective impairment of semantic memory. *Quarterly Journal of Experimental Psychology, 27*, 635–657.

Welbourne, S. R., & Lambon Ralph, M. A. (2005). Exploring the impact of plasticity-related recovery after brain damage in a connectionist model of single word reading. *Cognitive, Affective & Behavioral Neuroscience, 5*, 77–92.

Welbourne, S. R., & Lambon Ralph, M. A. (2007). Using PDP models to simulate phonological dyslexia: the key role of plasticity-related recovery. *Journal of Cognitive Neuroscience, 19*, 1125–1139.

Wilkins, A. J., & Moscovitch, M. (1978). Selective impairment of semantic memory after temporal lobectomy. *Neuropsychologia, 16*, 73–79.

Williams, G. B., Nestor, P. J., & Hodges, J. R. (2005). Neural correlates of semantic and behavioural deficits in frontotemporal dementia. *Neuroimage, 24*, 1042–1051.

Wise, R. (2003). Language systems in normal and aphasic human subjects: functional imaging studies and inferences from animal studies. *British Medical Bulletin, 65*, 95–119.

Woollams, A. M., Cooper-Pye, E., Hodges, J. R., & Patterson, K. (2007 revision). Anomia: a doubly typical signature of semantic dementia. Manuscript under revision.

Spatial Cognition and the Brain

NEIL BURGESS

Institute of Cognitive Neuroscience, University College London, United Kingdom

Recent advances in the understanding of spatial cognition are reviewed, focusing on memory for locations in large-scale space and on those advances inspired by single-unit recording and lesion studies in animals. Spatial memory appears to be supported by multiple parallel representations, including egocentric and allocentric representations, and those updated to accommodate self-motion. The effects of these representations can be dissociated behaviorally, developmentally, and in terms of their neural bases. It is now becoming possible to construct a mechanistic neural-level model of at least some aspects of spatial memory and imagery, with the hippocampus and medial temporal lobe providing allocentric environmental representations, the parietal lobe egocentric representations, and the retrosplenial cortex and parieto-occipital sulcus allowing both types of representation to interact. Insights from this model include a common mechanism for the construction of spatial scenes in the service of both imagery and episodic retrieval and a role for the remainder of Papez's circuit in orienting the viewpoint used. In addition, it appears that hippocampal and striatal systems process different aspects of environmental layout (boundaries and local landmarks, respectively) and do so using different learning rules (incidental learning and associative reinforcement, respectively).

Key words: parietal; hippocampal; striatal; fMRI; place cells; grid cells; allocentric; egocentric; computational modeling

Introduction

The explosion of interest in cognitive neuroscience derives from the ability of recent advances in neuroscience to shed new light on the mechanisms supporting cognition. Within this endeavor, the field of spatial cognition is particularly well placed due to the ease with which similar (spatial) experimental paradigms can be applied to both humans and animals. Thus neuroscientific findings in animals can be integrated with noninvasive (behavioral, neuropsychological, and neuroimaging) findings in humans. Accordingly, recent years have seen the reasonably direct application of insights from single-unit recording in freely moving animals to understanding the mechanisms of human cognition regarding memory for locations within large-scale space.

One theme to emerge, upon which I elaborate in this article, is the growing acceptance within the field of human spatial cognition of a long-held tenet of animal neuroscience (e.g., White & McDonald 2002) that multiple parallel systems are at play, making use of a variety of reference frames. Thus the emphasis of research has shifted from exclusive comparisons, for example, "Is spatial memory egocentric?" (Wang & Spelke 2002; Shelton & McNamara 1997), to addressing how the various systems combine to support behavior under different circumstances (Burgess 2006; Mou et al. 2004).

There has also been considerable recent progress in identifying the specific characteristics of neural representations of spatial location, including the startling recent discovery of an entirely new type of spatial representation "grid cells" (Hafting et al. 2005). These new findings are, in turn, beginning to feedback into cognitive models of spatial behavior. A crucial aid in relating neurophysiological findings to behavior is the use of computational modeling, which I touch upon where appropriate.

In this review I focus on the basic representations and mechanisms supporting spatial memory, navigation, and imagery. This necessarily leads to a focus on posterior parts of the brain: parietal, retrosplenial, and medial temporal neocortex as well as the hippocampal and striatal systems. Prefrontal cortex is only briefly mentioned, in the context of supplying simulated motor efference in the service of planning/imagining potential movements and in strategic mediation between hippocampal and striatal systems in controlling behavior. The review is structured according to different types of representations and processes and the

---

Address for correspondence: Neil Burgess, Institute of Cognitive Neuroscience, University College London, 17 Queen Square, London WC1N 3AR, U.K.
n.burgess@ucl.ac.uk

corresponding neural systems. I start at the more sensory end, with egocentric representations of location and their updating to accommodate self-motion, and move on to more abstract allocentric representations of location and their updating to accommodate self-motion. These issues, their neural bases, and their relationship to memory and imagery are treated within the framework of a model of medial temporal–parietal interactions in spatial cognition (Byrne et al. 2007; Burgess et al. 2001b; Becker & Burgess 2001). The second part of the review concerns the relationships between hippocampal and striatal systems in spatial memory and navigation: which aspects of environmental information they process; which learning rules they use; and how they combine to control behavior. The discussion focuses on the application of insights from spatial paradigms to more general issues such as the idea of a "geometric module" in the brain and the roles played by the hippocampal, parietal, and striatal systems in supporting declarative and procedural memory and imagery.

Multiple Parallel Reference Frames for Location

Egocentric Representations

Locations in the external world can be represented in a variety of ways. Sensory information is generally acquired in the coordinates of the corresponding receptor (e.g., retinotopic for vision and head-centered for audition), while actions must be specified in the appropriate body-centered coordinates for the corresponding effector. Sensorimotor integration, as in reaching for a visual target, requires translation between these various egocentric representations. Evidence for all of these egocentric representations can be found at the level of single neurons in sensory and motor cortices, and mechanisms for translation between them are suggested by "gain field" responses of neurons recorded in posterior parietal area 7a in primates. These neurons respond to visual stimuli at a specific retinotopic location, but their rate of firing is also modulated by the orientation of the monkey's gaze relative to the head (Andersen et al. 1987), by the orientation of the head relative to the trunk, or by the orientation of the monkey within the testing room (Snyder et al. 1998), see FIGURE 1. These gain-field responses are ideal for translating locations between the various egocentric reference frames (Zipser & Andersen 1988; Pouget & Sejnowski 1997; Deneve et al. 2001).

Of particular interest for the following sections, area 7a is the posterior parietal area most strongly connected with the medial temporal lobe, and the neurons there whose firing is modulated by the orientation of the monkey within the room can support translation between egocentric and allocentric representations of locations. These neurons potentially allow translation between allocentric representations of environmental layout in the medial temporal lobe and head-centered representations required for imagining spatial scenes in medial parietal areas, see below and (Byrne et al. 2007; Burgess et al. 2001b). In addition, the anterior bank of the parieto-occipital sulcus, which runs between the medial parietal and retrosplenial cortices, contains visually responsive neurons which respond to stimuli presented at a given location irrespective of the direction of gaze (Galletti et al. 1995).

Behavioral evidence for egocentric representations in human spatial memory includes "alignment effects" in retrieval of an array of objects that was studied from a specific viewpoint. Thus the time taken to correctly recognize the array in photographs from other viewpoints around the array increases with the size of the angular difference of the test viewpoint from the encoding viewpoint (see, e.g., Diwadkar & McNamara 1997). Equally, if people are asked to close their eyes and imagine being at a different location and orientation and then to point to where an object in the array would be (tasks sometimes referred to as judgments of relative direction), they are faster and more accurate when the imagined viewpoint has the same direction as the studied viewpoint (Shelton & McNamara 1997). These findings are consistent with storage of a viewpoint-dependent representation of the array, followed by a cumulative process of mental movement of viewpoint. (Note, however, that some findings can also be interpreted as interference between the imagined perspective and the participant's current perspective, rather than the stored perspective, e.g., May 2004).

Self-Motion and Egocentric Spatial Updating

An interesting puzzle implied by egocentric perceptual representations is that of the perceived stability of the external world despite the rapid and rapidly changing motion of our sensory receptors as we move. The problem of perceptual stability is beyond the scope of this review (see Ross et al. 2001; Bridgeman et al. 1994; Melcher 2007 for more on visual stability). Suffice it to say, following Helmholtz (1866), that a major component of the solution appears to be the automatic updating of sensory representations by information about intended movements, often referred to as "motor efference copy." In a recent parallel to the long history of behavioral studies of visual stability, electrophysiological studies in primate posterior parietal cortex have examined the effects of eye movements

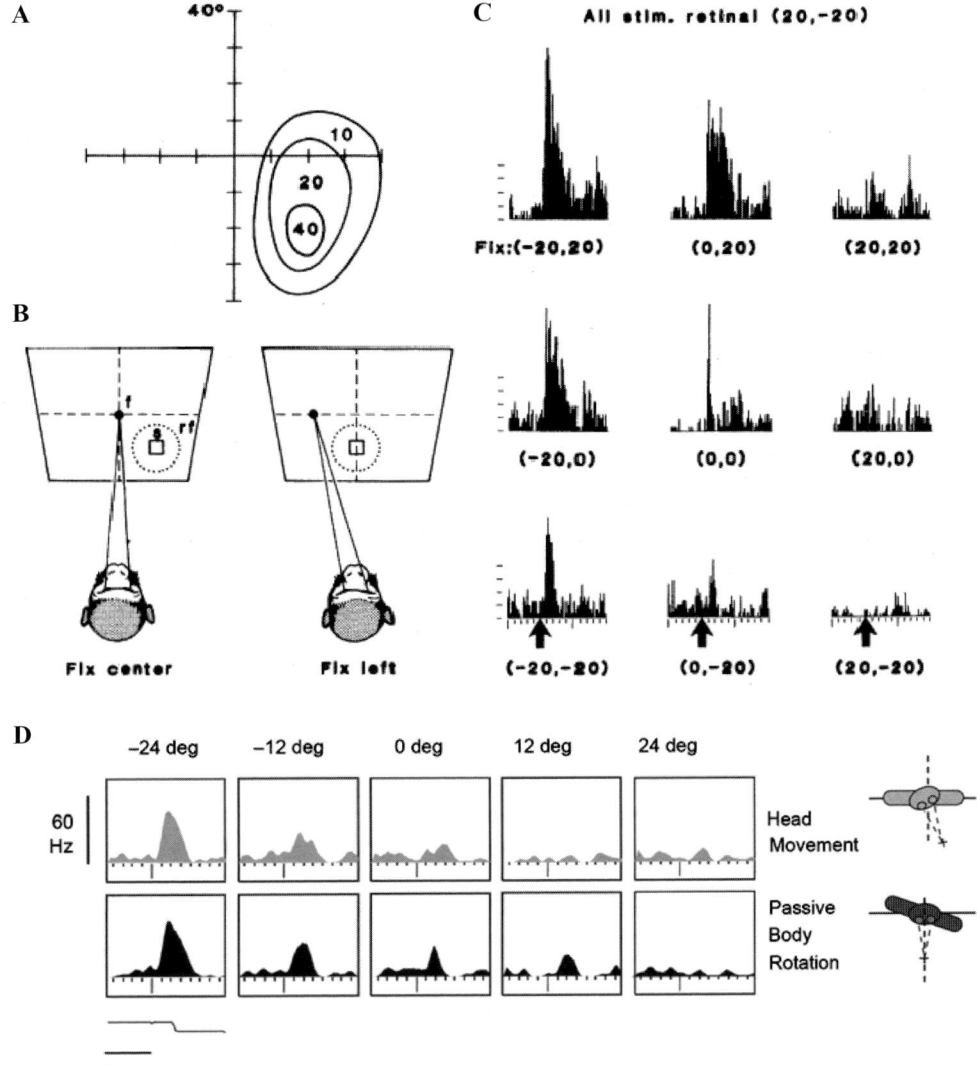

FIGURE 1. Parietal gain fields: encoding of the retinotopic location of a stimulus modulated by the angle of gaze relative to the head (B-C), the angle of the head relative to the trunk (D), or the angle of the trunk in the lab (not shown). **(A)** Example of a neuron in primate parietal area 7a with a retinotopic receptive field for visual stimuli, showing peak firing rate as a function of stimulus location relative to fixation at the center. **(B)** The angle of gaze relative to the head can be varied, modulating the amplitude of the response to a stimulus in the same retinotopic location. **(C)** Arrow indicates stimulus onset; the position of each plot and figures in brackets indicates the angle of fixation. **(D)** Retinotopic responses can also be modulated by the angle of the head relative to the trunk. Some neurons show the same modulation by angle for movement of the head or for passive rotation of the trunk (shown, cf. above and below). Others show modulation by the angle of gaze within the room for the same angles of gaze relative to the head and of the head relative to the trunk. Adapted from Andersen, Essick, & Siegel (1985) and Snyder, Grieve, Brotchie, & Andersen (1998).

on the responses of single neurons. Interestingly, neurons with retinotopic receptive fields, for example, in the lateral intraparietal area, can be seen to update their responses so as to respond to stimuli which will be in the receptive field after a saccadic eye movement, even though the stimulus has actually disappeared before the completion of the movement. These results indicate spatial updating of neuronal representations by motor efference copy (see e.g., Colby & Goldberg 1999 for a review).

Of course, the other potential mechanisms for spatial updating, aside from motor efference copy, should not be ignored. These include the integration of vestibular signals reflecting accelerations of the head, proprioceptive information regarding actual movements performed, and optic flow. All of these types of information can contribute to the processes of spatial updating and have been extensively studied within the more restricted context of "path integration": updating a representation of one's own displacement from the start of a movement trajectory by integrating the velocities experienced along the trajectory. We initially consider the likely egocentric processes supporting spatial updating in parietal areas and later consider likely allocentric processes supporting spatial updating in medial temporal areas. Note that, although spatial updating and path integration are regarded as egocentric processes in some treatments (e.g., Wang & Spelke 2002), categorization of these processes per se is arbitrary, depending on whether the object or start locations are updated relative to the participant or whether the location of the participant is updated relative to the locations of objects, start positions, or other aspects of the environment.

Following work from Rieser (1989) and others, Simons and Wang (Simons & Wang 1998; Wang & Simons 1999) introduced an elegant paradigm for dissociating the contributions to spatial memory of sensory-bound representations such as "visual snapshots" from representations of locations relative to the body which are automatically updated to accommodate self-motion. In this paradigm, people see five objects on a circular table and later have to indicate which one has been moved. In between presentation and test phases, with the table out of view, it is possible to have the person change his or her viewpoint, or for the table to be rotated. In four conditions, either the person's viewpoint or the table is rotated about the center of the table or both are rotated, or neither. The angle of rotation is the same for the viewpoint and for the table so that, if both are rotated, the egocentric locations of the objects relative to the viewer are unchanged. See FIGURE 2 conditions _, P, PT, and T. The consequence of these manipulations is a 2x2 factorial design in which the test array is either consistent or inconsistent with viewpoint-dependent representations of locations (consistent if both viewpoint and table are rotated together or if neither move) and also consistent or inconsistent with representations that are updated by self-motion (consistent if the viewpoint alone changes or if neither move). The results indicate a strong positive effect of consistency with representations updated by self-motion and a weaker effect of consistency with viewpoint-dependent sensory representations.

Another paradigm for investigating the presence of egocentric or allocentric representations in spatial memory concerns the distribution of errors in pointing to object locations, developed by Wang and Spelke (2000). In this paradigm, the participant views an array of objects scattered throughout a room and must then point to them from within a chamber in the center of the room (from which the objects can not longer be seen). Wang and Spelke reasoned that disorientating the participant by blindfolded rotation would have different effects upon egocentric and allocentric representations of the object locations. Namely, updating of individual egocentric representations will induce different amounts of error across the different locations, while updating of an integrated allocentric representation should induce similar amounts of error across the different locations. Consistent with their egocentric-only model (Wang & Spelke 2002), Wang and Spelke (2000) found that blindfolded rotation increased the variance in errors across object locations.

An interesting parallel to the effects of actual self-motion on spatial representations is provided by studies of imagined movement of viewpoint. In experiments on imagery, subjects study an array of objects and are subsequently blindfolded. They can then be asked to indicate the locations of objects following either imagined rotation of the array of objects or following imagined translocation of themselves to a new viewpoint around the array. In these situations performance is superior following imagined movement of the viewer than following an equivalent imagined movement of the array (e.g., Wraga et al. 2000). It is only when the array consists of a single location that performance for imagined array-rotation approaches that for imagined movement of the viewer.

Thus, there is strong evidence that egocentric representations of locations are maintained in the brain and that these are automatically updated by our own movements, intentions to move, or imagined movements. However, it is also possible that, where multiple locations or extended layouts are concerned, it is more efficient to maintain a cognitive representation of the world and to update our own location within it, rather than maintaining multiple egocentric representations each of which is affected differently by self-motion. In addition, having to retain information over prolonged self-motion increases the importance of knowledge of locations relative to environmental landmarks in avoiding the cumulative errors associated with egocentric updating. As we shall see in the next section, recent evidence points to the presence of these allocentric or world-centered representations in parallel to the egocentric representations discussed above.

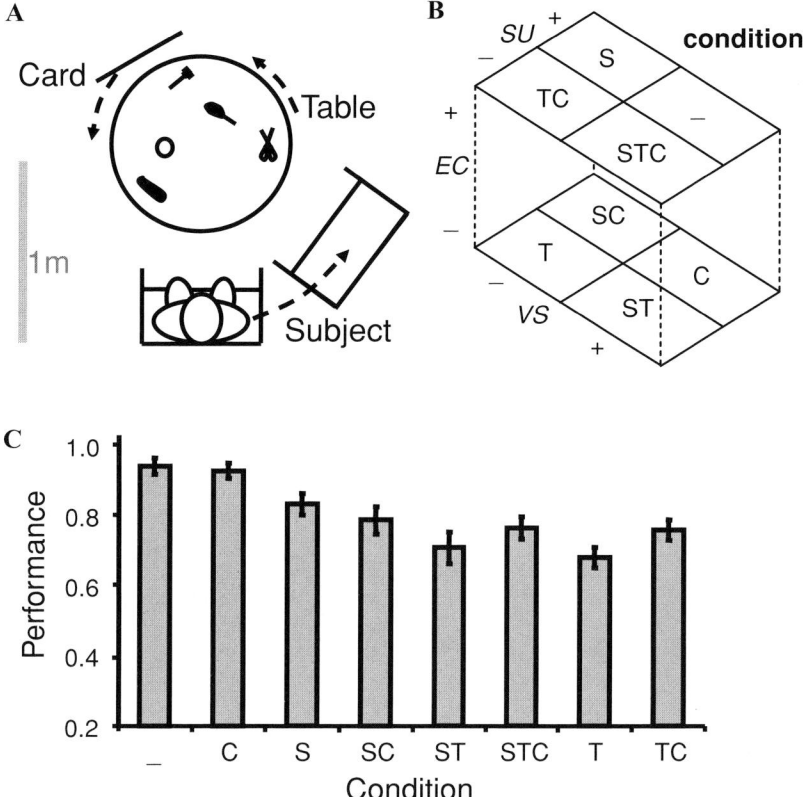

FIGURE 2. Paradigm for dissociating spatial reference frames, based on Simons and Wang (1998). **(A)** After initially seeing the array of objects and before being asked which one has moved, the position of the person (P), the table (T), or the external cue card (C) can be rotated about the center of the table. **(B)** These changes provide a fully factorial manipulation of the consistency (+ or −) of the test array with 3 different potential types of stored representation: visual snapshots (VS), representations spatially updated to accommodate the subject's movement (SU), representations of location relative to the external cue card (EC). **(C)** Performance benefits from consistency with any of these representations: the more the test array is consistent, the better performance is. Adapted from Burgess, Spiers, & Paleologou (2004).

Allocentric Representations

Although egocentric representations provide the obvious format for sensory perception and motor action, and transformations between such egocentric representations suffice for short-term sensorimotor integration, it has long been argued that memory over the longer term is likely better served by allocentric representations centered on environmental landmarks (e.g., Milner et al. 1999; O'Keefe & Nadel 1978). Updating of egocentric representations of location to accommodate self-motion (referred to as "path integration" when the location in question is the start of the path) will fall prey to cumulative error after relatively short paths (e.g., Etienne et al. 1996). Thus, when attempting to return to a previously visited location from a new direction after more than a few minutes of self-motion, representation of the location relative to the available environmental landmarks will often be of more use than egocentric representations. See Burgess (2006) for further discussion.

The idea of parallel representations (egocentric versus allocentric in the above discussion) with differential utility according to the amount of self-motion between presentation and test was recently investigated by Waller and Hodgson (2006). They reinterpreted the results of Wang and Spelke (2000), described above, arguing that increased variance in pointing errors after blindfolded rotation might result from a switch from using an accurate but transient representation to using a less accurate but more integrated enduring representation. In support of their interpretation, they found that, although variation in pointing errors increases

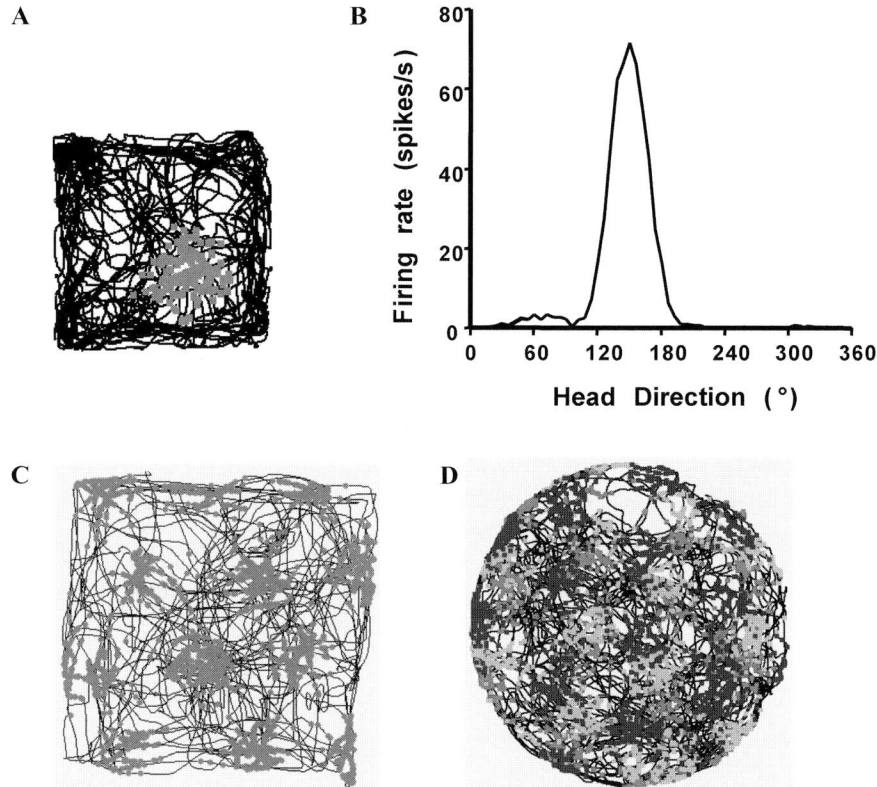

FIGURE 3. Place cells, head-direction cells, and grid cells. **(A)** Example of a place cell: the black line shows the rat's path in exploring a square enclosure, red squares show the locations at which a single neuron fired an action potential. **(B)** Example of a head-direction cell, showing firing rate as a function of head direction within the enclosure. **(C)** Example of a grid cell: firing occurs at an array of locations arranged in a regular triangular grid across the environment (same color scheme as A). **(D)** Example of three neighboring grid cells simultaneously recorded on the same tetrode, action potentials from the three cells shown in red, blue, and green. Adapted from Jeffery & Burgess (2006).

after disorientation (consistent with the use of a less accurate representation), variation in the errors made when judging the relative direction of one object from another actually reduced after disorientation (consistent with the use of a more integrated representation). Waller and Hodgson also found that the effect of "disorientation" on pointing error occurs in an all-or-none fashion after rotations of 135° or more, consistent with a switch from one representation to the other after movements of a certain magnitude. In addition, they found no disorientation-related increase in pointing error variation when pointing to objects within a very familiar environment, consistent with the development of more accurate enduring representations with exposure to an environment, and preferential use of them even over short movements and timescales. Here I interpret Waller and Hodgson's "enduring representation" as likely to be allocentric, see Burgess (2006) for further discussion. Below I briefly outline some of the neurophysiological evidence for allocentric representations in the mammalian brain and then describe some recent experiments indicating the presence of allocentric representations in human spatial cognition.

A neural representation of the animal's location relative to the surrounding environment can be seen in the firing of "place cells" in the hippocampus of rats (O'Keefe 1976) and primates (Ono et al. 1991), see Muller (1996) for a review. This representation is supported by representations of orientation (Taube 1998) and a grid-like representation suitable for path integration (Hafting et al. 2005) in nearby regions, both also environment centered. See FIGURE 3. The orientation of the firing patterns of these cells is primarily determined by distal visual cues, when available, with place cells specifically encoding location relative to extended boundaries in the environment, given this orientation (O'Keefe & Burgess 1996; Hartley et al. 2000). These representations appear to guide behavior in spatial memory paradigms in which simple egocentric representations do not suffice. In these situations, behavioral responses match the firing of the cells (Kubie et al. 2007; Lenck-Santini et al. 2005; O'Keefe & Speakman 1987). In addition, hippocampal lesions or inactivations impair performance in these tasks (e.g., Morris et al. 1982; Packard & McGaugh 1996).

Recent investigations of the neural bases of navigation in humans have made use of desk-top virtual reality (VR): allowing simulation of movement through large-scale space in stationary subjects, albeit without the vestibular and proprioceptive components. Using VR, neural responses resembling those of place cells have been found in the human brain, clustered in the hippocampus (Ekstrom et al. 2003), while functional neuroimaging (Maguire et al. 1998a; Hartley et al. 2003; Iaria et al. 2003) and neuropsychological (Abrahams et al. 1997; Spiers et al. 2001a; Spiers et al. 2001b) data confirm the involvement of the human hippocampus in accurate large-scale navigation. In addition, Hartley and colleagues (2004) used VR to investigate the effect of deformation of the environmental boundary on human search locations, finding results compatible with the assumption that place cells guide behavior, given how place cells respond to such manipulations (O'Keefe & Burgess 1996).

Direct evidence for allocentric representations in human spatial cognition has come from recent paradigms designed to replicate earlier experiments showing evidence of egocentric representations (discussed above), but also designed to probe any allocentric representations which might exist in parallel. Thus, memory for locations within an array has recently been found to show effects of the alignment of the testing perspective with directions defined by aspects of the external environment, as well as with those defined by the person's initial viewpoint (Mou & McNamara 2002; Schmidt & Lee 2006). When an array of objects contains an intrinsic axis (e.g., defined by symmetry), improved performance is found when pointing to objects from imagined viewpoints that are aligned with this axis or aligned with environmental features such as testing room walls (Mou & McNamara 2002; Schmidt & Lee 2006) and external landmarks (McNamara et al. 2003).

The use of allocentric and egocentric representations can also be dissociated within Simons and Wang's (1998) egocentric spatial updating paradigm (see above). In the original paradigm the conditions consistent with representations updated by self-motion, which all involve object locations that remain stationary within the testing room, are also consistent with allocentric representations centered on environmental cues. Thus, some of the effect ascribed to spatial updating may be due to the presence of allocentric representations. To pull apart these multiple influences, Burgess et al. (2004) included independent manipulation of environmental cues: testing effects of consistency with viewpoint-dependent, spatially updated, and allocentric representations within a $2 \times 2 \times 2$ design, see FIGURE 2. In this test, people viewed an array of fluorescent objects with an external fluorescent cue, in darkness, and subsequently indicated which object had moved. Between presentation and test, the person's viewpoint, the array, or the external cue could be rotated to change the consistency of the test array with either type of representation. In addition to replicating the effects of consistency with viewpoint-dependent and spatially updated representations (when the cue did not move), an effect of consistency with the orientation of the external cue was also found. For example, performance increased when the card and table moved together compared to when one or other moved alone. Thus, allocentric representations of object locations relative to environmental cues probably exist in parallel to egocentric representations of location relative to the subject.

The Simons and Wang–inspired paradigm of dissociating frames of reference by shifting the viewpoint and/or the array of objects has recently been successfully applied to developmental psychology. Thus, representations of locations within the testing room appear to be present as early as 3 years and to make a greater contribution to behavior than egocentric snapshots at this age (Nardini et al. 2006). Representations of location relative to the intrinsic frame of reference of the array appear to develop between years three and six. Although the relative dependence of room-related responding on allocentric representations or egocentric spatial updating is not clear, the results demand a rethink of Piagetian ideas of early egocentrism at least (Piaget & Inhelder 1956).

Temporo-Parietal Mechanisms of Spatial Memory, Imagery, and Motion-Related Updating

The nature of the representation of location by place cells has received much study over the several decades since their discovery. As a result, a neural-level model of spatial memory has begun to emerge from these findings, in combination with findings in related areas and in the parietal lobe. As a starting point, we briefly review some of the evidence concerning how environmental cues determine the spatial firing fields

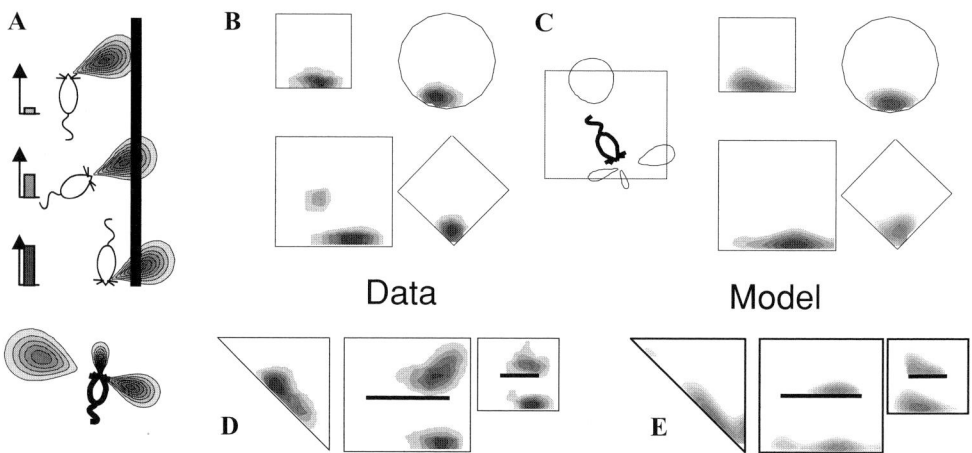

FIGURE 4. The boundary vector cell model of the sensory input to place cells. **(A)** Putative place cell inputs (boundary vector cells, BVCs) are assumed to be tuned to respond to the presence of a boundary at a given distance and allocentric direction (firing rate indicated by the bar on the left), with broader tuning at greater distances (below). **(B)** The firing of a place cell in four different enclosures can be modeled by an appropriate selection of BVC inputs. **(C)** The model can predict the firing of the cell in new configurations of the enclosure, including those with an internal barrier. **(E)** The actual firing of the cell in these environments reasonably matches the prediction. **(D)** Adapted from Burgess & Hartley (2002).

of place cells, and thus contribute to the rat's sense of self-location.

The relative independence of place cell firing from low-level sensory representations can be seen in the independence of place cell firing from the animal's orientation as it explores open environments (Muller & Kubie 1989) and in the robustness of the response to removal of the sensory cues controlling the orientation of the firing fields within the environment (O'Keefe & Conway 1978; O'Keefe & Speakman 1987; Pico et al. 1985; Fenton et al. 2000). In addition to cues to orientation (Taube 1998), place cell firing is strongly driven by any extended boundaries to motion within the environment. O'Keefe and Burgess (1996) recorded from the same cells across similar (rectangular) environments that differed in their dimensions. They observed that the location of peak firing of a given place cell typically remained in a constant position relative to the nearest walls, and in addition, several of the firing fields were stretched along the axes of the environment. They proposed that place cells received inputs that are tuned to respond to the presence of a barrier at a given distance along a given allocentric direction, with sharper tuning at shorter distances; this is the so-called boundary vector cell (BVC) model (Barry et al. 2006; Hartley et al. 2000), see FIGURE 4. The allocentric directions of BVC tuning are presumably defined relative to the head-direction cells, given that place cell and head-direction cells always seem to rotate consistently when external or internal orientation is manipulated.

In contrast to the robust effect of environmental boundaries on place cell firing, discrete landmarks within an environment have very little effect on place cell firing (Cressant et al. 1997). Equally, while removing individual distal cues to orientation does not have a marked effect on place cell firing (although the overall orientation of the representation may drift), removing environmental boundaries tends to lead to destruction of the place cell response (Barry et al. 2006; Barry et al. 2007). The BVC model has been used both to predict the pattern of place cell firing following deformation of the environmental boundaries to make an environment of different shape and size, including the addition of extended walls within the maze (Hartley et al. 2000). It has also been used to predict the search behavior of humans returning to a previously seen location, by assuming that they solve the task by moving to maximize the match between their current place cell representation and a stored place cell representation of the target location (Hartley et al. 2000; Hartley et al. 2004; O'Keefe & Burgess 1996).

The BVC model, in combination with models of the firing properties of neurons in the parietal lobe (Pouget & Sejnowski 1997; Salinas & Abbott 1995) suggest a computational model of memory and imagery for spatial scenes (Byrne et al. 2007; Burgess et al. 2001b; Becker & Burgess 2001). In this model,

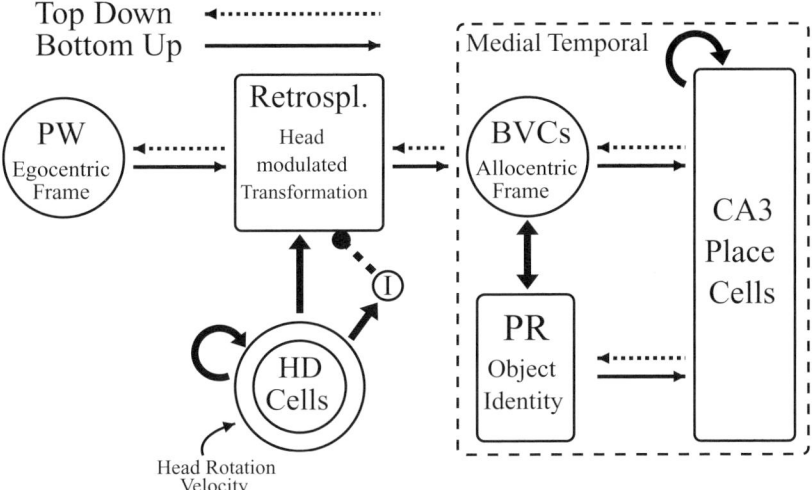

FIGURE 5. Schematic temporo-parietal model of spatial memory and imagery. Each box represents a set of neurons in a different brain region (PW: medial parietal "window" for visual perception and imagery; Retrospl: retroplenial cortex and parieto-occipital sulcus mediating ego-allo translation in conjunction with area 7a; HD cells: head-direction cells; BVCs: parahippocampal boundary vector cells; PR: perirhinal cortical encoding of visual identity). Thin solid arrows represent "bottom-up" connections from egocentric visual perception and imagery to allocentric medial temporal memory representations; thin dashed arrows represent "top-down" connections back again. Adapted from Byrne, Becker, & Burgess (2007).

connections between hippocampal place cells, parahippocampal boundary vector cells, and perirhinal cells encoding visual textures/features form an associative memory. Thus, within a familiar environment, a partial cue can reactivate the hippocampal representation of occupying a single location within an environment, which in turn reactivates the corresponding parahippocampal and perirhinal representations of environmental boundaries and visual features respectively. To be able to examine the products of this reconstructive process in visual imagery, the allocentric (North, South, East, West) parahippocampal representation must be translated into an egocentric (left, right, ahead, behind) medial parietal representation. This is assumed to occur via processing by gain-field neurons in posterior parietal cortex and representation of the intermediate stages of translation in retrosplenial cortex/parieto-occipital sulcus, making use of the representation of head direction found along Papez's circuit to dereference allocentric directions into egocentric ones, see FIGURE 5.

The model is able to simulate effects found in neuropsychological and single-unit recording experiments. For example, the effect of hemi-spatial neglect in imagery following right parietal damage can be simulated, as in the famous Milan Square experiment (Bisiach & Luzzatti 1978), in which patients could not describe the left-hand side of an imagined view of a famous piazza in their home town, whether imagining facing towards the cathedral or away from it. This is consistent with an intact medial temporal allocentric representation of the whole square along with damage to the parietal substrates of the egocentric representation or the allo-ego translation mechanism. In addition, experiments in which place cells are recorded while visual and path-integrative information are put into conflict (Gothard et al. 1996) can also be simulated.

As noted earlier in the review, it is important to bear in mind the multiple ways in which locations can be updated to accommodate self-motion. The model described above uses the translation from allocentric medial temporal representations to egocentric medial parietal representations to perform spatial updating of the egocentric locations, and translation back to the medial temporal representations to make sure the allocentric representation of self-location is also updated appropriately. However, it is also theoretically possible to directly update the allocentric representation of self-location given self-motion information. Again, both processes may exist in parallel, with egocentric updating most useful for keeping track of small numbers of locations over short durations and allocentric updating most useful where one's position must be maintained relative to larger amounts of environmental information and over longer durations.

The likely importance of task demands in determining whether egocentric or allocentric mechanisms for spatial updating are used to control behavior is illustrated by comparison of the studies by King et al. (2002; King et al. 2004) with that by Shrager et al. (2007). In this first group of studies, participants saw objects within a VR arena and were subsequently tested on their memory for the objects' locations from the same viewpoint as at presentation or from a shifted viewpoint. In the studies by King et al., the new viewpoint was imposed abruptly and, when different numbers of objects were used, the trials with different list lengths were intermingled. In these studies a developmental amnesic with focal hippocampal pathology was found to be specifically impaired from the shifted viewpoint, interpreted as consistent with hippocampal support of the allocentric mechanism. In the subsequent study (Shrager et al. 2007), participants watched as the virtual arena rotated in front of them between presentation and test and performed tasks with increasing list-lengths in order (i.e., spending several trials watching one location rotate, then two, then three). In this study, no specific effect of hippocampal damage upon performance from a shifted viewpoint was found, which was interpreted as an absence of evidence for hippocampal support of allocentric updating. However, a likely alternative interpretation, to my mind, is that the later study was solved by egocentric mental rotation.

It may be that the grid cells recently discovered in medial entorhinal cortex (Hafting et al. 2005) provide the neural substrate for allocentric updating of the place cell representation of one's own position within the environment, as follows. As a rat moves through its environment, each grid cell fires whenever the rat enters one of several locations which fall at the vertices of a regular triangular grid across the environment, see FIGURE 3. The grids of neighboring grid cells are simply shifted copies of each other, so that the relative positions of the firing locations of two grid cells remain constant across an environment and also remain constant across different environments (Fyhn et al. 2007). The nearby presubiculum, which contains head-direction cells, projects into medial (but not lateral) entorhinal cortex. This projection may allow the grid cells to perform path integration, allowing the grid cell activations to be updated in correspondence with the rat's movement. This could occur by each cell passing activity on to the appropriate neighbor (McNaughton et al. 2006; Sargolini et al. 2006; Fuhs & Touretzky 2006) or by each cell integrating movement information individually (Burgess et al. 2007). (See the original references for the details of these proposals.) In addition, the reciprocal connections between entorhinal cortex and the hippocampus might allow the place cell and grid-cell representations to combine both motion-related inputs (to grid cells) and environmental sensory information (the BVC inputs to place cells) in determining the animal's current location (Barry et al. 2007; O'Keefe & Burgess 2005; Burgess et al. 2007). A recent fMRI study in humans (Wolbers et al. 2007), in which they performed a path-integration task using only optic flow, showed performance to correlate with activation of the anterior hippocampus, possibly consistent with a role in allocentric spatial updating.

Parallel Hippocampo-Striatal Systems in Rats

The place cell data, summarized briefly above, seem to indicate that the hippocampus specifically processes the surface geometry of the rat's environment, with an important role also for the head-direction system, governed by distal cues to orientation. Hippocampal lesions dramatically impair performance on the classic version of the water maze, where rats must use distal landmark information as well as distance to the maze boundary to locate a hidden platform (Morris et al. 1982). Interestingly, the maze walls are powerful cues used to locate the platform even when they are transparent, illustrating the importance of continuous boundaries for navigation (Maurer & Derivaz 2000).

Distinct hippocampal and striatal contributions to spatial navigation can be seen in tests in the water maze. Hippocampal lesions do not disrupt the ability to navigate towards a location marked by a distinct visible landmark (or "beacon"). By contrast, striatal lesions impair navigation towards a location marked by a distinct visible landmark but not to an unmarked one defined relative to distal landmarks and boundaries (Packard & McGaugh 1992; McDonald & White 1994). When a location is defined by its distance and direction from an intramaze cue (given distal orienting cues), and not by the maze boundary, hippocampal damage does not impair navigation (Pearce et al. 1998), although lesions of the anterior thalamus (with presumed disruption of the head-direction system) do impair navigation (Wilton et al. 2001). Thus, the hippocampus may define locations relative to the boundary, while the striatum defines locations relative to local landmarks, and the head-direction system is required to derive a heading direction from distant landmarks.

The distinct contributions of hippocampal and striatal systems to spatial cognition can also be seen in the plus maze. In this task, rats are trained in an initial learning phase to retrieve food from the end of one arm (e.g., West), starting from another arm (e.g.,

South). This paradigm can be used to elegantly study whether rats learn to navigate to the food through learning a stereotyped response (turn left) or through learning the place within the test room (presumably defined by distal cues in the environment). The use of a response or a place strategy can be assessed during a probe trial in which rats start from a novel arm (e.g., North). The rat could either follow the learned response, that is, turning left and thus searching for food in the East arm (response strategy), or follow a place strategy and search in the arm in the West of the testing room. In probe trials after 8 and 16 days of training, healthy rats shifted from approaching the "place" associated with food after 8 days to making the turn "response" associated with food after 16 days. However, injections of lidocaine to inactivate the hippocampus abolished place learning, while injections into the striatum abolish response learning (Packard & McGaugh 1996).

We have described some of the different types of neural representation available to animals when solving spatial tasks. The head-direction system found throughout Papez's circuit may provide orientation, while the hippocampus has been identified with environment-centered representations of locations and the dorsal striatum has been associated with approach responses to a single landmark. In addition, the projections from the head-direction system to the nucleus accumbens imply that the striatal system might also allow navigation towards unmarked locations by using a visible local landmark in conjunction with external orienting cues. In the next section we consider recent evidence for a similar dissociation between right posterior hippocampal and right dorsal striatal substrates of spatial learning in the human brain.

Parallel Temporo-Striatal Systems in Humans

Study of the neural bases of large-scale navigation in humans has recently begun to take advantage of a combination of desk-top VR and functional neuroimaging. Several early studies revealed activation in parietal, retrosplenial, and parahippocampal areas as people find their way around (e.g., Aguirre & D'Esposito 1997; Maguire et al. 1998b; Ghaem et al. 1997), but interpretation of the functions of specific subregions remained difficult. In further experiments, some patterns began to emerge. Thus parahippocampal gyrus activation may reflect sensory (Epstein & Kanwisher 1998) or mnemonic (Janzen & van Turennout 2004) processing of spatial scenes and perhaps the use of peripheral vision in this (Levy et al. 2001), while hippocampal activation was found to reflect navigational accuracy and striatal (caudate) activation to reflect navigational speed (Maguire et al. 1998a). Recent advances in imaging technology, more realistic environments, and more sophisticated analyses of behavior (Spiers & Maguire 2007) have refined these interpretations further. Hartley et al. (2003) found that hippocampal activation corresponded to flexible wayfinding using new paths through previously explored environments, while striatal activation corresponded to following well-used routes (explaining the correlation with speed in the previous study). Wolbers and Buchel (2005) examined activation during the learning of a new environment and found hippocampal activation to correspond to increases in knowledge of the environmental layout, while retrosplenial activation corresponded to the absolute level of performance.

Iaria et al. (2003) adapted an elegant paradigm for identifying the use of distal cues in rat navigation for use with humans. In this task, subjects found objects in 4 arms in a virtual 8-arm maze with distal cues present around it to provide orientation. Their memory was then tested by asking them to revisit the same 4 arms again—entering the other arms counted as an error. In probe trials, the distal cues were removed during the test phase: an increase in the number of errors indicated that the subject was making use of the distal cues rather than, for example, remembering a sequence of turns. When the study was performed in an fMRI experiment, Iaria et al. found that the dependence on distal cues correlated with hippocampal activation, while distal cue–independent responding correlated with activation of the caudate nucleus. These results are consistent with hippocampal provision of an allocentric representation, requiring the distal cues, and striatal provision of route-like egocentric responses.

It seems that the hippocampal and striatal systems can act cooperatively in the context of adaptation to brain damage. Voermans et al. (2004) compared the activation provoked by remembering routes through houses (shown as video clips) between a group of patients with Huntington's disease and a group of healthy volunteers. They found reduced caudate activation corresponding to the progression of the disease (which attacks this part of the brain) in the patient group, but also increased hippocampal activation. Thus the more flexible hippocampal system may be able to take over some of the function of the striatal system in remembering routes. The extent to which the striatal system could accommodate for hippocampal damage is an interesting question for future research.

As well as the above dissociation between striatal support of overlearned route-like responses and hippocampal support of more flexible navigation, the

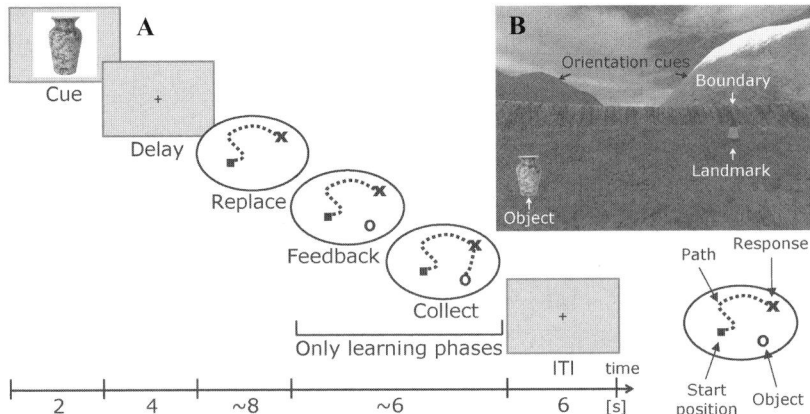

FIGURE 6. Experimental paradigm for comparing the relative contributions of local landmarks and boundaries to spatial memory. Participants play an adapted first-person perspective videogame in which they find objects within a virtual environment comprising a circular boundary and a landmark, with distal cues to orientation (rendered at infinity). **(A)** After collecting the objects in their respective locations, each subsequent trial has a cue phase (an object is shown) and a replace phase (the subject attempts to navigate to the object's location and presses a button). Learning trials, but not test trials, contain feedback from which subjects learn to improve their performance (i.e., replacement accuracy). Feedback consists of the object appearing in the correct location and being collected by the subject. A view of the virtual environment is shown in **(B)**. Adapted from Doeller and Burgess (2007).

animal studies reviewed above also suggest different neural bases for processing locations relative to local landmarks and environmental boundaries. This dissociation has recently been examined in humans (Doeller et al. 2007) using a VR object-location memory task, in which, without being distinguished by any explicit instructions, some objects maintained a fixed relation to the environmental boundary while others maintained a fixed relation to a single intramaze landmark. Participants explored a VR arena bounded by a circular wall, containing a single landmark and surrounded by distant orientation cues. Within this arena they encountered four objects in four different locations, see FIGURE 6. On each subsequent trial they saw a picture of one of the objects (the "cue phase") and indicated its location within the arena by navigating to it from a random start location and making a button-press response (the "replace" phase). The object then appeared in its correct location and was collected (the "feedback" phase). Each set of 16 trials (four per object) composed a block, with four blocks in the entire experiment. Critically, the landmark and boundary were moved relative to each other between blocks, with two objects maintaining their location relative to the boundary and two relative to the landmark.

Performance was measured in terms of the proximity of response location to the correct location, and learning during the feedback phase could be measured as the improvement in performance on the next trial with the same object. Once the two cues had been moved relative to each other, the relative influence of landmark or boundary on responding was reflected implicitly in the distance of the response location from the locations predicted by either cue. Both cues played functionally equivalent roles in the task and were not distinguished in the participants' instructions, and their relation to the distant orientation cues remained unchanged as these were projected at infinity.

Participants gradually learned locations relative to both types of cue at similar rates, with performance increasing similarly within and across blocks (FIG. 7). Inaccurate responses largely reflected use of the incorrect cue early in each block. Consistent with the predictions from animal studies, fMRI activation in the right dorsal striatum during the feedback phase correlated with learning for landmark-related objects, while activation in the right posterior hippocampus correlated with learning for boundary-related objects. In addition, the influence of the boundary on the replacement location correlated with right posterior hippocampal activation, while the influence of the landmark correlated with right dorsal striatal activation. Thus, differential activity seen in the hippocampus and caudate corresponded to the acquisition and expression of information about locations derived from environmental landmarks or boundaries respectively.

This analysis raises the question of what distinguishes a boundary from a landmark? A simple

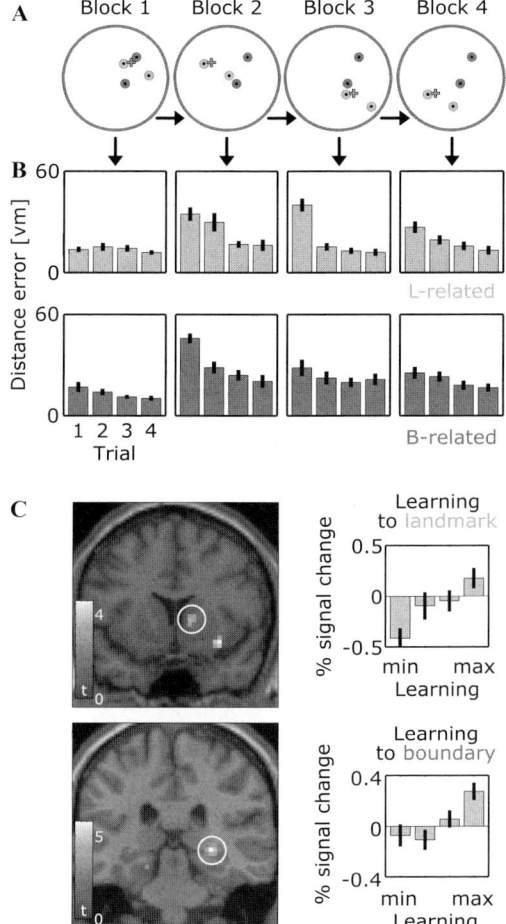

FIGURE 7. An fMRI study of the neural bases of learning locations relative to a local landmark or a local boundary; the paradigm is shown in FIGURE 6. **(A)** After four objects have been collected in their locations, participants completed blocks of four trials replacing each object, with feedback regarding their correct location, see FIGURE 6. At the end of each block, the landmark and boundary were moved relative to each other, with two objects moving with the landmark (shown in orange), and two with the boundary (shown in green). **(B)** Object locations were learned within and between blocks from the feedback provided. Average replacement error is shown separately for the landmark-related (orange) and boundary-related (green) objects. **(C)** Activation during the feedback phase corresponded to learning (improvement on the next trial with that object) in the right striatum for landmark-related objects and in the right posterior hippocampus for the boundary-related objects. Adapted from Doeller, King, & Burgess (2007).

potential answer comes from simulation of the firing of hippocampal place cells (Hartley et al. 2000; Burgess & Hartley 2002). In these simulations, place cells effectively perform a match to the distances to the nearest obstacle, integrating over distances in all directions around the rat. Thus, for place cells, any obstacle in the environment simply has an importance proportional to the horizontal angle it subtends at the rat. This potentially provides a measure of "boundaryness" in terms of proximity and extent. However, it is not clear what aspects of environmental stimuli correspond to "landmarkness" as reflected in their influence on striatal processing.

A final consideration of this study was the nature of the interaction between the two systems in controlling behavior after they had been put into conflict by the relative motion of the two cues. In this study, the levels of activation in hippocampus and striatum could be investigated trial-by-trial as both systems contributed to a single behavior. No evidence was found of a direct interaction between activation in the two systems, other than the variation reflected in behavior. Thus it seems that both systems operate in parallel, with their activation signaling their suitability to control behavior. Such an interpretation would be consistent with the effects of lidocaine injections in rats (Packard & McGaugh 1996) and extends previous studies of hippocampo-striatal interaction by looking at different tasks or different stages of the same task (Poldrack et al. 2001).

Incidental and Reinforcement Learning Rules in Hippocampus and Striatum

So far, I have concentrated on the representations supporting spatial cognition, but what of the rules underlying the learning of adaptive behavior? "Reinforcement learning" (Sutton & Barto 1988) provides the dominant model for learning from feedback over multiple trials. This model, derived from the Rescorla-Wagner law (Rescorla & Wagner 1972) and its development into associative learning theory (see e.g., Mackintosh 1975 and Dickinson 1980), associates cues to a measure of predicted feedback (see also, Dayan & Abbott 2002). This rule explains results in classical conditioning and also in "instrumental conditioning," or learning to act, by also associating cues to appropriate actions. In both cases, the learning rule for adjusting the strengths of these associations depends on the difference between the predicted and actual feedback (the "prediction error"). This simple and elegant model has provided a quantitative description of a great variety of behavioral data on learning and has received strong support from evidence that the prediction error signal can be seen in the striatal targets of the dopamine system (O'Doherty et al. 2004; Pessiglione et al. 2006; Schultz 2002).

However, there has been a long-standing but unproven hypothesis that spatial learning does not obey this type of error-correcting learning rule, but rather is incidental, occurring independently of performance, motivation, or prediction error (Tolman 1948). This type of learning was subsequently attributed to the hippocampus by O'Keefe and Nadel (1978). However, despite the many studies since, aimed at proving this hypothesis, the results have been mixed, with most finding results consistent with reinforcement learning.

A major prediction of reinforcement learning concerns the situation where, because the association from one cue already accurately predicts feedback, there will be no prediction error and no possibility of subsequent learning to a second cue (learning is said to be "blocked"). Similarly, where learning occurs to two cues concurrently, the learning to one will be reduced by the extent to which the other accurately predicts feedback (learning to it is said to be "overshadowed").

It is possible that the confounding of hippocampal and nonhippocampal contributions to spatial cognition may have contributed to the previous findings of blocking and overshadowing in spatial tasks (Hamilton & Sutherland 1999; Chamizo et al. 2003; Pearce et al. 2006). The above study (Doeller et al. 2007) indicates a way to dissociate the specifically hippocampal contribution to spatial learning. Under this view, learning to an environmental boundary, dependent on the hippocampus, would be incidental and would not show blocking or overshadowing, while learning to the landmark, dependent on the striatum, would conform to reinforcement learning.

Doeller and Burgess (2007) examined blocking between boundaries and landmarks within their virtual arena. Their blocking experiment consists of three phases. In a first "prelearning" phase, participants learn object locations while landmark and boundary are moved relative to each other at the beginning of each block: four objects maintaining a fixed location relative to the landmark and four other objects maintaining a fixed location relative to the boundary. In a second "compound learning" phase, both the landmark and the boundary remain in fixed positions, predicting the position of all eight objects. During the final "test" phase, memory performance is tested (without feedback) in the presence of either the landmark or the boundary alone.

If a given object is paired with cue 1 during prelearning, and the subject learns to accurately replace it on the basis of this association, then there should be little learning of the association to cue 2 during the compound learning phase. Thus performance should be poor when tested with cue 2 alone (compared to an object paired with cue 2 during prelearning). This provides a powerful test of reinforcement learning, since any effects of "learned irrelevance" or "super learning" (consequences of any association from the unpaired cue to the absence of reward) will be additive to the blocking effect.

Doeller and Burgess (2007) found that, although learning of objects to either type of cue occurred at similar rates and with similar levels of performance, there were different blocking effects for learning to the boundary and to the landmark. When tested with the landmark, performance was much worse for the object paired with the boundary during prelearning. By contrast, performance when tested with the boundary was equal for objects paired with either cue during prelearning. See FIGURE 8 for the results of the boundary–landmark blocking experiment. Consistent results were found when, again in the presence of the distal orientation cues, two landmarks were used as cues (each landmark blocking the other), when two opposing sections of the boundary were used (neither blocked the other), or when overshadowing was investigated (the boundary overshadowed the landmark, but not vice versa). Overall, the consistent finding was that learning to landmarks obeyed the predictions of reinforcement learning and learning to boundaries did not. Given the striatal and hippocampal activation corresponding to learning relative to landmarks and boundaries respectively (see above), it seems that, in this task, the striatum supports reinforcement learning relative to landmarks, while the hippocampus supports incidental learning to boundaries.

Discussion: Implications beyond Spatial Cognition

As noted in the Introduction, spatial cognition enjoys an advantage over some other fields of higher cognition in being able to share paradigms between human and animal research. This link allows some inferences regarding the actual neural representations and processes involved in human cognition to be drawn from invasive studies in animals. Given this advantage, are there more general implications that can be drawn for cognition beyond the spatial domain?

Memory and Imagery: Common Processes and Neural Bases?

Initial attempts to form a computational model of memory for spatial scenes, or for the spatial context of an event (Burgess et al. 2001b; Becker & Burgess 2001), force a consideration of the neural mechanisms involved. I briefly review these mechanisms and then discuss their more general implications for memory and imagery (see also Hartley et al. 2007).

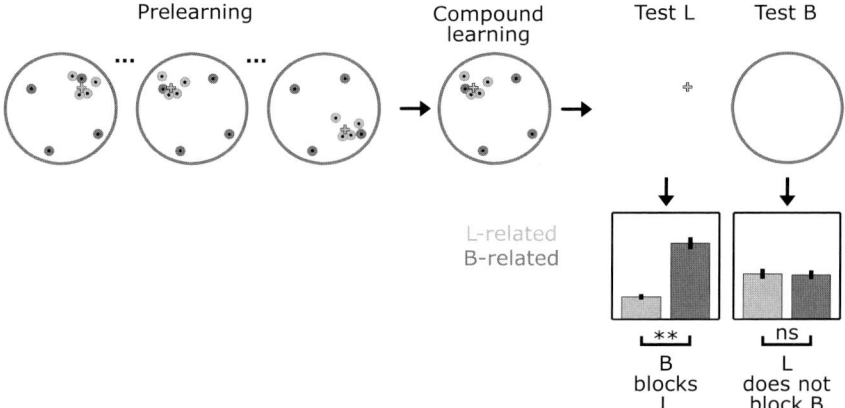

FIGURE 8. Learning to the boundary blocks learning to the landmark, but not vice versa. Participants learned eight object locations using the paradigm shown in FIGURE 6. During "prelearning" (eight blocks of two trials per object on average), the landmark and boundary moved relative to each other after each block, with four objects moving with the landmark (orange "+"; object locations are orange spots) and four with the boundary (green circle, object locations are green spots). During "compound learning" (one block of six trials per object), both types of cue (landmark and boundary) remained fixed, allowing them to become associated to the locations of objects previously paired with the other cue. Both learning phases included feedback at the end of each trial. Test phases (four objects tested with the landmark L; four with the boundary B) did not include feedback and showed little learning to the landmark for objects previously associated with the boundary (Test L) but unimpeded learning to the boundary of objects previously associated with the landmark (Test B). Adapted from Doeller and Burgess (2007).

The model by Byrne and colleagues (Byrne et al. 2007) makes use of the idea that the pattern of activation of place cells is constrained by the recurrent connections within area CA3 of the hippocampus to be consistent with the subject being at a single location. Other patterns of activation, involving place cells which normally fire in different environmental locations, can only be transient, that is, the place cells form a "continuous attractor" representation of location (Zhang 1996; Samsonovich & McNaughton 1997). The activation of place cells representing a single location can then reactivate the parahippocampal (BVC) representation of the distances and allocentric directions of environmental boundaries around that location. The retrieval of this information into visual imagery/working memory requires translation into an imaginable egocentric (head-centered) representation, involving retrosplenial/parieto-occipital sulcus and posterior parietal cortex, as well as the provision of current heading by Papez's circuit.

This model has implications for the way episodic memories or "events" are retrieved, or at least how the spatial context in which they occur is retrieved—a process thought to be specifically hippocampal dependent (Burgess et al. 2002; O'Keefe & Nadel 1978). Thus, the hippocampus provides a strong constraint on the subsets of information retrieval from the vast amount of abstract (allocentric) knowledge stored in the surrounding neocortical areas. Specifically, the hippocampus restricts retrieved subsets to be mutually consistent with perception from a single location. These products of retrieval are then capable of being put into a head-centered representation for imagery in medial parietal areas via (re)constructive mechanisms in retrosplenial/parieto-occipital and posterior parietal areas, including imposition of a viewing direction onto the allocentric medial temporal representation by the head-direction cells in Papez's circuit. As well as providing an outline for the functional roles of the various regions identified in episodic memory (Burgess et al. 2001a), the model explicitly highlights the close relationship between the mechanisms and neural bases of memory and imagery (Becker & Burgess 2001).

Recent work has verified the predicted link between memory and imagery. Similar effects of hippocampal lesions (known to affect episodic memory) have been found in spatial working memory (Hartley et al. 2007) and novel imagery (Hassabis et al. 2007). Similar patterns of activation have also been found in functional neuroimaging of memory for past events and for imagined "future" events (Addis et al. 2007). In addition, patients with hemispatial neglect in imagery, but not those with perceptual or motor neglect but unimpaired imagery, have also been found to have deficits in spatial navigation in tasks resembling the water maze (Guariglia et al. 2005). Given the close relationship between retrieval and imagery, and between their neural bases, it is possible that one of the hallmarks of episodic memory—that of subjective reexperience (Tulving 2001)—actually in large part reflects the success of the generation of a vivid internal image. And such imagery is of course not necessarily restricted to memory at all, although clearly implicated in much of the "reconstructive" process on which memory relies (Bartlett 1932; Addis et al. 2007).

Much future work is obviously required to identify the functional interactions between memory and imagery and between medial temporal and parietal areas, but hopefully the spatial model outlined above can provide some sort of initial framework.

Learning Rules, Procedural Versus Declarative Memory, and the "Geometric Module"

The finding of different learning rules in the processing associated with the hippocampal and striatal systems (Doeller & Burgess 2007; Doeller et al. 2007) suggests a different way of looking at the major suggested divisions of long-term memory. Thus, it has been suggested that the acquisition of consciously retrievable long-term knowledge (whether semantic or episodic in nature) depends on the hippocampus (Scoville & Milner 1957); this is termed "declarative" memory (Squire & Zola-Morgan 1991), in contrast to "procedural" memory (e.g., habits, motor learning), important aspects of which depend on the striatum (Yin & Knowlton 2006). Equally, it has been suggested that rapid one-shot encoding of events and their contexts (Tulving 1983) specifically depends on the hippocampus (Kinsbourne & Wood 1975; O'Keefe & Nadel 1978; Mishkin et al. 1997; Rugg & Yonelinas 2003; Fortin et al. 2002), as opposed to slowly acquired semantic knowledge acquired slowly over multiple exposures.

These traditional dissociations might arise from differences in the basic neurobiology of the two systems—leading each system to implement a different learning rule. Thus, synaptic plasticity in the striatum may be controlled by levels of dopamine locally released (see Redgrave & Gurney 2006) as a function of prediction error (Waelti et al. 2001; Montague et al. 2004; O'Doherty et al. 2004). By contrast, hippocampal synaptic plasticity simply reflects co-occurrence (in Doeller et al.'s study, co-ocurrence between the representation of the object and the place cell representation of location as a conjunction of bearings from the boundary).

Thus, the aspects of conscious awareness (which did not differ greatly between landmark and boundary learning) and rapidity of acquisition (which also did not differ between landmark and boundary learning) stressed by the declarative and episodic theories may be later consequences of a trial-and-error based learning rule on the one hand, and a Hebbian encoding of coincidences on the other (see also Hirsch 1974; O'Keefe & Nadel 1978).

The neuroscience literature reviewed here demonstrates that a variety of spatial representations are available for the purposes of controlling behavior. One of these, supported by the hippocampus, is specialized for processing location relative to environmental boundaries and appears to operate a distinct, incidental, learning rule. This view of the hippocampus has curious echoes of the idea of a "geometric module" (Cheng 1986; Gallistel 1990): a module for processing the surface geometry of the surrounding environment in an "encapsulated" way (i.e., its output concerns only this subset of the information available to the animal, independent from other, e.g., featural, information). The geometric module was proposed on purely behavioral grounds, independently of some of the above ideas of hippocampal processing already present in O'Keefe and Nadel's (1978) book. The main data for the geometric module were the preferential role played by environmental boundaries in reorienting a disoriented animal (or young child; Hermer & Spelke 1994) within a small rectangular enclosure.

The generality of the idea of a geometric module is restricted by its dependence on a single "reorientation" paradigm. For example, animals and young children do appear to be able to use featural cues to reorient in slightly different reorientation experiments, such as when using larger (Learmonth et al. 2002; Sovrano & Vallortigara 2006), rhombic (Hupbach & Nadel 2005), or symmetrical (Nardini et al. 2007; McGregor et al. 2004) enclosures, or learning over repeated trials (Cheng 1986; Vallortigara et al. 1990; Gouteux et al. 2001). They also routinely combine featural cues with geometric cues to navigate when not disoriented (e.g., Maurer & Derivaz 2000), indicating that the geometric module is not strictly "encapsulated." See Cheng and Newcombe (2005) for a recent review. The conflicting patterns of results from disorientation paradigms regarding both the presence or otherwise of geometric modules and the applicability or otherwise of reinforcement learning to spatial cognition may arise in part because so many types of cue interact to determine orientation, and do so within the head-direction system (e.g., Taube 1998), rather than the hippocampus. These include local cues, distal cues, and environmental geometry, and which cues actually determine orientation depends on many factors, including each cue's apparent stability (Jeffery et al. 1997; Jeffery & O'Keefe 1999), its distal or proximal location (Cressant et al. 1997), and the subject's history of disorientation (Knierim et al. 1995). By contrast, Doeller et al. (2007) attempted to dissociate a cleanly hippocampal contribution to spatial cognition, which may explain their more consistent results.

Conclusions

The field of spatial cognition has been evolving rapidly over the last few years, driven by convergence of results from the application of similar experimental paradigms in both humans and other animals. Here I have reviewed a small subset of these recent advances, focusing on the attempt to build a mechanistic understanding of how spatial behavior results from the actions of networks of neurons. In addition to the traditional strengths of cognitive science, of experimental dissociation of processes at the behavioral level, there have been vital contributions from other disciplines operating at different levels of description. These include the ability to link behavior to neural systems, for example, via neuropsychology or functional neuroimaging; the continued success of systems neuroscience, including the ability to examine the actual neural representations at play; and the ability to quantitatively integrate results at different levels by using computational modeling.

The picture which emerges of spatial cognition is one of multiple parallel systems using representations with different frames of reference, processing different aspects of the spatial scene, using different learning rules, and supported by a corresponding set of neural systems. A current challenge for the field is to begin to work out how these various neural systems, including medial temporal, parietal, and striatal regions, combine to produce the rich variety of spatial behavior underpinning our daily life. This in turn should lead to insights into the organization of other aspects of cognition and into the effects or causes of damage or dysfunction observable at the various levels of neurophysiology, systems neuroscience, and behavior.

Acknowledgments

I thank C. Bird and C.F. Doeller for commenting on this manuscript, and the UK Medical Research Council, Biotechnology and Biological Sciences Research Council and the Wayfinding project of the European Union for their support.

Conflict of Interest

The author declares no conflicts of interest.

References

Abrahams, S., Pickering, A., Polkey, C. E., & Morris, R. G. (1997). Spatial memory deficits in patients with unilateral damage to the right hippocampal formation. *Neuropsychologia, 35*(1), 11–24.

Addis, D. R., Wong, A. T., & Schacter, D. L. (2007). Remembering the past and imagining the future: Common and distinct neural substrates during event construction and elaboration. *Neuropsychologia, 45*(7), 1363–1377.

Aguirre, G. K., & D'Esposito, M. (1997). Environmental knowledge is subserved by separable dorsal/ventral neural areas. *J. Neurosci., 17*(7), 2512–2518.

Andersen, R. A., Essick, G. K., & Siegel, R. M. (1987). Neurons of area 7 activated by both visual stimuli and oculomotor behavior. *Exp. Brain Res., 67*(2), 316–322.

Barry, C., Hayman, R., Burgess, N., & Jeffery, K. J. (2007). Experience-dependent rescaling of entorhinal grids. *Nat. Neurosci., 10*(6), 682–684.

Barry, C., Lever, C., Hayman, R., Hartley, T., Burton, S., et al. (2006). The boundary vector cell model of place cell firing and spatial memory. *Rev. Neurosci., 17*, 71–97.

Bartlett, F. C. (1932). *Remembering, a study in experimental and social psychology*. New York: Macmillan.

Becker, S., & Burgess, N. (2001). A model of spatial recall, mental imagery and neglect. *Neural Information Processing Systems, 13*, 96–102.

Bisiach, E., & Luzzatti, C. (1978). Unilateral neglect of representational space. *Cortex, 14*, 129–133.

Bridgeman, B., Van Der Heijden, A. H. C., & Velichkovsky, B. M. (1994). A theory of visual stability across saccadic eye movements. *Behav. Brain Sci., 17*, 247–292.

Burgess, N. (2006). Spatial memory: How egocentric and allocentric combine. *Trends Cogn. Sci, 10*(12), 551–557.

Burgess, N., Barry, C., & O'Keefe, J. (2007). An oscillatory interference model of grid cell firing. *Hippocampus, 17*, 801–812.

Burgess, N., Becker, S., King, J. A., & O'Keefe, J. (2001). Memory for events and their spatial context: Models and experiments. *Philos. Trans. R. Soc. Lond B Biol. Sci., 356*, 1493–1503.

Burgess, N., & Hartley, T. (2002). Orientational and geometric determinants of place and head-direction. In *Neural information processing systems* (Vol. 14). Cambridge, MA: MIT Press.

Burgess, N., Maguire, E. A., & O'Keefe, J. (2002). The human hippocampus and spatial and episodic memory. *Neuron, 35*(4), 625–641.

Burgess, N., Maguire, E. A., Spiers, H. J., & O'Keefe, J. (2001). A temporoparietal and prefrontal network for retrieving the spatial context of lifelike events. *Neuroimage, 14*, 439–453.

Burgess, N., Spiers, H. J., & Paleologou, E. (2004). Orientational manoeuvres in the dark: Dissociating allocentric and egocentric influences on spatial memory. *Cognition, 94*(2), 149–166.

Byrne, P., Becker, S., & Burgess, N. (2007). Remembering the past and imagining the future: A neural model of spatial memory and imagery. *Psychol. Rev., 114*(2), 340–375.

Chamizo, V. D., Aznar-Casanova, J. A., & Artigas, A. A. (2003). Human overshadowing in a virtual pool: Simple guidance is a good competitor against locale learning. *Learn. Motiv.*, 34, 262–281.

Cheng, K. (1986). A purely geometric module in the rat's spatial representation. *Cognition*, 23(2), 149–178.

Cheng, K., & Newcombe, N. S. (2005). Is there a geometric module for spatial orientation? Squaring theory and evidence. *Psychon. Bull. Rev.*, 12(1), 1–23.

Colby, C. L., & Goldberg, M. E. (1999). Space and attention in parietal cortex. *Annu. Rev. Neurosci.*, 22, 319–349.

Cressant, A., Muller, R. U., & Poucet, B. (1997). Failure of centrally placed objects to control the firing fields of hippocampal place cells. *J. Neurosci.*, 17(7), 2531–2542.

Dayan, P., & Abbott, L. F. (2002). *Computational neuroscience*. Cambridge, MA: MIT Press.

Deneve, S., Latham, P. E., & Pouget, A. (2001). Efficient computation and cue integration with noisy population codes. *Nat. Neurosci.*, 4(8), 826–831.

Dickinson, A. (1980). *Contemporary animal learning theory*. Cambridge, UK: Cambridge University Press.

Diwadkar, V. A., & McNamara, T. P. (1997). Viewpoint dependence in scene recognition. *Psychological Science*, 8(4), 302–307.

Doeller, C. F., & Burgess, N. (2007). Distinct error-correcting and incidental learning of location relative to landmarks and boundaries. Submitted for publication.

Doeller, C. F., King, J. A., & Burgess, N. (2007). Parallel striatal and hippocampal systems for landmarks and boundaries in spatial memory. Submitted for publication.

Ekstrom, A. D., Kahana, M. J., Caplan, J. B., Fields, T. A., Isham, E. A., et al. (2003). Cellular networks underlying human spatial navigation. *Nature*, 425(6954), 184–188.

Epstein, R., & Kanwisher, N. (1998). A cortical representation of the local visual environment. *Nature*, 392(6676), 598–601.

Etienne, A. S., Maurer, R., & Seguinot, V. (1996). Path integration in mammals and its interaction with visual landmarks. *J. Exp. Biol.*, 199(Pt 1), 201–209.

Fenton, A. A., Csizmadia, G., & Muller, R. U. (2000). Conjoint control of hippocampal place cell firing by two visual stimuli. I. The effects of moving the stimuli on firing field positions. *J. Gen. Physiol.*, 116(2), 191–209.

Fortin, N. J., Agster, K. L., & Eichenbaum, H. B. (2002). Critical role of the hippocampus in memory for sequences of events. *Nat. Neurosci.*, 5(5), 458–462.

Fuhs, M. C., & Touretzky, D. S. (2006). A spin glass model of path integration in rat medial entorhinal cortex. *J. Neurosci.*, 26(16), 4266–4276.

Fyhn, M., Hafting, T., Treves, A., Moser, M. B., & Moser, E. I. (2007). Hippocampal remapping and grid realignment in entorhinal cortex. *Nature*, 446(7132), 190–194.

Galletti, C., Battaglini, P. P., & Fattori, P. (1995). Eye position influence on the parieto-occipital area PO (V6) of the macaque monkey. *Eur. J. Neurosci.*, 7(12), 2486–2501.

Gallistel, R. (1990). *The organization of learning*. Cambridge, MA: MIT Press.

Ghaem, O., Mellet, E., Crivello, F., Tzourio, N., Mazoyer, B., et al. (1997). Mental navigation along memorized routes activates the hippocampus, precuneus, and insula. *Neuroreport*, 8(3), 739–744.

Gothard, K. M., Skaggs, W. E., & McNaughton, B. L. (1996). Dynamics of mismatch correction in the hippocampal ensemble code for space: Interaction between path integration and environmental cues. *J. Neurosci.*, 16(24), 8027–8040.

Gouteux, S., Thinus-Blanc, C., & Vauclair, J. (2001). Rhesus monkeys use geometric and nongeometric information during a reorientation task. *J. Exp. Psychol. Gen.*, 130(3), 505–519.

Guariglia, C., Piccardi, L., Iaria, G., Nico, D., & Pizzamiglio, L. (2005). Representational neglect and navigation in real space. *Neuropsychologia*, 43(8), 1138–1143.

Hafting, T., Fyhn, M., Molden, S., Moser, M. B., & Moser, E. I. (2005). Microstructure of a spatial map in the entorhinal cortex. *Nature*, 436, 801–806.

Hamilton, D. A., & Sutherland, R. J. (1999). Blocking in human place learning: Evidence form virtual navigation. *Psychobiol.*, 27, 453–461.

Hartley, T., Bird, C. M., Chan, D., Cipolotti, L., Husain, M., et al. (2007). The hippocampus is required for short-term topographical memory in humans. *Hippocampus*, 17, 34–48.

Hartley, T., Burgess, N., Lever, C., Cacucci, F., & O'Keefe, J. (2000). Modeling place fields in terms of the cortical inputs to the hippocampus. *Hippocampus*, 10(4), 369–379.

Hartley, T., Maguire, E. A., Spiers, H. J., & Burgess, N. (2003). The well-worn route and the path less traveled: Distinct neural bases of route following and wayfinding in humans. *Neuron*, 37(5), 877–888.

Hartley, T., Trinkler, I., & Burgess, N. (2004). Geometric determinants of human spatial memory. *Cognition*, 94, 39–75.

Hassabis, D., Kumaran, D., Vann, S. D., & Maguire, E. A. (2007). Patients with hippocampal amnesia cannot imagine new experiences. *Proc. Natl. Acad. Sci. U.S.A.*, 104(5), 1726–1731.

Hermer, L., & Spelke, E. S. (1994). A geometric process for spatial reorientation in young children. *Nature*, 370(6484), 57–59.

Hirsch, R. (1974). The hippocampus and contextual retrieval of information from memory: A theory. *Behav. Biol.*, 12(4), 421–444.

Hupbach, A., & Nadel, L. (2005). Reorientation in a rhombic environment: No evidence for an encapsulated geometric module. *Cognitive Development*, 20, 279–302.

Iaria, G., Petrides, M., Dagher, A., Pike, B., & Bohbot, V. D. (2003). Cognitive strategies dependent on the hippocampus and caudate nucleus in human navigation: Variability and change with practice. *J. Neurosci.*, 23(13), 5945–5952.

Janzen, G., & van Turennout, M. (2004). Selective neural representation of objects relevant for navigation. *Nat. Neurosci.*, 7(6), 673–677.

Jeffery, K. J., Donnett, J. G., Burgess, N., & O'Keefe, J. M. (1997). Directional control of hippocampal place fields. *Exp. Brain Res.*, 117(1), 131–142.

Jeffery, K. J., & O'Keefe, J. M. (1999). Learned interaction of visual and idiothetic cues in the control of place field orientation. *Exp. Brain Res.*, 127(2), 151–161.

King, J. A., Burgess, N., Hartley, T., Vargha-Khadem, F., & O'Keefe, J. (2002). Human hippocampus and viewpoint dependence in spatial memory. *Hippocampus*, *12*(6), 811–820.

King, J. A., Trinkler, I., Hartley, T., Vargha-Khadem, F., & Burgess, N. (2004). The hippocampal role in spatial memory and the familiarity-recollection distinction: A single case study. *Neuropsychology*, *18*, 405–417.

Kinsbourne, M., & Wood, F. (1975). Short-term memory and the amnesic syndrome. In D. Deutsch & J. A. Deutsch (Eds.), *Short term memory* (pp. 257–291). New York: Academic.

Knierim, J. J., Kudrimoti, H. S., & McNaughton, B. L. (1995). Place cells, head direction cells, and the learning of landmark stability. *J. Neurosci.*, *15*(3 Pt 1), 1648–1659.

Kubie, J. L., Fenton, A., Novikov, N., Touretzky, D., & Muller, R. U. (2007). Changes in goal selection induced by cue conflicts are in register with predictions from changes in place cell field locations. *Behav. Neurosci.*, *121*(4), 751–763.

Learmonth, A. E., Nadel, L., & Newcombe, N. S. (2002). Children's use of landmarks: Implications for modularity theory. *Psychol. Sci.*, *13*(4), 337–341.

Lenck-Santini, P. P., Rivard, B., Muller, R. U., & Poucet, B. (2005). Study of CA1 place cell activity and exploratory behavior following spatial and nonspatial changes in the environment. *Hippocampus*, *15*(3), 356–369.

Levy, I., Hasson, U., Avidan, G., Hendler, T., & Malach, R. (2001). Center-periphery organization of human object areas. *Nat. Neurosci.*, *4*, 533–539.

Mackintosh, N. J. (1975). A theory of attention: Variations in the associability of stimuli with reinforcement. *Psychol. Rev.*, *82*, 276–298.

Maguire, E. A., Burgess, N., Donnett, J. G., Frackowiak, R. S., Frith, C. D., et al. (1998a). Knowing where and getting there: A human navigation network. *Science*, *280*(5365), 921–924.

Maguire, E. A., Burgess, N., Donnett, J. G., O'Keefe, J., & Frith, C. D. (1998b). Knowing where things are: Parahippocampal involvement in encoding object locations in virtual large-scale space. *J. Cogn. Neurosci.*, *10*(1), 61–76.

Maurer, R., & Derivaz, V. (2000). Rats in a transparent morris water maze use elemental and configural geometry of landmarks as well as distance to the pool wall. *Spatial Cognition and Computation*, *2*, 135–156.

May, M. (2004). Imaginal perspective switches in remembered environments: Transformation versus interference accounts. *Cognit. Psychol.*, *48*(2), 163–206.

McDonald, R. J., & White, N. M. (1994). Parallel information processing in the water maze: Evidence for independent memory systems involving dorsal striatum and hippocampus. *Behav. Neural Biol.*, *61*(3), 260–270.

McGregor, A., Hayward, A. J., Pearce, J. M., & Good, M. A. (2004). Hippocampal lesions disrupt navigation based on the shape of the environment. *Behav. Neurosci.*, *118*(5), 1011–1021.

McNamara, T. P., Rump, B., & Werner, S. (2003). Egocentric and geocentric frames of reference in memory of large-scale space. *Psychon. Bull. Rev.*, *10*(3), 589–595.

McNaughton, B. L., Battaglia, F. P., Jensen, O., Moser, E. I., & Moser, M. B. (2006). Path integration and the neural basis of the "cognitive map." *Nat. Rev. Neurosci.*, *7*(8), 663–678.

Melcher, D. (2007). Predictive remapping of visual features precedes saccadic eye movements. *Nat. Neurosci.*, *10*(7), 903–907.

Milner, A. D., Dijkerman, H. C., & Carey, D. P. (1999). Visuospatial processing in a case of visual form agnosia. In N. Burgess, K. J. Jeffery, & J. O'Keefe (Eds.), *The hippocampal and parietal foundations of spatial cognition* (pp. 443–466). Oxford, UK: Oxford University Press.

Mishkin, M., Suzuki, W. A., Gadian, D. G., & Vargha-Khadem, F. (1997). Hierarchical organization of cognitive memory. *Philos. Trans. R. Soc. Lond B Biol. Sci.*, *352*(1360), 1461–1467.

Montague, P. R., Hyman, S. E., & Cohen, J. D. (2004). Computational roles for dopamine in behavioural control. *Nature*, *431*(7010), 760–767.

Morris, R. G. M., Garrud, P., Rawlins, J. N., & O'Keefe, J. (1982). Place navigation impaired in rats with hippocampal lesions. *Nature*, *297*(5868), 681–683.

Mou, W., & McNamara, T. P. (2002). Intrinsic frames of reference in spatial memory. *J. Exp. Psychol. Learn. Mem. Cogn.*, *28*(1), 162–170.

Mou, W., McNamara, T. P., Valiquette, C. M., & Rump, B. (2004). Allocentric and egocentric updating of spatial memories. *J. Exp. Psychol. Learn Mem. Cogn.*, *30*(1), 142–157.

Muller, R. U. (1996). A quarter of a century of place cells. *Neuron*, *17*(5), 813–822.

Muller, R. U., & Kubie, J. L. (1989). The firing of hippocampal place cells predicts the future position of freely moving rats. *J. Neurosci.*, *9*(12), 4101–4110.

Nardini, M., Atkinson, J., & Burgess, N. (2007). Children reorient using the left/right sense of coloured landmarks at 18–24 months. *Cognition*. Epub ahead of print. DOI:10.1016/j.cognition.2007.02.007.

Nardini, M., Burgess, N., Breckenridge, K., & Atkinson, J. (2006). Differential developmental trajectories for egocentric, environmental and intrinsic frames of reference in spatial memory. *Cognition*, *101*(1), 153–172.

O'Doherty, J., Dayan, P., Schultz, J., Deichmann, R., Friston, K., et al. (2004). Dissociable roles of ventral and dorsal striatum in instrumental conditioning. *Science*, *304*(5669), 452–454.

O'Keefe, J. (1976). Place units in the hippocampus of the freely moving rat. *Exp. Neurol.*, *51*(1), 78–109.

O'Keefe, J., & Burgess, N. (1996). Geometric determinants of the place fields of hippocampal neurons. *Nature*, *381*(6581), 425–428.

O'Keefe, J., & Burgess, N. (2005). Dual phase and rate coding in hippocampal place cells: Theoretical significance and relationship to entorhinal grid cells. *Hippocampus*, *15*, 853–866.

O'Keefe, J., & Conway, D. H. (1978). Hippocampal place units in the freely moving rat: Why they fire where they fire. *Exp. Brain Res.*, *31*(4), 573–590.

O'Keefe, J., & Nadel, L. (1978). *The hippocampus as a cognitive map*. Oxford, UK: Oxford University Press.

O'Keefe, J., & Speakman, A. (1987). Single unit activity in the rat hippocampus during a spatial memory task. *Exp. Brain Res., 68*(1), 1–27.

Ono, T., Nakamura, K., Fukuda, M., & Tamura, R. (1991). Place recognition responses of neurons in monkey hippocampus. *Neurosci. Lett., 121*(1–2), 194–198.

Packard, M. G., & McGaugh, J. L. (1992). Double dissociation of fornix and caudate nucleus lesions on acquisition of two water maze tasks: Further evidence for multiple memory systems. *Behav. Neurosci., 106*(3), 439–446.

Packard, M. G., & McGaugh, J. L. (1996). Inactivation of hippocampus or caudate nucleus with lidocaine differentially affects expression of place and response learning. *Neurobiol. Learn. Mem., 65*(1), 65–72.

Pearce, J. M., Graham, M., Good, M. A., Jones, P. M., & McGregor, A. (2006). Potentiation, overshadowing, and blocking of spatial learning based on the shape of the environment. *J. Exp. Psychol. Anim. Behav. Process, 32*(3), 201–214.

Pearce, J. M., Roberts, A. D., & Good, M. (1998). Hippocampal lesions disrupt navigation based on cognitive maps but not heading vectors. *Nature, 396*(6706), 75–77.

Pessiglione, M., Seymour, B., Flandin, G., Dolan, R. J., & Frith, C. D. (2006). Dopamine-dependent prediction errors underpin reward-seeking behaviour in humans. *Nature, 442*(7106), 1042–1045.

Piaget, J., & Inhelder, B. (1956). *The child's conception of space*. London: Routledge.

Pico, R. M., Gerbrandt, L. K., Pondel, M., & Ivy, G. (1985). During stepwise cue deletion, rat place behaviors correlate with place unit responses. *Brain Res., 330*(2), 369–372.

Poldrack, R. A., Clark, J., Pare-Blagoev, E. J., Shohamy, D., Creso, M. J., et al. (2001). Interactive memory systems in the human brain. *Nature, 414*(6863), 546–550.

Pouget, A., & Sejnowski, T. J. (1997). A new view of hemineglect based on the response properties of parietal neurones. *Philos. Trans. R. Soc. Lond B Biol. Sci., 352*(1360), 1449–1459.

Redgrave, P., & Gurney, K. (2006). The short-latency dopamine signal: A role in discovering novel actions? *Nat. Rev. Neurosci., 7*(12), 967–975.

Rescorla, R. A., & Wagner, A. R. (1972). A theory of Pavlovian conditioning: Variations in the effectiveness of reinforcement and non-reinforcement. In A. H. Black & W. F. Prokasy (Eds.), *Classical conditioning II. Current research and theory* (pp. 64–99). New York: Appleton-Century-Crofts.

Rieser, J. J. (1989). Access to knowledge of spatial structure at novel points of observation. *J. Exp. Psychol.-Learn. Mem. Cogn., 15*(6), 1157–1165.

Ross, J., Morrone, M. C., Goldberg, M. E., & Burr, D. C. (2001). Changes in visual perception at the time of saccades. *Trends Neurosci, 24*(2), 113–121.

Rugg, M. D., & Yonelinas, A. P. (2003). Human recognition memory: A cognitive neuroscience perspective. *Trends Cogn. Sci., 7*(7), 313–319.

Salinas, E., & Abbott, L. F. (1995). Transfer of coded information from sensory to motor networks. *J. Neurosci., 15*(10), 6461–6474.

Samsonovich, A., & McNaughton, B. L. (1997). Path integration and cognitive mapping in a continuous attractor neural network model. *J. Neurosci., 17*(15), 5900–5920.

Sargolini, F., Fyhn, M., Hafting, T., McNaughton, B. L., Witter, M. P., et al. (2006). Conjunctive representation of position, direction, and velocity in entorhinal cortex. *Science, 312*(5774), 758–762.

Schmidt, T., & Lee, E. Y. (2006). Spatial memory organized by environmental geometry. *Spatial Cognition & Computation, 6*(4), 347–369.

Schultz, W. (2002). Getting formal with dopamine and reward. *Neuron, 36*(2), 241–263.

Scoville, W. B., & Milner, B. (1957). Loss of recent memory after bilateral hippocampal lesions. *J. Neurol. Neurosurg. Psychiatry, 20*, 11–21.

Shelton, A. L., & McNamara, T. P. (1997). Multiple views of spatial memory. *Psychon. Bull. Rev., 4*(1), 102–106.

Shrager, Y., Bayley, P. J., Bontempi, B., Hopkins, R. O., & Squire, L. R. (2007). Spatial memory and the human hippocampus. *Proc. Natl. Acad. Sci. U.S.A., 104*(8), 2961–2966.

Simons, D. J., & Wang, R. F. (1998). Perceiving real-world viewpoint changes. *Psychological Science, 9*, 315–320.

Snyder, L. H., Grieve, K. L., Brotchie, P., & Andersen, R. A. (1998). Separate body- and world-referenced representations of visual space in parietal cortex. *Nature, 394*(6696), 887–891.

Sovrano, V. A., & Vallortigara, G. (2006). Dissecting the geometric module: A sense linkage for metric and landmark information in animals' spatial reorientation. *Psychological Science, 17*(7), 616–621.

Spiers, H. J., Burgess, N., Hartley, T., Vargha-Khadem, F., & O'Keefe, J. (2001a). Bilateral hippocampal pathology impairs topographical and episodic memory but not visual pattern matching. *Hippocampus, 11*, 715–725.

Spiers, H. J., Burgess, N., Maguire, E. A., Baxendale, S. A., Hartley, T., et al. (2001b). Unilateral temporal lobectomy patients show lateralised topographical and episodic memory deficits in a virtual town. *Brain, 124*, 2476–2489.

Spiers, H. J., & Maguire, E. A. (2007). A navigational guidance system in the human brain. *Hippocampus, 17*(8), 618–626.

Squire, L. R., & Zola-Morgan, S. (1991). The medial temporal lobe memory system. *Science, 253*(5026), 1380–1386.

Sutton, R. S., & Barto, A. G. (1988). *Reinforcement learning: An introduction*. Cambridge, MA: MIT Press.

Taube, J. S. (1998). Head direction cells and the neuropsychological basis for a sense of direction. *Prog. Neurobiol., 55*, 225–256.

Tolman, E. C. (1948). Cognitive maps in rats and men. *Psychol. Rev., 55*, 189–208.

Tulving, E. (1983). *Elements of episodic memory*. Oxford, UK: Clarendon Press.

Tulving, E. (2001). Episodic memory and common sense: How far apart? *Philos. Trans. R. Soc. Lond. B Biol. Sci., 356*(1413), 1505–1515.

Vallortigara, G., Zanforlin, M., & Pasti, G. (1990). Geometric modules in animals' spatial representations: A test with chicks (Gallus gallus domesticus). *J. Comp. Psychol., 104*(3), 248–254.

Voermans, N. C., Petersson, K. M., Daudey, L., Weber, B., Van Spaendonck, K. P., et al. (2004). Interaction between the human hippocampus and the caudate nucleus during route recognition. *Neuron, 43*(3), 427–435.

von Helmholtz, H. (1866). *Handbuch der physiologischen optik.* Hamburg, Germany: Leopold Voss.

Waelti, P., Dickinson, A., & Schultz, W. (2001). Dopamine responses comply with basic assumptions of formal learning theory. *Nature, 412*(6842), 43–48.

Waller, D., & Hodgson, E. (2006). Transient and enduring spatial representations under disorientation and self-rotation. *J. Exp. Psychol. Learn Mem. Cogn., 32*(4), 867–882.

Wang, R. F., & Simons, D. J. (1999). Active and passive scene recognition across views. *Cognition, 70*(2), 191–210.

Wang, R. F., & Spelke, E. (2000). Updating egocentric representations in human navigation. *Cognition, 77*, 215–250.

Wang, R. F., & Spelke, E. S. (2002). Human spatial representation: Insights from animals. *Trends Cogn. Sci., 6*(9), 376–382.

White, N. M., & McDonald, R. J. (2002). Multiple parallel memory systems in the brain of the rat. *Neurobiol. Learn Mem., 77*(2), 125–184.

Wilton, L. A., Baird, A. L., Muir, J. L., Honey, R. C., & Aggleton, J. P. (2001). Loss of the thalamic nuclei for "head direction" impairs performance on spatial memory tasks in rats. *Behav. Neurosci., 115*(4), 861–869.

Wolbers, T., & Buchel, C. (2005). Dissociable retrosplenial and hippocampal contributions to successful formation of survey representations. *J. Neurosci., 25*(13), 3333–3340.

Wolbers, T., Wiener, J. M., Mallot, H. A., & Buchel, C. (2007). Differential recruitment of the hippocampus, medial prefrontal cortex, and the human motion complex during path integration in humans. *J. Neurosci., 27*(35), 9408–9416.

Wraga, M., Creem, S. H., & Proffitt, D. R. (2000). Updating displays after imagined object and viewer rotations. *J. Exp. Psychol. Learn. Mem. Cogn., 26*(1), 151–168.

Yin, H. H., & Knowlton, B. J. (2006). The role of the basal ganglia in habit formation. *Nat. Rev. Neurosci., 7*(6), 464–476.

Zhang, K. (1996). Representation of spatial orientation by the intrinsic dynamics of the head-direction cell ensemble: A theory. *J. Neurosci., 16*(6), 2112–2126.

Zipser, D., & Andersen, R. A. (1988). A back-propagation programmed network that simulates response properties of a subset of posterior parietal neurons. *Nature, 331*(6158), 679–684.

Multisensory-based Approach to the Recovery of Unisensory Deficit

ELISABETTA LÀDAVAS

Dipartimento di Psicologia, Università di Bologna, Bologna, Italy
Centro Studi e Ricerche in Neuroscienze Cognitive, Cesena, Italy

This chapter reviews several highly convergent behavioral findings that provide strong evidence for the existence of multimodal integration systems subserving spatial representation in humans. These systems generally function through the multisensory coding of visuoauditory and visuotactile events but vary in their specific functional and anatomical characteristics. The chapter will also consider the adaptive advantages of multisensory integration systems; these systems might modulate the level of activation in cortical areas in short- and long-term ways, thereby providing a mechanism for permanent recovery from sensory and spatial deficits.

Key words: multisensory integration; spatial orienting; neurorehabilitation

Introduction

Perception of the external world often depends on integrating different sensory information. When the primary modality of information is weak—for example, when viewing a dimly lit scene or when listening to speech in a noisy environment—we can benefit from the information derived from our other senses. Indeed, we typically receive a rich and simultaneous flow of information from all our senses, so our comprehension of objects in the world is always the product of an integrated, multisensory perception. This integration of multiple sensory cues provides animals with enormous response flexibility, so that their reaction to the presence of one stimulus can be altered by the presence of another. Compelling evidence now exists that information represented in each of the primary sensory systems—visual, auditory, somatosensory, and olfactory—is highly susceptible to influence from the other senses (Calvert et al. 2004).

Although the prevailing view is that modality-specific cortical areas are unaffected by other sensory inputs, a growing body of evidence now suggests that their exclusivity may have been overestimated (Schroeder & Foxe 2004; Cohen & Andersen 2004; Calvert & Lewis 2004). Beyond the principal modality-specific regions, many areas outside the primary projection pathways are also known to contain both neurons receptive to one sensory modality and neurons that receive converging inputs from multiple modalities; thus, both primary regions and their downstream targets can be substantially multisensory.

Multisensory integration can be clearly beneficial—for example, in producing response enhancement, when the signal from a single modality is weak, or when a sensory system is deprived of its modality-specific brain area (Calvert et al. 2004). Multisensory areas normally associated with both the deprived and nondeprived senses will continue to respond to stimuli of the intact sense, preventing total stimulus deprivation in those areas. Indeed, this may allow multisensory cells to retain their responsiveness to cross-modal stimuli. This ensures that the additional information provided by cross-modal stimuli can be used to maximum advantage when the information provided by one modality is weak.

In animal studies, the effectiveness of unimodal signals, at the single-unit level, is a major determinant of the advantage resulting from some form of multisensory integration (Stein & Meredith 1993). For example, the electrophysiological responses of multisensory cells in the superior colliculus of nonhuman mammals, which can be considered the major neural structure for integrative spatial processing (Stein et al. 2004), show proportionately greater enhancement with progressively less effective (e.g., lower intensity) stimuli, a phenomenon called the inverse effectiveness rule. Thus, the loss of input to one sensory system can enable cross-modal activation in multimodal brain structures. As a consequence, the activation of multisensory systems might represent the neural correlate of sensory compensation after damage to one sensory system. For

---

Address for correspondence: Elisabetta Làdavas, PhD, Dipartimento di Psicologia, Viale Berti Pichat 5, 40127 Bologna, Italy.
elisabetta.ladavas@unibo.it

example, an undetectable visual stimuli can be detected by presenting an auditory stimulus.

This article will develop this hypothesis by considering the results of studies on normal subjects, in whom unimodal sensory information has been rendered ineffective at a perceptual level, and on clinical subjects, in whom unimodal sensory information has been damaged by a cerebral lesion. In the first part, I will provide evidence of the existence in humans of integrated visuoauditory systems, and I will examine the relevance of those systems for the temporary recovery from visual and auditory deficits; multisensory information can potentially enable patients with a sensory deficit to detect "bimodal" stimuli for which one sensory component has been damaged by the lesion. Then, I will present findings in humans supporting the pivotal role of the superior colliculus in mediating multisensory spatial integration when making spatial orienting responses. I will also discuss the important adaptive role of multisensory integration, including a discussion of how multisensory systems might modulate the level of activation in cortical areas in a long-lasting way, ultimately offering a unique opportunity for permanent recovery from sensory and spatial deficits. For instance, I will show how a systematic audiovisual stimulation of the visual field, activating multisensory neurons in the superior colliculus (SC), might affect orientation toward the blind hemifield and improve oculomotor exploration with long-lasting effects.

Finally, in the second part of the article, I will present evidence supporting the notion that visual information related to the body affects tactile sensation. The mechanism underlying this effect is functionally different from the previous one, but it is nevertheless important for showing the relevance of multisensory information on normal and impaired behavior and on rehabilitation of sensory deficits. For visuotactile interaction related to the body, visual information can be used to boost sensation through the modulation of responses in primary somatosensory cortex (SI) (Taylor-Clarke et al. 2002; Fiorio & Haggard 2005). I will discuss how the effect of this visuotactile integration might facilitate recovery from tactile deficits in patients with lesions of the somatosensory cortices.

An Integrated Visuoauditory System Responsible for Spatial Orienting

Cross-modal Visual Enhancement: The Influence of Audition on Visual Detection

The neurophysiological basis of visual enhancement through multisensory integrative processing was first demonstrated by Stein et al. (Stein & Meredith 1993) in nonhuman primates. This type of enhancement of visual processing is based on an important and adaptive property of multisensory integration: The secondary auditory input will enhance the multisensory response to unseen primary visual inputs because multisensory interaction is modulated by the efficacy of the primary unimodal stimuli. Whereas the pairing of weakly effective stimuli results in a vigorous enhancement of the multisensory neuronal activity, the combination of highly effective stimuli results in little increase in the neural response (a phenomenon called the *inverse effectiveness rule*). Multisensory enhancement in space is also determined by the *spatial* and *temporal* characteristics of the stimuli. When multiple sensory cues are provided by the same event, those cues will be in temporal and spatial proximity, and their integration can be of substantial value in enhancing detection, identification, and orientation. By manipulating these spatial and temporal parameters, a given combination of stimuli (e.g., visual and auditory) can produce either response enhancement or depression in the same neurons (Stein & Meredith 1993). According to the spatial principle governing this type of multisensory integration (the *spatial rule*), visual and auditory stimuli originating from the same position in space will fall within the excitatory receptive fields of a visuoauditory multisensory neuron. The physiological result of this pairing is an enhancement in the multisensory neuron's response. The maximum angular distance that can separate paired visual and auditory stimuli while still producing a facilitating effect depends on the size of the visual and auditory receptive fields. Auditory receptive fields are larger than visual receptive fields (Knudsen 1982; King & Hutchings 1987), so any auditory stimulus will excite neurons over a large spatial region, including regions excited by the paired visual stimulus. If a sound comes from a spatial position outside the excitatory receptive field of a bimodal neuron, that neuron's response to the paired visual stimulus is no longer enhanced.

A second crucial aspect of multisensory integration concerns the relative timing of the two sensory events (the *temporal rule*). Maximal multisensory interactions are achieved when the peak activities of the unimodal discharge trains overlap. This situation is usually achieved when stimuli are presented simultaneously, although a temporal window for multisensory interactions allows for small temporal discrepancies between stimuli.

The evidence that multisensory systems obey the three rules highlighted so far (the inverse effectiveness rule, the spatial rule, and the temporal rule) comes

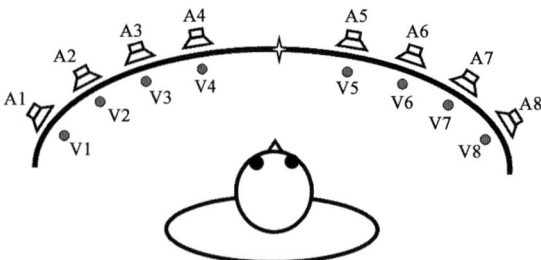

FIGURE 1. Experimental apparatus. Bird's eye schematic view of the position of loudspeakers and light displays.

mainly from animal studies. Whether systems with those particular characteristics are present in humans remains an open question. That question has been addressed in the last year in our laboratory, and here I will present the results of studies both in normal subjects and in patients suffering visual disorders due to cortical lesions. The logic underlying these studies is the following: The existence of this specific multisensory system in humans can be proved by showing an amelioration on visual detection when the audiovisual (AV) stimuli are presented according to the rules highlighted above. That is, visual detectability should be maximized when two stimuli, of which at least one is weak, are presented at the same position and time.

Studies on Normal Subjects

To investigate whether the integrative effects observed in SC in animals could be found in humans at a level of behavioral responses, our laboratory conducted an experiment using signal detection measures and visual masking to degrade visual stimuli beyond the threshold for unimodal detection (Frassinetti et al. 2002).

Subjects fixated on a central point and were asked to detect masked visual targets displayed horizontally at 8°, 24°, 40° and 56°, in both the left and right visual fields (FIG. 1).

The task was performed either in a unimodal condition (i.e., only visual or auditory stimuli were presented) or in one of two cross-modal conditions (i.e., a sound was presented together with the visual target). In the cross-modal conditions, sounds could be presented either at the same spatial position as the visual target (the spatially coincident cross-modal condition) or at one of the remaining seven spatial positions (the spatially disparate cross-modal conditions). Moreover, to determine the effect of the temporal proximity on auditory–visual interaction, the acoustic and the visual stimuli could either be presented simultaneously or the acoustic stimulus could precede the visual stimulus by 500 ms. The subjects were instructed to ignore the auditory cue, which was not predictive of the visual location, and to indicate the presence of the visual target by pressing a button.

The results show that auditory stimuli may enhance the efficiency of the visual system in a difficult detection task: Perceptual sensitivity (d') to subthreshold masked visual stimuli, reflecting subject's accuracy to discern a sensory event from its background (perceptual level), was indeed improved by concurrent acoustic stimuli. No difference was found on the β parameter, reflecting the subject's decision criterion of response (decision level). Moreover, perceptual sensitivity to the visual stimulus increased when temporally overlapping visual and acoustic stimuli were presented in the same rather than different spatial positions. Thus, when multiple weak sensory cues are provided by the same event, integration can be of substantial value in enhancing detection and orientation.

Studies on Patients with Visual Deficits

In another study (Frassinetti et al. 2005), we used a similar paradigm to investigate cross-modal audio–visual integration in patients with visual impairments due either to a visual field deficit (e.g., hemianopia) or to a visuospatial attentional deficit (e.g., neglect). These patients usually fail to report, respond, or orient to visual stimuli presented contralaterally to the lesioned hemisphere (Halligan et al. 2003).

The results of this study showed that when a sound was associated with a visual stimulus, patients' ability to consciously perceive the visual stimuli in their blind or neglected fields increased. Moreover, the sound improved the detection of the visual target only when it was presented in the same spatial position as the visual target, but not when there was a spatial disparity between the stimuli (i.e., 16° and 32° [FIG. 2]).

These results are in accordance with the functional characteristics of multisensory neurons in the SC—multisensory responses are enhanced only when stimuli from different sensory modalities are spatially coincident.

Another interesting finding of this study was the correlation between multisensory integration and unimodal visual impairment. Patients exhibited multisensory enhancement when detection of the visual stimulus alone was difficult, as evidenced by the negative correlation between patients' performance in the unimodal visual condition and the magnitude of multisensory enhancement. That is, the improvement observed in the cross-modal spatially aligned condition was greater when the visual stimuli in the unimodal condition were less effective.

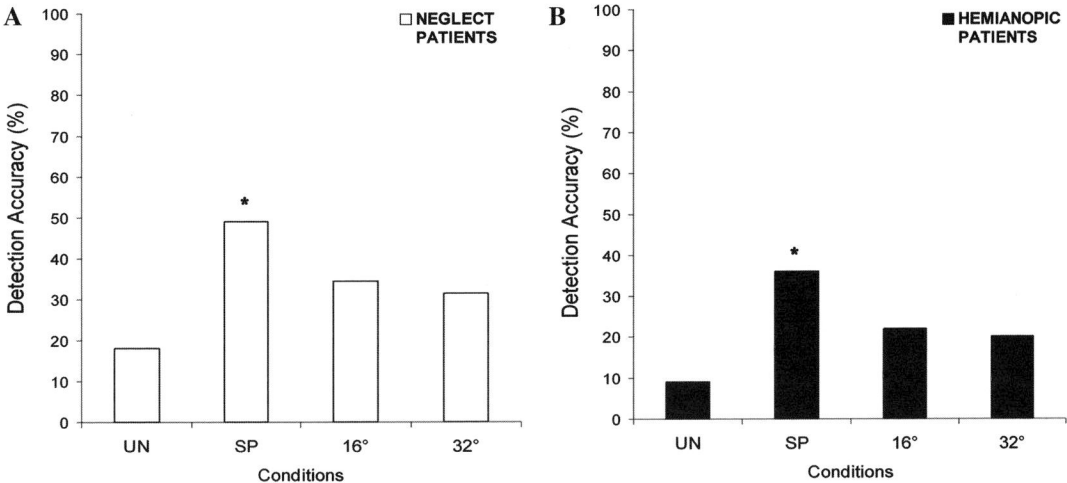

FIGURE 2. Mean percentage of correct visual detection in neglect **(A)** and hemianopic **(B)** patients for unimodal visual condition (UN) and cross-modal visual–auditory conditions. Auditory stimulus was presented either in the same position (SP) or at a disparity of 16° or 32° from the visual stimulus. Asterisks indicate statistically significant pairwise comparisons between unimodal and cross-modal conditions. *, $P < .01$.

This behavioral feature of cross-modal processing in humans appears to have parallels in the electrophysiological response properties of multisensory cells in the SC of nonhuman mammals (i.e., the inverse effectiveness rule).

Cross-modal Auditory Localization: Influence of Vision on Auditory Localization

So far, this article examined the effects of audition on vision; now I will review evidence for the influence of vision on audition both in normal subjects (Bolognini et al. in press) and in patients with auditory localization deficits (Bolognini et al. 2005a). These studies demonstrate that visual cues can affect auditory processing in a spatially and temporally specific way.

Normal Subjects

Bolognini et al. (in press) demonstrated the powerful effect of multisensory integration in maximizing sensitivity to sensory events by examining the effects of multisensory integration on auditory localization in healthy human subjects. Our specific objective was to test whether the relative intensity and location of a seemingly irrelevant visual stimulus would influence auditory localization in accordance with the inverse effectiveness and spatial rules of multisensory integration (Stein & Meredith 1993).

Subjects were asked to localize a sound during trials in which a neutral visual stimulus was presented either at or above threshold. In both types of trials, the spatial disparity between the visual and auditory stimuli was systematically varied. The results reveal that stimulus salience is a critical factor in determining the effect of a neutral visual cue on auditory localization. Visual capture, and hence perceptual translocation of the auditory stimulus, occurred when the visual stimulus was suprathreshold, regardless of its location. However, this was not the case when the visual stimulus was at threshold. In those trials, the influence of the visual cue was apparent only when the two cues were spatially coincident and resulted in an enhancement of stimulus localization.

The visual capture, observable when the two stimuli are well detected by the two sensory (visual and auditory) systems, is also consistent with the parallels among perspectives guiding our understanding of visual dominance. For example, Heron et al. (2004) proposed that when the nervous system deems visual information most reliable, as is generally the case in normal conditions, vision dominates auditory localization judgments. As a consequence, we observe a perceptual translocation of the auditory stimulus regardless of its location. Instead, multisensory integration occurs when at least one of the two modalities is weak. Here we observed an integration between the two modalities, and the effects are following the temporal and the spatial rules governing multisensory integration in the SC.

These data suggest that the brain uses multiple strategies to integrate multisensory information, depending on the salience of the stimulus. A likely explanation of these differences is that enhancement and visual bias depend on different neural pathways, with the former dependent on circuits involving the SC

(Leh et al. 2006), a structure involved in the integration of cues from multiple senses to facilitate orientation/localization (Stein & Meredith 1993), and the latter dependent on geniculostriate circuits that facilitate more detailed analyses of the visual scene (for more details, see the next section).

Patients with Auditory Localization Deficits

Patients with lesions in the right hemisphere often exhibit deficits in auditory representations of space (Clarke et al. 2000; Pavani et al. 2003). Several studies have reported selective mislocalization within the hemispace contralateral to the brain lesion, after left hemispheric lesions (Pinek & Bouchon 1992), or within the whole auditory field after unilateral right brain lesion (Bisiach et al. 1984).

We explored a possible beneficial effect of the multisensory integration system in improving auditory localization performance in a patient with a right hemispheric lesion, without neglect, and a subsequent localization deficit across her whole auditory field (Bolognini et al. 2005a). In this study, the patient was asked to verbally indicate the spatial position where a sound was presented. The task was performed in either a unisensory condition (i.e., only sounds were presented) or in multisensory conditions (i.e., a visual stimulus was presented simultaneous with the auditory target). In the multisensory conditions, the visual cue was presented either at the same spatial position as the sound or at 16° or 32° nasally or temporally from the auditory target.

The results of this study clearly show that a visual cue, spatially and temporally coincident with a sound, improves auditory localization in a patient with a selective deficit in auditory localization (FIG. 3).

Because of the absence of significant differences between the percentages of sound displacement in the unisensory auditory condition and those in the multisensory spatially disparate conditions, the patient's improvement in sound localization cannot be ascribed to a simple "visual capture" of the sound location (Bertelson & Aschersleben 1998). We observed an increase in correct responses only in the spatially coincident cross-modal conditions, without significant improvement in the spatially disparate cross-modal conditions, a result in direct accordance with the spatial and temporal rules of multisensory integration in the SC.

Another example of the important adaptive role of multisensory integration, that is, the ability to use information deriving from other multisensory systems to detect the presence of a stimuli, can be found in a recent study (Leo, Bolognini, et al. in press) on hemianopic patients.

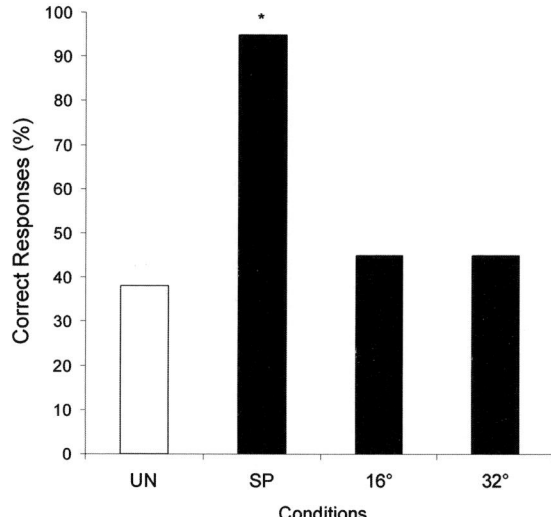

FIGURE 3. Mean percentage of correct responses in auditory localization task. White bars, unimodal auditory condition (UN); black bars, cross-modal conditions (auditory stimulus was presented either in the same position [SP] or at a disparity of 16° or 32° from the visual stimulus). Asterisks indicate statistically significant pairwise comparisons between unimodal and cross-modal conditions. *, $P < .0002$.

Patients with Visual Field Deficits

Some patients with lesions in the primary visual cortex (V1) demonstrate residual visual capacity without conscious perceptual awareness, a phenomenon known as "blindsight" (Ro et al. 2004; Rafal et al. 1990). Blindsight is an example of implicit processing in the absence of explicit knowledge (Weiskrantz 1996). Given the involvement of the midbrain in some aspects of blindsight (Weiskrantz 1996), we asked whether the SC might subserve not only covert processing within the visual modality but also cross-modal covert processing in hemianopia.

We examined cross-modal localization in hemianopic patients by comparing the effects of visual stimuli presented in the blind and the normal hemifields on these patients' ability to locate hard-to-localize sounds. Auditory targets were presented alone (unimodal condition) or with a visual stimulus (cross-modal condition) in either hemifield and at various spatial (0°, 16°, 32°) and temporal (0 ms, 500 ms) disparities.

The results of this study showed that visual information in the blind hemifield of hemianopic patients can significantly improve their auditory localization performance but can do so critically only when the two stimuli are presented in the same position and time. Surprisingly, this multisensory benefit was as great as it was in their intact hemifield. Nevertheless, patients remained unaware of the presence of the visual stimulus and of its effects on their auditory responses. Despite the retention of this important visual–auditory integration in the contralesional hemifield, the full range of multisensory interactions was not retained. In particular, the visual capture that normally occurs with spatially disparate cross-modal stimuli was lost. Though evident in the intact hemifield, there was no evidence that the auditory stimulus was perceptually translocated by a visual stimulus in the damaged hemifield. These observations suggest that the neural circuitry underlying the visual influences on auditory localization differs depending on whether the stimuli are likely to be derived from the same event (i.e., are spatially coincident) or from different events. Apparently, the damaged visual cortices were critical for the latter but not for the former. This proposal is indeed supported by a recent finding showing that the ventriloquism illusion is directly related to the visual influences on the auditory cortex responses to sound (Bonath et al. 2007). The absence of a visual bias in the hemianopic field when the two stimuli are spatially separated supports the key role of the visual cortex for such an effect; when the visual cortex has been damaged, no visual bias is observed (see also a related study by Phan et al. 2000).

In contrast, the lesion of the visual cortex does not prevent the integration of the two auditory and visual stimuli when they are simultaneously presented in the same spatial position. Instead, a temporal interval of 500 ms abolished the integration effect. On the basis of an analogous visual–auditory localization paradigm, neurophysiological findings in animals with reversible or permanent lesions of the association cortex support our results. The ability of SC neurons to integrate cross-modal inputs in cats involves descending inputs from specific regions of the association cortex (the anterior ectosylvian sulcus and rostral lateral suprasylvian sulcus) and not from primary or secondary cortices (Stein 2005). Presumably, whatever the homologous regions are in humans, they would be distant from the hemianopia-inducing lesions in the patients studied here. Jiang and coworkers (Jiang et al. 2002; Jiang & Stein 2003) suggest that although the enhancement of spatially coincident visual–auditory stimuli is eliminated in cats by anterior ectosylvian sulcus and rostral lateral suprasylvian sulcus lesions, the depression normally induced by disparate visual–auditory stimuli is degraded only because these competitive or depressive SC functions involve contributions from other brain areas. Thus, a likely interpretation of our results is that the enhancement of the auditory localization in the blind field reflects the activation of the extrageniculate pathway, leading directly from the retina to the SC, a structure that plays an important role in orientation, localization behaviors, and multisensory integration (Stein & Meredith 1993).

Multisensory Integration and the SC

In recent years, comparative research has identified several brain structures that receive and combine information from different modalities, including the SC (Stein & Meredith 1993; Kadunce et al. 2001). However, evidence supporting the role of the SC comes mainly from lesion studies in animals, and, more compellingly, from single-unit recordings in the cat (Stein & Meredith 1993; Burnett et al. 2007). The questions of whether this region is necessary for the observed multisensory integration behaviors in humans, and whether these effects critically depend on other multisensory areas of the brain, remain open. Consistent with this latter possibility, neuroimaging studies have revealed several cortical areas (among others, the insula, the superior temporal sulcus, the intraparietal sulcus, and several frontal regions; Calvert 2001; Calvert & Thesen 2004; Macaluso & Driver 2005) that are involved in the detection and integration of multisensory stimuli based on their shared spatial location, thereby suggesting that this process does not necessarily involve the SC.

However, physiological evidence in the cat indicates that multisensory integration in cortical association areas (i.e., the anterior ectosylvian fissure and the lateral sulcus) is less restrained by the precise temporal and spatial congruency of the multisensory stimuli (Wallace et al. 1992) and therefore may not directly mediate the behavioral consequences of multisensory integration.

In our laboratory, we recently tested the hypothesis that multisensory AV spatial integration is mediated by the SC in healthy adults (Leo, Bertini, et al. in press). We exploited the fact that neurophysiological studies have reported that short-wave S cones in the retina send few or no projections to the SC (Marrocco & Li 1977; Sumner et al. 2004). As well, S-cone stimuli cannot reach the SC via corticotectal projections (i.e., projections running from the visual cortex to the SC) because S-cone stimuli are invisible also to the magnocellular pathway, which feeds these projections. Therefore, stimuli uniquely detected by S cones should remain invisible to the SC. If the SC is a critical neural substrate for mediating multisensory spatial integration, then we predicted an effect of spatial congruency (i.e., faster response times [RTs] for spatially coincident than for spatially disparate audiovisual stimuli) when using bimodal stimulation comprising a red monochromatic stimulus (i.e.,

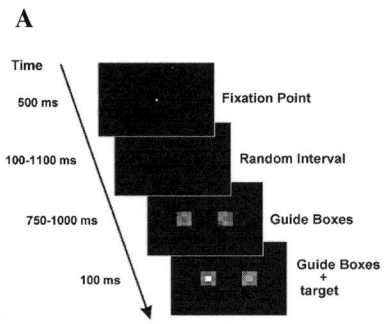 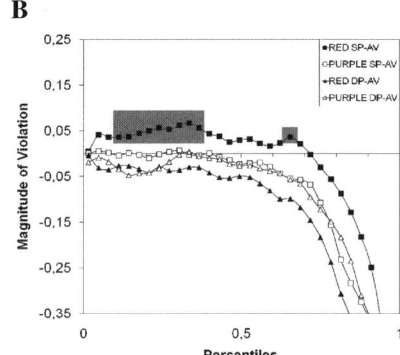

FIGURE 4. **(A)** Schematic diagram of a typical trial requiring a spatial orienting response. The white square in the center of the guide box represents the visual target. Loudspeakers (not reported in the figure) were placed immediately below the guide boxes. **(B)** Violation of the race inequality test for the four bimodal AV conditions. Gray rectangles mark the areas in which the violation is statistically significantly different from zero, as assessed by one-sample t test.

a stimulus visible to the SC) and a concurrent auditory stimulus, presented on the same or opposite side as the visual stimulus. Conversely, multisensory spatial integration was not expected when using bimodal stimulation comprising a purple monochromatic stimulus (i.e., a stimulus invisible to the SC) accompanied by a spatially congruent or incongruent auditory stimulus.

To provide evidence for multisensory spatial integration, we used a "redundant signals" paradigm for simple reaction time, in which the observer must initiate a response as quickly as possible after the detection of any stimulus onset (auditory, visual, or bimodal audiovisual; FIG. 4A). Since the pioneering study by Todd (Todd 1912), it has been known that responses to bimodal stimuli are faster, on average, than responses to unimodal ones. This phenomenon is known as the redundant target effect (RTE), and the difference in response time (RT) between single and double targets is called the redundancy gain. Two alternative models have been suggested to explain the RTE: the *race model* (*statistical facilitation*) and the *neural coactivation model*. According to the race model, both elements of a bimodal stimulus are processed by independent channels, and the one that reaches the output stage first triggers the response; this model suggests that RTE is generated by statistical facilitation. If the limit predicted by the race model inequality is violated, then a statistical facilitation explanation is no longer tenable, and the RTE can be ascribed to a mechanism that is commonly referred to as *neural coactivation*. This mechanism would transform the separate sensory inputs by a nonlinear summation into an integrated product (i.e., multisensory integration).

Using this model, we recently showed a reliable RTE in all AV conditions and, more interestingly, we demonstrated that responses in the multisensory conditions varied as a function of the color of visual stimuli. When red, long-wavelength stimuli were used, RTs to spatially coincident AV stimuli were significantly faster than RTs to the spatially disparate AV stimuli. In striking contrast, when purple, short-wavelength stimuli were used, no significant RT difference was evident between coincident and disparate audiovisual conditions. This finding demonstrates a specific spatial audiovisual integration effect for red but not for purple visual stimuli.

Moreover, a second analysis based on Miller's race inequality model (Miller 1982) showed a significant violation of the race model only for the long wavelength, spatially coincident condition; therefore, the RTE found under other conditions can be explained simply in terms of statistical facilitation (FIG. 4B).

In summary, the neural coactivation mechanism can be observed only when two conditions are satisfied: First, visual information must reach the SC (as occurs with red, long-wavelength visual stimuli); second, concurrent auditory and visual stimuli must be presented in the same spatial position. Indeed, the violation of the race model occurred only when auditory stimuli were accompanied by red, spatially congruent visual stimuli. These findings are entirely consistent with previously reported neurophysiological findings. and it is therefore justified to conclude that nonlinear, multisensory integration for spatial orienting cannot be reliably found with visual inputs to which the SC is blind.

Some authors (Holmes & Spence 2005) have questioned the validity of Stein's model because some examples of the multisensory integration, such as the McGurk illusion, are unaffected by the relative locations of visual and auditory signals. However, there is

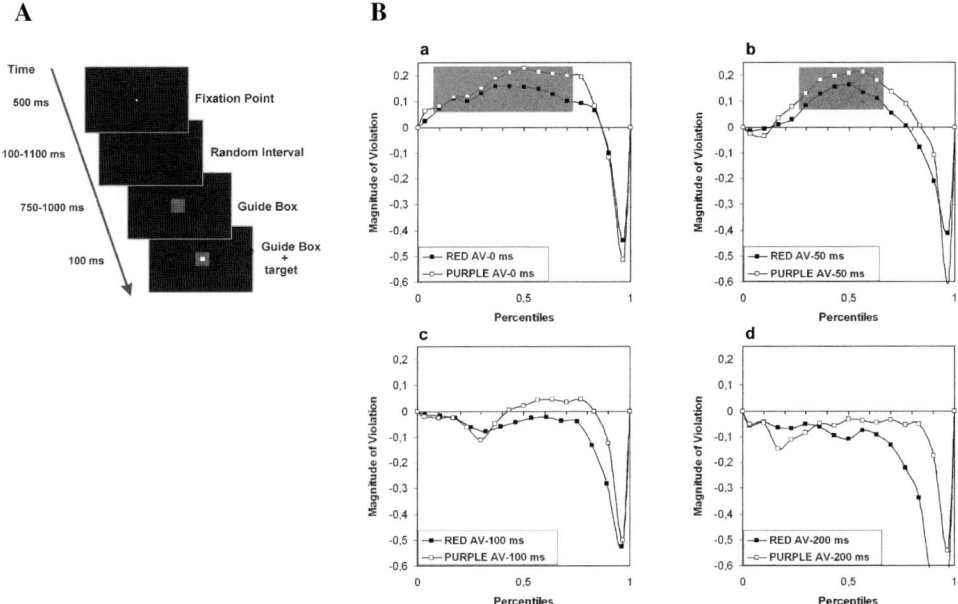

FIGURE 5. (A) Schematic diagram of a typical trial when the stimuli are presented at fixation. The white square in the center of the guide box represents the visual target. Loudspeaker (not reported in the figure) was placed immediately below the guide box. **(B)** Violation of the race inequality test for the eight bimodal AV conditions. Gray rectangles in **A** and **B** mark the areas in which the violation is statistically significantly different from zero, as assessed by one-sample *t* test.

no reason to expect an activation of SC in tasks that do not require an overt or covert orienting response. Several neurophysiological studies in both animals and humans support the hypothesis that the SC is critically involved in coding spatial locations for guiding saccades and shifts of attention (Kustov & Robinson 1996; Ignashchenkova et al. 2004).

To clarify this position, we tested in the same study whether SC involvement in multisensory integration strictly depends on whether the perceptual task requires spatial orienting responses. Participants responded to both unimodal and bimodal audiovisual stimuli presented at fixation (FIG. 5A). If the SC integrates multisensory stimuli for guiding gaze or attention shifts across space, then presenting AV stimuli at fixation should reduce the contribution of the SC to the task, because orienting responses are minimized. Therefore, the different effects of visual stimuli, visible or invisible to the SC, should be significantly reduced or abolished. To measure multisensory integration, bimodal AV stimuli either occurred at the same time as, or at different time from, the auditory stimulus always preceding the visual one. Indeed, previous studies have shown that temporally coincident AV stimuli produce enhanced performance (faster RTs and increased perceptual sensitivity) relative to temporally disparate stimuli (Frassinetti et al. 2002).

The results of this latter study (Leo, Bertini, et al. in press) are perfectly consistent with this view. They demonstrate that when the reorienting of gaze or attention is not required, multisensory spatial integration can occur without direct access to the SC or to the magnocellular pathway (FIG. 5B). Although undetectable by the SC, short-wavelength visual stimuli are visible to several cortical areas with strong parvocellular inputs (Mullen et al. 2007), indicating that the AV integration effect observed at fixation, when the two sensory events are temporally coincident, may have a cortical origin, probably within cortical temporal areas (Miller & D'Esposito 2005).

Although our findings demonstrate that the SC is a critical neural substrate underlying multisensory spatial integration in humans, they do not rule out the possibility that other brain areas in the magnocellular system (including frontal or parietal eye fields, which may also be blind to short-wavelength stimuli) have a role in spatially synthesizing audiovisual stimuli. However, lesion studies in humans have shown that cortical damage separately affecting the frontotemporoparietal areas (in neglect patients) or the occipital areas (in hemianopic patients) does not alter the synthesis of spatially coincident audiovisual stimuli (Frassinetti et al. 2005). That finding indicates that these cortical areas may not be strictly necessary for the behavioral effects of multisensory spatial integration. However, a simultaneous lesion of areas involved in visuospatial attention (frontotemporoparietal areas) and areas involved in primary sensory visual processing (occipital areas) prevents cross-modal integration, demonstrating the influence of these cortical areas on the SC. In line with these results, evidence in the cat suggests that deactivation of the cortical association cortex eliminates the characteristic multisensory response enhancement in the SC (Jiang et al. 2007). Thus, although the SC is essential for the enhanced performance in response to spatially coincident multimodal stimuli (Leo, Bertini, et al. in press), it may also require modulatory influences from other cortical regions. More studies are needed to clarify the nature of the influence of cortical areas in modulating the activity of the SC in humans.

On the basis of the results discussed so far, multisensory integration might offer a unique approach for the stimulation of the SC, which is often spared in lesions causing neglect and hemianopia. Thus, systematic bimodal stimulation, affecting orientation toward the blind hemifield and modulating the processing of visual events, might improve visual exploration, possibly with long-lasting effects. A cross-modal training regimen might reinforce the innate ability of our brain to perceive multisensory events, an ability normally hidden when unimodal processing of the sensory events is sufficient for their perception.

Cognitive Neurorehabilitation: Cross-modal Stimulation as a Tool for Long-Lasting Amelioration of Hemianopia

On the basis of this body of research, we tried to take advantage of the AV integration system to rehabilitate patients with visual field defects (Bolognini et al. 2005b). We hypothesized that systematic AV stimulation of the visual field, activating multisensory neurons in the SC, affects orientation toward the blind hemifield and improves oculomotor exploration with long-lasting effects.

In this study, patients with chronic visual field defects were trained to detect the presence of visual targets that could be presented alone, that is, in a unisensory condition, or together with an acoustic stimulus, that is, multisensory conditions. In the multisensory conditions, the spatial disparity between the visual and the acoustic stimuli were systematically varied (between $0°$, $16°$, and $32°$). Patients underwent the treatment for 4 h daily, for nearly 2 weeks.

After the treatment, patients were assessed with a battery of tests that showed a progressive improvement in visual detection and an improvement in visual search time. These gains allowed patients to efficiently compensate for the loss of their vision. The improvement in patients' performance was highly consistent across all tests assessing visual exploration, both for accuracy and search times, as evidenced in some tests by nearly error-free performances and reduced visual scanning times after treatment. Moreover, the improvement in visual detection and exploration was stable at both the 1-month (Bolognini et al. 2005b) and 3-month (Passamonti et al. 2007) follow-up sessions. One important feature of this result was that the increased accuracy in the blind area was evident only when patients were allowed to use eye movements during visual detection. In contrast, either weak or no amelioration was found in the same tests when patients were instructed to keep their eye positions fixed.

The discrepancy between the two eye movement conditions suggests that the amelioration in visual perception induced by training is not due to an enlargement of the visual field but rather to an increase in the visual responsiveness of the oculomotor system, possibly mediated by the intact SC. The SC is an important oculomotor structure, involved in both the execution and initiation of saccades and in target selection (Krauzlis et al. 2004); moreover, because sensory maps within the SC are in register with premotor maps, multisensory information can be translated directly into an appropriate orientation response toward the blind hemifield. Indeed, studies of healthy subjects suggest that AV stimulation improves saccade accuracy and saccadic timing responses (Corneil et al. 2002).

To directly assess the effect of multisensory training on oculomotor scanning behavior, we studied the oculomotor responses during both a visual search task and a reading task both before and after an AV training regimen, in a group of 12 patients with chronic visual field defects (Passamonti et al. 2007). Eye movements were recorded using an infrared recording technique, with respect to a range of spatial and temporal variables. The results showed that patients' performance before the treatment was significantly different from that of healthy subjects in relation to fixation and saccade parameters: After the training, all patients demonstrated improvements in ocular exploration, characterized by fewer fixations and refixations (FIG. 6), quicker and larger saccades in the blind field, and reduced length in the scan path, reducing the total exploration time.

Similarly, reading measures were significantly improved by the training, with respect to the specific impairments observed in both left- and right-hemisphere–damaged patients. These findings provide evidence that AV integration training may encourage a more organized pattern of visual exploration because of implementing efficient oculomotor strategies. The

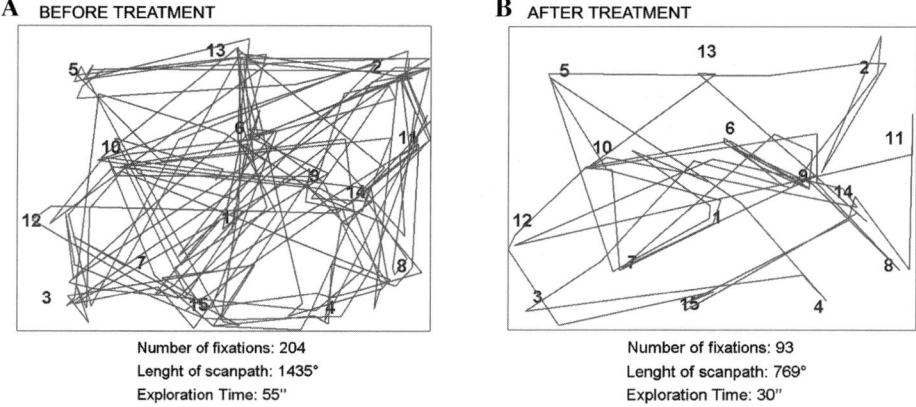

FIGURE 6. Oculomotor scanning patterns before **(A)** and after **(B)** the treatment in the visual search task.

most novel aspect of the AV training used in this study was that it was based on the innate ability to integrate information from different sensory modalities.

An Integrated Visual–Tactile System Responsible for the Enhancement of Somatosensory Processing

So far I have reviewed evidence showing the existence of an AV integration system and its relevance for the recovery of visual and auditory unisensory deficits. Here I will focus on how vision can influence primary levels of tactile processing and, in particular, on how visual information pertaining to the body affects tactile sensation.

Several lines of evidence suggest that visual and tactile information are integrated to affect primary tactile processing. First, viewing the body accelerates tactile processing. Tipper et al. (1998) showed that reaction times to tactile stimuli on the hand were faster when subjects could see their stimulated hand on a video monitor, even when the tactile stimuli themselves were invisible. Further studies have demonstrated that visual information related to the body also improves tactile acuity. Kennett et al. (2001) assessed tactile acuity on healthy participants' forearms with the two-point discrimination (2pd) threshold, administered while subjects viewed either their own forearms or a neutral object presented in the same spatial location or while they were blindfolded. Tactile acuity improved when subjects viewed their stimulated arm, compared with viewing the neutral object or when blindfolded. These results clearly show that viewing the body during invisible tactile stimulation improves tactile processing; this effect has been called the "visual enhancement of touch" (VET), and the basic effect has been replicated several times (Taylor-Clarke et al. 2002; Press et al. 2004; Serino et al. in press).

Several results indicate that touch enhancement due to vision of the body acts at the level of the primary somatosensory cortex. Taylor-Clarke et al. (2002) used event-related potentials to compare cortical activity in somatosensory regions during the 2pd task while subjects viewed either their own stimulated arm or a neutral object. They found that viewing the stimulated arm was associated with an increase in early somatosensory event-related potentials. Consistent with these results, Schaefer et al. have recently used a magnetoencephalograph to demonstrate that viewing the index finger being touched while receiving a corresponding tactile stimulation results in a differential activation of the SI region representing the index finger, compared with conditions of no visual stimulation (Schaefer et al. 2005a) or of asynchronous visuotactile stimulation (Schaefer et al. 2005b). A causal role of SI modulation in VET was suggested by Fiorio and Haggard (2005); the VET effect was abolished by transcranial magnetic stimulation over primary but not secondary somatosensory cortex.

An indirect confirmation that VET occurs within primary somatosensory cortex comes from a recent psychophysical study by Serino et al. (in press). This work addressed the issue of whether VET acts according to a somatotopic principle, that is, whether VET is specific for the viewed body part or extends to body parts not directly viewed. In this study, subjects viewed either their own hand or a neutral object while performing 2pd tasks on the hand, the face, and the foot. These body parts were chosen on the basis of their location in the SI body representation: The hand and face representations lie adjacent to each other on the lateral aspect of the postcentral gyrus, whereas the foot representation is distant and more medial. When viewing the hand, 2pd threshold scores improved on the hand and the face but not on the foot (Penfield & Bolderey 1937; Sato et al. 2005). This pattern of results can be explained on the basis of the corepresentation of hand and face in the lateral aspect of SI. These findings confirm that visual modulation of tactile processing occurs within SI and further suggest that VET primarily acts on the SI representation of the viewed body part, here the hand, and secondarily extends *locally* to the adjacent region of SI, here the face, even when the relevant neurons have receptive fields on distant body surfaces.

Another recent study elucidates a possible functional mechanism underlying VET. I have established so far that visual information related to the body modulates neural activity in a local portion of SI and that tactile acuity depends on the receptive field size of SI neurons. The effect of vision on tactile acuity suggests that viewing the body influences somatosensory neurons by reducing their receptive field size. This prediction has been directly tested (Haggard et al. 2007). The effectiveness of vibrotactile maskers positioned at different distances from a tactile target stimulus was used as a behavioral proxy for SI receptive field size. The assumption was that maskers interfered with the tactile task only if they fell within the receptive field of the putative population of somatosensory neurons responsible for spatial representation of the target. The results showed that viewing the body reduced the effect of distant maskers and enhanced the effect of close maskers, compared with viewing a neutral object, suggesting that tactile receptive fields were sharpened when viewing the body.

Therefore, the visuotactile interaction underlying VET seems to function in improving tactile acuity. This suggestion is supported by another interesting property of VET described by Press et al. (2004), namely, that the benefit of vision on touch occurs only when spatial discrimination tasks are close to their perceptual limits. Press et al. showed that viewing the arm improved reaction time in a 2pd task only if the spatial separation between tactile stimuli was close to the participant's discrimination threshold—not when stimuli were widely separated. This finding suggests that visual information related to the body is used only to increase the spatial sensitivity of touch. This property resembles the inverse effectiveness rule described for other multisensory systems. According to the inverse effectiveness principle, signals from different modalities are more strongly integrated when modality-specific signals are individually less effective in producing a unisensory response. For visuotactile interactions related to the body, visual information is used to boost tactile sensation only when touch alone cannot provide enough spatial discriminations close to perceptual limits. When better tactile information is available and tactile tasks are easy, the benefit of visuotactile integration is no longer apparent. This conclusion has been confirmed in a recent study by Serino et al. (2007), who showed that the VET effect varies among individuals in inverse proportion to their tactile acuity. Subjects showing poor tactile ability when viewing a neutral baseline stimulus showed greater improvements when viewing the stimulated body part.

Taken together, these findings indicate that multisensory integration might improve the sensitivity of a unisensory modality in situations of deficit, and, again, favor a possible functional role for multisensory integration in ameliorating the performance deficits of perceptual systems.

Moreover, we further showed that viewing the body was effective in improving tactile functioning in patients whose tactile sensitivity was reduced after brain lesions (Serino et al. 2007). In these patients, selected for the presence of somatosensory deficits, tactile thresholds on the arm were improved by viewing their own arms but not by viewing a natural object or another body part. This finding might have important and new significance for rehabilitation: Multisensory stimulation may represent an alternative means of enhancing somatosensory performance after brain damage. In contrast to this claim, most current treatments for the rehabilitation of somatosensory deficits *prevent* the patient from seeing the relevant body part. For instance, patients typically lie supine during physiotherapy, with their eyes closed, or while looking at the ceiling, while physiotherapists stimulate their affected limbs. Instead, our data suggest that looking at the stimulated body part itself positively boosts somatosensory recovery.

Performance enhancement due to the sight of the body might involve two distinct processes. The first is a short-term functional improvement in its own right, as shown in Serino et al.'s study. This process might also initiate the long-term recovery of somatosensation. When brain lesions affect the SI, continuous visual reinforcement of tactile experience might be effective in promoting a long-term reorganization of the affected areas. This process might contribute to the recovery of somatosensation after stroke, and indeed a case study has recently shown that somatosensory recovery is strictly associated with the reemergence of activity in somatosensory cortices (Carey et al. 2002).

Conclusions

The neural synergy shown in the SC by spatially concordant AV cues and the antagonism that results from spatially disparate cues have their behavioral counterparts in the increased or decreased probability of evoking overt orientation responses. This finding is not surprising, given the well-known role of the SC in the generation of such behavior. Integration in the SC ensures that the information provided by cross-modal stimuli can be used to maximum advantage for both temporary and long-lasting compensation for sensory loss, as for visual filed deficits, visual neglect, and impairment in auditory localization tasks. Also, the integration of vision and touch can be extremely important in modulating tactile deficits, as manifest in VET when the tactile system is close to perceptual limits. The work reviewed in this article makes it clear that multisensory interactions are commonplace rather than exceptional. The challenge is now to achieve a better understanding of the nature of normal multisensory interactions, of their specific role during sensory deprivation, and of the mechanisms that reinforce the innate ability of our brains to perceive multisensory events.

Acknowledgments

I wish to thank Caterina Bertini, Fabrizio Leo, and Claudia Passamonti for their helpful comments on this manuscript.

Conflicts of Interest

The author declares no conflicts of interest.

References

Bertelson, P. & Aschersleben, G. (1998). Automatic visual bias of perceived auditory localization. *Psychon. Bull. Rev., 5,* 482–489.

Bisiach, E., Cornacchia, L., Sterzi, R., et al. (1984). Disorders of perceived auditory lateralization after lesions of the right hemisphere. *Brain, 107,* 37–52.

Bolognini, N., Rasi, F. & Làdavas, E. (2005a). Visual localization of sounds. *Neuropsychologia, 43,* 1655–1661.

Bolognini, N., Rasi, F., Coccia, M., et al. (2005b). Visual search improvement in hemianopic patients after audio-visual stimulation. *Brain, 128,* 2830–2842.

Bolognini, N., Leo, F., Passamonti, C., et al. (in press). Multisensory-mediated auditory localization. *Perception.*

Bonath, B., Noesselt, T., Martinez, A., et al. (2007). Neural basis of the ventriloquist illusion. *Curr. Biol., 17,* 1697–1703.

Burnett, L. R., Stein, B. E., Perrault, J. T., et al. (2007). Excitotoxic lesions of the superior colliculus preferentially impact multisensory neurons and multisensory integration. *Exp. Brain Res., 179,* 325–338.

Calvert, G. A. (2001). Crossmodal processing in the human brain: insights from functional neuroimaging studies. *Cereb. Cortex, 11,* 1110–1123.

Calvert, G. A. & Thesen, T. (2004). Multisensory integration: methodological approaches and emerging principles in the human brain. *J. Physiol. Paris, 98,* 191–202.

Calvert, G. A., Spence, C. & Stein, B. E. (Eds.). (2004). *The Handbook of Multisensory Processing.* Cambridge, MA: MIT Press.

Calvert, G. A. & Lewis, J. W. (2004). Hemodynamic studies of audiovisual interactions. In G. A. Calvert, C. Spence & B. E. Stein (Eds.), *The Handbook of Multisensory Processing.* Cambridge, MA: MIT Press.

Carey, L. M., Abbott, D. F., Puce, A., et al. (2002). Reemergence of activation with poststroke somatosensory recovery: a serial fMRI case study. *Neurology, 59,* 749–752.

Clarke, S., Bellmann, A., Meuli, R. A., et al. (2000). Auditory agnosia and auditory deficits following left hemispheric lesions: evidence for distinct processing pathways. *Neuropsychologia, 38,* 797–807.

Cohen, Y. E. & Andersen, R. A. (2004). Multisensory representation of space in the posterior parietal cortex. In G. A. Calvert, C. Spence & B. E. Stein (Eds.), *The Handbook of Multisensory Processing.* Cambridge, MA: MIT Press.

Corneil, B. D., VanWanrooij, M., Munoz, D. P., et al. (2002). Auditory-visual interactions subserving goal-directed saccades in a complex scene. *J. Neurophysiol., 88,* 438–454.

Fiorio, M. & Haggard, P. (2005). Viewing the body prepares the brain for touch: effects of TMS over somatosensory cortex. *Eur. J. Neurosci., 22,* 773–777.

Frassinetti, F., Bolognini, N. & Làdavas, E. (2002). Enhancement of visual perception by crossmodal audio-visual interaction. *Exp. Brain Res., 147,* 332–342.

Frassinetti, F., Bolognini, N., Bottari, D., et al. (2005). Audiovisual integration in patients with visual deficit. *J. Cogn. Neurosci., 17,* 1442–1452.

Haggard, P., Christakou, A. & Serino, A. (2007). Viewing the body modulates tactile receptive fields. *Exp. Brain Res., 180,* 187–93.

Halligan, P. W., Fink, G. R., Marshall, J. C., et al. (2003). Spatial cognition: evidence from visual neglect. *Trends Cogn. Sci., 7,* 125–133.

Heron, J., Whitaker, D. & McGraw, P. V. (2004). Sensory uncertainty governs the extent of audio-visual interaction. *Vision Res., 44,* 2875–2884.

Holmes, N. P. & Spence, C. (2005). Multisensory integration: space, time and superadditivity. *Curr. Biol. 15,* R762–R764.

Ignashchenkova, A., Dicke, P. W., Haarmeier, T., et al. (2004). Neuron-specific contribution of the superior colliculus to overt and covert shifts of attention. *Nat. Neurosci., 7,* 56–64.

Jiang, W., Jiang, H. & Stein, B. E. (2002). Two corticotectal areas facilitate multisensory orientation behavior. *J. Cogn. Neurosci., 14,* 1240–1255.

Jiang, W. & Stein, B. E. (2003). Cortex controls multisensory depression in superior colliculus. *J. Neurophysiol., 90,* 2123–35.

Jiang, W., Jiang, H., Rowland, B. A., et al. (2007). Multisensory orientation behavior is disrupted by neonatal cortical ablation. *J. Neurophysiol., 97*, 557–562.

Kadunce, D. C., Vaughan, J. W., Wallace, M. T., et al. (2001). The influence of visual and auditory receptive field organization on multisensory integration in the superior colliculus. *Exp. Brain Res., 139*, 303–310.

Kennett, S., Taylor-Clarke, M. & Haggard, P. (2001). Noninformative vision improves the spatial resolution of touch in humans. *Curr. Biol., 11*, 1188–1191.

King, A. J. & Hutchings, M. E. (1987). Spatial response properties of acoustically responsive neurons in the superior colliculus of the ferret: a map of auditory space. *J. Neurophysiol., 57*, 596–624.

Knudsen, E. I. (1982). Auditory and visual maps of space in the optic tectum of the owl. *J. Neurosci., 2*, 1177–1194.

Krauzlis, R. J., Liston, D. & Carello, C. D. (2004). Target selection and the superior colliculus: goals, choices and hypothesis. *Vis. Res., 44*, 1445–1451.

Kustov, A. A. & Robinson, D. L. (1996). Shared neural control of attentional shifts and eye movements. *Nature, 384*, 74–77.

Leh, S. E., Johansen-Berg, H. & Ptito, A. (2006). Unconscious vision: new insights into the neuronal correlate of blindsight using diffusion tractography. *Brain, 129*, 1822–1832.

Leo, F., Bertini, C., di Pellegrino, G., et al. (in press). Multisensory spatial integration in humans requires the activation of the superior colliculus. *Exp. Brain Res.*

Leo, F., Bolognini, N., Passamonti, C., et al. (in press). Crossmodal localization in hemianopia: new insights on multisensory integration. *Brain.*

Macaluso, E. & Driver, J. (2005). Multisensory spatial interactions: a window onto functional integration in the human brain. *Trends Neurosci., 28*, 264–271.

Marrocco, R. T. & Li, R. H. (1977). Monkey superior colliculus: properties of single cells and their afferent inputs. *J. Neurophysiol., 40*, 844–860.

Miller, J. (1982). Divided attention: evidence for coactivation with redundant signals. *Cognit. Psychol., 14*, 247–279.

Miller, L. M. & D'Esposito, M. (2005). Perceptual fusion and stimulus coincidence in the cross-modal integration of speech. *J. Neurosci., 25*, 5884–5893.

Mullen, K. T., Dumoulin, S. O., McMahon, K. L., et al. (2007). Selectivity of human retinotopic visual cortex to S-cone-opponent, L/M-cone-opponent and achromatic stimulation. *Eur. J. Neurosci., 25*, 491–502.

Passamonti, C., Bertini, C. & Làdavas, E. (2007). Audio-visual stimulation improves oculomotor patterns in patients with hemianopia. Manuscript in preparation.

Pavani, F., Farnè, A., & Làdavas, E. (2003). Task dependent visual coding of sound position in visuo-spatial neglect patients. *Neuroreport, 14*, 99–103.

Penfield, W. & Boldrey, E. (1937). Somatic motor and sensory representation in the cerebral cortex of man as studied by electrical stimulation. *Brain, 60*, 389–433.

Phan, M. L., Schendel, K. L., Recanzone, G. H., et al. (2000). Auditory and visual spatial localization deficits following bilateral parietal lobe lesions in a patient with Balint's syndrome. *J. Cogn. Neurosci., 12*, 583–600.

Pinek, B. & Bouchon, M. (1992). Head turning versus manual pointing to auditory in normal subjects and in subjects with right parietal damage. *Brain Cogn., 18*, 1–11.

Press, C., Taylor-Clarke, M., Kennett, S., et al. (2004). Visual enhancement of touch in spatial body representation. *Exp. Brain Res., 154*, 238–245.

Rafal, R., Smith, J., Krantz, J., et al. (1990). Extrageniculate vision in hemianopic humans: saccade inhibition by signals in the blind field. *Science, 250*, 118–121.

Ro, T., Shelton, D., Lee, O. L., et al. (2004). Extrageniculate mediation of unconscious vision in transcranial magnetic stimulation-induced blindsight. *Proc. Natl. Acad. Sci. USA, 101*, 9933–9935.

Sato, K., Nariai, T., Tanaka, Y., et al. (2005). Functional representation of the finger and face in the human somatosensory cortex: intraoperative intrinsic optical imaging. *NeuroImage, 25*, 1292–1301.

Schaefer, M., Heinze, H. J. & Rotte, M. (2005a). Task-relevant modulation of primary somatosensory cortex suggests a prefrontal-cortical sensory gating system. *NeuroImage, 27*, 130–5.

Schaefer, M., Flor, H., Heinze, H. J., et al. (2005b). Dynamic shifts in the organization of primary somatosensory cortex induced by bimanual spatial coupling of motor activity. *NeuroImage, 25*, 395–400.

Schroeder, C. E. & Foxe, J. J. (2004). Multisensory convergence in early cortical processing. In G. A. Calvert, C. Spence & B. E. Stein (Eds.), *The Handbook of Multisensory Processing.* Cambridge, MA: MIT Press.

Serino, A., Farnè, A., Rinaldesi, M. L., et al. (2007). Can vision of the body ameliorate impaired somatosensory function? *Neuropsychologia, 45*, 1101–1107.

Serino, A., Padiglioni, S., Haggard, P., et al. (in press). Seeing the hand boosts feeling on the cheek. *Cortex.*

Stein, B. E. & Meredith, M. A. (1993). *Merging of the Senses.* Cambridge, MA: MIT Press.

Stein, B. E., Stanford, T. R., Wallace, M. T., et al. (2004). Crossmodal spatial interactions in subcortical and cortical circuits. In C. Spence & J. Driver (Eds.), *Crossmodal Space and Crossmodal Attention.* Oxford, UK: Oxford University Press.

Stein, B. E. (2005). The development of a dialogue between cortex and midbrain to integrate multisensory information. *Exp. Brain Res., 166*, 305–315.

Sumner, P., Nachev, P., Vora, N., et al. (2004). Distinct cortical and collicular mechanisms of inhibition of return revealed with S cone stimuli. *Curr. Biol., 14*, 2259–2263.

Taylor-Clarke, M., Kennett, S. & Haggard, P. (2002). Vision modulates somatosensory cortical processing. *Curr. Biol., 12*, 233–236.

Tipper, S. P., Lloyd, D., Shorland, B., et al. (1998). Vision influences tactile perception without proprioceptive orienting. *Neuroreport, 9*, 1741–1744.

Todd, J. W. (1912). *Reaction to Multiple Stimuli.* Oxford, UK: Science Press.

Wallace, M. T., Meredith, M. A. & Stein, B. E. (1992). Integration of multiple sensory modalities in cat cortex. *Exp. Brain Res., 91*, 484–488.

Weiskrantz, L. (1996). Blindsight revisited. *Curr. Opin. Neurobiol., 6*(2), 215–220.

The Adolescent Brain

B.J. Casey,[a] Rebecca M. Jones,[a] and Todd A. Hare[b]

[a]*Sackler Institute, Weill Medical College of Cornell University, New York, New York, USA*
[b]*California Institute of Technology, Pasadena, California, USA*

Adolescence is a developmental period characterized by suboptimal decisions and actions that are associated with an increased incidence of unintentional injuries, violence, substance abuse, unintended pregnancy, and sexually transmitted diseases. Traditional neurobiological and cognitive explanations for adolescent behavior have failed to account for the nonlinear changes in behavior observed during adolescence, relative to both childhood and adulthood. This review provides a biologically plausible model of the neural mechanisms underlying these nonlinear changes in behavior. We provide evidence from recent human brain imaging and animal studies that there is a heightened responsiveness to incentives and socioemotional contexts during this time, when impulse control is still relatively immature. These findings suggest differential development of bottom-up limbic systems, implicated in incentive and emotional processing, to top-down control systems during adolescence as compared to childhood and adulthood. This developmental pattern may be exacerbated in those adolescents prone to emotional reactivity, increasing the likelihood of poor outcomes.

Key words: adolescence; prefrontal cortex; nucleus accumbens; amygdala; limbic; impulsivity; reward; development; risk taking; emotion

Introduction

Adolescence is the period between childhood and adulthood encompassed by changes in physical, psychological, and social development (Ernst et al. 2006). These alterations make this period a time of vulnerability and adjustment (Steinberg 2005). According to the National Center for Health Statistics, there are over 13,000 adolescent deaths in the United States each year. Approximately 70% of these deaths result from motor vehicle crashes, unintentional injuries, homicide, and suicide (Eaton et al. 2006). Results from the 2005 National Youth Risk Behavior Survey (YRBS) show that adolescents engage in behaviors that increase their likelihood of death or illness by driving a vehicle after drinking or without a seat belt, carrying weapons, using illegal substances, and engaging in unprotected sex resulting in unintended pregnancies and STDs, including HIV infection (Eaton et al. 2006). These statistics underscore the importance of understanding risky choices and behavior in adolescents.

Adolescence is also a time of increased emotional reactivity. During this period, the social environment is changing such that more time is spent with peers versus adults, and more conflicts arise between the adolescent and his/her parents (Csikszentmihalyi et al. 1977; Steinberg 1989). These changes in social interactions may influence the rise of emotional reactivity. In addition, given the increase in risky choices and behavior during adolescence, it appears the value of positive and negative information may be exaggerated. Greater emotional reactivity and sensitivity during adolescence may play a role in the higher incidence of affective disorder onset and addiction during this developmental period (Pine et al. 2001; Silveri et al. 2004; Steinberg 2005).

A number of cognitive and neurobiological hypotheses have been postulated to explain why adolescents engage in suboptimal choice behavior. In a recent review of the literature on human adolescent brain development, Yurgelun-Todd (2007) suggests that cognitive development during adolescence is associated with progressively greater efficiency of cognitive control and affective modulation. An increase in activity in the prefrontal regions as an indication of maturation (Rubia et al. 2000; Rubia et al. 2006; Tamm et al. 2002) and diminished activity in irrelevant brain regions (Brown et al. 2005; Durston et al. 2006; Monk

Address for correspondence: BJ Casey, Sackler Institute, Weill Cornell Medical College, 1300 York Avenue, Box 140, New York, NY 10021, Voice: +212-746-5832 fax: 212-746-5755 USA.
bjc2002@med.cornell.edu

et al. 2003) are described as the neurobiological explanation for the behavioral changes associated with adolescence. This general pattern, of improved cognitive control and emotion regulation with maturation of the prefrontal cortex, suggests a linear increase in development from childhood to adulthood.

As evidenced by the National Center for Health Statistics on adolescent behavior and mortality, suboptimal choices and actions observed during adolescence represent a nonlinear change in behavior, distinct from childhood and adulthood. If immaturity of prefrontal cortex were the basis for suboptimal choice behavior and heightened emotional reactivity in adolescence, then children who have less developed prefrontal cortex and cognitive abilities should look remarkably similar or even worse than adolescents. Thus, immature prefrontal function alone cannot account for adolescent behavior.

This review will provide evidence from developmental animal and human neuroimaging studies that may account for nonlinear changes in behavior and development during adolescence. A model of adolescent brain development is presented in the context of risk factors including suboptimal decision making and heightened emotional reactivity.

Development of Goal-directed Behavior: Risk versus Impulse

An accurate conceptualization of cognitive and neurobiological changes during adolescence must treat adolescence as a transitional developmental period (Spear 2000), rather than a single snapshot in time (Casey et al. 2005). In other words, to understand this developmental period, transitions into and out of adolescence are necessary for distinguishing distinct attributes of this stage of development. Adolescent behavior has been described as impulsive and risky, almost synonymously, yet these behaviors rely on different cognitive and neural processes (Casey et al. in press), which suggest distinct constructs with different developmental trajectories.

A cornerstone of cognitive development is the ability to suppress inappropriate thoughts and actions in favor of goal-directed ones, especially in the presence of compelling incentives (Casey et al. 2005; Casey et al. 2000; Casey et al. 2002). A number of classic developmental studies have shown that this ability develops throughout childhood and adolescence (Case 1972; Flavell et al. 1966; Keating & Bobbitt 1978; Pascual-Leone 1970). Several theorists (e.g., Bjorkland 1985, 1987; Case 1985) have argued that cognitive development is due to increases in processing speed and efficiency and not due to an increase in mental capacity. Other theorists have included the construct of "inhibitory" processes in their account of cognitive development (Harnishfeger & Bjorkland 1993). According to this account, immature cognition is characterized by susceptibility to interference from competing sources that must be suppressed (e.g., Brainerd & Reyna 1993; Dempster 1993) (Casey et al. 2002; Diamond 1985; Munakata & Yerys 2001). Thus goal-directed behavior requires the control of impulses or delay of gratification for optimization of outcomes, and this ability appears to mature across childhood and adolescence.

On a cognitive or behavioral level, the immature cognition of adolescence is characterized as impulsive (i.e., lacking cognitive control) and risk taking, with these constructs used synonymously and without appreciation for distinct developmental trajectories for each. Human imaging and animal studies suggest distinct neurobiological and developmental trajectories for the neural systems that underlie these separate constructs of impulse control and risky decisions. Specifically, a review of the literature suggests that impulsivity diminishes with age across childhood and adolescence (Casey et al. 2005; Casey et al. 2002; Galvan et al. 2007) and is associated with protracted development of the prefrontal cortex (Casey et al. 2005; Casey et al. 2002; Galvan et al. 2007) and is associated with protracted development of the prefrontal cortex (Casey et al. 2005). However, there are individual differences in the degree of impulsivity, regardless of age.

In contrast to the linear increase with age associated with impulse control, risk taking appears greater during adolescence relative to childhood and adulthood and is associated with subcortical systems known to be involved in evaluation of incentives and affective information. Human imaging studies that are reviewed here suggest an increase in subcortical activation (accumbens and amygdala) when making risky choices and processing emotional information (Ernst et al. 2005; Monk et al. 2003; Montague & Berns 2002) (Kuhnen & Knutson 2005; Matthews et al. 2004) that is exaggerated in adolescents, relative to children and adults (Ernst et al. 2005; Galvan et al. 2006).

These findings suggest distinct neurobiological trajectories for impulse versus risk taking behavior. The limbic subcortical systems appear to be developed by adolescence in contrast to control systems that show a protracted and linear developmental course into young adulthood. The prefrontal cortical control systems are necessary for overriding inappropriate choices and actions in favor of goal-directed ones.

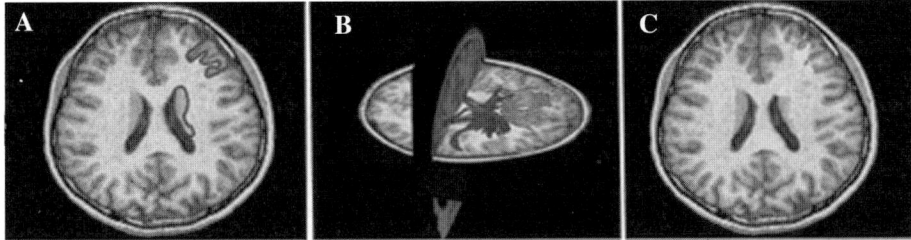

FIGURE 1. Illustrations of the most common magnetic resonance methods used in the study of human development. **(A)** Structural magnetic resonance imaging (MRI) to produce structural images of the brain useful for anatomical and morphometric studies, **(B)** diffusion tensor imaging (DTI) measures myelination and directionality of fiber tracts between anatomical structures, and **(C)** functional MRI (fMRI) measures patterns of brain activity within those structures (from Casey et al. 2005).

Animal Studies of Adolescent Brain Development

Until recently, much of our understanding of the adolescent brain has come from animal studies. These experiments have been critical for obtaining information about the neurochemical and cellular changes that occur as a function of age. The validity of animal models to study adolescence has been questioned, since it is argued that only humans undergo the psychological stress of adolescence (e.g., Bogin 1994). However, animals including rodents and nonhuman primates exhibit increased social interactions during adolescence (Primus & Kellogg 1989) as well as novelty-seeking and risk-taking behaviors (Adriani et al. 1998; Spear 2000). These behavioral findings suggest that animal models are appropriate for studying neurobiological changes during adolescence.

Studies in rodents have shown at the cellular level that there are distinct changes in limbic and prefrontal regions during adolescence. During early puberty, there is an overproduction of axons and synapses, followed by rapid pruning in later adolescence (Crews et al. 2007). Specifically, there is dendritic pruning in the amygdala (Zehr et al. 2006), nucleus accumbens (Teicher et al. 1995), and prefrontal cortex (Andersen & Teicher 2004; Andersen et al. 2000) and continual growth in the density of the fibers connecting the amygdala and prefrontal cortex into early adulthood (Cunningham et al. 2002). There is more prolonged pruning throughout adolescence in the prefrontal cortex versus the accumbens (Andersen et al. 2000; Teicher et al. 1995). These differences in pruning in rodents are consistent with our model suggesting that the accumbens matures earlier than the prefrontal cortex.

Consistent with the cellular changes in animals, there are alterations in neurotransmission in these subcortical and cortical areas. Animal studies have shown that dopamine is crucial for communication between the accumbens, amygdala, and prefrontal cortex and that signaling between these regions relies upon the fine balance between excitatory and inhibitory dopamine transmission (Floresco & Tse 2007; Grace et al. 2007; Jackson et al. 2001). There are significant peaks in dopamine expression during adolescence. Dopamine projections to the prefrontal cortex continue to develop into early adulthood, with dopamine levels peaking in the prefrontal cortex during adolescence versus earlier or later in life in nonhuman primates (Rosenberg & Lewis 1994, 1995) and in rats (Kalsbeek et al. 1988). Dopamine receptor expression is highest in the accumbens during early adolescence (Tarazi et al. 1998). These findings in rodents suggest that there are specific regions undergoing structural changes, and therefore, connections and communication between subcortical and cortical regions are in transition and in flux during adolescence. Significant evidence suggests that the neuroanatomical changes described above are also occurring during adolescence in humans, but our methods for studying humans only provide an approximate index of such changes.

Neuroimaging Studies of Human Brain Development

Our current understanding of the human adolescent brain has come from advances in neuroimaging methodologies that can be used with developing human populations. These methods depend on magnetic resonance imaging (MRI) methods (see FIG. 1) and include structural MRI, which is used to measure the size and shape of structures; diffusion tensor imaging (DTI), which is used to index connectivity of white matter fiber tracts; and functional MRI which is used to measure patterns of brain activity. These methods have

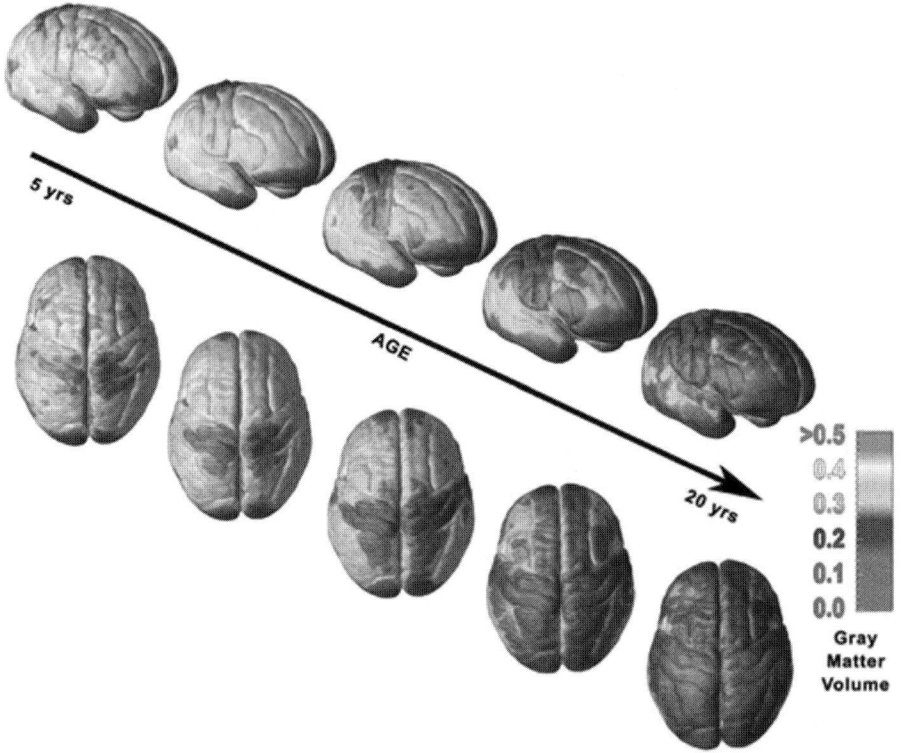

FIGURE 2. Illustration of gray matter volume maturation over the cortical surface from 5 to 20 years of age (from Lenroot & Giedd 2006).

furthered our understanding of the neurobiological basis and development of reward or incentive behavior relative to goal-directed behavior.

MRI Studies of Human Brain Development

Several studies have used structural MRI to map the developmental course of the normal brain (for review, see Durston et al. 2001). Although the brain reaches approximately 90% of its adult size by age six, the gray and white matter subcomponents of the brain continue to undergo dynamic changes throughout adolescence. Data from recent longitudinal MRI studies indicate that the change in gray matter volume over time has an inverted U-shape pattern and has greater regional variation than white matter (Giedd 2004; Gogtay et al. 2004, Sowell et al. 2003, 2004). In general, regions that involve primary functions, such as motor and sensory systems, mature earliest compared to the higher-order association areas that integrate these primary functions (Gogtay et al. 2004; Sowell et al. 2004). MRI studies show loss of cortical gray matter first in primary sensorimotor areas, followed by that in the dorsolateral prefrontal and lateral temporal cortices (Gogtay et al. 2004) (see FIG. 2). This pattern of change is consistent with nonhuman primate (Bourgeois et al. 1994) and human postmortem studies (Huttenlocher 1979) indicating that the prefrontal cortex is one of the last brain regions to mature. In contrast to gray matter, white matter volume increases in a roughly linear pattern throughout development and into adulthood (Gogtay et al. 2004). These changes most likely reflect ongoing myelination of axons by oligodendrocytes enhancing neuronal conduction and communication.

When examining neuroanatomical changes across development, the subcortical regions are often overlooked, however, it is important to note that these areas have some of the largest changes during development in the brain, particularly in the basal ganglia (Sowell et al. 1999) and specifically in males (Caviness et al. 1996; Giedd et al. 1996; Reiss et al. 1996). Developmental changes in structural volume within basal ganglia and prefrontal regions are interesting in light of the previously mentioned animal work showing pruning in these regions during adolescence. These processes allow for the fine tuning and strengthening of connections between prefrontal and subcortical regions during development and learning that may correspond to greater cognitive control.

How do these changes in structure relate to differences in cognition? A number of studies have related frontal lobe structural maturation and cognitive function using neuropsychological and cognitive measures (e.g., Sowell et al. 2003). Specifically, these studies showed associations between MRI-based regional volumes of the prefrontal cortex and basal ganglia with measures of cognitive control (i.e., ability to override an inappropriate response in favor of another or to suppress attention toward irrelevant stimulus attribute in favor of relevant stimulus attribute) (Casey et al. 1997, 1997). These findings suggest that cognitive changes are reflected in structural brain changes and underscore the importance of subcortical (basal ganglia) as well as cortical (e.g., prefrontal cortex) development. While these findings showed associations between structure and function, a more in-depth discussion of functional imaging evidence for changes in activity that more directly coincide with behavior across development is presented in the fMRI section.

DTI Studies of Human Brain Development

The MRI-based morphometry studies previously reviewed suggest that during development, cortical connections are fine tuned via elimination of an overabundance of synapses and by strengthening of relevant connections, although these measures do not have the resolution to visualize or measure synapses. Recent advances in MRI technology, like DTI, provide a potential tool for examining the role of specific white matter tracts in the development of the brain and behavior (for review, see Cascio et al. 2007). Examining white matter tracts can provide knowledge about pathways of connectivity in the brain, and presumably it is via these pathways that information is able to travel from one region of the brain to another (Cascio et al. 2007). Relevant to this paper are the neuroimaging studies that have linked the development of white matter fiber tracts with improvements in cognitive ability with age.

Recently, associations have been shown between DTI-based measures of prefrontal white matter development and cognition in children. Nagy and colleagues showed a positive correlation between maturation of prefrontal–parietal fiber tracts and working memory in children (Nagy et al. 2004), which is consistent with functional neuroimaging studies showing differential recruitment of these regions in children relative to adults. Using a similar approach, Liston and colleagues (2006) have shown that white matter tracts between prefrontal–basal ganglia and posterior fiber tracts continue to develop across childhood into adulthood, but only tracts between the prefrontal cortex and basal ganglia are correlated with impulse control, as measured by performance on a go/no-go task. The prefrontal fiber tracts were defined by regions of interests, which were identified in an fMRI study using the go/no-go task. In developmental DTI studies, fiber tract measures were correlated with age, but specificity of particular fiber tracts with cognitive performance were shown by dissociating the particular tract (Liston et al. 2006) or cognitive ability (Nagy et al. 2004). These findings highlight the importance of examining not only regional, but also related circuitry changes, when making inferences about neural changes in cognition across development.

Functional MRI Studies of Human Brain Development

Compared to MRI and DTI, fMRI is a more direct approach for examining behavior changes during development and for establishing structure–function relationships. Using fMRI to measure functional changes in the developing brain has significant potential for the field of developmental science and provides a means for constraining interpretations of adolescent behavior.

As stated previously, the development of the prefrontal cortex is believed to play an important role in the maturation of higher cognitive abilities such as decision making and cognitive control (Casey et al. 2002; Casey et al. 1997; Hare & Casey 2005). Many behavioral paradigms, together with fMRI, have assessed the neurobiological basis of these abilities, including flanker, Stroop, and go/no-go tasks (Casey et al. 1997; Casey et al. 2000; Durston et al. 2003). Collectively, these studies show that children recruit distinct but often larger and more diffuse prefrontal regions when performing these tasks than do adults. The patterns of brain activity that are important for task performance, such as those regions that correlate with cognitive performance, become more fine tuned with age. Regions that are not correlated with task performance diminish in activity with age. This pattern has been observed across both cross-sectional (Brown et al. 2005) and longitudinal studies (Durston et al. 2006) and across a variety of paradigms. Neuroimaging studies cannot definitively characterize the mechanism of such developmental changes as dendritic arborization or synaptic pruning. However, these studies suggest that change over a period of time results in both refinement within brain regions as well as fine tuning of projections from these regions (Brown et al. 2005; Bunge et al. 2002; Casey et al. 1997; Casey et al. 2002; Luna et al. 2001; Moses et al. 2002; Schlaggar et al. 2002; Tamm et al. 2002; Thomas et al. 2004; Turkeltaub et al. 2003).

Functional MRI Studies of Behavior during Adolescence

The question remains how can fMRI studies help explain whether adolescents, compared to children or adults, are 1) lacking sufficient cognitive control (impulsive), 2) risky in their choices and actions, and 3) more sensitive to affective information when required to exert cognitive control than children or adults.

Impulse control, as measured by cognitive control tasks like the go/no-go task, shows a linear pattern of development across childhood and adolescence, as described above. However, we were interested in understanding changes across development in top-down control regions and subcortical reward-seeking regions. It is only recently that risk taking in adolescents has been examined with neuroimaging techniques (Ernst et al. 2005; May et al. 2004). These studies have focused primarily on the region of the accumbens, a portion of the basal ganglia involved in predicting reward outcomes. Although two recent reports showed less ventral prefrontal activity (Eshel et al. 2007) and posterior mesofrontal activity (Bjork et al. 2007) in adolescents versus adults on risk-taking behavior, the goal of our studies was to characterize the development of limbic subcortical regions involved in motivation and emotional reactivity in conjunction with top-down control regions (prefrontal cortex). Many studies have examined the neural response in children and adolescents to affective information (e.g., emotional faces) (Baird et al. 1999; Killgore et al. 2001; Monk et al. 2003; Thomas et al. 2001b; Yurgelun-Todd & Killgore 2006) but typically have used passive viewing or attention tasks (Monk et al. 2003) unrelated to processing of the affective information. Our studies examine how affect influences cognitive control across development and characterizes the activation of the subcortical systems (amygdala) involved in affect regulation relative to the cortical (prefrontal) regions associated with cognitive control.

A Neurobiological Model of Adolescence

How do neural changes in subcortical regions (e.g., accumbens and amygdala) associated with reward-seeking and emotion coincide with development of the prefrontal regions and do they relate to impulsivity and risk-taking behaviors? We have developed a neurobiological model of adolescent development within this framework that builds on rodent models (Laviola et al. 1999; Spear 2000) and recent imaging studies of children, adolescents, and adults (Ernst

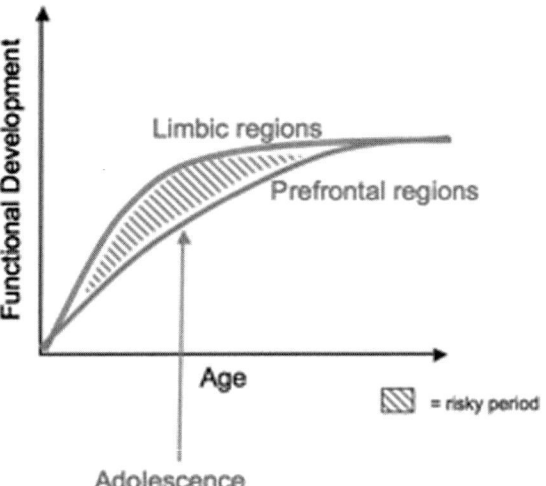

FIGURE 3. The traditional explanation of adolescent behavior has been that it is due to the protracted development of the prefrontal cortex. Our model takes into consideration the development of the prefrontal cortex together with subcortical limbic regions (e.g., nucleus accumbens and amygdala) that have been implicated in risky choices and emotional reactivity.

et al. 2005; Galvan et al. 2007; Galvan et al. 2006; Hare & Casey, in press). FIGURE 3 depicts this model illustrating how bottom-up limbic and prefrontal top-down control regions should be considered together. The graph shows different developmental trajectories for these systems, with limbic systems developing earlier than prefrontal control regions. According to this model, the individual is biased more by functionally mature limbic regions during adolescence (i.e., imbalance of limbic relative to prefrontal control), compared to children, for whom these systems are both still developing, and compared to adults, for whom these systems are fully mature. This perspective provides a basis for nonlinear shifts in behavior across development, due to earlier maturation of this limbic system relative to the less mature top-down prefrontal control region. Furthermore, with development and experience, the functional connectivity between these regions provides a mechanism for top-down control of these regions (Hare & Casey, in press). Our model reconciles the contradiction between health statistics of risky behavior during adolescence and the astute observation by Reyna and Farley (2006) that adolescents are able to reason and understand risks of behaviors in which they engage.

According to our model, in emotionally salient situations, the more mature limbic system will win over the prefrontal control system. In other words, when a poor decision is made in an emotional context, the adolescent may know better, but the salience of the emotional context biases his or her behavior in opposite direction of the optimal action.

Our neurobiological model proposes that the combination of heightened responsiveness to rewards and immaturity in behavioral control areas may bias adolescents to seek immediate rather than long-term gains, perhaps explaining their increase in risky decision making and emotional reactivity. Tracking subcortical (e.g., accumbens and amygdala) and cortical (e.g., prefrontal) development of decision making and emotional reactivity across childhood and through adulthood provides additional clarification on whether changes reported in adolescence are specific to this period of development or, rather, reflect maturation that is steadily occurring in a somewhat linear pattern from childhood to adulthood.

Two recent fMRI studies spanning from childhood to adulthood provide empirical evidence consistent with our neurobiological model. In the first study (Galvan et al. 2006), we examined behavioral and neural responses to reward manipulations across development, focusing on brain regions implicated in reward-related learning and behavior in animal (Hikosaka & Watanabe 2000; Pecina et al. 2003; Schultz 2006) and adult imaging studies (e.g., Knutson et al. 2001; O'Doherty et al. 2001; Zald et al. 2004) and in studies of addiction (Hyman & Malenka 2001; Volkow & Li 2004). Based on rodent models (Laviola et al. 1999; Spear 2000) and previous imaging work (Ernst et al. 2005), we hypothesized that relative to children and adults, adolescents would show exaggerated responses to reward as indexed by elevated accumbens activity in concert with less mature recruitment of top-down prefrontal control regions.

Our findings were consistent with rodent models (Laviola et al. 2003) and previous imaging studies during adolescence (Ernst et al. 2005), which show enhanced accumbens activity to rewards. Adolescents, as compared to children and adults, showed an exaggerated accumbens response in anticipation of reward. However, both children and adolescents showed a less mature response in prefrontal control regions than adults. These findings suggest that there are different developmental trajectories for these regions. The enhancement in accumbens activity during adolescence may relate to the increase in impulsive and risky behaviors observed during this period of development (see FIG. 4).

In the second study, we examined the development of behavioral and neural responses in performance of an emotional go/no-go paradigm (Hare & Casey,

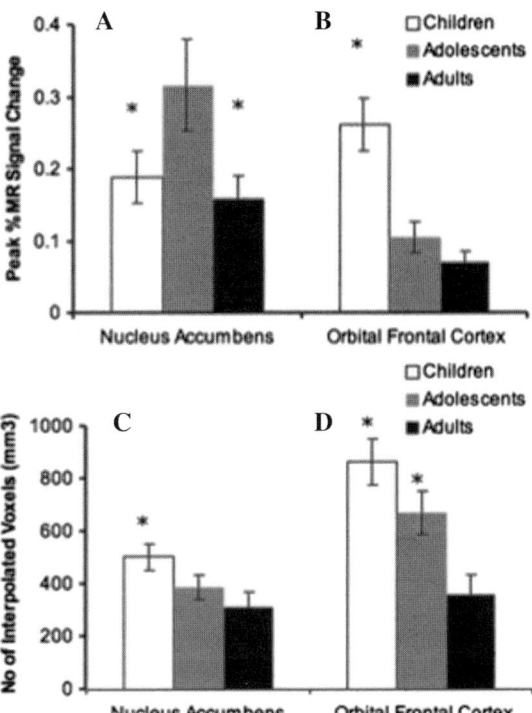

FIGURE 4. Magnitude and extent of accumbens and OFC activity to reward. Adolescents (13–17 years) showed greater percent signal change to large rewards than either children (aged 7–11 years) or adults (23–29 years) in the accumbens **(A)**. Children had the greatest percent signal change in the OFC compared to adolescents and adults **(B)**. Children had the greatest volume of activity in the accumbens relative to adolescents and adults **(C)** Children and adolescents showed greater volume of activity in the OFC than adults **(D)**. Adapted from Galvan et al. (2006).

in press; Hare et al. 2005). During the experiment, participants were presented with two emotional facial expressions (fearful, neutral, or happy) and were asked to respond to one of the emotions (e.g., fear) and suppress their response to the other emotion (e.g., neutral). In the context of negative emotional information (fearful faces), reaction times improved with age but were longer when detecting fearful faces relative to a neutral or happy face. This slowing in reaction time was correlated with greater amygdala activity (Hare & Casey, in press). Activity in the orbital frontal cortex increased with age, and greater orbital frontal activity relative to amygdala was associated with more efficiency in suppressing emotional reactivity (longer reaction times and greater amygdala activity). These findings are in accordance with animal studies (Baxter et al. 2000) which show connectivity between the

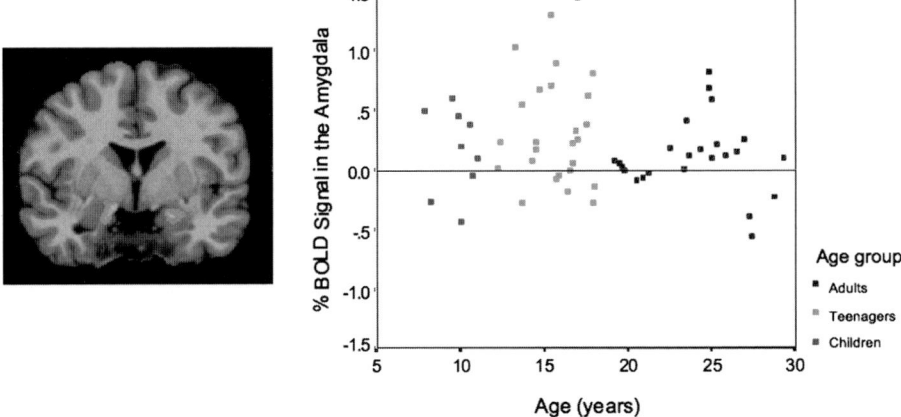

FIGURE 5. Bilateral amygdala activation (left). Graph depicts amygdala activity in adults, teenagers, and children. Adapted from Hare et al. (in press).

amgydala and orbital frontal cortex are important for assessing changes in emotional value of an object and adapting behavior accordingly.

Differential recruitment of prefrontal and subcortical regions has been reported across a number of developmental fMRI studies (Casey et al. 2002; Monk et al. 2003; Thomas et al. 2004). These findings were typically interpreted in terms of immature prefrontal regions rather than as an imbalance between prefrontal and subcortical regional development. Given evidence of prefrontal regions in guiding appropriate actions in different contexts (Miller & Cohen 2001), immature prefrontal activity might hinder appropriate estimation of future outcomes, especially when making a decision within an emotional context (i.e., heat of the moment). This interpretation is consistent with previous research showing elevated subcortical, relative to cortical, activity when decisions are biased by immediate versus long-term gains (McClure et al. 2004). Further, fMRI studies have shown limbic subcortical activity positively correlates with suboptimal choice behaviors (Kuhnen & Knutson 2005).

In sum, during adolescence, relative to childhood or adulthood, an immature ventral prefrontal cortex may not provide sufficient top-down control of robustly activated reward and affect processing regions (e.g., accumbens and amygdala). This imbalance in development of these regions and relative top-down control results in less influence of prefrontal systems (orbitofrontal cortex) relative to the accumbens and amygdala in reward valuation and emotional reactivity.

Why Would the Adolescent Brain Be Programmed This Way?

Adolescence can be described as a progressive transition from childhood into adulthood with an indefinable ontogenetic time course (Spear 2000) yet often co-occurring with puberty, which is defined by specific biological markers. The significant neuroendocrinological changes associated with puberty, such as increases in adrenal and gonadal hormones, are correlated with the development of secondary sexual characteristics and can influence brain function (for a review see Spear 2000). The onset and hormone fluctuations of puberty may provide an explanation for the observed functional differences in subcortical activity between children and adolescents, versus activity in the prefrontal region, which reflects a linear change with age.

From an evolutionary perspective, adolescence is the period in which independence skills are acquired in order to increase the success of separating from the protective influence of the family. It is also a period when there is an increase in the likelihood of harm such as injury, depression, anxiety, drug use, and addiction (Kelley et al. 2004). However, our neurobiological model suggests that risky behavior and emotional reactivity are the products of a biologically driven imbalance between increased novelty and positive sensation seeking in conjunction with immature "self-regulatory competence" (Steinberg 2004).

As previously mentioned, during adolescence, independence-seeking behaviors are prevalent across species, such as increases in peer-directed social interactions and intensifications in novelty seeking and risk-taking behaviors. In other species such as rodents, nonhuman primates, and birds, behaviors like seeking out same-age peers and fighting with parents are also observed and may be important adaptive skills to remove the adolescent from the home territory in order to mate (Spear 2000). Relative to adults, periadolescent rats show increased novelty-seeking behaviors in a free-choice novelty paradigm (Laviola et al. 1999). Neurochemical evidence indicates that the balance in the adolescent brain between cortical and subcortical dopamine systems begins to shift toward greater cortical dopamine levels during adolescence (Spear 2000). And as previously described, in the nonhuman primate there is an increase in dopamine enervation of the prefrontal cortex into early adulthood (Rosenberg & Lewis 1995). Thus this elevated risk-taking behavior appears to occur across species and have important adaptive functions.

It is possible that this developmental pattern is an evolutionary feature. One needs to engage in high-risk behavior in order to leave the family and village to find a mate. This risk behavior occurs simultaneously with an increase in sexual hormones, resulting in adolescents seeking sexual partners and is seen in other species. In conjunction with this novelty-seeking behavior, there would need to be some mechanism for detecting cues of safety or danger. The increase in emotional reactivity during this period may allow adolescents to be more vigilant and aware of threat, to ensure their survival as they move from a safe environment to a novel one. In today's society when adolescence may extend indefinitely—with individuals well into their 20s living with their parents, remaining financially dependent, and choosing mates later in life—these behaviors may be deemed inappropriate.

Biological Predispositions, Development, and Risky Behavior

The recognition of individual differences in impulse control and taking risks is not new in the field of psychology (Benthin et al. 1993). Perhaps one of the classic examples of individual differences in the social, cognitive, and developmental psychology literatures is delay of gratification (Mischel et al. 1989). Delay of gratification is typically assessed in 3- to 4-year-old toddlers. A toddler is seated in a room with two cookies and a bell. The child is then told that the experimenter will leave the room in order to prepare for upcoming activities and explains to the child that if she remains in her seat and does not eat a cookie, she will receive the large reward (2 cookies). If the child cannot wait, she should ring a bell to summon the experimenter and thereby receive the smaller reward (1 cookie). Distractions in the room are minimized, with no toys, books, or pictures. The experimenter returns after 15 minutes or after the child has rung the bell, eaten the rewards, or shown any signs of distress. Mischel (1989) showed that children typically behave in one of two ways: 1) either they ring the bell almost immediately in order to have the cookie, which means they only get one; or 2) they wait and optimize their gains to receive both cookies. This observation suggests that some individuals are better than others in their ability to control impulses in the presence of highly salient incentives, and this bias can be detected in early childhood (Mischel et al. 1989). This differential in impulse control appears to remain throughout adolescence and young adulthood (Eigsti et al. 2006).

What might explain individual differences in decision making and behavior? Some theorists have postulated that the dopaminergic mesolimbic circuitry, implicated in reward processing, underlies risky behavior (Blum et al. 2000), and that individual differences in this circuitry might relate to the propensity to engage in risky behavior (O'Doherty 2004). A number of studies have shown increases in activity in the nucleus accumbens immediately prior to making risky choices on monetary-risk paradigms (Kuhnen & Knutson 2005; Matthews et al. 2004; Montague & Berns 2002), and as described previously, adolescents show exaggerated accumbens activity to rewarding outcomes relative to children or adults (Ernst et al. 2005; Galvan et al. 2006). Collectively, these data suggest that as a group adolescents may be more likely to engage in risky choices (Gardener & Steinberg 2005). However, some adolescents will be more prone than others to engage in risky behaviors, putting them at potentially greater risk for negative outcomes. Therefore it is important to consider individual variability when examining complex brain–behavior relationships related to risk taking and reward processing in developmental populations.

To explore individual differences in risk-taking behavior, Galvan and colleagues (2007) recently examined the association between activity in reward-related neural circuitry in anticipation of a large monetary reward with behavioral measures of risk taking and impulsivity in adolescence. Specifically, Galvan and colleagues used functional magnetic resonance imaging and anonymous self-report rating scales of risky behavior, risk perception, and impulsivity in individuals between the ages of 7 and 29 years (see FIG. 6). There was a positive association between accumbens

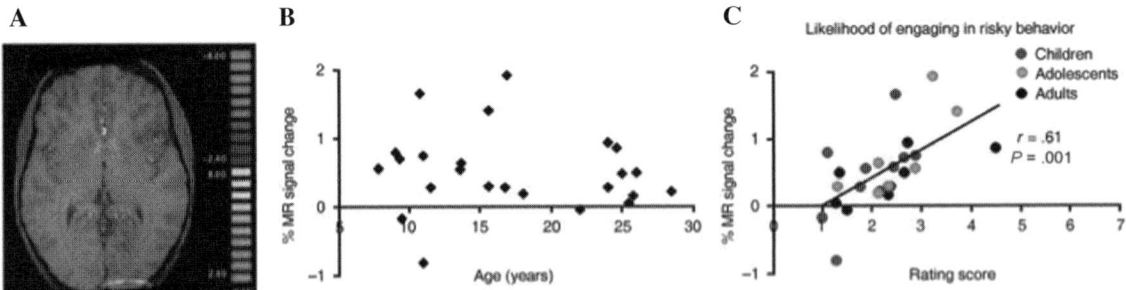

FIGURE 6. Activity in the nucleus accumbens in anticipation of reward **(A)**. Percent change in fMRI signal in the accumbens in anticipation of reward as a function of age **(B)**. The association between accumbens activity to reward and the likelihood of engaging in risky behavior in three age groups **(C)** (Adapted from Galvan et al. 2007).

activity and the likelihood of engaging in risky behavior across development. In other words, those individuals, who perceived risky behaviors as leading to dire consequences, activated the accumbens less to reward. Impulsivity ratings were not associated with accumbens activity, but rather with age, further dissociating impulse control from incentive-based risky behaviors. These findings suggest that during adolescence, some individuals have a predisposition to engage in risky behaviors due to developmental neural changes.

Adolescent behavior is repeatedly characterized as impulsive and risky, yet this review of the imaging literature suggests different neurobiological substrates and developmental trajectories for these two types of behavior. Specifically, impulsivity is associated with immature ventral prefrontal development and gradually diminishes from childhood to adulthood (Casey et al. 2005). The negative correlation between impulsivity ratings and age in the study by Galvan and colleagues (2007) further supports this notion. In contrast, risk taking is associated with an increase in accumbens activity (Kuhnen & Knutson 2005; Matthews et al. 2004; Montague & Berns 2002) that is exaggerated in adolescents, relative to both children and adults (Ernst et al. 2005; Galvan et al. 2006). Thus adolescent choices and behavior cannot be explained by impulsivity or protracted development of the prefrontal cortex alone, as children would then be predicted to be greater risk takers. The findings provide a neural basis for why some adolescents are at greater risk than others, but also demonstrate a basis for why adolescent risk-taking behavior in general is different from risk taking in children and adults.

Adolescence, Individual Differences, and Affective Disorders

Adolescence is a time of greater emotional reactivity and a period when symptoms of many psychiatric disorders (e.g., schizophrenia, depression, anxiety) manifest. Normal adolescent development can be interpreted as the coordination of emotions and behavior in the social and intellectual environment, and the development of psychopathology during adolescence can be seen as resulting from a difficulty in balancing these factors (Steinberg 2005). We have previously described enhanced bottom-up emotional processing in subcortical regions relative to less effective top-down modulation in prefrontal regions to affective information during adolescence. It is possible that this imbalance may play a role in the increased risk for affective disorders during adolescence (Steinberg 2005). Clearly, not all adolescents develop psychopathology; there must be individual variability in emotional reactivity and the ability to modulate these behaviors. Individual differences may predispose a person to be at greater risk for poorer outcomes.

The amygdala has been implicated as a key neural region in emotional dysregulation in psychiatric disorders. This region is essential to learning the emotional significance of cues in the environment (see Maren & Quirk 2004 for review). In animal studies, amygdala lesions result in a reduction of fear behavior (Anglada-Figueroa & Quirk 2005; Davis & Whalen 2001; Kalin et al. 2004), and human neuroimaging studies have shown increases in activity in the amygdala to fearful stimuli in adults (Breiter et al. 1996; Morris et al. 1998) and in children (Thomas et al. 2001b). There is evidence for dysregulation of amygdala activity in anxious and depressed children (Thomas et al. 2001a) and adults (Leppanen 2006; Rauch et al. 2003; Thomas et al. 2001a).

In a recent study, we examined individual differences in anxiety levels as measured by the Spielberger State Trait Anxiety Index and neural responses to affective information in adolescents and adults during an emotional go/no-go task (Hare et al. in press). Adolescents showed greater initial amygdala activity than

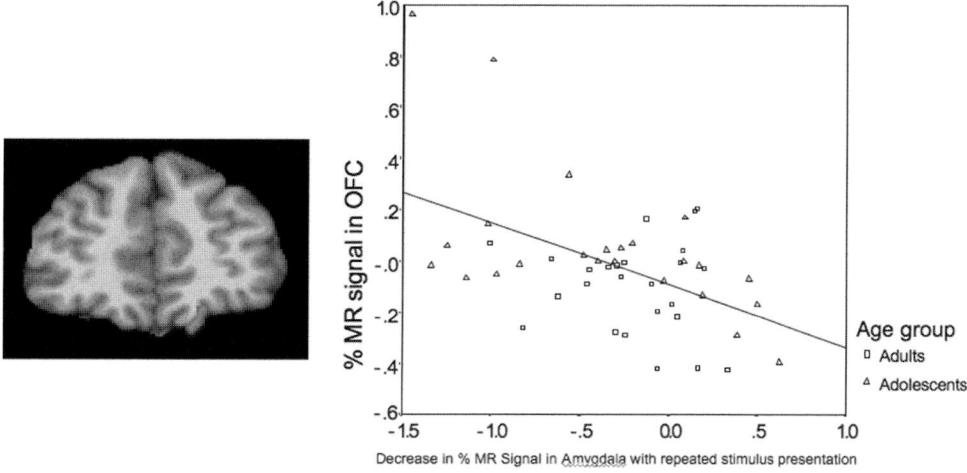

FIGURE 7. Picture depicts left orbitofrontal activity. Graph illustrates correlation of activity in the OFC and in the amygdala in both adults and adolescents (adapted from Hare et al. in press).

adults, and sustained amygdala activity was correlated with trait anxiety. Increased activity in orbitofrontal regions correlated with a decrease in amygdala activity over time (i.e., repeated presentation of a fearful face, see FIG. 7), suggesting dampening of emotional reactivity due to top-down control from prefrontal regions. These findings are consistent with animal studies showing the importance of the orbitofrontal cortex (OFC) in extinction of fear conditioning in animals with repeated exposure to empty threat (Gallagher et al. 1999).

Our results are consistent with previous fMRI studies in clinically anxious adults and children that have shown unregulated amygdala activity to negative emotional information and less activity in the prefrontal cortex (McClure et al. 2007; Shin et al. 2004; Thomas et al. 2001b) in adolescents at risk for anxiety disorders (Perez-Edgar et al. 2007). Together these findings suggest that prefrontal regions serve to regulate emotional reactivity and that individual differences in emotion regulation may be due to an imbalance in activity between these regions that is exacerbated during adolescence.

Conclusions

Human imaging studies show structural and functional changes in frontolimbic regions (Jernigan et al. 1991; Giedd et al. 1999; Giedd et al. 1996; Sowell et al. 1999; for review, Casey et al. 2005; Jernigan et al. 1991; Giedd et al. 1999; Giedd et al. 1996; Sowell et al. 1999) for review, (Casey et al. 2005) that seem to parallel increases in cognitive control and self-regulation (Casey et al. 1997; Luna & Sweeney 2004; Luna et al. 2001; Rubia et al. 2000; Steinberg 2004). These changes appear to show a shift in activation of prefrontal regions from diffuse to more focal recruitment over time (Brown et al. 2005; Bunge et al. 2002; Casey et al. 1997; Durston et al. 2006; Moses et al. 2002) and elevated recruitment of subcortical regions during adolescence (Casey et al. 2002; Durston et al. 2006; Luna et al. 2001). Although neuroimaging studies cannot definitively characterize the mechanism of such developmental changes, these changes in volume and structure may reflect development within, and refinement of, projections to and from these brain regions during maturation suggestive of fine tuning of the system with development.

We have discussed the importance of considering individual variability when examining complex brain–behavior relationships related to risk taking, reward processing, and emotional reactivity in developmental populations. Using an approach that looks at developmental trajectories, rather than snapshots in time, allows one to comprehensively study these behaviors during development and examine individual differences. It is not possible to fully explain the emergence of affective disorders or atypical development by simply examining one time point. Longitudinal studies across development would be the best methodology to address these issues.

Taken together, the findings synthesized here indicate that increased risk-taking behavior and greater emotional reactivity in adolescence are associated with different developmental trajectories of subcortical limbic regions relative cortical control regions. These developmental changes can be exacerbated by individual differences (e.g., genetic risk) in baseline activity of limbic systems.

This model of development reconciles a number of contradictions and myths about adolescence. First, there have been many reports that suggest that adolescent behavior is due to protracted development of prefrontal cortex. However, if this were the case, then children would engage in similar or worse behavior than adolescents. The National Center for Health Statistics on adolescent behavior and mortality shows that suboptimal choices and actions observed during adolescence represent a nonlinear change in behavior, distinct from childhood and adulthood. Adolescents, unlike children, may be in situations (e.g., driving a car) that may put them at greater risk for mortality, but even when taking these conditions into account, there is still a significant elevation of risky behavior in adolescents in comparison to children. Furthermore, experimental studies have shown that when risk is held constant, such as in the appraisal of risky vignettes, children perceive greater risk in hypothetical scenarios than do adolescents (reviewed in Furby & Beyth-Marom 1992). Our neurodevelopmental model provides an explanation for these nonlinear changes in behavior.

Reyna and Farley (2006) have reconciled the second myth by showing that adolescents are able to reason and understand risks of behaviors in which they engage and do not consider themselves invincible. Prior research has also shown that adolescents knowingly engage in risky behavior, and this is often due to influences of feelings, emotions, and peers (Gardener & Steinberg 2005; Steinberg 2004, 2005). The observation that adolescents know that they are engaging in risky behavior is not supported by the sole explanation of a less developed prefrontal cortex. In this context, our model suggests that the adolescent is capable of making rational decisions, but in emotionally charged situations the more mature limbic system will win over the prefrontal control system.

When faced with an immediate personal decision, adolescents will rely less on intellectual capabilities and more on feelings. Nevertheless, when reasoning about a hypothetical, moral dilemma, the adolescent will rely more on logical information (Steinberg 2005). In other words, when a poor decision is made in the heat of the moment, the adolescent may know better, but the salience of the emotional context biases his or her behavior in opposite direction of the optimal action. This work coincides with studies of social cognition showing that adolescents make more rational decisions about hypothetical scenarios versus real-life situations (Sobesky 1983). The environmental context and emotional significance of the decision greatly influence the adolescent (Steinberg 2005).

Our findings and model have significant implications for heated debates on public policy and the treatment of minors in our judicial system. Adolescents show adult levels of intellectual capability earlier than they show evidence of adult levels of impulse control (Reyna & Farley 2006). As such, adolescents may be capable of making informed choices about their future (e.g., terminating a pregnancy) but do not yet have full capacity to override impulses in emotionally charged situations that require decisions in the heat of the moment. Unfortunately, judges, politicians, advocates, and journalists are biased toward drawing a single line between adolescence and adulthood for different purposes under the law that is at odds with developmental cognitive neuroscience (Steinberg et al. in press). Our neurodevelopmental model of adolescence will hopefully help to make strides in moving this single line to multiple lines that consider developmental changes across both context (emotionally charged or not) and time (in the moment or in the future).

Acknowledgments

This work was supported in part by grants from the National Institute of Drug Abuse R01 DA18879 and the National Institute of Mental Health R01 MH73175 and P50 MH62196 to BJC.

Conflict of Interests

The authors declare no conflicts of interest.

References

Adriani, W., Chiarotti, F., & Laviola, G. (1998). Elevated novelty seeking and peculiar d-amphetamine sensitization in periadolescent mice compared with adult mice. *Behav Neurosci*, *112*(5), 1152–1166.

Andersen, S. L., & Teicher, M. H. (2004). Delayed effects of early stress on hippocampal development. *Neuropsychopharmacology*, *29*(11), 1988–1993.

Andersen, S. L., Thompson, A. T., Rutstein, M., Hostetter, J. C., & Teicher, M. H. (2000). Dopamine receptor pruning in prefrontal cortex during the periadolescent period in rats. *Synapse*, *37*(2), 167–169.

Anglada-Figueroa, D., & Quirk, G. J. (2005). Lesions of the basal amygdala block expression of conditioned fear but not extinction. *J Neurosci*, *25*(42), 9680–9685.

Baird, A. A., Gruber, S. A., Fein, D. A., Maas, L. C., Steingard, R. J., Renshaw, P. F., et al. (1999). Functional magnetic resonance imaging of facial affect recognition in children and adolescents. *J Am Acad Child Adolesc Psychiatry, 38*(2), 195–199.

Baxter, M. G., Parker, A., Lindner, C. C., Izquierdo, A. D., & Murray, E. A. (2000). Control of response selection by reinforcer value requires interaction of amygdala and orbital prefrontal cortex. *J Neurosci, 20*(11), 4311–4319.

Benthin, A., Slovic, P., & Severson, H. (1993). A psychometric study of adolescent risk perception. *J Adolesc, 16*(2), 153–168.

Bjork, J. M., Smith, A. R., Danube, C. L., & Hommer, D. W. (2007). Developmental differences in posterior mesofrontal cortex recruitment by risky rewards. *J Neurosci, 27*(18), 4839–4849.

Bjorkland, D. F. (1985). The role of conceptual knowledge in the development of organization in children's memory. In C. J. Brainerd & M. Pressley (Eds.), *Basic Processes in Memory Development: Progress in Cognitive Development Research* (pp. 103–142). New York: Springer-Verlag.

Bjorkland, D. F. (1987). How age changes in knowledge base contribute to the development of children's memory: An interpretive review. *Developmental Review, 7*, 93–130.

Blum, K., Braverman, E. R., Holder, J. M., Lubar, J. F., Monastra, V. J., Miller, D., et al. (2000). Reward deficiency syndrome: a biogenetic model for the diagnosis and treatment of impulsive, addictive, and compulsive behaviors. *J Psychoactive Drugs, 32 Suppl*, i–iv, 1–112.

Bogin, B. (1994). Adolescence in evolutionary perspective. *Acta Paediatr Suppl, 406*, 29–35; discussion 36.

Bourgeois, J. P., Goldman-Rakic, P. S., & Rakic, P. (1994). Synaptogenesis in the prefrontal cortex of rhesus monkeys. *Cereb Cortex, 4*(1), 78–96.

Brainerd, C. J., & Reyna, V. F. (1993). Memory independence and memory interference in cognitive development. *Psychol Rev, 100*(1), 42–67.

Breiter, H. C., Etcoff, N. L., Whalen, P. J., Kennedy, W. A., Rauch, S. L., Buckner, R. L., et al. (1996). Response and habituation of the human amygdala during visual processing of facial expression. *Neuron, 17*(5), 875–887.

Brown, T. T., Lugar, H. M., Coalson, R. S., Miezin, F. M., Petersen, S. E., & Schlaggar, B. L. (2005). Developmental changes in human cerebral functional organization for word generation. *Cereb Cortex, 15*(3), 275–290.

Bunge, S. A., Dudukovic, N. M., Thomason, M. E., Vaidya, C. J., & Gabrieli, J. D. (2002). Immature frontal lobe contributions to cognitive control in children: evidence from fMRI. *Neuron, 33*(2), 301–311.

Cascio, C. J., Gerig, G., & Piven, J. (2007). Diffusion tensor imaging: Application to the study of the developing brain. *J Am Acad Child Adolesc Psychiatry, 46*(2), 213–223.

Case, R. (1972). Balidation of a neo-Piagetian capacity construct. *Journal of Experimental Child Psychology, 14*, 287–302.

Case, R. (1985). *Intellectual Development Birth to Adulthood*. New York: Academic Press.

Casey, B. J., Castellanos, F. X., Giedd, J. N., Marsh, W. L., Hamburger, S. D., Schubert, A. B., et al. (1997a). Implication of right frontostriatal circuitry in response inhibition and attention-deficit/hyperactivity disorder. *J Am Acad Child Adolesc Psychiatry, 36*(3), 374–383.

Casey, B. J., Galvan, A., & Hare, T. A. (2005a). Changes in cerebral functional organization during cognitive development. *Curr Opin Neurobiol, 15*(2), 239–244.

Casey, B., Getz, S., & Galvan, A. (in press). *Developmental Review*.

Casey, B. J., Giedd, J. N., & Thomas, K. M. (2000a). Structural and functional brain development and its relation to cognitive development. *Biol Psychol, 54*(1–3), 241–257.

Casey, B. J., Thomas, K. M., Davidson, M. C., Kunz, K., & Franzen, P. L. (2002a). Dissociating striatal and hippocampal function developmentally with a stimulus-response compatibility task. *J Neurosci, 22*(19), 8647–8652.

Casey, B. J., Thomas, K. M., Welsh, T. F., Badgaiyan, R. D., Eccard, C. H., Jennings, J. R., et al. (2000b). Dissocaiation of response conflict, attentional selection, and expectancy with functional magnetic resonance imaging. *Proc Natl Acad Sci, USA, 97*(18), 8728–8733.

Casey, B. J., Tottenham, N., & Fossella, J. (2002b). Clinical, imaging, lesion, and genetic approaches toward a model of cognitive control. *Dev Psychobiol, 40*(3), 237–254.

Casey, B. J., Tottenham, N., Liston, C., & Durston, S. (2005b). Imaging the developing brain: what have we learned about cognitive development? *Trends in Cognitive Science, 9*(3), 104–110.

Casey, B. J., Trainor, R. J., Orendi, J. L., Schubert, A. B., Nystrom, L. E., Giedd, J. N., et al. (1997b). A developmental functional MRI study of prefrontal activation during performance of a go-no-go task. *Journal of Cognitive Neuroscience, 9*, 835–847.

Caviness, V., Kennedy, D., Richelme, C., Rademacher, J., & Filipek, P. (1996). The human brain age 7–11 years: a volumetric analysis based on magnetic resonance images. *Cereb Cortex, 6*(5), 726–736.

Crews, F., He, J., & Hodge, C. (2007). Adolescent cortical development: a critical period of vulnerability for addiction. *Pharmacol Biochem Behav, 86*(2), 189–199.

Csikszentmihalyi, M., Larson, R., & Prescott, S. (1977). The ecology of adolescent activity and experience. *Journal of Youth and Adolescence, 6*, 281–294.

Cunningham, M. G., Bhattacharyya, S., & Benes, F. M. (2002). Amygdalo-cortical sprouting continues into early adulthood: implications for the development of normal and abnormal function during adolescence. *J Comp Neurol, 453*(2), 116–130.

Davis, M., & Whalen, P. J. (2001). The amygdala: vigilance and emotion. *Mol Psychiatry, 6*(1), 13–34.

Dempster, F. N. (Ed.) (1993). *Resistance to Interference: Developmental Changes in a Basic Processing Mechanism*. (Vol. 1). New York: Springer-Verlag.

Diamond, A. (1985). Development of the ability to use recall to guide action, as indicated by infants' performance on AB. *Child Development, 56*, 868–883.

Durston, S., Davidson, M. C., Thomas, K. M., Worden, M. S., Tottenham, N., Martinez, A., et al. (2003). Parametric manipulation of conflict and response competition using rapid mixed-trial event-related fMRI. *Neuroimage, 20*(4), 2135–2141.

Durston, S., Davidson, M. C., Tottenham, N., Galvan, A., Spicer, J., Fossella, J. A., et al. (2006). A shift from diffuse to focal cortical activity with development. *Dev Sci, 9*(1), 1–8.

Durston, S., Hulshoff, H. E., Casey, B. J., Giedd, J. N., Buitelaar, J. K., & Van Engeland, H. (2001). Anatomical MRI of the developing human brain: What have we learned? *J Am Acad Child Adolesc Psychiatry, 40*(9), 1012–1020.

Eaton, L. K., Kinchen, S., Ross, J., Hawkins, J., Harris, W. A., Lowry, R., et al. (2006). Youth risk behavior surveillance-United States, 2005, surveillance summaries. *Morbidity and Mortality Weekly Report, 55*(SS-5), 1–108.

Eigsti, I. M., Zayas, V., Mischel, W., Shoda, Y., Ayduk, O., Dadlani, M. B., et al. (2006). Predicting cognitive control from preschool to late adolescence and young adulthood. *Psychol Sci, 17*(6), 478–484.

Ernst, M., Nelson, E. E., Jazbec, S., McClure, E. B., Monk, C. S., Leibenluft, E., et al. (2005). Amygdala and nucleus accumbens in responses to receipt and omission of gains in adults and adolescents. *Neuroimage, 25*(4), 1279–1291.

Ernst, M., Pine, D. S., & Hardin, M. (2006). Triadic model of the neurobiology of motivated behavior in adolescence. *Psychol Med, 36*(3), 299–312.

Eshel, N., Nelson, E. E., Blair, R. J., Pine, D. S., & Ernst, M. (2007). Neural substrates of choice selection in adults and adolescents: development of the ventrolateral prefrontal and anterior cingulate cortices. *Neuropsychologia, 45*(6), 1270–1279.

Flavell, J. H., Feach, D. R., & Chinsky, J. M. (1966). Spontaneous verbal rehearsal in a memory task as a function of age. *Child Development, 37*, 283–299.

Floresco, S. B., & Tse, M. T. (2007). Dopaminergic regulation of inhibitory and excitatory transmission in the basolateral amygdala-prefrontal cortical pathway. *J Neurosci, 27*(8), 2045–2057.

Furby, L., & Beyth-Marom, R. (1992). Risk taking in adolescence: A decision-making perspective. *Developmental Review, 12*(1), 1–44.

Gallagher, M., McMahan, R. W., & Schoenbaum, G. (1999). Orbitofrontal cortex and representation of incentive value in associative learning. *J Neurosci, 19*(15), 6610–6614.

Galvan, A., Hare, T., Voss, H., Glover, G., & Casey, B. J. (2007). Risk-taking and the adolescent brain: who is at risk? *Dev Sci, 10*(2), F8–F14.

Galvan, A., Hare, T. A., Parra, C. E., Penn, J., Voss, H., Glover, G., et al. (2006). Earlier development of the accumbens relative to orbitofrontal cortex might underlie risk-taking behavior in adolescents. *J Neurosci, 26*(25), 6885–6892.

Gardener, M., & Steinberg, L. (2005). Peer influence on risk taking, risk preference, and risky decision making in adolescence and adulthood: an experimental study. *Developmental Psychology, 41*, 625–635.

Giedd, J. N. (2004). Structural magnetic resonance imaging of the adolescent brain. *Ann N Y Acad Sci, 1021*, 77–85.

Giedd, J. N., Blumenthal, J., Jeffries, N. O., Castellanos, F. X., Liu, H., Zijdenbos, A., et al. (1999). Brain development during childhood and adolescence: a longitudinal MRI study. *Nat Neurosci, 2*(10), 861–863.

Giedd, J. N., Snell, J. W., Lange, N., Rajapakse, J. C., Casey, B. J., Kaysen, D., et al. (1996). Quantitative magnetic resonance imaging of human brain development: ages 4–18. *Cereb Cortex, 6*, 551–560.

Gogtay, N., Giedd, J. N., Lusk, L., Hayashi, K. M., Greenstein, D., Vaituzis, A. C., et al. (2004). Dynamic mapping of human cortical development during childhood through early adulthood. *Proc Natl Acad Sci U S A, 101*(21), 8174–8179.

Grace, A. A., Floresco, S. B., Goto, Y., & Lodge, D. J. (2007). Regulation of firing of dopaminergic neurons and control of goal-directed behaviors. *Trends Neurosci, 30*(5), 220–227.

Hare, T., & Casey, B. (in press). *Biological Psychiatry*.

Hare, T. A., & Casey, B. J. (2005). The neurobiology and development of cognitive and affective control. *Cognition, Brain, Behavior, 9*(3), 273–286.

Hare, T. A., Tottenham, N., Davidson, M. C., Glover, G. H., & Casey, B. J. (2005). Contributions of amygdala and striatal activity in emotion regulation. *Biol Psychiatry, 57*(6), 624–632.

Hare, T. A., Tottenham, N., Voss, H. U., Glover, G. H., & Casey, B. J. (in press). The adolescent brain and potential risk for anxiety and depression. *Biological Psychiatry*.

Harnishfeger, K. K., & Bjorkland, F. (1993). The ontogeny of inhibition mechanisms: A renewed approach to cognitive development. In M. L. Howe & R. Pasnek (Eds.), *Emerging Themes in Cognitive Development* (Vol. 1, pp. 28–49). New York: Springer-Verlag.

Hikosaka, K., & Watanabe, M. (2000). Delay activity of orbital and lateral prefrontal neurons of the monkey varying with different rewards. *Cereb Cortex, 10*(3), 263–271.

Huttenlocher, P. R. (1979). Synaptic density in human frontal cortex - developmental changes and effects of aging. *Brain Res, 163*(2), 195–205.

Hyman, S. E., & Malenka, R. C. (2001). Addiction and the brain: the neurobiology of compulsion and its persistence. *Nat Rev Neurosci, 2*(10), 695–703.

Jackson, M. E., Frost, A. S., & Moghaddam, B. (2001). Stimulation of prefrontal cortex at physiologically relevant frequencies inhibits dopamine release in the nucleus accumbens. *J Neurochem, 78*(4), 920–923.

Jernigan, T. L., Zisook, S., Heaton, R. K., Moranville, J. T., Hesselink, J. R., & Braff, D. L. (1991). Magnetic resonance imaging abnormalities in lenticular nuclei and cerebral cortex in schizophrenia. *Arch Gen Psychiatry, 48*, 881–890.

Kalin, N. H., Shelton, S. E., & Davidson, R. J. (2004). The role of the central nucleus of the amygdala in mediating fear and anxiety in the primate. *J Neurosci, 24*(24), 5506–5515.

Kalsbeek, A., Voorn, P., Buijs, R. M., Pool, C. W., & Uylings, H. B. (1988). Development of the dopaminergic innervation in the prefrontal cortex of the rat. *J Comp Neurol, 269*(1), 58–72.

Keating, D. P., & Bobbitt, B. L. (1978). Individual and developmental differences in cognitive processing components of mental ability. *Child Development, 49*, 155–167.

Kelley, A. E., Schochet, T., & Landry, C. F. (2004). Risk taking and novelty seeking in adolescence: introduction to part I. *Ann N Y Acad Sci, 1021*, 27–32.

Killgore, W. D., Oki, M., & Yurgelun-Todd, D. A. (2001). Sex-specific developmental changes in amygdala responses to affective faces. *Neuroreport, 12*(2), 427–433.

Knutson, B., Adams, C. M., Fong, G. W., & Hommer, D. (2001). Anticipation of increasing monetary reward selectively recruits nucleus accumbens. *J Neurosci, 21*(16), RC159.

Kuhnen, C. M., & Knutson, B. (2005). The neural basis of financial risk taking. *Neuron, 47*(5), 763–770.

Laviola, G., Adriani, W., Terranova, M. L., & Gerra, G. (1999). Psychobiological risk factors for vulnerability to psychostimulants in human adolescents and animal models. *Neurosci Biobehav Rev, 23*(7), 993–1010.

Laviola, G., Macri, S., Morley-Fletcher, S., & Adriani, W. (2003). Risk-taking behavior in adolescent mice: psychobiological determinants and early epigenetic influence. *Neurosci Biobehav Rev, 27*(1–2), 19–31.

Lenroot, R. K., & Giedd, J. N. (2006). Brain development in children and adolescents: insights from anatomical magnetic resonance imaging. *Neurosci Biobehav Rev, 30*(6), 718–729.

Leppanen, J. M. (2006). Emotional information processing in mood disorders: a review of behavioral and neuroimaging findings. *Curr Opin Psychiatry, 19*(1), 34–39.

Liston, C., Watts, R., Tottenham, N., Davidson, M. C., Niogi, S., Ulug, A. M., et al. (2006). Frontostriatal microstructure modulates efficient recruitment of cognitive control. *Cereb Cortex, 16*(4), 553–560.

Luna, B., & Sweeney, J. A. (2004). The emergence of collaborative brain function: FMRI studies of the development of response inhibition. *Ann N Y Acad Sci, 1021*, 296–309.

Luna, B., Thulborn, K. R., Munoz, D. P., Merriam, E. P., Garver, K. E., Minshew, N. J., et al. (2001). Maturation of widely distributed brain function subserves cognitive development. *Neuroimage, 13*(5), 786–793.

Maren, S., & Quirk, G. J. (2004). Neuronal signalling of fear memory. *Nat Rev Neurosci, 5*(11), 844–852.

Matthews, S. C., Simmons, A. N., Lane, S. D., & Paulus, M. P. (2004). Selective activation of the nucleus accumbens during risk-taking decision making. *Neuroreport, 15*(13), 2123–2127.

May, J. C., Delgado, M. R., Dahl, R. E., Stenger, V. A., Ryan, N. D., Fiez, J. A., et al. (2004). Event-related functional magnetic resonance imaging of reward-related brain circuitry in children and adolescents. *Biol Psychiatry, 55*(4), 359–366.

McClure, E. B., Monk, C. S., Nelson, E. E., Parrish, J. M., Adler, A., Blair, R. J., et al. (2007). Abnormal attention modulation of fear circuit function in pediatric generalized anxiety disorder. *Arch Gen Psychiatry, 64*(1), 97–106.

McClure, S. M., Laibson, D. I., Loewenstein, G., & Cohen, J. D. (2004). Separate neural systems value immediate and delayed monetary rewards. *Science, 306*(5695), 503–507.

Miller, E. K., & Cohen, J. D. (2001). An integrative theory of prefrontal cortex function. *Annu Rev Neurosci, 24*, 167–202.

Mischel, W., Shoda, Y., & Rodriguez, M. I. (1989). Delay of gratification in children. *Science, 244*(4907), 933–938.

Monk, C. S., McClure, E. B., Nelson, E. E., Zarahn, E., Bilder, R. M., Leibenluft, E., et al. (2003). Adolescent immaturity in attention-related brain engagement to emotional facial expressions. *Neuroimage, 20*(1), 420–428.

Montague, P. R., & Berns, G. S. (2002). Neural economics and the biological substrates of valuation. *Neuron, 36*(2), 265–284.

Morris, J. S., Friston, K. J., Buchel, C., Frith, C. D., Young, A. W., Calder, A. J., et al. (1998). A neuromodulatory role for the human amygdala in processing emotional facial expressions. *Brain, 121*(Pt 1), 47–57.

Moses, P., Roe, K., Buxton, R. B., Wong, E. C., Frank, L. R., & Stiles, J. (2002). Functional MRI of global and local processing in children. *Neuroimage, 16*(2), 415–424.

Munakata, Y., & Yerys, B. E. (2001). All together now: when dissociations between knowledge and action disappear. *Psychol Sci, 12*(4), 335–337.

Nagy, Z., Westerberg, H., & Klingberg, T. (2004). Maturation of white matter is associated with the development of cognitive functions during childhood. *J Cogn Neurosci, 16*(7), 1227–1233.

O'Doherty, J., Kringelbach, M. L., Rolls, E. T., Hornak, J., & Andrews, C. (2001). Abstract reward and punishment representations in the human orbitofrontal cortex. *Nat Neurosci, 4*(1), 95–102.

O'Doherty, J. P. (2004). Reward representations and reward-related learning in the human brain: insights from neuroimaging. *Curr Opin Neurobiol, 14*(6), 769–776.

Pascual-Leone, J. A. (1970). A mathematical model for transition in Piaget's developmental stages. *Acta Psychologica, 32*, 301–345.

Pecina, S., Cagniard, B., Berridge, K. C., Aldridge, J. W., & Zhuang, X. (2003). Hyperdopaminergic mutant mice have higher "wanting" but not "liking" for sweet rewards. *J Neurosci, 23*(28), 9395–9402.

Perez-Edgar, K., Roberson-Nay, R., Hardin, M. G., Poeth, K., Guyer, A. E., Nelson, E. E., et al. (2007). Attention alters neural responses to evocative faces in behaviorally inhibited adolescents. *Neuroimage, 35*(4), 1538–1546.

Pine, D. S., Cohen, P., & Brook, J. S. (2001). Emotional reactivity and risk for psychopathology among adolescents. *CNS Spectr, 6*(1), 27–35.

Primus, R. J., & Kellogg, C. K. (1989). Pubertal-related changes influence the development of environment-related social interaction in the male rat. *Dev Psychobiol, 22*(6), 633–643.

Rauch, S. L., Shin, L. M., & Wright, C. I. (2003). Neuroimaging studies of amygdala function in anxiety disorders. *Ann N Y Acad Sci, 985*, 389–410.

Reiss, A., Abrams, M., Singer, H., Ross, J., & Denckla, M. (1996). Brain development, gender and IQ in children. A volumetric imaging study. *Brain, 119*, 1763–1774.

Reyna, V., & Farley, F. (2006). Risk and rationality in adolescent decision making: implications for theory, practice, and public policy. *Psychological Science in the Public Interest, 7*(1), 1–44.

Rosenberg, D. R., & Lewis, D. A. (1994). Changes in the dopaminergic innervation of monkey prefrontal cortex during late postnatal development: a tyrosine hydroxylase immunohistochemical study. *Biol Psychiatry, 36*(4), 272–277.

Rosenberg, D. R., & Lewis, D. A. (1995). Postnatal maturation of the dopaminergic innervation of monkey prefrontal and motor cortices: a tyrosine hydroxylase immunohistochemical analysis. *J Comp Neurol, 358*(3), 383–400.

Rubia, K., Overmeyer, S., Taylor, E., Brammer, M., Williams, S. C., Simmons, A., et al. (2000). Functional frontalisation with age: mapping neurodevelopmental trajectories with fMRI. *Neurosci Biobehav Rev, 24*(1), 13–19.

Rubia, K., Smith, A. B., Woolley, J., Nosarti, C., Heyman, I., Taylor, E., et al. (2006). Progressive increase of frontostriatal brain activation from childhood to adulthood during event-related tasks of cognitive control. *Hum Brain Mapp, 27*(12), 973–993.

Schlaggar, B. L., Brown, T. T., Lugar, H. M., Visscher, K. M., Miezin, F. M., & Petersen, S. E. (2002). Functional neuroanatomical differences between adults and school-age children in the processing of single words. *Science, 296*(5572), 1476–1479.

Schultz, W. (2006). Behavioral theories and the neurophysiology of reward. *Annual Reviews of Psychology, 57*, 87–115.

Shin, L. M., Orr, S. P., Carson, M. A., Rauch, S. L., Macklin, M. L., Lasko, N. B., et al. (2004). Regional cerebral blood flow in the amygdala and medial prefrontal cortex during traumatic imagery in male and female Vietnam veterans with PTSD. *Arch Gen Psychiatry, 61*(2), 168–176.

Silveri, M. M., Tzilos, G. K., Pimentel, P. J., & Yurgelun-Todd, D. A. (2004). Trajectories of adolescent emotional and cognitive development: effects of sex and risk for drug use. *Ann N Y Acad Sci, 1021*, 363–370.

Sobesky, W. (1983). The effects of situational factors on moral judgements. *Child Development, 54*, 575–584.

Sowell, E. R., Peterson, B. S., Thompson, P. M., Welcome, S. E., Henkenius, A. L., & Toga, A. W. (2003). Mapping cortical change across the human life span. *Nat Neurosci, 6*(3), 309–315.

Sowell, E. R., Thompson, P. M., Holmes, C. J., Jernigan, T. L., & Toga, A. W. (1999). In vivo evidence for post-adolescent brain maturation in frontal and striatal regions. *Nat Neurosci, 2*(10), 859–861.

Sowell, E. R., Thompson, P. M., & Toga, A. W. (2004). Mapping changes in the human cortex throughout the span of life. *Neuroscientist, 10*(4), 372–392.

Spear, L. P. (2000). The adolescent brain and age-related behavioral manifestations. *Neurosci Biobehav Rev, 24*(4), 417–463.

Steinberg, L. (1989). Pubertal maturation and parent-adolescent distance: an evolutionary perspective. In G. Adams, R. Montemayor & T. Gullotta (Eds.), *Advances in Adolescent Behavior and Development* (pp. 71–97). Newbury Park, CA: Sage Publications.

Steinberg, L. (2004). Risk taking in adolescence: what changes, and why? *Ann N Y Acad Sci, 1021*, 51–58.

Steinberg, L. (2005). Cognitive and affective development in adolescence. *Trends Cogn Sci, 9*(2), 69–74.

Steinberg, L., Cauffman, E., Woolard, J., Graham, S., & Banich, M. (in press). Are adolescents less mature than adults? Minors' access to abortion, the juvenile death penalty, and the alleged APA "Flip-Flop".

Tamm, L., Menon, V., & Reiss, A. L. (2002). Maturation of brain function associated with response inhibition. *J Am Acad Child Adolesc Psychiatry, 41*(10), 1231–1238.

Tarazi, F. I., Tomasini, E. C., & Baldessarini, R. J. (1998). Postnatal development of dopamine and serotonin transporters in rat caudate-putamen and nucleus accumbens septi. *Neurosci Lett, 254*(1), 21–24.

Teicher, M. H., Andersen, S. L., & Hostetter, J. C., Jr. (1995). Evidence for dopamine receptor pruning between adolescence and adulthood in striatum but not nucleus accumbens. *Brain Res Dev Brain Res, 89*(2), 167–172.

Thomas, K. M., Drevets, W. C., Dahl, R. E., Ryan, N. D., Birmaher, B., Eccard, C. H., et al. (2001a). Amygdala response to fearful faces in anxious and depressed children. *Arch Gen Psychiatry, 58*(11), 1057–1063.

Thomas, K. M., Drevets, W. C., Whalen, P. J., Eccard, C. H., Dahl, R. E., Ryan, N. D., et al. (2001b). Amygdala response to facial expressions in children and adults. *Biol Psychiatry, 49*(4), 309–316.

Thomas, K. M., Hunt, R. H., Vizueta, N., Sommer, T., Durston, S., Yang, Y., et al. (2004). Evidence of developmental differences in implicit sequence learning: an FMRI study of children and adults. *J Cogn Neurosci, 16*(8), 1339–1351.

Turkeltaub, P. E., Gareau, L., Flowers, D. L., Zeffiro, T. A., & Eden, G. F. (2003). Development of neural mechanisms for reading. *Nat Neurosci, 6*(7), 767–773.

Volkow, N. D., & Li, T. K. (2004). Drug addiction: the neurobiology of behaviour gone awry. *Nat Rev Neurosci, 5*(12), 963–970.

Yurgelun-Todd, D. (2007). Emotional and cognitive changes during adolescence. *Curr Opin Neurobiol, 17*(2), 251–257.

Yurgelun-Todd, D. A., & Killgore, W. D. (2006). Fear-related activity in the prefrontal cortex increases with age during adolescence: a preliminary fMRI study. *Neurosci Lett, 406*(3), 194–199.

Zald, D. H., Boileau, I., El-Dearedy, W., Gunn, R., McGlone, F., Dichter, G. S., et al. (2004). Dopamine transmission in the human striatum during monetary reward tasks. *J Neurosci, 24*(17), 4105–4112.

Zehr, J. L., Todd, B. J., Schulz, K. M., McCarthy, M. M., & Sisk, C. L. (2006). Dendritic pruning of the medial amygdala during pubertal development of the male Syrian hamster. *J Neurobiol, 66*(6), 578–590.

Cognitive Neuroscience of Aging

CHERYL L. GRADY

Rotman Research Institute at Baycrest, University of Toronto, Toronto, Ontario, Canada

The number of reports on the cognitive neuroscience of aging has increased in recent years, and most of these studies have found many similarities in the patterns of activity in young and old adults, indicating that basic neural mechanisms are maintained into older age. Despite these overall similarities, older adults often have less activity in some regions, such as medial temporal areas during memory processing and visual regions across a variety of cognitive domains. It seems clear that age reductions in cognitive function can be tied, at least in part, to these reductions in brain activity. On the other hand, older adults typically also overrecruit some brain areas, mainly the ventral or dorsal prefrontal cortex during memory tasks, as well as both the frontal and parietal regions during tasks engaging cognitive control processes, such as attention. Sometimes this overrecruitment appears to be in response to altered function in other brain regions and is often seen in those older adults who perform better on the task at hand. These findings have provided rather convincing support for the idea that overrecruitment can be compensatory in the elderly. Nevertheless, not all age increases can be interpreted as compensatory, and some are more indicative of neural inefficiency. The challenge facing future research will be to understand the task conditions that promote compensation in older adults, the role of the various brain areas in aiding cognitive function, and how these compensatory mechanisms can be elicited to enhance quality of life in the elderly.

Key words: memory; attention; functional magnetic resonance imaging; frontal lobes; compensation, plasticity

The past few years have seen a dramatic increase in the number of reports using functional magnetic resonance imaging (fMRI) to explore brain function (Bandettini 2007). Although still a small proportion of the total, the number of articles on the cognitive neuroscience of aging also has increased in recent years (Cabeza et al. 2005). Work in this area has focused primarily on memory, which reflects the large behavioral literature on memory changes in older adults. Behavioral studies typically show reductions in memory function in older adults, particularly in terms of episodic memory (e.g., Balota et al. 2000) and working memory (e.g., Foos & Wright 1992; Hasher & Zacks 1988). Consistent with these behavioral data, reduced brain activity in older adults, compared with that in younger adults, has been noted during a variety of memory tasks, in regions such as the left prefrontal cortex (PFC) during encoding, or learning new material (Cabeza et al. 1997; Grady et al. 1995; Logan et al. 2002) and medial temporal areas during memory encoding and retrieval (Cabeza et al. 2004; Grady et al. 1995; Gutchess et al. 2005).

However, reports of increased brain activity in older adults, compared with that in young adults, have attracted more interest from researchers in this field. This "overrecruitment" typically is found in the frontal lobes, either in areas of the PFC not active in young adults or in homologous regions in the opposite hemisphere from regions active in the young. These age-related increases have been seen in episodic memory tasks (Cabeza 2002), working memory tasks (Grady et al. 1998; Reuter-Lorenz et al. 2000), and even in perceptual tasks (Grady et al. 1994). Because this pattern of overrecruitment in older adults has been reported in those who perform better on the task (Cabeza et al. 2002; Grady et al. 2005), there have been suggestions that additional recruitment of brain activity compensates for age-related changes in brain structure and function. On the other hand, some of this increased prefrontal activity in the elderly may reflect greater need or use of frontally mediated executive functions at lower levels of task demand than would be necessary for activation of this area in young adults. In this case, the increased activity in the PFC might not be related to performance on the particular experimental task but would reflect a type of nonselective recruitment in older adults, perhaps related to task difficulty (Logan et al. 2002). Thus, although additional recruitment of PFC in older

Address for correspondence: Cheryl L. Grady, PhD, Rotman Research Institute at Baycrest, 3560 Bathurst St., Toronto, Ontario M6A 2E1, Canada.
cgrady@rotman-baycrest.on.ca

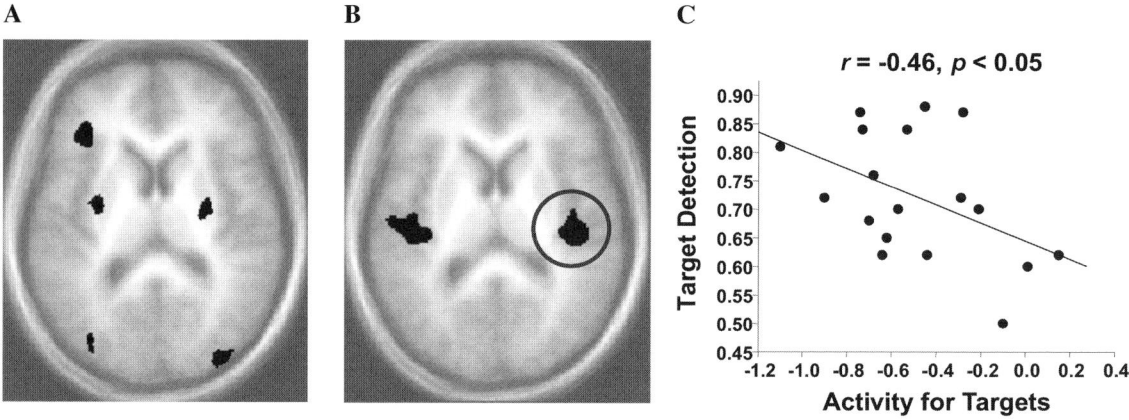

FIGURE 1. Age differences in brain activity during auditory working memory are shown (adapted from Grady et al. 2008). **(A)** Areas with more sustained activity in older adults than younger adults during the nonspatial task (blue), the spatial task (red), and both tasks (yellow, regions shown on an average MRI slice). **(B)** Regions of auditory cortex bilaterally (in blue) where older adults showed less adaptation to one-back targets than did younger adults. The degree of adaptation in the right auditory cortex (circled) was related to working memory performance in the older adults **(C)**. That is, the ability to reduce activity in this region for targets was associated with better target detection.

adults may be compensatory, it is not necessarily so.

The recent reports published in cognitive neuroscience of aging have continued to examine the issue of compensation but have also extended this work to begin to examine the influence of structural changes with age on functional measures. This review will group the past year's work on the basis of four broad themes that characterize the research foci emerging in the past year. These are (1) studies focusing primarily on the effects of age on specific cognitive processes, (2) studies that address the relation of activation to underlying structure or vasculature, (3) the elucidation of cognitive networks by using analytic approaches that emphasize functional connectivity, and (4) studies whose main aim is the exploration of the relation between activation and behavior in older adults to find evidence for or against the compensation hypothesis.

Specific Cognitive Processes

Memory

Recent work has continued to focus on memory mechanisms, as did many of the earlier studies in this field. Two experiments have used the mixed block–event type of fMRI design (Donaldson et al. 2001) to look at both sustained and transient activity in young and older adults during memory processing. Dennis et al. (2007) examined brain activity during a semantic encoding task by using words, and measures of both trial-related transient activity and block-related sustained activity were obtained. In the analysis, both transient and sustained activity were weighted by whether each stimulus was remembered and the participant's confidence in the memory judgment. Transient activity during encoding showed a reduction with age in the hippocampus and visual regions but increased activity in the left dorsolateral PFC. In contrast, sustained activity in the right dorsolateral PFC was lower in older adults, and no areas showed sustained increases. The authors suggested that during semantic classification, older adults show less spontaneous engagement of hippocampally mediated encoding processes but greater use of semantic processes mediated by the left PFC. Also, the decline in sustained right PFC activity may involve age-related deficits in sustained attention that affect encoding processes. A somewhat different result was reported by Grady et al. (2008), who used environmental sounds and a mixed block–event fMRI design to examine working memory for spatial and nonspatial auditory information by using one-back tasks. Sustained activity during blocks of the two types of task was assessed, along with transient activity to targets. In this experiment, older adults had more sustained activity in the left inferior PFC, as well as left parietal and bilateral occipital activity, during both tasks (FIG. 1A). Age increases in transient activity were seen only during the nonspatial task in the parietal and subcortical regions. There were many differences between the design of these two experiments, so they cannot be compared directly, but the different results in the PFC indicate that additional recruitment of PFC-mediated executive functions in older adults can be either sustained throughout performance of a memory task or engaged transiently for processing of specific items. In both cases, this overrecruitment of the left PFC supported performance in the elderly, because it was found during successful encoding events or during performance of a working memory task on which no age difference in accuracy was seen.

Two other studies reported age differences in both PFC and hippocampal activity during memory processing. These studies also attempted to remove any confounders of performance differences in older adults by studying conditions under which older adults can perform as well as do younger adults. Daselaar et al. (2006) used a verbal recognition task to assess recollection and familiarity in young and older adults, and the group matched performance on a subject-by-subject basis in the two age groups. They found a dissociation within the medial temporal lobes between recollection-related activity in the hippocampus, which was reduced in older adults, and familiarity-related activity in the rhinal cortex, which was increased in older adults, relative to the younger group. Older adults also showed reduced functional connectivity within a hippocampal–parietotemporal network but increased connectivity within a rhinal–frontal network. The authors interpreted these findings as evidence that older adults compensate for hippocampal deficits by relying more on the rhinal cortex, possibly through a top-down frontal modulation. Fernandes et al. (2006) compared young and old adults on verbal recognition memory tasks under both full and divided attention, in which the secondary task was making animacy judgments on words. Older adults showed the same amount of memory interference as young adults during the divided-attention condition. Younger adults in the divided condition showed an increase in the left inferior PFC, coupled with a decrease in right hippocampal activity; these effects were diminished in older adults, who also showed an increase in anterior frontal activity bilaterally. Fernandes et al. concluded that the equivalent memory interference seen in the older adults was due to both a dampening of the hippocampal and left inferior PFC responses to divided attention and the increased anterior PFC activity. Also, it seems unlikely that the age differences in PFC and hippocampal activity seen in these two experiments reflected task difficulty or simple performance differences, because behavioral measures were equivalent in younger and older groups.

Performance issues also were a focus of recent work on working and semantic memory in older adults. A study by Mattay et al. (2006) examined the effect of increased working memory load, using a series of n-back tasks, on brain activity, and clarified some of the limits of overrecruitment in older adults. They found a similar distribution of cortical activity between younger and older groups during the n-back tasks; however, there was a significant group difference in dorsolateral PFC bilaterally. In the one-back task, when the older group performed as well as the younger group, the older group showed greater PFC activity. At higher working memory loads, when they performed worse than the younger adults, this relative increase was absent. The authors suggested that compensatory mechanisms, such as additional prefrontal activity, can be called upon to maintain proficiency in task performance, but as cognitive demand increases, compensation cannot be maintained and performance declines. Nielson et al. (2006) looked at a task tapping semantic memory for famous people, in which there were no group differences in accuracy, and both young and old adults scored at better than 90% accuracy levels. Both groups engaged several regions during the task, including the posterior cingulate, right hippocampus, temporal lobe, and left prefrontal regions. Older adults had more extensive and greater magnitude of activation in the left PFC, right medial temporal regions, bilateral lateral temporal cortex, and the right fusiform gyrus. In both studies, overrecruitment of PFC was seen in the context of good performance in older adults, consistent with the idea that older adults recruit additional frontal executive resources to compensate for reductions in other cognitive processes. This additional recruitment also can be found when the task is a relatively easy one for both young and older adults to perform.

Several recent studies looked at source memory, or the influence of source information on memory, which is typically impaired in older adults even if memory for items is not (e.g., Glisky et al. 1995; Hashtroudi et al. 1989; Schacter et al. 1991). Mitchell et al. (2006) used a somewhat unusual working memory approach to source memory and compared source memory judgments for stimulus format, that is, either picture or word, in young and older adults. Young adults showed activation of an area in the left dorsolateral PFC during source judgments, similar to that reported in previous work (Mitchell et al. 2004), but older adults did not. Older adults also were less accurate at these source judgments. The authors posited that older adults' source memory deficits may be related, in part, to reduced function of the left PFC region engaged by young adults. A different result was obtained by Morcom et al. (2007), who equated overall source memory between groups of healthy younger and older adults by manipulating the number of study presentations and took the additional step of analyzing only those trials in which the source was correctly identified. Contrasts of the activity associated with correct source judgments and correctly identified new items revealed that the two groups recruited many of the same brain regions. However, in older adults, retrieval-related increases in the bilateral anterior PFC and parietal cortex were more widespread and of greater magnitude than that in the young. Given that older adults performed the same as younger adults but had more activation of task-related regions, these findings were interpreted as evidence that there is an age-related decline in the efficiency with which neural populations support cognitive function. Also, comparing the overrecruitment of PFC in this study with the underrecruitment reported by Mitchell et al. emphasizes that age differences in memory performance can influence how one interprets age differences in brain activity. Another study by Gutchess et al. (2007) involved the incidental encoding of pictures of objects presented in meaningful contexts, followed by a memory test for the objects presented in identical or new contexts. The elderly group showed more false alarms than young when new objects were presented in familiar contexts, showing a greater influence of context, or source, on their memory decisions. This behavioral effect was accompanied by reduced activity in cognitive control regions, such as the anterior cingulate, dorsolateral PFC, and parietal regions. However, those older adults who performed better on the task had more right anterior and bilateral ventral PFC activity, an increase not seen in those older adults who performed worse on the task.

Executive Functions

Executive functions, such as attention and inhibition, have not been studied to the same extent as memory, but the experiments done in this area have shown the same basic pattern of results as has been found for memory, that is, that older adults have both decreased and increased activity compared with that of young adults. One early study found that older adults had less PFC activity during tasks requiring inhibition of responses (Jonides et al. 2000), whereas a second study found more frontal activity in older adults (Nielson et al. 2002), with the primary difference being that the latter study examined only successful inhibition trials. Other studies have shown failures to suppress brain activity that were attributed to failure to inhibit irrelevant information (Gazzaley et al. 2005; Milham et al. 2002).

More recent work has tended to find increased activity in older than in younger adults. Madden and colleagues (2007) used visual search tasks requiring detection of specific letter targets in an array and extracted functional measures from regions of interest collapsed across hemispheres. They found increased activity in frontal regions, including frontal eye fields, and parietal regions. When the task involved top-down control of the search, performance was correlated with activation in frontal eye fields and superior parietal cortex in the older group, whereas activity in the fusiform gyrus correlated with performance in the young. This age difference in the relation between activation and search performance supported the hypothesis of age differences in how top-down attention is instantiated in neural activity. Townsend et al. (2006) also studied top-down control by using tasks requiring shifting of attention between auditory and visual stimuli. Both young and older adults had increased activity in bilateral frontal and parietal regions associated with cognitive control during the shifting condition, but these regions were activated to a greater degree in older adults, similar to the result of Madden et al. Because the areas with age increases overlapped with areas of activation in young adults, they were interpreted as greater reliance on brain regions typically used by younger adults when task demands are greater, rather than a reorganization of the attention networks.

A third study used a different approach to studying cognitive control by focusing on default mode regions (Persson et al. 2007). The default mode is thought to be the type of cognitive activity that people engage in when not carrying out externally driven tasks and includes monitoring of both internal and external milieus (Raichle et al. 2001). Default activity is suspended when effort is expended on a task, which in turn engages a different set or sets of brain areas. This task-related reduction of activity in default mode regions is smaller in older adults (Grady et al. 2006; Lustig et al. 2003). Persson et al. used verb generation tasks varying in selection demands to examine default mode activity in young and older adults. They found equivalent deactivations in young and older adults in a task requiring minimal selection demands, but age reductions in the magnitude of deactivation emerged with increasing demands on selection. These findings are consistent with the previously reported age reductions in the ability to suppress default mode activity, and the results further suggest that this ability is particularly compromised in older adults when tasks demand a high degree of cognitive control. These three studies show that there are age differences in the neural resources underlying attentional control, and that, for a given level of demand, older adults engage attentional processes in frontal/parietal regions to a greater degree than do young adults.

Emotion

A recent trend in cognitive neuroscience research is the study of emotion and emotional memory. Young adults consistently show better memory for emotional than for nonemotional material (Bradley & Baddeley 1990; M. M. Bradley et al. 1992; Carstensen & Turk-Charles 1994; Charles et al. 2003; Dewhurst & Parry 2000; Kensinger et al. 2002; Ochsner 2000), particularly negatively valenced items. Consistent with these behavioral findings, young adults have increased activity in the amygdala when viewing negative emotional stimuli (Anderson et al. 2003; Canli et al. 2000; Critchley et al. 2000; Morris et al. 1998), and this activity is related to later memory for this material (Cahill et al. 1996; Canli et al. 2000; Dolcos et al. 2004; Kensinger & Corkin 2004). Older adults may fail to show better memory for negative stimuli (Charles et al. 2003; Grady et al. 2007) and may make more errors in labeling the specific negative emotions in faces than do young adults (Calder et al. 2003; Keightley et al. 2006; MacPherson et al. 2002; McDowell et al. 1994; Oscar-Berman et al. 1990; Phillips et al. 2002). Several studies have looked at the neural mechanisms of these age differences in processing negative stimuli, and all have reported lower activity in the amygdala in older adults when viewing negative stimuli than that in young adults (Fischer et al. 2005; Gunning-Dixon et al. 2003; Iidaka et al. 2002; Mather et al. 2004; Tessitore et al. 2005). One study recently reported no age difference in amygdala activity to negative stimuli, fearful faces in this case (Wright et al. 2006), although there was less activation of the fusiform gyrus in older adults than in the younger group. One potential confounder in this result, however, is that the fearful faces were not only negatively valenced but also were new, whereas the control faces were both neutral and familiar. The amygdala response was probably influenced both by familiarity and valence (Gobbini & Haxby 2007; Gobbini et al. 2004), making it difficult to know which effect had the greater influence on activity in the older adults.

Other recent studies have pursued this line of research from the viewpoint of age deficits as well as aspects of emotional function that are unchanged with age. One experiment (Keightley et al. 2007) used fMRI to explore brain activity in young and old adults while they viewed and labeled faces expressing all the standard emotions as well as neutral expressions. Older adults had significantly greater difficulty identifying negative expressions than did young adults, as noted in earlier studies, but both groups performed at ceiling for happy expressions. Consistent with the superior identification of happy faces, both young and old adults recruited a pattern of brain activity that distinguished happy expressions from all others, but the patterns were age specific. Older adults showed increased activity in the ventromedial PFC, lingual gyrus, and premotor cortex for happy expressions, whereas younger adults recruited a more widely distributed set of regions, including the amygdala, ventromedial PFC, lateral PFC, and bilateral inferior parietal areas. Conversely, younger adults showed more activity in the dorsal anterior cingulate for other types of expressions, and older adults had more activity in the dorsal cingulate, as well as the middle and inferior frontal gyri, somatosensory cortex, and insula. These results support previous research demonstrating age differences in brain activity during emotional processing, including age reductions in the amygdala, and suggest possible age-related differences in cognitive strategy during identification of happy faces, despite no effect of age on this ability.

In another study (Urry et al. 2006) older participants carried out a task that required them to either increase or decrease their emotional response to negatively valenced pictures. This type of task in younger adults results in modulation of the amygdala and medial PFC such that decreasing one's emotional response results in decreased amygdala activity and increased activity in the PFC, indicative of a top-down influence on emotional processing. The older group showed a similar response in the amygdala, where activity was increased above control levels for the "increase" condition and decreased below control levels for the "decrease" condition. However, unlike young adults, the older group had medial and lateral PFC activation for the increase condition, but not the decrease condition. Nevertheless, the inverse relation between the ventromedial PFC and the amygdala was maintained in the older adults. Also, those older adults who were better able to decrease activity in the amygdala and increase activity in the medial PFC showed better diurnal cortisol patterns, indicating a link between regulation of stress responses and modulation of brain regions representing emotional responses.

Another study looking at emotion regulation, but in the context of life span changes in regulation, was reported by Williams et al. (2006). In this study, emotion regulation, as measured by self-reported neuroticism, and brain responses to emotional faces were measured in a sample of individuals ranging from 12 to 79 years of age. Levels of neuroticism were linearly and negatively correlated with age, as was activity in the medial PFC during viewing of happy faces. In contrast, viewing fearful faces was associated with a linear increase of activity in the medial PFC. Activity in the amygdala showed nonlinear changes with age;

fear-related amygdala activity was greater in young and middle-aged adults than in older adults, whereas happiness-related activity was greater in young adults and teenagers than in middle-aged and old adults. These findings provide evidence that emotional stability improves from adolescence into older age and is predicted by an increase in controlled processing through the medial PFC of negative emotion, with a corresponding reduction for positive emotion. The authors proposed that changes in motivational priorities and accumulated life experience of older age bring greater selectivity in the perception of positive versus negative emotion, as well as influencing plasticity in the medial prefrontal systems that participate in emotional regulation.

Although not directly addressing emotion per se, a recent study by Samanez Larkin et al. (2007) examined behavioral and brain responses to anticipation of monetary gains and losses. This work was based on the idea that older adults have preserved positive affective experience relative to younger adults but reduced sensitivity to negative affect (Carstensen et al. 2003), so that their anticipatory responses to gains (representing positive affect) would be the same, but age differences should emerge for losses (negative affect). Indeed, they found no age differences in activation of areas representing reward, that is, the striatum and insula, during gain anticipation, but a relative reduction in activation during loss anticipation. These findings show an asymmetry in the processing of gains and losses in older adults that may have implications for decision making and the role of emotion in decision making.

Perception

Finally, two studies looked at the effects of age on visual perceptual function. Such studies have been relatively few but have generally shown a pattern of over-recruitment of activity in some brain areas by older adults, as well as reduced activity in visual cortices (Grady et al. 1994; Madden et al. 2004). These studies have indicated that older adults may place relatively greater emphasis on the attentional control of response regulation, in compensation for the age-related decline in visual processing efficiency. In one of the recent studies, Chee et al. (2006) used the phenomenon of fMRI adaptation, which reflects the decrease in activity seen in sensory cortices when a stimulus is repeated (similar to priming and repetition suppression; Buckner et al. 1998; Desimone 1996; Grill-Spector & Malach 2001). Adaptation is an increasingly popular way to determine the response of brain regions to specific stimulus features. In this particular study, older and younger adults viewed objects placed in background scenes, both of which were either repeated or new. In young adults, there was adaptation to objects in the fusiform and inferior occipital gyri, to background scenes in the parahippocampal gyrus, and contextual binding (adaptation to specific object–scene pairs) in the fusiform, parahippocampus, and hippocampus. Older adults showed neither adaptation to objects in any brain area nor adaptation responses corresponding to binding in the medial temporal areas. They did show adaptation to background scenes in the parahippocampal gyri, as did the young adults. These findings suggest that the elderly have difficulty with simultaneous visual processing of objects and backgrounds that, in turn, could contribute to deficient contextual binding. The auditory working memory study by Grady et al. discussed above (2008) also found less adaptation in older adults; there the adaptation deficit was seen in the auditory cortex to targets in the one-back working memory task (FIG. 1B). Also, the level of adaptation achieved by the older adults was related to their performance on the task; those older adults who were better able to reduce activity in the auditory cortex to targets showed better detection of the targets (FIG. 1C). Both experiments indicate that age differences in adaptation might reflect differences in the basic processing of stimulus features that could influence higher-order processes, such as memory.

Payer et al. (2006) examined brain activity during processing of faces and houses to examine the relation between altered activity in the visual cortex and prefrontal activity in older adults. These tasks were used because young adults typically have selective activation for faces and houses in different parts of ventral visual cortex (e.g., Haxby et al. 2001; Maurer et al. 2007). Although both groups showed selective activity for faces and houses, this selectivity was reduced with age, which was interpreted as a type of dedifferentiation of visual function. Also, older adults showed bilateral activation in the prefrontal region, whereas younger adults had right hemisphere activity, although no direct group comparisons were reported. The finding that apparently greater prefrontal activations for the old were concurrent with reduced visual selectivity led the authors to suggest that prefrontal activity may compensate for dedifferentiated object recognition mechanisms in the visual cortex. This supposition is similar to an earlier suggestion (Grady et al. 1994) that increased activity in frontal regions occurs in response to decreased activity in visual areas in older adults.

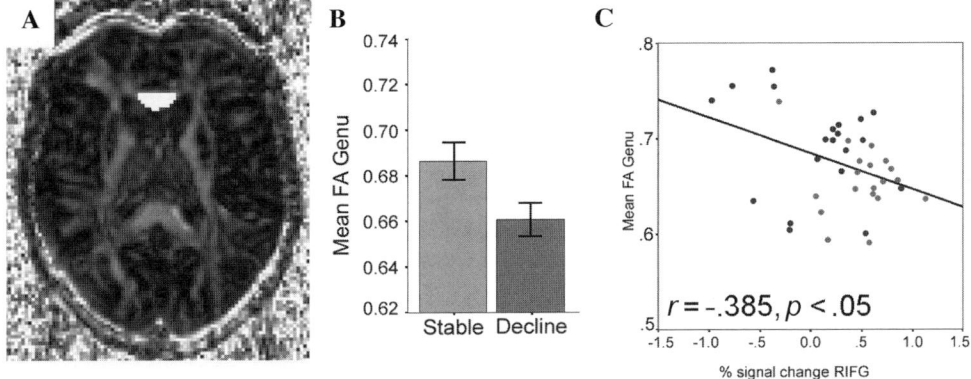

FIGURE 2. Data are from Persson et al. (2006). **(A)** The area of the genu of the corpus callosum assessed in this study is highlighted in white on a transverse DTI slice showing fractional anisotropy (FA), a measure of white matter integrity. Higher signal intensity (brightness) in this image reflects higher FA. **(B)** Mean FA as a function of longitudinal memory performance in the subgroup of older adults with stable memory and in the subgroup with declining memory. **(C)** Scatterplot shows the increase in right PFC activation with lower FA in the genu. Error bars show SEM. Figure used with permission.

Brain Structure and Function

Most evidence from studies of brain structure indicates that age differences in both gray and white matter are distributed throughout the brain but are more prominent in frontal than posterior brain areas (Buckner 2004; Raz 2000). Activity in cortical regions as measured by the blood oxygen level–dependent (BOLD) effect from fMRI could be reduced or altered in older adults because the neurons in the regions themselves are dysfunctional or because the fibers that connect them to other areas are damaged or less efficient. Indeed, the predominant functional changes in the PFC indicate that structural changes seen there might influence activity in widespread areas of the brain that are connected anatomically to frontal regions. The effect of structural changes with age on cognition has been documented (e.g., DeCarli et al. 1995; Garde et al. 2000; Gunning-Dixon & Raz 2000; Pfefferbaum et al. 2000), and a few studies have recently looked at the effect of these structural changes on functional activation. The results of these studies are not entirely consistent, but they shed some interesting light on brain structure–function relations. In one study, brain activity was measured with fMRI during a flanker task that required inhibition of conflicting information adjacent to a cue indicating the correct response. Gray and white matter density were assessed from structural MRIs (Colcombe et al. 2005). Older adults had more activation of the left inferior PFC than did younger adults, and this increase was larger in those older adults performing worse on the inhibitory task. The older adults also had lower gray and white matter density in the PFC than those of the young group. There were no differences between good and poor performers in the older group in gray matter density, but the good performers had a higher density of white matter in the corpus callosum and underlying the frontal lobes than did the poor performers. These data suggest that age changes in white matter underlying cortical regions have a greater influence on executive function than changes in the cortex itself—consistent with the idea that integrity of the white matter connecting cortical regions is critical for both cognitive ability and brain function.

Two other studies looked at white matter integrity using diffusion tensor imaging (DTI), which provides a measure of the structural integrity of myelinated white matter tracts (Moseley 2002). In one of these studies, Persson et al. (2006) studied groups of older adults who were followed up for several years and scanned during a verbal semantic task (abstract/concrete judgment). They found that white matter integrity of the genu of the corpus callosum was reduced in seniors who also showed a decline in memory function over the follow-up period, compared with those whose memory function was stable over this period. Also, activation in the right PFC increased with lower measures of white matter integrity in this region (FIG. 2), similar to the results of Colcombe et al. The authors suggested that increased cortical activation either is caused by white matter disruption or is a compensatory response to such disruption. Madden et al. (2007) examined brain activity and white matter integrity with DTI during visual search tasks (the previous section also cites this study). They found that white matter measures were reduced in older adults relative to younger adults in several areas, including the genu of the corpus callosum and regions underlying the PFC and parietal cortex. However, these measures did not mediate the age-related increase in activation of the frontal and parietal regions that was observed. A similar result was found by Langenecker et al. (2007), who obtained both structural volumes and functional measures of the basal ganglia to examine the contribution of these structures to age differences on an inhibitory go–no-go task. Older adults had more activity in the putamen and less in the caudate than did the young adults, but older adults had smaller volumes in both areas. Critically for the question at hand, activation and volumetric measures were not significantly correlated, suggesting that loss of volume in these subcortical regions does not explain the age differences in functional activity or task performance.

Using a somewhat different approach, Nordahl et al. (2006) used structural MRI in older adults to quantify the extent of white matter hyperintensities (WMHs), which are common in the elderly (Soderlund et al. 2003) and have some deleterious effects on cognition (DeCarli et al. 1995). In this experiment, the investigators tested whether WMH burden predicted the magnitude of PFC activity observed during performance of episodic and working memory tasks. Increases in dorsal prefrontal WMH volume were associated with *decreases* in frontal task related activity, unlike the increased activity associated with loss of white matter integrity found in the studies by Persson et al. and Colcombe et al. discussed earlier. Also, frontal WMH volume was associated with decreased activity not only in the PFC but also in areas such as the medial temporal lobe and posterior parietal cortex. The authors posited that disruption of white matter tracts, especially within the PFC, may be a mechanism for age-related reductions in both memory functioning and brain activation.

In addition to age differences in white and gray matter integrity, there is some evidence that age is associated with changes in the vascular system (Hillary & Biswal 2007) and that these vascular changes may influence the hemodynamic BOLD response (Aizenstein et al. 2004; Buckner et al. 2000; D'Esposito et al. 1999; Huettel et al. 2001). A recent study examining this variability (Handwerker et al. 2007) used a breath-holding condition as a challenge to estimate the vascular response to hypercapnia. The BOLD responses were measured in young and older adults during a visuomotor saccade task, and the relation between the task-related response and the change in activity during breath holding was assessed. The BOLD response was significantly decreased in the older adults in several areas that mediate saccades, including the frontal eye fields and primary visual cortex. The signal change during the saccade task was linearly related to the change during hypercapnia in both age groups. Also, when the BOLD response during the task was adjusted by dividing it by the signal change during hypercapnia, the only significant age decrease remaining was that in the visual cortex. This result suggests that the BOLD signal decrease with age in this region is neural in origin, whereas the age difference in signal in other regions may be due, in part, to vascular changes. This experiment also provides a relatively simple way of assessing the role of age-related vascular changes in fMRI studies.

The results of these studies, taken together, indicate that there is probably some influence of age-related structural and vascular changes on functional measures obtained from the cortex of older adults, but the strength of this influence or whether it is task- or region specific remain to be determined. It is apparent, however, that age reductions in gray or white matter integrity do not necessarily translate into functional reductions. Perhaps the type of change, particularly in the white matter, is critical for the effect seen on the BOLD response. For example, changes in the myelin that are detected with DTI may result in subtle alterations in neural function that can be compensated for by increased activity, whereas disruptions caused by WMH underlying specific cortical regions may be more severe and lead to alterations of function that are more difficult to adapt to. Damage to white matter in the corpus callosum may have a different effect on brain activity than does damage to white matter fibers underlying the cortex. Also, some of the differences in the results noted earlier may be due to the use of a longitudinal rather than a cross-sectional study design. More work on the assessment of change in white matter integrity and functional capacity in older adults will be needed to understand this complex relationship.

Cognitive Networks and Aging

Recently there has been increasing interest in assessing cognitive brain networks by using analytic techniques that facilitate the multivariate identification of whole-brain patterns of activity or that directly assess functional connectivity between brain areas (e.g., Horwitz et al. 1992; Lee et al. 2006; McIntosh 1999). Functional brain networks show evidence of "small-world properties" (Achard et al. 2006; He et al. 2007), meaning that they are characterized by dense local connectivity with relatively few long-range connections, resulting in a short path length between any pair of regions in the network. Earlier studies had shown age differences in such neural networks, even when no differences were apparent in behavioral measures or simple task contrasts of brain activity (Della-Maggiore et al. 2000; Grady et al. 2003). Recently, Achard and Bullmore (2007) examined the efficiency of human brain functional networks in young and older adults scanned in a resting state. Functional connectivity between many cortical and subcortical regions was estimated, and efficiency was defined as a function of the minimum path length between regions. The older adults showed reduced global and local efficiency of these networks, with the local changes seen primarily in orbitofrontal, lateral temporal, and medial temporal regions. Because these cortical regions are thought to be "hubs," or highly interconnected areas, these data suggest that aging reduces the effectiveness of brain function by reducing the efficiency with which these hubs can operate.

Two other recent studies examined the effects of older age on motor networks. Taniwaki et al. (2007) examined activity in two previously identified motor loops, one consisting of the basal ganglia, thalamus, and motor cortex and the other involving the cerebellum and its cortical connections. In a prior study, the authors had demonstrated functional interactions within the basal ganglia–thalamus–motor cortex loop during self-initiated movements in young adults and cerebellum–cortical connections loop connectivity during externally triggered movements (Taniwaki et al. 2006). Interestingly, older adults showed decreased connectivity in both loops during their respective tasks but increased connectivity within motor cortices and between hemispheres during both tasks. These results were interpreted as evidence for an age-related decline of cortico–subcortical connectivity with increased interactions between motor cortices, possibly due to a reduction in interhemispheric inhibitory processes.

Wu et al. (2007) also examined motor system networks but did so using connectivity measured during the resting state (Biswal et al. 1995). A network of regional nodes was specified, based on previous work, and the total amount of connectivity for each region was estimated and compared between young and older adults. Older adults showed a decrease in the amount of functional connectivity in two of the network nodes, the right cingulate motor area and left premotor cortex, compared with young adults. Both this study and that by Taniwaki et al. suggest that aging is associated with reduced function of individual nodes in the motor networks, as well as altered connectivity among the nodes, both of which could be related to reduced motor function in the elderly.

Finally, a recent study by Stern et al. (in press) demonstrates a unique approach to the study of cognitive networks and aging. This group has been exploring the concept of cognitive reserve (CR), which some individuals can use to mitigate the effects of aging on cognitive function. For indices of CR, these investigators used vocabulary and IQ scores and determined whether groups of young and old adults would show a common neural network for CR during the performance of two recognition tasks with different cognitive demands (a verbal and a spatial task). A multivariate analysis was used to identify networks of brain regions where activity was associated with the CR measure in the two age groups. During stimulus presentation, there was a pattern of activity that was differently expressed in young and old adults during the verbal task. There also was a common pattern that was related to CR variables in both the verbal and nonverbal tasks in the young group, but it was expressed only in the verbal task by the older group. The authors posited that this latter pattern could represent a general neural network mediating CR that is affected by the aging process and that the former pattern, which was expressed differently by young and old adults, may represent a reorganization of this set of brain areas in compensation for the disruption of the common network brought on by aging.

Thus, all the studies summarized in this section found that aging alters distributed networks of brain activity, either by reducing the efficiency or function of networks seen in young adults or by leading to recruitment of new and perhaps compensatory networks. Also, age-related changes in white matter integrity will affect network connectivity, as well as activation per se, so that the issues discussed earlier regarding structural brain changes will need to be addressed with network approaches.

Brain–Behavior Correlations in Older Adults

This last section of the review will focus on one of the most important questions in the cognitive neuroscience of aging, that is, to determine the effect of age differences in brain activity, such as overrecruitment in older adults, on behavior. Although all studies in this field attempt to interpret their imaging results in terms of the observed behavior, only some of them have *directly* addressed the relation between brain activity and task performance. Before one reviews the

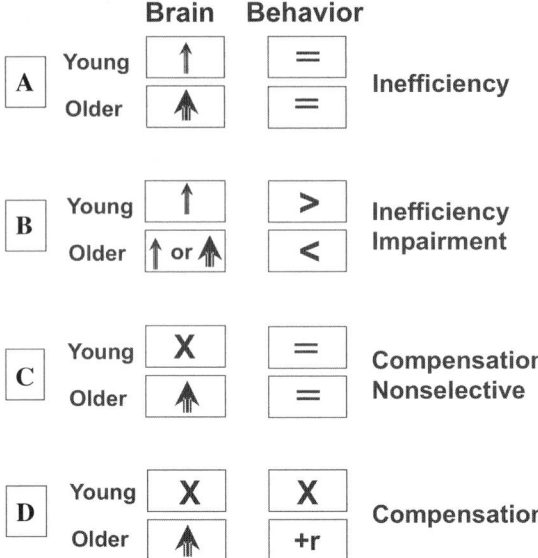

FIGURE 3. Three current explanations for age differences in brain activity are represented schematically. In model **A**, older adults show more brain activity but the same performance level as younger adults. In model **B**, the older adults have equal or greater brain activity but worse performance. Both patterns have been interpreted as evidence of less efficient neural processing in the elderly, although Model **B** could also reflect activity that impairs performance. Model **C** shows a pattern of effects that is often interpreted as compensatory but might also reflect nonselective brain activity in older adults. Model **D** presents the strongest evidence for compensation in older adults (see text for fuller explanation of these models). Up-arrows, increase in brain activity, with the magnitude indicated by the size of the arrow; =, equivalent performance in young and old; >, better performance in the younger adults; <, worse performance in the older adults; X, no reliable effect; +r, positive correlation between brain activity and behavior.

recent studies that have addressed this issue, it is useful to summarize the explanations for age differences in brain activity that have been invoked most often to date (FIG. 3). Two types of result have been considered evidence of inefficient use of brain activity in older adults. One is when there is no age difference in behavior but older adults have more activity in task-related brain regions than do younger adults (FIG. 3, model A). Equal or more brain activity in older adults but poorer performance also could be considered an example of inefficiency, although more activity in the context of poorer performance could indicate that the additional activity impairs performance in the elderly (FIG. 3, model B). In both cases, the areas activated in young and old would be similar, but older adults are getting "less bang for the buck." When older adults recruit a brain region that is not active in younger adults but have performance equivalent to that seen in young adults, the overrecruitment is generally considered compensatory (FIG. 3, model C). However, the possibility that this engagement of a new region represents nonselective recruitment or dedifferentiation in the elderly cannot be ruled out entirely. Finally, perhaps the strongest evidence for compensation is the situation in which older adults recruit brain activity that is not seen in younger adults, and the engagement of this area or areas is directly correlated with better performance only in the older adults and not in the young (FIG. 3, model D). This finding would indicate the recruitment of a unique pattern of neural activity that supports task performance in an age-specific manner. Examples of these patterns have already been noted, such as recruitment of additional PFC regions in the elderly with no age differences in behavior reported by Fernandes et al. (2006) and Daselaar et al. (2006), consistent with model C in FIGURE 3, and the reduced neural efficiency found by Morcom et al. (2007), consistent with model A.

To address these various possibilities, Zarahn et al. (2007) carried out a study using a recognition task for visually presented letters, with various set sizes. In this experiment there was a pattern of activity expressed by both younger and older adults, but because the older adults had lower mean performance on the task, the use of activation in these regions was considered less efficient (model B). Also, activity in the right parahippocampal gyrus distinguished older from younger adults, with those older adults who performed the slowest on the task showing the most activity in this area (also consistent with model B). A similar result was found by Colcombe et al. (2005), in that overrecruitment of the left PFC was seen in those adults who performed worse on an inhibitory task. Because the better-performing elderly in both studies had brain activation more similar to that seen in young adults, these data would not be consistent with the notion of compensation as it is considered typically and, indeed, might even indicate that age-related differences in brain activity impair performance. On the other hand, Zarahn et al. (2007) posited that there might be a type of compensation that could have a beneficial effect on performance, relative to what performance would have been without engagement of an age-specific pattern, even if this pattern is not associated with better task performance in a particular study. That is, those lower-performing older adults who show the largest expression of an age-specific pattern of brain activity would do even worse on the task without this engagement.

Rypma et al. (2007) also used a letter recognition task, with various set sizes (similar to that used by

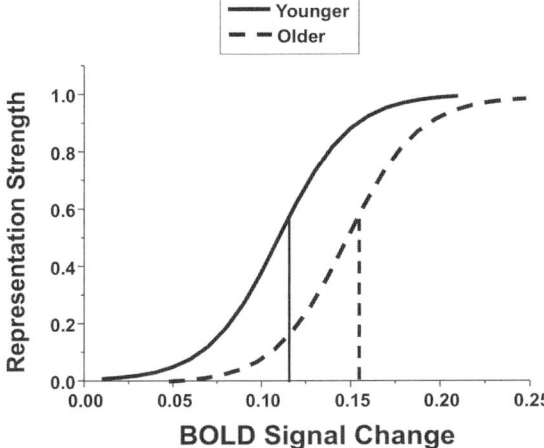

FIGURE 4. The sigmoid model of age-related differences in brain–behavior relationships proposed by Rypma et al. (2007). In this model (axes are hypothetical), the strength of a stimulus representation is related to the degree of PFC activity in a sigmoid fashion, with the maximal difference in representation strength occurring in the midpoint of the curve. This function is right-shifted in older adults, such that more prefrontal activation would be required for older adults to achieve optimum levels of performance (dashed vertical line) than for younger adults (solid vertical line). That is, as neural activity increases, discriminability moves into the optimal range for older adults but into a less optimal range for younger adults.

Zarahn et al. 2007), to examine neural efficiency in older adults. Activity in the PFC increased in response to memory load in both young and older adults, although the older adults were less accurate on the task—consistent with an age reduction in neural efficiency (model B in FIG. 3, also similar to the result of Zarahn et al.). However, older adults had better accuracy and faster reaction times with increasing activity in the dorsal PFC, whereas younger adults had better performance with lower levels of activity. This work was interpreted as support for the idea that there is a sigmoid relation between neural activation and the ability to make a decision on the basis of stimulus representations (FIG. 4). The sigmoid relationship between PFC activation and representation strength means that middle ranges of neural activation result in large differences in signal and easy discrimination between representations. However, the sigmoid function relating neural activation to response may be shifted to the right for older adults compared with younger adults, so that lower levels of activation lead to optimum stimulus discriminability for younger adults but higher levels of activation are needed for optimum discriminability in older adults.

Other recent studies have reported evidence consistent with the idea of compensatory activity in older adults. Davis et al. (in press) studied younger and older adults during verbal recognition and visual perceptual tasks. The hypothesis was that older adults would show reduced activity in the occipital cortex (as others have reported, e.g., Grady et al. 1994), increased activity in the PFC, and critically that the overrecruitment of the PFC would be correlated with the degree of underrecruitment of visual areas. The results supported this hypothesis. Older adults had more activity in a region of the PFC than did younger adults, who did not reliably activate this region. Not only was activity in the PFC negatively correlated with occipital activity in older adults but also was positively correlated with performance on the tasks—consistent with the idea that activity in this region was compensating for reduced activity in visual areas (FIG. 3, model D).

Also, one should not focus exclusively on the PFC when examining age differences in brain activity and its relation to behavior. Wierenga et al. (2006) studied naming ability with age, using a task that typically activates the left frontal regions in young adults. Although there was no difference in overall naming accuracy between groups, older adults had more activity in the right inferior frontal gyrus than did the young. Activity in this area positively correlated with greater naming accuracy only in the older group (FIG. 3, model D), consistent with the idea that recruitment of the bilateral PFC can be compensatory in older adults (Cabeza 2002). However, age increases of activity in other right hemisphere regions were not related to better naming, indicating that additional activity per se is not necessarily compensatory in older adults. In contrast, a study by Van der Veen et al. (2006) indicated that activity outside the PFC may be more strongly related to performance in older adults than PFC activity. These investigators examined recognition memory in young and old adults and found that successful retrieval was accompanied by activation in the left inferior frontal gyrus, left precentral gyrus, and right cerebellum regardless of age. Older participants showed additional activity in the bilateral medial PFC and right parahippocampal gyrus. Further analyses showed that only the additional parahippocampal activation correlated positively with task performance in the older group (again consistent with FIG. 3, model D), suggesting that activation in this area served the purpose of functional compensation even though PFC activity did not.

Now one might wonder how compensation in the elderly actually works and which cognitive processes are engaged. A recent model of how compensation

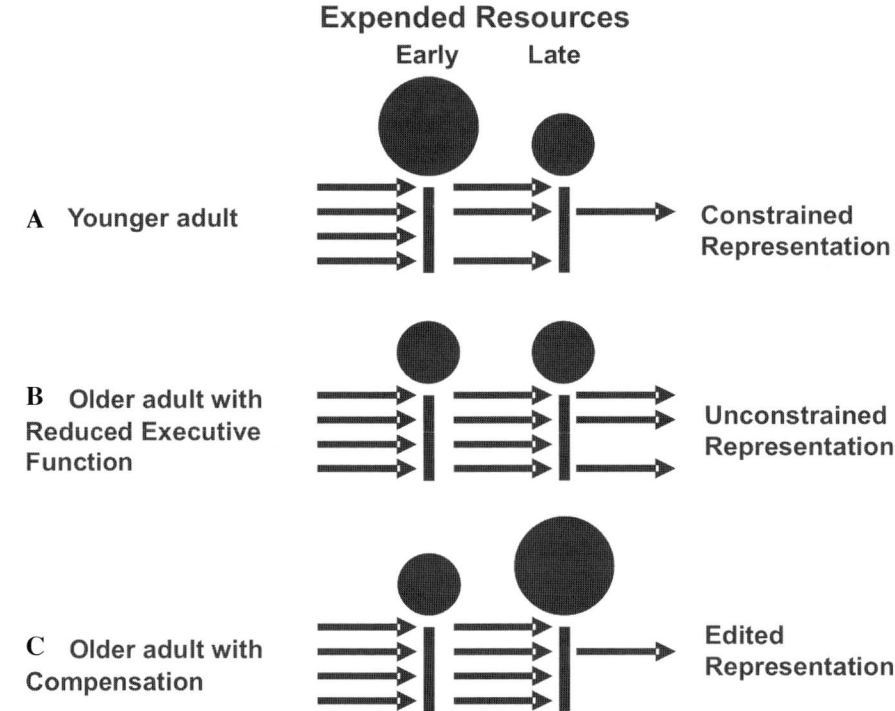

FIGURE 5. The load-shift model of cognitive aging proposed by Velanova et al. (2007). Memory retrieval is considered to be a set of processes automatically elicited by a cue that are constrained by early-selection processes and edited by late-selection processes. Resources, represented by circles, can be expended at early- and late-selection stages to aid effective memory retrieval. **(A)** Young adults are hypothesized to rely on a combination of early- and late-selection processes, with more resources used to constrain processing through top-down mechanisms at early-selection stages. **(B)** Because of compromise in executive function, older adults fail to constrain processing at the early-selection stage. As a result, representations are poorly constrained. **(C)** To compensate, older adults expend greater resources to edit the retrieval event at late-selection stages.

might evolve during memory retrieval was proposed by Velanova et al. (2007). According to this model, executive and cognitive control resources are required both early in the retrieval process and late in retrieval (FIG. 5). Young adults can engage early resources to constrain the amount of information necessary to determine whether a stimulus is old or new, and hence there is less demand on later processes. However, with aging there is a reduction in these early resources so that more reliance on later resources, so called backend processing, is needed to compensate. Support for this model was found in two experiments of word recognition in which an age-related increase was found in both the ventral and dorsal PFC that appeared to occur after parietal activity that indicated that a successful retrieval decision had been reached. This is an interesting hypothesis that would account for some of the results reviewed here, although it will need further testing. For example, the proposed age deficit in early top-down processing will need to be distinguished from any age differences in early bottom-up attentional changes.

Finally, a critical question is whether age differences in brain activity thought to be compensatory can be elicited through training of specific cognitive processes in older adults. That is, if overrecruitment of the PFC is compensating for some age decline in brain structure or function, then in older adults who are trained on a particular task, and thereby improve their performance, prefrontal activity should increase accordingly. This process would increase age differences in prefrontal activity when scanning is done after training. On the other hand, training may reduce the effort needed for older adults to perform the task or result in older adults using behavioral strategies more like those used by younger adults, thus reducing age differences in brain activity. These alternatives have not been studied yet to any great degree, but one recent study examined this issue in the context of training on a dual-task paradigm. In this study, participants carried out two visual tasks (color detection and letter detection) either singly or simultaneously (Erickson et al. 2007). A subset of young and older adults then received 5 h of training on the tasks over several weeks. Both young and old trained groups showed improved performance on the tasks, both in accuracy and reaction times. In pretraining brain activity, young adults had more activity in the left ventral PFC than the older group, and older adults had more activity in the dorsal PFC bilaterally than did the young. After training, older adults showed an increase in left ventral PFC activity and a decrease in dorsal PFC activity, such that age differences in these regions were no longer apparent. Also, these changes in prefrontal activity were correlated with improved reaction time on the dual task in the older adults. This result does not support the idea that behavioral improvement after training on these tasks was associated with compensatory increases of frontal activity to levels above that seen in younger adults. Instead, activity in the older adults after training was more similar to that seen in the young group. One explanation for these findings is that older adults before training needed more cognitive control to perform the dual tasks, indicated by more dorsal prefrontal activity, and that the training allowed them to reduce their dependence on these control processes.

The studies reviewed here showed a variety of brain–behavior correlations, similar to those reported in earlier studies, ranging from inefficiency to compensation in the elderly. Unfortunately, it is proving difficult to precisely determine in older adults the effect of overrecruitment of the PFC, or engagement of different patterns of brain activity, using cross-sectional comparisons with younger adults. This difficulty could be due to relatively small samples chosen from a heterogeneous older population, task, or regional specificity of brain–behavior relations; the influence of unmeasured factors such as genotype or personality; or perhaps a combination of these factors. Also, some studies have assessed the relation between brain activity and reaction times, whereas others have looked at accuracy, and these two behavioral measures do not necessarily show the same relation with brain activity (e.g., Lenartowicz & McIntosh 2005). More studies will need to be done to address this issue by using other kinds of tasks, as well as to determine more precisely the effects of training on brain activity in young and older adults.

Conclusions

Over the past two decades, we have learned quite a bit about how cognitive aging is reflected in the brain, and the studies published in the past year have supported the basic conclusions drawn from earlier ones. In general, studies done to date find many similarities in the patterns of activity in young and old adults, indicating that basic neural mechanisms are maintained into older age. Despite these overall similarities, older adults often have less activity in some regions, such as medial temporal areas during memory encoding or retrieval and visual regions across a variety of cognitive domains. It seems clear that age reductions in cognitive function can be tied, at least in part, to these reductions in brain activity. For example, reduced hippocampal activity could result in less effective encoding as well as reduced levels of recollection at retrieval, because the hippocampus has been tied to both processes (e.g., Nadel et al. 2000; Squire 1992). On the other hand, older adults typically also overrecruit some brain areas, mainly the ventral or dorsal PFC during memory tasks, and both frontal and parietal regions during tasks engaging cognitive control processes, such as attention. Sometimes this overrecruitment appears to be in response to altered function in other brain regions, such as the hippocampus or sensory cortices, and is often seen in those older adults who perform better on the task at hand. These findings have provided rather convincing support for the idea that overrecruitment can be compensatory in the elderly. Nevertheless, not all age increases can be interpreted as compensatory, and some are more indicative of neural inefficiency. Also, the recent training study reviewed here (Erickson et al. 2007) indicates that improving performance through training does not necessarily lead to increased activity in the PFC but may actually result in less activity, thereby reducing age differences. The result of training will probably depend on whether the training leads to greater automaticity, in which case PFC activity would be expected to decrease, or learning of a new way to apply cognitive control, in which case PFC activity would be expected to increase.

It is worth considering whether the evidence accumulated so far has indicated any *specific* prefrontal region or regions as being major players in compensatory mechanisms. A recent review of episodic and working memory experiments (Rajah & D'Esposito 2005) concluded that aging results in the dedifferentiation of function, or loss of task selectivity, in bilateral ventral prefrontal regions and deficits in function in the right dorsal PFC. The authors further suggested that even when older adults recruit the right dorsal frontal area that this does not help them perform the task but that activity in the left dorsal and anterior PFC may be compensatory. The studies reviewed here are broadly consistent with these conclusions. For example, most found greater activation of the left PFC in older than in younger adults that was often associated with good performance in the older group, although this was seen in both the left dorsolateral and ventrolateral areas. The regional and hemispheric differences that have been reported in this field probably reflect the engagement of different cognitive processes, but what these exact processes are or what one must do to elicit them still is not clear. Models of how compensation might take place, such as the one by Velanova et al. (2007) reviewed here, are a welcome addition to the field and will, it is hoped, stimulate more research into the timing and mechanisms of compensation, as well as the regions mediating these effects.

An important methodological consideration is that most of the studies of cognitive aging and brain activity have used cross-sectional designs and contrasted younger and older adults. Only a few have reported longitudinal data, although the advantages of this approach in avoiding cohort effects and examining within-subject age-related declines are obvious. One group that has been able to take a longitudinal approach to brain function in aging is the group examining data from the Baltimore Longitudinal Study of Aging. In this large longitudinal study, a group of older adults who maintained good physical and cognitive health were followed up for 8 years and underwent five scanning sessions (every other year) during rest and delayed verbal and figural recognition memory tasks (Beason-Held et al. in press-a, in press-b). Although memory performance remained stable over the 8 years, longitudinal changes in brain activity were seen. Longitudinal decreases common to all scan conditions were seen in the anterior cingulate, superior temporal, and subcortical regions, whereas increases were seen in the PFC and hippocampus. Some of these changes were linear (e.g., the superior temporal gyrus), and others appeared as step changes in one year or another (e.g., the PFC). Task-specific changes also were noted. These data, in view of the stable memory performance, suggest that there are distinctive patterns of age-related functional decline and compensatory activity over time. PFC activity increased over time in this older sample, consistent with the cross-sectional increases seen in PFC activity relative to young adults. Data such as these can be valuable, although difficult to obtain, so it is not clear that many such longitudinal studies will be done.

Finally, activity reductions and/or increases in older adults are unlikely to be the whole story. The few studies that have examined functional networks indicate that distributed patterns of brain activity also are altered in older adults. Functional and anatomical connectivity will have to be taken into account before we fully understand the brain mechanisms underlying cognitive aging. This type of approach, although more difficult to carry out and interpret than univariate contrasts of brain activity across tasks or conditions, nevertheless holds promise for capturing the complexity of brain function. Also, the influence of structural changes is far from clear and will need further work to determine whether there is an influence, which structural measure (e.g., white matter or gray matter) is most closely related to activation, and what form the influence will take (i.e., leading to an increase or decrease of activity). So, despite the wealth of data accumulated over the past decade on the aging brain, we still have a long way to go. One challenge facing future research will be to understand the task conditions that promote compensation in older adults, the role of the various brain areas in aiding cognitive function, and how these compensatory mechanisms can be elicited to enhance quality of life in the elderly.

References

Achard, S., & Bullmore, E. (2007). Efficiency and cost of economical brain functional networks. *PLoS Computational Biology*, 3, 174–183.

Achard, S., Salvador, R., Whitcher, B., Suckling, J., & Bullmore, E. (2006). A resilient, low-frequency, small-world human brain functional network with highly connected association cortical hubs. *Journal of Neuroscience*, 26, 63–72.

Aizenstein, H. J., Clark, K. A., Butters, M. A., Cochran, J., Stenger, V. A., Meltzer, C. C., et al. (2004). The BOLD hemodynamic response in healthy aging. *Journal of Cognitive Neuroscience*, 16, 786–793.

Anderson, A. K., Christoff, K., Panitz, D., De Rosa, E., & Gabrieli, J. D. (2003). Neural correlates of the automatic processing of threat facial signals. *Journal of Neuroscience*, 23, 5627–5633.

Balota, D. A., Dolan, P. O., & Duchek, J. M. (2000). Memory changes in healthy older adults. In E. Tulving & F. Craik (Eds.), *The Oxford Handbook of Memory* (pp. 395–410). New York: Oxford University Press.

Bandettini, P. (2007). Functional MRI today. *International Journal of Psychophysiology*, 63, 138–145.

Beason-Held, L. L., Kraut, M. A., & Resnick, S. M. (in press-a). I. Longitudinal changes in aging brain function. *Neurobiology of Aging*.

Beason-Held, L. L., Kraut, M. A., & Resnick, S. M. (in press-b). II. Temporal patterns of longitudinal change in aging brain function. *Neurobiology of Aging*.

Biswal, B., Yetkin, F. Z., Haughton, V. M., & Hyde, J. S. (1995). Functional connectivity in the motor cortex of resting human brain using echo-planar MRI. *Magnetic Resonance in Medicine*, 34, 537–541.

Bradley, B. P., & Baddeley, A. D. (1990). Emotional factors in forgetting. *Psychological Medicine*, 20, 351–355.

Bradley, M. M., Greenwald, M. K., Petry, M. C., & Lang, P. J. (1992). Remembering pictures: pleasure and arousal in memory. *Journal of Experimental Psychology: Learning, Memory, and Cognition, 18*, 379–390.

Buckner, R. L. (2004). Memory and executive function in aging and AD: multiple factors that cause decline and reserve factors that compensate. *Neuron, 44*, 195–208.

Buckner, R. L., Goodman, J., Burock, M., Rotte, M., Koutstaal, W., Schacter, D., et al. (1998). Functional-anatomic correlates of object priming in humans revealed by rapid presentation event-related fMRI. *Neuron, 20*, 285–296.

Buckner, R. L., Snyder, A. Z., Sanders, A. L., Raichle, M. E., & Morris, J. C. (2000). Functional brain imaging of young, nondemented, and demented older adults. *Journal of Cognitive Neuroscience, 12*, 24–34.

Cabeza, R. (2002). Hemispheric asymmetry reduction in older adults: The HAROLD model. *Psychology and Aging, 17*, 85–100.

Cabeza, R., Anderson, N. D., Locantore, J. K., & McIntosh, A. R. (2002). Aging gracefully: compensatory brain activity in high-performing older adults. *NeuroImage, 17*, 1394–1402.

Cabeza, R., Daselaar, S. M., Dolcos, F., Prince, S. E., Budde, M., & Nyberg, L. (2004). Task-independent and task-specific age effects on brain activity during working memory, visual attention and episodic retrieval. *Cerebral Cortex, 14*, 364–375.

Cabeza, R., Grady, C. L., Nyberg, L., McIntosh, A. R., Tulving, E., Kapur, S., et al. (1997). Age-related differences in neural activity during memory encoding and retrieval: a positron emission tomography study. *Journal of Neuroscience, 17*, 391–400.

Cabeza, R., Nyberg, L., & Park, D. (Eds.). (2005). *Cognitive Neuroscience of Aging*. Oxford, UK: Oxford University Press.

Cahill, L., Haier, R. J., Fallon, J., Alkire, M. T., Tang, C., Keator, D., et al. (1996). Amygdala activity at encoding correlated with long-term, free recall of emotional information. *Proceedings of the National Academy of Science USA, 93*, 8016–8021.

Calder, A. J., Keane, J., Manly, T., Sprengelmeyer, R., Scott, S., Nimmo-Smith, I., et al. (2003). Facial expression recognition across the adult life span. *Neuropsychologia, 41*, 195–202.

Canli, T., Zhao, Z., Brewer, J., Gabrieli, J. D. E., & Cahill, L. (2000). Event-related activation in the human amygdala associates with later memory for individual emotional experience. *Journal of Neuroscience, 20:RC99*, 1–5.

Carstensen, L. L., Fung, H. F., & Charles, S. T. (2003). Socioemotional selectivity theory and the regulation of emotion in the second half of life. *Motivation and Emotion, 27*, 103–123.

Carstensen, L. L., & Turk-Charles, S. (1994). The salience of emotion across the adult life span. *Psychology and Aging, 9*, 259–264.

Charles, S. T., Mather, M., & Carstensen, L. L. (2003). Aging and emotional memory: the forgettable nature of negative images for older adults. *Journal of Experimental Psychology: General, 132*, 310–324.

Chee, M. W., Goh, J. O., Venkatraman, V., Tan, J. C., Gutchess, A., Sutton, B., et al. (2006). Age-related changes in object processing and contextual binding revealed using fMR adaptation. *Journal of Cognitive Neuroscience, 18*, 495–507.

Colcombe, S. J., Kramer, A. F., Erickson, K. I., & Scalf, P. (2005). The implications of cortical recruitment and brain morphology for individual differences in inhibitory function in aging humans. *Psychology of Aging, 20*, 363–375.

Critchley, H., Daly, E., Phillips, M., Brammer, M., Bullmore, E., Williams, S., et al. (2000). Explicit and implicit neural mechanisms for processing of social information from facial expressions: a functional magnetic resonance imaging study. *Human Brain Mapping, 9*, 93–105.

Daselaar, S. M., Fleck, M. S., Dobbins, I. G., Madden, D. J., & Cabeza, R. (2006). Effects of healthy aging on hippocampal and rhinal memory functions: an event-related fMRI study. *Cerebral Cortex, 16*, 1771–1782.

Davis, S. W., Dennis, N. A., Daselaar, S. M., Fleck, M. S., & Cabeza, R. (in press). Que PASA? The posterior anterior shift in aging. *Cerebral Cortex*.

DeCarli, C., Murphy, D. G., Tranh, M., Grady, C. L., Haxby, J. V., Gillette, J. A., et al. (1995). The effect of white matter hyperintensity volume on brain structure, cognitive performance, and cerebral metabolism of glucose in 51 healthy adults. *Neurology, 45*, 2077–2084.

Della-Maggiore, V., Sekuler, A. B., Grady, C. L., Bennett, P. J., Sekuler, R., & McIntosh, A. R. (2000). Corticolimbic interactions associated with performance on a short-term memory task are modified by age. *Journal of Neuroscience, 20*, 8410–8416.

Dennis, N. A., Daselaar, S., & Cabeza, R. (2007). Effects of aging on transient and sustained successful memory encoding activity. *Neurobiology of Aging, 28*, 1749–1758.

Desimone, R. (1996). Neural mechanisms for visual memory and their role in attention. *Proceedings of the National Academy of Sciences USA, 93*, 13494–13499.

D'Esposito, M., Zarahn, E., Aguirre, G. K., & Rypma, B. (1999). The effect of normal aging on the coupling of neural activity to the BOLD hemodynamic response. *NeuroImage, 10*, 6–14.

Dewhurst, S. A., & Parry, L. A. (2000). Emotionality, distinctiveness, and recollective experience. *European Journal of Cognitive Psychology, 12*, 541–551.

Dolcos, F., LaBar, K. S., & Cabeza, R. (2004). Interaction between the amygdala and the medial temporal lobe memory system predicts better memory for emotional events. *Neuron, 42*, 855–863.

Donaldson, D. I., Petersen, S. E., Ollinger, J. M., & Buckner, R. L. (2001). Dissociating state and item components of recognition memory using fMRI. *NeuroImage, 13*, 129–142.

Erickson, K. I., Colcombe, S. J., Wadhwa, R., Bherer, L., Peterson, M. S., Scalf, P. E., et al. (2007). Training-induced plasticity in older adults: effects of training on hemispheric asymmetry. *Neurobiology of Aging, 28*, 272–283.

Fernandes, M. A., Pacurar, A., Moscovitch, M., & Grady, C. L. (2006). Neural correlates of auditory recognition under full and divided attention in young and old adults. *Neuropsychologia, 44*, 2452–2464.

Fischer, H., Sandblom, J., Gavazzeni, J., Fransson, P., Wright, C. I., & Backman, L. (2005). Age-differential patterns of brain activation during perception of angry faces. *Neuroscience Letters, 386*, 99–104.

Foos, P. W., & Wright, L. (1992). Adult age differences in the storage of information in working memory. *Experimental Aging Research, 18*, 51–57.

Garde, E., Mortensen, E. L., Krabbe, K., Rostrup, E., & Larsson, H. B. (2000). Relation between age-related decline in intelligence and cerebral white-matter hyperintensities in healthy octogenarians: a longitudinal study. *Lancet, 356*, 628–634.

Gazzaley, A., Cooney, J. W., Rissman, J., & D'Esposito, M. (2005). Top-down suppression deficit underlies working memory impairment in normal aging. *Nature Neuroscience, 8*, 1298–1300.*

Glisky, E. L., Polster, M. R., & Routhieaux, B. C. (1995). Double dissociation between item and source memory. *Psychology and Aging, 9*, 229–235.

Gobbini, M. I., & Haxby, J. V. (2007). Neural systems for recognition of familiar faces. *Neuropsychologia, 45*, 32–41.

Gobbini, M. I., Leibenluft, E., Santiago, N., & Haxby, J. V. (2004). Social and emotional attachment in the neural representation of faces. *NeuroImage, 22*, 1628–1635.

Grady, C. L., Hongwanishkul, D., Keightley, M. L., Lee, W. S. C., & Hasher, L. (2007). The effect of age on memory for emotional faces. *Neuropsychology, 21*, 371–380.

Grady, C. L., Maisog, J. M., Horwitz, B., Ungerleider, L. G., Mentis, M. J., Salerno, J. A., et al. (1994). Age-related changes in cortical blood flow activation during visual processing of faces and location. *Journal of Neuroscience, 14*, 1450–1462.

Grady, C. L., McIntosh, A. R., Bookstein, F., Horwitz, B., Rapoport, S. I., & Haxby, J. V. (1998). Age-related changes in regional cerebral blood flow during working memory for faces. *NeuroImage, 8*, 409–425.

Grady, C. L., McIntosh, A. R., & Craik, F. (2005). Task-related activity in prefrontal cortex and its relation to recognition memory performance in young and old adults. *Neuropsychologia, 43*, 1466–1481.

Grady, C. L., McIntosh, A. R., & Craik, F. I. (2003). Age-related differences in the functional connectivity of the hippocampus during memory encoding. *Hippocampus, 13*, 572–586.

Grady, C. L., McIntosh, A. R., Horwitz, B., Maisog, J. M., Ungerleider, L. G., Mentis, M. J., et al. (1995). Age-related reductions in human recognition memory due to impaired encoding. *Science, 269*, 218–221.

Grady, C. L., Springer, M. V., Hongwanishkul, D., McIntosh, A. R., & Winocur, G. (2006). Age-related changes in brain activity across the adult lifespan. *Journal of Cognitive Neuroscience, 18*, 227–241.

Grady, C. L., Yu, H., & Alain, C. (2008). Age-related differences in brain activity underlying working memory for spatial and nonspatial auditory information. *Cerebral Cortex, 18*, 189–199.

Grill-Spector, K., & Malach, R. (2001). fMR-adaptation: a tool for studying the functional properties of human cortical neurons. *Acta Psychologia (Amsterdam), 107*, 293–321.

Gunning-Dixon, F. M., Gur, R. C., Perkins, A. C., Schroeder, L., Turner, T., Turetsky, B. I., et al. (2003). Age-related differences in brain activation during emotional face processing. *Neurobiology of Aging, 24*, 285–295.

Gunning-Dixon, F. M., & Raz, N. (2000). The cognitive correlates of white matter abnormalities in normal aging: a quantitative review. *Neuropsychology, 14*, 224–232.

Gutchess, A. H., Hebrank, A., Sutton, B. P., Leshikar, E., Chee, M. W., Tan, J. C., et al. (2007). Contextual interference in recognition memory with age. *NeuroImage, 35*, 1338–1347.

Gutchess, A. H., Welsh, R. C., Hedden, T., Bangert, A., Minear, M., Liu, L. L., et al. (2005). Aging and the neural correlates of successful picture encoding: frontal activations compensate for decreased medial temporal activity. *Journal of Cognitive Neuroscience, 17*, 84–96.

Handwerker, D. A., Gazzaley, A., Inglis, B. A., & D'Esposito, M. (2007). Reducing vascular variability of fMRI data across aging populations using a breathholding task. *Human Brain Mapping, 28*, 846–859.

Hasher, L., & Zacks, R. T. (1988). Working memory, comprehension, and aging: A review and a new view. In G. H. Bower (Ed.), *The Psychology of Learning and Motivation* (Vol. 22, pp. 193–225). San Diego, CA: Academic Press.

Hashtroudi, S., Johnson, M. K., & Chrosniak, L. D. (1989). Aging and source monitoring. *Psychology and Aging, 4*, 106–112.

Haxby, J. V., Gobbini, M. I., Furey, M. L., Ishai, A., Schouten, J. L., & Pietrini, P. (2001). Distributed and overlapping representations of faces and objects in ventral temporal cortex. *Science, 293*, 2425–2430.

He, Y., Chen, Z. J., & Evans, A. C. (2007). Small-world anatomical networks in the human brain revealed by cortical thickness from MRI. *Cerebral Cortex, 17*, 2407–2419.

Hillary, F. G., & Biswal, B. (2007). The influence of neuropathology on the fMRI signal: a measurement of brain or vein? *Clinical Neuropsychology, 21*, 58–72.

Horwitz, B., Soncrant, T. T., & Haxby, J. V. (1992). Covariance analysis of functional interactions in the brain using metabolic and blood flow data. In F. Gonzalez-Lima, T. Finkenstaedt & H. Scheich (Eds.), *Advances in Metabolic Mapping Techniques for Brain Imaging of Behavioral and Learning Functions* (pp. 189–217). Dordrecht, The Netherlands: Kluwer Academic Publishers.

Huettel, S. A., Singerman, J. D., & McCarthy, G. (2001). The effects of aging upon the hemodynamic response measured by functional MRI. *NeuroImage, 13*, 161–175.

Iidaka, T., Okada, T., Murata, T., Omori, M., Kosaka, H., Sadato, N., et al. (2002). Age-related differences in the medial temporal lobe responses to emotional faces as revealed by fMRI. *Hippocampus, 12*, 352–362.

Jonides, J., Marshuetz, C., Smith, E. E., Reuter-Lorenz, P. A., Koeppe, R. A., & Hartley, A. (2000). Age differences in behavior and PET activation reveal differences in interference resolution in verbal working memory. *Journal of Cognitive Neuroscience, 12*, 188–196.

Keightley, M. L., Chiew, K., Winocur, G., & Grady, C. L. (2007). Age-related differences in brain activity underlying identification of emotional expressions in faces. *Social, Cognitive, and Affective Neuroscience, 2*, 292–302.

Keightley, M. L., Winocur, G., Burianova, H., Hongwanishkul, D., & Grady, C. (2006). Age effects on social cognition: faces tell a different story. *Psychology and Aging, 21*, 558–572.

Kensinger, E. A., Brierley, B., Medford, N., Growdon, J. H., & Corkin, S. (2002). Effects of normal aging and Alzheimer's disease on emotional memory. *Emotion, 2*, 118–134.

Kensinger, E. A., & Corkin, S. (2004). Two routes to emotional memory: distinct neural processes for valence and arousal. *Proceedings of the National Academy of Sciences USA, 101*, 3310–3315.

Langenecker, S. A., Briceno, E. M., Hamid, N. M., & Nielson, K. A. (2007). An evaluation of distinct volumetric and functional MRI contributions toward understanding age and task performance: a study in the basal ganglia. *Brain Research, 1135*, 58–68.

Lee, L., Friston, K., & Horwitz, B. (2006). Large-scale neural models and dynamic causal modelling. *NeuroImage, 30*, 1243–1254.

Lenartowicz, A., & McIntosh, A. R. (2005). The role of anterior cingulate cortex in working memory is shaped by functional connectivity. *Journal of Cognitive Neuroscience, 17*, 1026–1042.

Logan, J. M., Sanders, A. L., Snyder, A. Z., Morris, J. C., & Buckner, R. L. (2002). Under-recruitment and nonselective recruitment: dissociable neural mechanisms associated with aging. *Neuron, 33*, 827–840.

Lustig, C., Snyder, A. Z., Bhakta, M., O'Brien, K. C., McAvoy, M., Raichle, M. E., et al. (2003). Functional deactivations: change with age and dementia of the Alzheimer type. *Proceedings of the National Academy of Sciences USA, 100*, 14504–14509.

MacPherson, S. E., Phillips, L. H., & Della Sala, S. (2002). Age, executive function, and social decision making: a dorsolateral prefrontal theory of cognitive aging. *Psychology and Aging, 17*, 598–609.

Madden, D. J., Spaniol, J., Whiting, W. L., Bucur, B., Provenzale, J. M., Cabeza, R., et al. (2007). Adult age differences in the functional neuroanatomy of visual attention: a combined fMRI and DTI study. *Neurobiology of Aging, 28*, 459–476.

Madden, D. J., Whiting, W. L., Provenzale, J. M., & Huettel, S. A. (2004). Age-related changes in neural activity during visual target detection measured by fMRI. *Cerebral Cortex, 14*, 143–155.

Mather, M., Canli, T., English, T., Whitfield, S., Wais, P., Ochsner, K., et al. (2004). Amygdala responses to emotionally valenced stimuli in older and younger adults. *Psychological Science, 15*, 259–263.

Mattay, V. S., Fera, F., Tessitore, A., Hariri, A. R., Berman, K. F., Das, S., et al. (2006). Neurophysiological correlates of age-related changes in working memory capacity. *Neuroscience Letters, 392*, 32–37.

Maurer, D., O'Craven, K. M., Le Grand, R., Mondloch, C. J., Springer, M. V., Lewis, T. L., et al. (2007). Neural correlates of processing facial identity based on features versus their spacing. *Neuropsychologia, 45*, 1438–1451.

McDowell, C. L., Harrison, D. W., & Demaree, H. A. (1994). Is right hemisphere decline in the perception of emotion a function of aging? *International Journal of Neuroscience, 79*, 1–11.

McIntosh, A. R. (1999). Mapping cognition to the brain through neural interactions. *Memory, 7*, 523–548.

Milham, M. P., Erickson, K. I., Banich, M. T., Kramer, A. F., Webb, A., Wszalek, T., et al. (2002). Attentional control in the aging brain: insights from an fMRI study of the stroop task. *Brain and Cognition, 49*, 277–296.

Mitchell, K. J., Johnson, M. K., Raye, C. L., & Greene, E. J. (2004). Prefrontal cortex activity associated with source monitoring in a working memory task. *Journal of Cognitive Neuroscience, 16*, 921–934.

Mitchell, K. J., Raye, C. L., Johnson, M. K., & Greene, E. J. (2006). An fMRI investigation of short-term source memory in young and older adults. *NeuroImage, 30*, 627–633.

Morcom, A. M., Li, J., & Rugg, M. D. (2007). Age effects on the neural correlates of episodic retrieval: Increased cortical recruitment with matched performance. *Cerebral Cortex, 17*, 2491–2506.

Morris, J. S., Friston, K. J., Buchel, C., Frith, C. D., Young, A. W., Calder, A. J., et al. (1998). A neuromodulatory role for the human amygdala in processing emotional facial expressions. *Brain, 121*, 47–57.

Moseley, M. (2002). Diffusion tensor imaging and aging—a review. *NMR in Biomedicine, 15*, 553–560.

Nadel, L., Samsonovich, A., Ryan, L., & Moscovitch, M. (2000). Multiple trace theory of human memory: computational, neuroimaging, and neuropsychological results. *Hippocampus, 10*, 352–368.

Nielson, K. A., Douville, K. L., Seidenberg, M., Woodard, J. L., Miller, S. K., Franczak, M., et al. (2006). Age-related functional recruitment for famous name recognition: an event-related fMRI study. *Neurobiology of Aging, 27*, 1494–1504.

Nielson, K. A., Langenecker, S. A., & Garavan, H. (2002). Differences in the functional neuroanatomy of inhibitory control across the adult life span. *Psychology and Aging, 17*, 56–71.

Nordahl, C. W., Ranganath, C., Yonelinas, A. P., Decarli, C., Fletcher, E., & Jagust, W. J. (2006). White matter changes compromise prefrontal cortex function in healthy elderly individuals. *Journal of Cognitive Neuroscience, 18*, 418–429.

Ochsner, K. N. (2000). Are affective events richly recollected or simply familiar? The experience and process of recognizing feelings past. *Journal of Experimental Psychology: General, 129*, 242–261.

Oscar-Berman, M., Hancock, M., Mildworf, B., Hutner, N., & Weber, D. A. (1990). Emotional perception and memory in alcoholism and aging. *Alcoholism Clinical and Experimental Research, 14*, 383–393.

Payer, D., Marshuetz, C., Sutton, B., Hebrank, A., Welsh, R. C., & Park, D. C. (2006). Decreased neural specialization in old adults on a working memory task. *Neuroreport, 17*, 487–491.

Persson, J., Lustig, C., Nelson, J. K., & Reuter-Lorenz, P. A. (2007). Age differences in deactivation: a link to cognitive control? *Journal of Cognitive Neuroscience, 19*, 1021–1032.

Persson, J., Nyberg, L., Lind, J., Larsson, A., Nilsson, L. G., Ingvar, M., et al. (2006). Structure-function correlates of cognitive decline in aging. *Cerebral Cortex, 16*, 907–915.

Pfefferbaum, A., Sullivan, E. V., Hedehus, M., Lim, K. O., Adalsteinsson, E., & Moseley, M. (2000). Age-related decline in brain white matter anisotropy measured with spatially corrected echo-planar diffusion tensor imaging. *Magnetic Resonance in Medicine, 44*, 259–268.

Phillips, L. H., MacLean, R. D., & Allen, R. (2002). Age and the understanding of emotions: neuropsychological and sociocognitive perspectives. *Journal of Gerontology B: Psychological Science and Social Science, 57*, 526–530.

Raichle, M. E., MacLeod, A. M., Snyder, A. Z., Powers, W. J., Gusnard, D. A., & Shulman, G. L. (2001). A default mode of brain function. *Proceedings of the National Academy of Sciences USA, 98*, 676–682.

Rajah, M. N., & D'Esposito, M. (2005). Region-specific changes in prefrontal function with age: a review of PET and fMRI studies on working and episodic memory. *Brain, 128*, 1964–1983.

Raz, N. (2000). Aging of the brain and its impact on cognitive performance: integration of structural and functional findings. In F. I. M. Craik & T. A. Salthouse (Eds.), *Handbook of Aging and Cognition—II* (pp. 1–90). Mahwah, NJ: Lawrence Erlbaum.

Reuter-Lorenz, P. A., Jonides, J., Smith, E. E., Hartley, A., Miller, A., Marshuetz, C., et al. (2000). Age differences in the frontal lateralization of verbal and spatial working memory revealed by PET. *Journal of Cognitive Neuroscience, 12*, 174–187.

Rypma, B., Eldreth, D. A., & Rebbechi, D. (2007). Age-related differences in activation-performance relations in delayed-response tasks: a multiple component analysis. *Cortex, 43*, 65–76.

Samanez Larkin, G. R., Gibbs, S. E., Khanna, K., Nielsen, L., Carstensen, L. L., & Knutson, B. (2007). Anticipation of monetary gain but not loss in healthy older adults. *Nature Neuroscience, 10*, 787–791.

Schacter, D. L., Kaszniak, A. W., Kihlstrom, J. F., & Valdiserri, M. (1991). The relation between source memory and aging. *Psychology and Aging, 6*, 559–568.

Soderlund, H., Nyberg, L., Adolfsson, R., Nilsson, L. G., & Launer, L. J. (2003). High prevalence of white matter hyperintensities in normal aging: relation to blood pressure and cognition. *Cortex, 39*, 1093–1105.

Squire, L. R. (1992). Memory and the hippocampus: A synthesis from findings with rats, monkeys, and humans. *Psychological Review, 99*, 195–231.

Stern, Y., Zarahn, E., Habeck, C., Holtzer, R., Rakitin, B. C., Kumar, A., et al. (in press). A common neural network for cognitive reserve in verbal and object working memory in young but not old. *Cerebral Cortex*.

Taniwaki, T., Okayama, A., Yoshiura, T., Togao, O., Nakamura, Y., Yamasaki, T., et al. (2006). Functional network of the basal ganglia and cerebellar motor loops in vivo: different activation patterns between self-initiated and externally triggered movements. *NeuroImage, 31*, 745–753.

Taniwaki, T., Okayama, A., Yoshiura, T., Togao, O., Nakamura, Y., Yamasaki, T., et al. (2007). Age-related alterations of the functional interactions within the basal ganglia and cerebellar motor loops in vivo. *Neuroimage, 36*, 1263–1276.

Tessitore, A., Hariri, A. R., Fera, F., Smith, W. G., Das, S., Weinberger, D. R., et al. (2005). Functional changes in the activity of brain regions underlying emotion processing in the elderly. *Psychiatry Research, 139*, 9–18.

Townsend, J., Adamo, M., & Haist, F. (2006). Changing channels: an fMRI study of aging and cross-modal attention shifts. *NeuroImage, 31*, 1682–1692.

Urry, H. L., van Reekum, C. M., Johnstone, T., Kalin, N. H., Thurow, M. E., Schaefer, H. S., et al. (2006). Amygdala and ventromedial prefrontal cortex are inversely coupled during regulation of negative affect and predict the diurnal pattern of cortisol secretion among older adults. *Journal of Neuroscience, 26*, 4415–4425.

van der Veen, F. M., Nijhuis, F. A., Tisserand, D. J., Backes, W. H., & Jolles, J. (2006). Effects of aging on recognition of intentionally and incidentally stored words: an fMRI study. *Neuropsychologia, 44*, 2477–2486.

Velanova, K., Lustig, C., Jacoby, L. L., & Buckner, R. L. (2007). Evidence for frontally mediated controlled processing differences in older adults. *Cerebral Cortex, 17*, 1033–1046.

Wierenga, C. E., Benjamin, M., Gopinath, K., Perlstein, W. M., Leonard, C. M., Rothi, L. J., et al. (2006). Age-related changes in word retrieval: role of bilateral frontal and subcortical networks. *Neurobiology of Aging*.

Williams, L. M., Brown, K. J., Palmer, D., Liddell, B. J., Kemp, A. H., Olivieri, G., et al. (2006). The mellow years?: neural basis of improving emotional stability over age. *Journal of Neuroscience, 26*, 6422–6430.

Wright, C. I., Wedig, M. M., Williams, D., Rauch, S. L., & Albert, M. S. (2006). Novel fearful faces activate the amygdala in healthy young and elderly adults. *Neurobiology of Aging, 27*, 361–374.

Wu, T., Zang, Y., Wang, L., Long, X., Hallett, M., Chen, Y., et al. (2007). Aging influence on functional connectivity of the motor network in the resting state. *Neuroscience Letters, 422*, 164–168.

Zarahn, E., Rakitin, B., Abela, D., Flynn, J., & Stern, Y. (2007). Age-related changes in brain activation during a delayed item recognition task. *Neurobiology of Aging, 28*, 784–798.

Can Neurological Evidence Help Courts Assess Criminal Responsibility? Lessons from Law and Neuroscience

EYAL AHARONI,[a] CHADD FUNK,[a] WALTER SINNOTT-ARMSTRONG,[b] AND MICHAEL GAZZANIGA[a]

[a]*University of California, Santa Barbara, Santa Barbara, California, USA*
[b]*Dartmouth College, Hanover, New Hampshire, USA*

Can neurological evidence help courts assess criminal responsibility? To answer this question, we must first specify legal criteria for criminal responsibility and then ask how neurological findings can be used to determine whether particular defendants meet those criteria. Cognitive neuroscience may speak to at least two familiar conditions of criminal responsibility: intention and sanity. Functional neuroimaging studies in motor planning, awareness of actions, agency, social contract reasoning, and theory of mind, among others, have recently targeted a small assortment of brain networks thought to be instrumental in such determinations. Advances in each of these areas bring specificity to the problems underlying the application of neuroscience to criminal law.

Key words: neuroscience; neuroimaging; fMRI; law; ethics; responsibility; excuse; defense; insanity; diminished capacity; mens rea; free will; determinism

By the time the battery acid had circulated through his bloodstream, Pablo Ortiz was quickly slipping away. The perpetrators of this vicious act, Simon and Heriberto Pirela, then instructed their accomplices to "finish him off" or face the same fate (Weichselbaum 2004). In 1982, a Pennsylvania judge sentenced Simon Pirela to death for murder in the first degree.

Twenty-one years later, an appellate court reduced Pirela's punishment to life in prison on account of new evidence. What kind of evidence could possibly mitigate this killer's crime? Pictures of Pirela's brain. Neuroimaging data successfully convinced the judge that Pirela was not eligible for the death penalty because he suffered from aberrations in his frontal lobes, diminishing his ability to function normally (*Commonwealth of Pennsylvania v. Pirela*, 2007). It seems that when the mind is on trial, pictures of brains are worth a thousand words.

In the time since Pirela's victim took his final breath, unprecedented advances have been made in cognitive neuroscience. As the science has become available, defense attorneys have inevitably tried to use this science to help their clients. The best-known use of neuroscience in criminal trials may be found in the Supreme Court case of *Roper v. Simmons* (2005), which ruled out the death penalty for crimes committed by adolescents younger than 18 years. Since then, the use of imaging data as a tool to reduce responsibility or completely exculpate criminal offenders has become a familiar target for hopes, jokes, and contention.

Can the best neuroscientific evidence available today reduce or even rule out criminal responsibility? Many scientists, lawyers, defendants, and media representatives are already eagerly answering "yes." Others are enthusiastic that such evidence could be used by prosecutors to *establish* criminal responsibility. However, the utmost caution must be taken in making these claims because false conclusions are likely to cost real lives and livelihoods. As some of us have argued previously, the worth of neuroscience in criminal decisions is far from obvious, in part because there is not, and will never be, a brain correlate of responsibility (Gazzaniga & Steven 2005; Grafton et al. 2006–2007). Rather than being an independent neutral property of an individual, legal responsibility also requires a normative judgment that depends on the social purposes of those who ascribe it. Neuroscience can offer us only descriptive models of brain organization and function; ascriptions of responsibility, on the other hand, are unequivocally

Address for correspondence: Eyal Aharoni, M.A., Department of Psychology, University of California, Santa Barbara, Santa Barbara, CA 93106. Voice: 805-893-2791; fax: 805-893-4303.
aharoni@psych.ucsb.edu

prescriptive. This is one reason why to explain, by itself, is not to excuse.

To examine whether neuroscience can inform determinations of responsibility, we need to begin by examining how neuroscience fits into a larger philosophical debate about responsibility in general and then identify the legal criteria for criminal responsibility in particular. Finally we must ask whether and how current neuroscientific findings can be used to determine whether particular individuals meet these criteria.

This task might seem relatively straightforward, but the language of law is vastly different from the language of neuroscience. Matching neurological data to legal criteria can be much like performing a chemical analysis of a cheesecake to find out whether it was baked with love. To span the divide between the way neuroscientists describe mental states and the way the law applies them, we must develop a set of rules for evaluating when a defendant's neurological profile meets or fails a particular legal requirement. Too liberal, and the guilty run free; too strict, and the ill and innocent suffer imprisonment or death. These rules would have to reconcile probabilistic findings about continuous mental states with categorical legal decisions about guilt and punishment. These rules also need to apply findings about groups to particular defendants. Though difficult to devise, such a system of rules could reveal when, if ever, neuroscientific techniques will become of adequate use for criminal trials.

To accomplish this feat in our lifetime would take nothing short of a miracle. A humbler goal, which we adopt here, is to (1) outline key philosophical issues, (2) identify how the law determines when a defendant is considered responsible, and (3) apply rigorous exemplars of modern neuroscience to these criteria in hopes of providing useful models for future scientific research and legal decision making. We have no guarantee that neuroscientific models, in all their detail, will make responsibility determinations easier rather than harder. Hence, another of our goals is to evaluate how well this technology can contribute in the coming years to the ongoing challenge of improving the criminal justice system.

Philosophical Background

Our task would be relatively easy if responsibility could be ruled out simply by finding any old neural cause of action. The resulting temptation is to proclaim, "*I* didn't do it—my *brain* made me do it." This move is supported by a classic philosophical argument:

(1) Every act is determined.
(2) If an act is determined, then its agent is not responsible for the act.
(3) Therefore, no agent is responsible for any act.

If a cause of an action does not just make that action likely but determines that the action definitely will be done, then any action that is caused is also determined. Neural causes would determine their effects just as much as any other causes. Then, if we can trace an act to a neural cause, its agent is not responsible, according to this argument.

This argument seems to have special force when we can trace an action to causes beyond its agent's control. The neural connections that affect actions developed long before the actions (perhaps during childhood) and were caused by external circumstances or prior events that were beyond the agent's control. Moreover, most agents do not know what is going on in their brains, so they cannot choose certain neural events rather than others with any specificity. In that way, the neural causes of an action are beyond the agent's control. Such considerations, among others, lead some philosophers to deny that agents are responsible for anything they do (see, e.g., Greene & Cohen 2004; Pereboom 2001).

Most philosophers, however, are not hard determinists. Many reject the conclusion that agents should not be held responsible and contest one of the argument's premises. The result is an array of positions (see Table 1).

Some indeterminists defend responsibility by denying determinism and claiming instead that many human actions are uncaused. However, critics charge that uncaused actions, if there were any, would be random, and random actions do not merit responsibility. Many philosophers have argued that randomness removes responsibility. By analogy, a robot programmed to shoot a gun as an output of a random outcome generator is no more free than one programmed by a fixed-outcome generator. Both robots' actions are unfit for responsibility. And, of course, robots that appear random can really have causes that we don't detect. Likewise, human volition that is truly random would not lead to responsible action, and human volition that appears random might really be caused.

Instead of claiming that human actions are not caused at all, most libertarians claim that human actions are self-caused or caused by the agent rather than by any prior event. In the jargon, they deny event causation and then invoke agent causation to avoid randomness (Kane 1996; van Inwagen 1983). There are several problems with this view. First, the denial of

TABLE 1. Philosophical positions on responsibility

	Accept premise (1): determinism	**Deny premise (1): indeterminism**
Accept premise (2): incompatibilism	Accept conclusion (3): hard determinism	Deny conclusion (3): libertarianism
Deny premise (2): compatibilism	Deny conclusion (3): soft determinism	Deny conclusion (3): soft indeterminism

event causation becomes less and less defensible in light of contemporary neuroscience, genetics, behaviorism, and every other science that models antecedents of human behavior. Second, it is difficult to make sense of the notion of agent causation (Pereboom 2001, chaps. 2–3). The most basic problem is that the agent exists equally before the action is done, while it is done, and after it is done, so citing the agent as a cause cannot explain why the act was done at the particular time when it was done. Only prior events can explain that.

Problems like these lead many philosophers toward compatibilism. They claim that determinism can be reconciled with freedom and responsibility. But how? One popular approach interprets freedom in terms of responsiveness to reasons, and agents can respond to reasons even if they are determined to do so (Fischer & Ravizza 1998; Wolf 1990).

Compatibilism has also been embraced by various legal scholars. Morse and Hoffman, for example, warn on both logical and practical grounds that we should not infer from the bare descriptive fact that an act is caused to the prescriptive claim that its agent ought to be free of responsibility (Morse & Hoffman 2007, 80–81). According to these authors, "My genes made me do it," "My upbringing made me do it," and "My Twinkie made me do it" are not popularly compelling excuses in modern jurisdictions, so "My brain made me do it" should not be exculpatory either (Morse & Hoffman 2007, 82). In their view, causal explanations by themselves provide insufficient grounds to excuse.

Moreover, neuroscience cannot demonstrate that all acts are determined. One reason is that most neuroscientific studies reveal only correlations rather than causation. Even studies that find neural causes do not prove that those causes are deterministic, and they clearly do not generalize to all actions of all sorts. To the confusion of many, neuroscience might then be used to both support and undermine determinism. Neuroscience is not independently qualified to prove either that all actions are caused or that any actions are entirely spontaneous. These are ancient and enduring debates that science or philosophy will not soon solve.

So let's leave determinism behind. Neuroscience still might raise separate problems for freedom and responsibility. Regardless of what, if anything, causes our wills, we also need to ask what, if anything, our wills cause. To see why, imagine that someone plans to kill a rival by running him over as the rival jogs in the park. As the driver backs out of his driveway on the way to commit the murder, the jogger unexpectedly appears and is run over and killed by accident. The driver consciously and did freely will to kill the jogger and had that will at the time when he killed the jogger. Nonetheless, the driver's will did not cause the accident or the death in a normal or expected way. Hence, the driver might not be guilty of either reckless driving or attempted murder. Even if the driver were reckless, this particular act of killing was not done *from* free will, and the driver is not responsible for murder. What this case shows, then, is that freedom and responsibility for an act require more than just a will or intention to do the act. They seem to require that the act results from the conscious will in a normal way.

Moreover, many views of freedom and responsibility focus on conscious will. Libertarians who invoke agent causation often cite the agent's conscious reasons or will as the crucial part of the agent that makes the agent responsible. Compatibilists who analyze freedom in terms of responsiveness to reasons usually refer to conscious reasons, because it is not clear how we could be expected to respond to reasons that we are not aware of. Some laws explicitly require conscious intentions as elements of crimes. This focus on consciousness is supposed to seem plausible in examples. Imagine that someone cooks some soup for a friend, and the cook's only conscious goal is to make the friend happy. Unfortunately, the soup contains peanuts—to which the friend is allergic. If the cook is not negligent, then he does not seem responsible for the friend's allergic reaction. But suppose that a prosecutor or an enemy argues that the cook has some kind of unconscious desire, plan, or will to hurt his friend. Such an unconscious will does not seem enough to make the cook responsible on several common views. After all, if the cook is not conscious of deciding to hurt his friend, how can he control whether he does hurt his friend? Without such control, how can he be responsible for hurting his friend?

Such examples and lines of thought give some initial plausibility to the principle that an agent is free and responsible only for acts that result from that agent's conscious will. This view does not deny that our actions often result from unconscious processes that guide our actions better than conscious thought or decision would. The claim is only that we are not responsible when our acts result from unconscious processes with no input from conscious will. This thesis has been questioned, but the point here is only that it is popular and persuasive.

Neuroscience raises doubts about this common assumption. In classic experiments, Libet (2004) and his collaborators developed a clever method for determining precisely when participants become conscious of choosing to flex their wrists or fingers. They then used electroencephalograms to determine the onset of activity in the supplementary motor area (SMA), called the "readiness potential," that begins the process that leads to flexing. Surprisingly, this neural activity in the motor strip starts, on average, about 350 ms *earlier* than the consciousness of making a choice. But if the conscious choice to flex one's finger comes later than the neural initiation of action, then the conscious choice cannot independently cause the action in the way that most people assume.

Libet denied that his results rule out free will or responsibility because he thought that, through conscious processes, we still have time to stop the neural activation from causing motion in the finger. Critics respond, however, that the decision to stop that process is itself a consequence of unconscious neural processes. If so, it is hard to see how the decision to stop the action could be any more free or effective than the apparent conscious choice to start it. It is then unclear how free will could play a causal role in action (Wegner 2002).

Of course, defenders of freedom and responsibility have many responses. One common objection is that subjects consciously chose to cooperate in the study, so they willed to flex their fingers long before the brain potential that Libet measured. Nonetheless, this earlier general intention to flex a finger at one time or another did not cause subjects to flex a finger at the precise time that they did, so that intention did not cause the particular action that they performed. The above example of driving over the jogger shows that particular proximate intentions rather than such distal intentions determine responsibility. Hence, Libet's results challenge traditional views of freedom and responsibility, even if our acts are preceded by some general intentions.

Another common objection is that Libet's experiments used simple actions, so more complex actions still might result from conscious intentions. When criminals rob banks according to their plans, their conscious intentions do seem to cause them to do what they do. However, such more complex actions are made up of smaller actions like flexing body parts, and it is not clear how the whole can be free if its parts are not. It is possible for freedom to apply only at the higher level of generality, but it is a challenge to explain how this works. Besides, acts like raising a hand are exactly the kind of case that defenders of free will use to show that they are free: "See. I can raise it or lower it, as I wish." If Libet's findings show that these supposed exemplars of freedom do not result from conscious intentions, that would seem to cast doubt on a larger range of cases. And even if Libet's claim applied only to simple actions, it would still be surprising and important that those actions do not result from conscious will, since they seem to.

More technical objections are also raised. Some critics chide Libet for sometimes describing readiness potentials as intentions or decisions when they are more like urges (Mele 2006). Others question the precision of subjects' post-hoc reports about when they made decisions. Still others point out that similar neural activations can occur when the subject does not intend to act or when the subject only watches someone else (Kilner et al. 2004). All these objections need to be taken seriously. Although Libet's results are not conclusive, they do point toward one direction in which neuroscience might challenge our traditional views of freedom and responsibility without even mentioning determinism.

Ultimately, a keen knowledge of why people break the law might gain leverage from understanding not how free agents make choices but how causal brains influence people to follow some rules and not others. However, we are a long way away from predictive models of how people adhere to legal rules, so until that time, it is important that neuroscience still be compatible with the subjective appearance of freedom. A human action can be both determined, possibly by readiness potentials before conscious willing, and still subjectively free at the same time (see Gazzaniga 2005, and Gazzaniga & Steven 2005 for similar arguments). Choosing to raise one's hand results from physical causes, but it also *feels* free. Even if this feeling of free will is a mere construction of the brain, this does not mean that such a construction is useless or ineffectual. The felt experience of free will, and the ability to attribute free will to others, seems to be integral for human beings to navigate our complex social landscape. Our intuitions about free will enable us to make predictions about human action that are as good as or better than our best neuroscientific models. They cannot then be dismissed merely as misleading illusions.

In these ways, although neuroscience is not equipped to resolve the ancient philosophical debates, the application of neuroscience can illuminate those debates. Moreover, although modern neuroscience is far from becoming a direct mechanism of exculpation, neuroscientific studies may potentially help to clarify when agents are responsible by testing accusations and excuses against systematic observations of real human behavior. This possibility becomes especially important when neuroscience is applied to legal decisions.

How the Law Determines Whether a Defendant Is Responsible

In determining who is responsible, the law is where the rubber meets the road. However, it is not easy to define how the law determines responsibility. One reason is that different legal jurisdictions have different criteria for responsibility. This variation itself is an indication of the inherent difficulties in defining criteria of responsibility. Furthermore, determinations of responsibility can play many roles in a trial.

The relevance of neuroscientific evidence has been implicated in at least two of these roles: defenses that deny intentions and affirmative defenses, such as insanity. Other variants of mens rea, such as recklessness and negligence, and other excuses, such as duress, coercion, irresistible impulse, and automatism, also bear on criminal responsibility and are intriguing candidates for neuroscientific investigation. However, several recent neuroscientific studies seem directly relevant to intention and insanity. Examining these studies and concepts will provide substantial room for our discussion on the future of criminal responsibility.

We will focus on the extent to which neuroscience could be used to *reduce* responsibility, not to *establish* it. This is because (1) establishing responsibility seems to require the ability to decipher the content of particular mental states, which is a much harder problem for neuroscience to solve than ruling these states out by furnishing evidence that a defendant lacked the capacity for a certain mental state, and (2) establishing responsibility is likely to rely on mandatory neuroimaging, which might violate the defendant's right to privacy, right against search and seizure, and right against self-incrimination—all complex debates that have been reviewed elsewhere (Tovino 2007).

Hence, our topic will be how denials of intentions and of sanity can be used to reduce or remove responsibility. We will begin by outlining the legal concepts of intention and insanity. Then we will discuss some relevant scientific studies.

Mens Rea

A criminal act is standardly divided into the actus reus and the mens rea, which are, respectively, roughly the physical act and the mental element. Theft, for example, might require taking property (the actus reus) with the knowledge that it belongs to someone else and the intention to deprive that person of it (the mens rea). Both elements of a crime must be proven beyond reasonable doubt for the prosecution to convict a defendant of that crime.

Different crimes require different mental states, or mens rea, for conviction. The crime of first-degree murder usually requires an intention to kill (except in cases of felony murder, depraved indifference, and Pinkerton liability), whereas manslaughter can often be committed without any intention to kill. The mens rea required for a given crime can also vary between jurisdictions and over time.

Mens rea commonly includes at least four variants: intention or purpose, knowledge that the act is done, recklessness, and negligence (Model Penal Code § 2.01 1962). These refer to specific mental states required for an act to qualify as an instance of a particular crime. Some crimes require intent, such as an intention to kill, harm, or deprive of property. Other crimes do not require intention but do require knowledge, such as knowledge that the harm will occur. Still other crimes do not require knowledge that a harm or offense will definitely occur but, instead, require only knowledge of a risk of the harm or offense. Unjustified disregard of that known risk then constitutes recklessness, as in some cases of drunk driving. Finally, some crimes do not require actual knowledge even of risk but are committed when an agent should have known about the harm or the risk. The act or agent is then called negligent. A successful defense against any of these variants results in a reduced charge to a less serious offense or, sometimes, an acquittal.

Neuroscience might in principle be used to determine when any of these mental conditions is met. However, current neuroscience speaks most strongly to matters of intention, so we will focus on that form of mens rea.

Intention is commonly defined as a commitment to a plan of action. In normal cases, an act is done intentionally when the actor commits to a plan that includes that action as an essential part. For an act to be intentional, the actor must also know that he is planning and performing it. People kill intentionally in this sense when they know that death is a likely consequence of their acts and when the resulting death is also part of what they need to accomplish to fulfill their plans (Bratman 1987; Perkins 1969, 747). Although long-range premeditation sometimes may be present, it is not necessary to establish intention.

When a crime requires intention of this kind, the prosecution needs to show that the defendant had sufficient knowledge and relevant plans. The defense can respond that the defendant lacked one of these mental states. One way to show this lack might be to show that the defendant has abnormalities in the brain that prevent the defendant from forming or committing to plans of action. Many jurisdictions recognize this as a defense of diminished capacity (e.g., *Kansas v. Wilburn* 1991). These jurisdictions usually regard the diminished capacity defense as a challenge to intention or other culpable states, different from an insanity defense, which we will discuss in the next section.

If it can be empirically demonstrated that a defendant has difficulties forming intentional actions, there might be some probability that he lacked the capacity to act intentionally at the time of the offense. If this case can be made, he might be acquitted of the greater crime and charged with a lesser crime if one is available. In this way, neuroscience could become relevant to the criminal charge. The burden is then placed on neuroscientists to identify and measure abnormalities associated with these functions and dysfunctions. This is a tall order that we will examine below.

Insanity

Neuroscientific evidence also seems applicable to the insanity defense. A successful insanity defense acquits the defendant "by reason of insanity" and usually results in commitment to a mental hospital as long as the defendant is a danger to himself or others.

How insanity is defined could have important implications for how neuroscience evidence is used. The definition varies quite a bit among the United States. It also takes different forms in case law from that in statutes. Still, some formulations are common. Some states still adhere to the M'Naghten Rule, according to which a person is legally insane if

> ...at the time of the committing of the act, the party accused was laboring under such a defect of reason, from disease of mind, as not to know the nature and quality of the act he was doing; or if he did know it, that he did not know what he was doing was wrong. (1843)

This test is purely cognitive insofar as only lack of knowledge can support a verdict of not guilty by reason of insanity.

What counts as knowledge is not clear, so some later laws required defendants not only to know but also to "appreciate" what they were doing and that it was wrong in order to be found guilty. Some jurisdictions also added a volitional prong, so that defendants could be found not guilty by reason of insanity if they had a mental illness that either removed their capacity to resist impulses or created an impulse so strong that nobody could resist it. Either of these conditions would destroy the defendant's capacity to abide by law.

These developments culminated in the insanity defense of the Model Penal Code of the American Law Institute:

> A person is not responsible for criminal conduct if at the time of such conduct as a result of mental disease or defect he lacks substantial capacity either to appreciate the wrongfulness of his conduct or to conform his conduct to the requirements of the law.

So that psychopaths and sociopaths would not be excused, another clause in the Model Penal Code added, "the terms 'mental disease or defect' do not include an abnormality manifested only by repeated criminal or otherwise antisocial conduct."

The Model Penal Code test of insanity was accepted in most U.S. jurisdictions until John Hinckley was found not guilty by reason of insanity after trying to assassinate President Ronald Reagan (*U.S. v. Hinckley* 1982). Many commentators criticized that decision and blamed it on the broad insanity defense in that jurisdiction. As a result, most states removed the conformity prong of the Model Penal Code test and adopted purely cognitive insanity defenses closer to the old M'Naghten rule. Some jurisdictions also shifted the burden of proof, so that the defense would have to prove insanity and the prosecution would not have to prove sanity.

After these changes, defendants could still be found not guilty by reason of insanity if they showed that they could not know what they were doing or that they could not know that what they were doing was wrong. Such lack of knowledge could result from delusion, retardation, and possibly sleepwalking or automatism in some jurisdictions.

Neuroscientific evidence then becomes useful if it can establish such lack of capacity to know. As with challenges to the existence of mens rea, neuroscientists who want their research to be legally relevant face the challenge of designing a method of measuring an individual's capacity to know. In the next section, we discuss the advances and difficulties in operationalizing these constructs at a neural level.

Comparing Current Neurological Data to Legal Standards

As suggested, an effective neuroscience of responsibility might begin by showing a neurological basis for a reduced capacity to fulfill the mens rea and sanity requirements. We begin by evaluating some recent evidence related to intention formation and then the two chief conditions of legal insanity.

Defense against Mens Rea

How might neuroscience determine whether a particular person performed a particular act intentionally? Unfortunately, modern neuroscience is in no position to demonstrate a lack of intention for the particular crime charged because of course there is no known way to retroactively observe the state of the brain as it was during the commission of the offense.

It still might be possible to answer this question indirectly and probabilistically by showing that the individual probably lacked the ability to form plans or intentions. To support such a defense, neuroscientists would need (1) to identify some network in the brain that is necessary for forming "intentions" and then (2) to show that this network in the defendant's brain is dysfunctional during attempts at planned action, preventing him from reliably forming intentions but leaving intact the ability to perform the prohibited action (the actus reus).

To localize an "intention" mechanism in the brain, an ideal approach would be to measure the neural activation of an intended act as well as the neural activation of the same act performed unintentionally and then to subtract the latter from the former. Unfortunately, it is no easy task to systematically elicit specific unintentional actions, especially within the confines of a brain scanning apparatus. That might be why this direct approach has not been used.

An alternative approach could be to have participants intentionally perform simple motor behaviors such as a button press and to then instruct them to attend either to the experience of the act or to the experience of intending itself, and subtract the activation in the action condition from the activation in the intention condition. The fundamental assumption underlying this design is that attention directly modulates the activity of brain networks responsible for intention formation. Specifically, by attending to intention formation, there should be enhanced activity in the networks responsible for intention formation relative to conditions in which intention is formed less attentively.

Lau et al. (2004) did precisely this in a penetrating article in *Science*. They identified unique activation in the pre-SMA when participants attended to their intentions. This finding led the authors to conclude that this area of the brain generates intentions for motor behavior. They also observed an interaction with the dorsolateral prefrontal cortex, leading them to believe that this area was responsible for the ability to attend to these intentions. They concluded that this "attention to intention may be one mechanism by which effective conscious control of actions becomes possible" (1210).

Data like those of Lau et al. might seem to suggest that intention has been found in the brain and that observable abnormality in this area is proof of impairment in forming an intention. However, as with any study, such tempting inferences must be qualified. One limitation arises from the initial assumption that attention positively modulates activity in areas implicated in intention. A plausible alternative, for instance, might be that when attending to intention, this metacognitive task produces cognitive load for the attention processor, perhaps even *reducing* intentional capacities, and that the resulting increased activation is actually evidence of this attentional load, not of intention per se.

More evidence for the involvement of the medial frontal cortex in intention is reported by Haynes and colleagues (2007). They used a clever experimental design in which they had subjects freely decide whether they would add or subtract a subsequently presented pair of numbers. However, before these numbers were displayed, there was a time lag. This required subjects to maintain their intention for the length of the lag (which varied across trials). The numbers were displayed, and then four answers were displayed in random positions. This prevented subjects from forming habitual motor responses, enabling the researchers to isolate intention formation from motor planning. The authors found areas in the anterior medial frontal cortex that could be used to decode which intention the subjects were maintaining. Each intention was predicted by a separate pattern of activity within this region. Also, the authors noted activity in the posterior medial frontal cortex that was associated with action execution during the response phase. Like Lau et al., the investigators seem to have dissociated intention formation and maintenance from action execution, providing more evidence for the involvement of the medial frontal cortex in intention.

Others have attempted to isolate intention in the brain by comparing an intentional action task, such as a button press, to a task in which the same action has been previously conditioned as an almost automatic response to a stimulus such as an aural tone (Cunnington et al. 2002). The logic is that, if one subtracts the more "exogenous," reflexive action from the more "endogenous," effortful one, an activation profile for intention will manifest. However, this design suffers from the criticism that conditioned responses do not necessarily lack intentional regulation and conversely that the intention to act was not entirely endogenous but was prompted by instruction. Thus, it may come as no surprise that this design has yielded mixed results.

Additional evidence suggests that pre-SMA activity decays when subjects repeat a simple motor response (Sakai et al. 1999), but it is difficult to determine that this initial activation actually reflects intention and not effort. It is also difficult to show that performing practiced actions under experimental conditions is driven by the intention to perform a specific repeated behavior and not simply by the intention to follow the experimenter's instructions. It is certainly possible that these two operations are neurally distinct. For instance, work by Hoshi and Tanji indicates that the pre-SMA may be involved with specific motor intentions (Hoshi and Tanji 2004), whereas the cingulate motor area may be involved in the more general decision to cooperate with the experimenter (Hoshi, Sawamura, & Tanji 2005). This supposition is far from established but helps us to appreciate the subtle controls required for making general claims about intention.

A more central problem to overcome in studies of intentionality, and the application of neuroscience to law in general, is the homunculus problem. Indeed, one of the most fundamental asymmetries between the law and cognitive neuroscience is that while the law seeks to analyze the guilt of an *agent*, cognitive neuroscience has largely exiled the existence of a "homunculus," or an agent who resides at the top of top-down processes and makes decisions and exerts free will. Typical cognitive neuroscience models, and even the rare few that defend the notion of a homunculus with strictly limited powers (Roepstorff & Frith 2004), approach brain function in terms of a series of interacting mechanisms forming various computations in convergent, divergent, and parallel fashions. To understand how voluntary or intentional actions emerge from neural activity, one provocative theory posits the notion of competition between neural systems.

Recent efforts have had success applying this notion to activity of the pre-SMA (Nachev et al. 2005; Sumner et al. 2007). In this view, the neural correlates of self-generated, voluntary actions arise from automatic action plans originating in the pre-SMA. But even as intentions are formed, there are many competing action plans being formed in various cortical and subcortical brain areas preconsciously, in response to the environment. These include the SMA (Grèzes & Decety 2002). Competition between these conflicting plans is thought to determine which intentions become selected. Consequently, the enhanced activity of the pre-SMA may represent the neural events necessary for the selection and execution of "intentional" rather than "unintentional" action plans.

It is possible that this competition, regulated by cortical regions like the pre-SMA, takes place largely subcortically. The pre-SMA has projections to the putamen (Johansen-Berg et al. 2004; Wolbers et al. 2006) and the subthalamic nucleus (Aron et al. 2007) that may be important for motor selection and inhibition, respectively. Without the pre-SMA to provide well-orchestrated positive and negative bias to these subcortical areas, action plans that normally would have been outcompeted would be victorious. This consequence of the mechanism is crucial for assessing the selection of actions.

As the conflict hypothesis might predict, patients with an inability to perform intentional actions *are not* paralyzed. They can still perform motor actions based on environmental cues and other nonintentional sources of action. For example, patient A.G., who has damage to the pre-SMA but not the SMA proper, has difficulty voluntarily initiating action or voluntarily making online changes in the middle of an act. Nonetheless, she can perform cued behaviors with response times comparable to those of control subjects (Nachev et al. 2007).

Thus, there are two important points to glean from the neural framework outlined here: (1) There is an emerging case to be made that the pre-SMA reflects a neural basis of intention and that it displays the functional connectivity necessary for cognitive influence on intention formation and thereby on the execution of action; (2) when the neural areas responsible for intention are dysfunctional, an imbalance in competition between various automatic action plans allows complex actions to be performed in the absence of intention.

Once the neural mechanisms of intention have been implicated, a defendant's brain would have to yield evidence of dysfunction in these networks during attempts at planned action along with behavioral indicators of difficulty forming such plans. The above-mentioned research suggests that this goal might be achieved by searching for pre-SMA dysfunction in qualified defendants during intention formation.

However, even if we are looking at "intention" in the brain, it does not necessarily follow that abnormalities in this region imply an inability to form intentions. In general, abnormal activation could manifest as hypoactivation, hyperactivation, positive or negative activation, or some erratic pattern. It is not now known which of these patterns indicates dysfunction, but we do know that it will almost certainly depend on the neural area in question. This is one reason why examining the behavioral correlates of brain dysfunction is so essential. After all, the law cares about the brain only insofar as it can tell us something about its effect on actual behavior.

Another reason that abnormalities in the pre-SMA area do not imply difficulty forming intentions lies in the ample evidence of brain redundancy and distributed processing. It is plausible that when the pre-SMA area is dysfunctional, other areas "take up the slack." Other as yet undetected brain networks might supplant the computations underlying intention formation so that the procedures required for intention formation can still be normally executed. Thus, whether a particular brain network is useful does not imply that it is necessary (Halgren & Marinkovic 1996; Price et al. 1999). Second, for hypoactivity, maybe reduced activity in the intention areas simply indicates that this individual's pre-SMA requires less activation to function normally. Reduced activation in the pre-SMA, although encouraging and important, leaves many questions about intention formation unanswered.

Moreover, even if normal pre-SMA activation is necessary to form intentions, the fact that a defendant shows abnormal activation in the pre-SMA after being arrested does not show that the same area was dysfunctional when the crime was committed. It is also not clear that dysfunction in the pre-SMA for one kind of action, which is tested in the lab after arrest, shows that the defendant's pre-SMA would also be dysfunctional for other kinds of actions in real circumstances. Such questions about whether lab findings during trials establish mental states during real crimes are a recurring problem when applying neuroscience in the law.

Insanity Defense

Can neuroscience help us determine whether a defendant is insane? That depends on how insanity is defined. According to the laws discussed above, insanity seems to depend at least in part on an inability to know the nature and quality of the act and to know that the act is wrong. Neuroscience is potentially relevant to each of these conditions.

Knowing the Nature and Quality of an Act

What constitutes "knowing" something? How is the "nature" of an act different from its "quality"? Legal theorists have examined these questions in detail (Robinson, 2 Crim. L. Def. § 173, West, 2007). However, legal concepts almost always rely on intuitive explanations without clear operational scientific definitions. To apply neuroscience to legal issues, we must eventually jump the divide between legal concepts and scientific ones.

The "nature and quality of an act" (in the M'Naghten rule) includes the consequences and circumstances of the act. To know that an act has the nature and quality of killing, its agent must know that the act will have death as a consequence. To know that an act is theft, its agent must know, or at least truly believe, that the taken object belongs to someone else. If an agent cannot know such essential consequences or circumstances, that agent cannot know the nature and quality of the act. The agent then fails this cognitive part of the insanity defense.

It is still not clear what counts as *knowing*. One operational way to define "know[ing] the nature and quality of the act" is having an explicit, declarative representation of an instrumental action, including its consequences, circumstances, and means. By this definition, a defense relying on neuroscience would have to show that an individual lacks the capacity to build such representations because of dysfunction in the brain networks responsible for this operation.

At least two kinds of information are used by the brain to gain knowledge of action: efferent information governed by motor planning and afferent information such as somatosensory and proprioceptive feedback. Interestingly, afferent feedback is not required for successful execution of actions (Farrer et al. 2003). Hence, selective damage to these feedback mechanisms might not provide sufficient reason to excuse offenders with this type of damage. In contrast, motor planning and initiation do seem to be necessary for successful execution of actions. Above, we discussed the automatic, nonreflective processes underlying intention formation, but the law is concerned not just with intention formation but also with awareness, or knowledge, of planned actions, as the M'Naghten rule illustrates. Indeed, there is some evidence that these two operations are neurally distinct.

Research has shown that the angular gyrus, an area within the parietal cortex, may house mechanisms that allow us to reflect on the intentions being formed in the frontal cortex (Sirigu et al. 2004). Subjective awareness of intentions may rely on predictive models that project what the execution and consequences of the action will be like—a known function of the parietal cortex (Desmurget & Grafton 2000). These predictions are formed before sensory feedback about the action arrives. If indeed these predictive models are the correlates of awareness of motor intention, and because this awareness precedes action initiation in control subjects (Sirigu et al. 2004), one function of this awareness may be inhibition of automatically generated intentions. Evidence from at least one study suggests that it is possible to inhibit intended actions when subjective awareness of intention precedes the execution of the action (Brass & Haggard 2007). This view relegates awareness to the indirect role of moderating the relationship between forming intentions and inhibiting them.

If the angular gyrus is dysfunctional, we may not become subjectively aware of an intention until we become aware of the resulting action through sensory feedback, after the action has already commenced (Sirigu et al. 2004). Consequently, for quick actions, such as a simple pull of a trigger, it should be possible for people with damage to this area to complete the action before becoming aware of it. However, such damage may be of little exculpatory use for someone guilty of more complex actions such as loading and aiming a gun or robbing a bank because, in such complex cases, enough time exists for sensory feedback to reach awareness before the action is complete.

The sequence of intention awareness followed by perceptual awareness of action is also important in another way. The ability to become aware of one's intentions before they have resulted in action seems necessary for a sense of agency—the experience of being the causal source of one's actions. To "know the nature and quality of [his] act," an individual would presumably have to recognize that these actions were caused by him- or herself rather than someone else.

Recent developments by Farrer and colleagues (in press) have advanced our understanding of the neural correlates of a sense of agency. In one study, participants were asked to perform a simple motor task that was visually recorded and played back to them after a short delay. Participants were led to believe that half of the delayed-feedback videos were of acts authored by someone else and that their presentation order was random. Participants then had to decide on which trials the feedback was self-authored, without the benefit of direct feedback from intentional systems. The tendency to attribute actions to an external agent correlated with increased bilateral angular gyrus activity relative to self-attribution. These results indicate that the angular gyrus may control the subjective experience of agency and that it is modulated by the synchrony between predicted (intentional) and actual (sensory) feedback. (See Moore and Haggard [2007] for a compelling theory of how the experience of agency arises from the dynamic interactions between predictive and inferential processes.)

Translating the results from these studies into the courtroom would require structural and functional imaging of the angular gyrus. If it is dysfunctional, the defendant may have diminished awareness of his motor intentions before they are actually realized. This supposition could be verified with behavioral tasks involving temporal judgment of the experiences of intention and the initiation of actions. If the angular gyrus is abnormally active at times when it should not be or if it is not modulated by delayed-feedback conditions, then it is possible that the defendant misattributes his own actions to other agents. In both cases, action awareness is diminished in such a way that the defendant could not, or would not, attempt to prevent the actions from occurring.

Once again, it is dangerously tempting to conclude that damage to this brain area necessarily implies that an individual cannot consciously represent his own actions. As we mentioned, there may be conditions under which this is possible, but we have also indicated that "awareness" may not be a unitary phenomenon and its degree of plasticity as well as its functional significance remain largely unknown. Consequently, the angular gyrus should be a starting point, not a destination, in our understanding of the different aspects of awareness and how they interact.

Knowing that an Act Is Wrong

Knowledge of rules against the act. Even if a defendant is aware of "the nature and quality of the act," he still might not be aware that it was wrong (either legally or morally). Much research has been done recently on the neural basis of moral judgments (see Greene & Haidt 2002 and Moll et al. 2005; see also Sinnott-Armstrong 2008). If neuroscientists could determine which brain circuits are necessary to form moral judgments, then dysfunctions in those circuits might be used as evidence that defendants cannot know that their acts are wrong.

To illustrate some problems for this strategy, consider a recent study (Koenigs et al. 2007). This group presented several types of moral dilemmas to six subjects with damage to the ventromedial prefrontal cortex (VMPFC). In each case, subjects chose whether to perform a hypothetical act that saves more lives by killing fewer. These dilemmas varied both in the personal involvement demanded of the subject (such as either pulling a switch or pushing someone off a bridge) and the aggregate utility of the outcome (the proportion of people saved). The investigators compared their moral judgments to those of typical subjects as well as subjects with brain damage outside the VMPFC. Subjects without VMPFC damage were relatively unwilling to endorse highly personal acts even when those acts resulted in high aggregate utility. The VMPFC subjects, in contrast, showed a relatively increased willingness to endorse such acts. This finding suggests that an intact VMPFC weighs personal involvement as a factor in moral reasoning. The authors are the first to point out that the specificity of this finding does not suggest that these subjects lack a general capacity to judge moral wrongness, because their judgments were normal in the other conditions. Thus, such studies, while sometimes illuminating, do not yet have clear implications for the legal issue of whether defendants can know that their acts are wrong under general conditions.

Other brain studies become relevant if we assume that knowing whether something is wrong requires an ability to understand and apply social rules. Research into the neural correlates of reasoning about rules has been particularly fruitful in recent years.

In a functional magnetic resonance imaging (fMRI) experiment, Fiddick et al. (2005) had participants use both precautionary reasoning about hazardous situations and social contract reasoning about obligations to others. Participants were presented with various rules from both categories, followed by brief descriptions about people who may or may not have followed these rules. The precautionary category included items like "if you go hang gliding, then you must stay away from power lines." The social contract category included items like "if you order the buffet dinner, then you must eat the food yourself." Using only the information provided, participants had to decide whether the person could have broken the rule. Social contract reasoning but not precautionary reasoning was associated with increased activity in the bilateral ventrolateral prefrontal cortex and the medial frontal gyrus, as well as the left angular gyrus and the left orbitofrontal cortex. Interestingly, two of these areas, the medial frontal gyrus and the angular gyrus, are thought to be involved in generating emotional responses that inform some kinds of moral judgments among other things (Greene et al. 2004; Greene et al. 2001).

If dysfunction in areas associated with social contract reasoning reduces the capacity to reason about social contract rules, then this reduced capacity may in turn hinder one's ability to judge any particular social contract violation as wrong. If so, defendants with such deficits might become eligible for the insanity defense under some common formulations.

A lack of moral knowledge also might seem to excuse psychopaths (Fine & Kennett 2004). Though this conclusion might sound troubling, there is some evidence that psychopaths do not know or at least appreciate that their acts are morally wrong. First, psychopaths show reduced startle and skin-conductance responses to pictures of people harmed by violent assaults (Blair et al. 1997; Kiehl 2008; Levenston et al. 2000). This finding seems to underscore their notorious lack of empathy and may plausibly hinder their ability to appreciate the wrongness of immoral acts. Second, when psychopaths talk about moral wrongness, they often show confusion about what makes acts wrong and what it means for acts to be wrong (Kennett & Fine 2008). Third, at least one study (Blair et al. 1995) found that psychopaths fail to distinguish moral from conventional violations, oddly overclassifying conventional violations as moral ones. It is, of course, still controversial to claim that psychopaths do not know that their acts are wrong. Indeed, the ability to persuade and deceive others may profit from an ability to entertain others' notions of moral wrongness. However, even if psychopathic offenders tend to have a poor understanding of the wrongness of their acts, this would not necessarily imply that they *lack the ability* to understand wrongness. Only if this latter criterion can be met could neuroscience become legally relevant to psychopathy.

Some studies have suggested that psychopaths display a distinctive pattern in electroencephalograms (Kiehl 2008) and event-related potentials tests (Raine 1989a, 1989b). Those patterns, if they prove to be highly predictive of psychopathic behavior, might then be used to determine which defendants are psychopaths. This diagnosis could then be used to argue that these defendants are eligible for the insanity defense if psychopaths in general were shown to be incapable of appreciating wrongfulness and if that incapacity suffices for the insanity defense in the relevant jurisdiction. Although neuroscientific methods have never been considered necessary for psychopathy diagnoses, these methods might carry the potential to influence how we interpret psychopathy by showing that psychopathic brains are physically abnormal in ways relevant to crime and responsibility.

Of course, acquitted psychopaths would not be let back on the streets to commit more crimes. They would, instead, be institutionalized in a secure mental hospital rather than a prison, possibly for longer than the time they would have spent in prison. As mentioned above, the Model Penal Code added a special clause to its insanity test to avoid acquitting or freeing psychopaths. However, that special exclusion would no longer apply if the diagnosis of psychopathy can be established by neuroscientific evidence rather than by repeated criminal behavior. Although this concern remains entirely conjectural, the question of whether psychopaths are responsible needs to be faced, and it is one area where neuroscience might become relevant to legal decisions regarding insanity.

Knowledge of others' mental states. A sense of moral wrongness might also depend on the ability to anticipate that other people may be averse to the consequences of one's actions. When an act offends other people or makes them suffer or distrust the agent, those consequences provide some reason to judge the act wrong. Defendants may be unable to know that such acts are wrong if they cannot reason normally about others' mental states—that is, if they do not have an intact Theory of Mind.

Recent cognitive neuroscience literature has implicated a network of brain areas thought to be required for a Theory of Mind (Saxe 2006). One particularly important area is the right temporoparietal junction (RTPJ). Saxe and Wexler (2005) provide strong evidence that the RTPJ is involved in belief attribution, a fundamental component of Theory of Mind. They had participants read statements about an individual's background, desires, and the outcome of a related story, and they then asked participants to decide if the character would be pleased with the outcome. To respond to this question, participants had to develop a model of the character's desires and predict the preferred outcome on the basis of that model. They found that relative to reading the background statement, reading the desire statement induced increased activity in the RTPJ. Thus, the RTPJ was active during the segment of the experiment in which participants had to attribute beliefs and desires to another person. This role of the RTPJ has been replicated in a recent study of moral judgments (Young et al. 2007).

Interestingly, the RTPJ has been identified as an area that is hypoactive relative to that in control subjects when high-functioning autistic and Asperger syndrome patients perform tasks that require a Theory of Mind (Castelli et al. 2002). A leading theory regarding the nature of autism and Asperger syndrome is that affected individuals cannot form an adequate Theory of Mind. Taken together, the results from the above studies indicate that hypoactivity in the RTPJ could result in inadequate belief attribution and, therefore, Theory of Mind. This finding lends itself to a related hypothesis, that other abnormal forms of activation in the RTPJ may result in overattributions of others' mental states—perhaps the frightening delusion that others want to harm you (a common symptom of paranoid schizophrenia). Some studies have already shown a correspondence between positive symptoms of schizophrenia and hyperactivation in other brain areas (Dierks et al. 1999). Psychotic delusions could potentially motivate an actor to deploy a defensive assault that is entirely justified within the logic of that actor's delusion.

If a defendant could be shown to have dysfunction in the RTPJ and to lack the ability to make judgments about others' beliefs and desires, a case could be made that this individual has an improper understanding of others' mental states and, consequently, lacks sufficient capacity to judge the wrongness of his own acts.

Importantly, however, even if social contract reasoning and Theory of Mind are shown to be functionally impaired, there easily could be other cues to assessments of wrongness that typical brains compute for which we simply have not accounted. It is widely accepted, for instance, that people model their behavior after other social agents (Bandura 1977). It could be that individuals can extract moral information from the behavior of others, even when social contract reasoning and Theory of Mind are dysfunctional. This is just one of many alternative hypotheses that awaits thorough psychological and neuroscientific investigation.

Future of the Neuroscience of Criminal Responsibility

Thus far we have argued that the significant advances made in the neuroscience of mental states do not yet provide compelling evidence that associated brain regions are necessary or sufficient for normal functioning of these mental states. Even our most thorough descriptions of abnormal brain activity do not necessarily imply dysfunction (Pinker 2002, 184). Moreover, if strong evidence of specific brain dysfunction is found, this alone does not necessarily imply innocence or impunity because, after all, most individuals with similar dysfunction never commit crimes (Gazzaniga & Steven 2005; Grafton et al. 2006–2007). As we discussed above, there are several missing links in the connection between neuroscience and responsibility.

How can these problems be solved? Where do we go from here? The field of law and neuroscience is changing quickly. It is hard to predict what will come next or where the field is headed. Still, we can say a little about what is needed and likely in the law and in neuroscience.

What Do We Need from Law?

The legal issues outlined above are all filled with uncertainty. Even the best neuroscientific evidence will leave us unsure whether some particular defendants meet the conditions for criminal responsibility. Mistakes can have devastating effects in criminal justice. If the scientific interpretations of neurological results are accurate, say, 90% of the time, these interpretations will be misleading 10 of 100 times. Defendants then face a considerable risk to liberty or life if they (or prosecutors) rely on neuroscientific evidence. Scientific claims must attain impeccable accuracy when lives and livelihoods are on the line.

The importance of such claims means, first, that we need to determine the error rates of various methods in neuroscience. It is not clear how we can determine error rates to begin with. What are the average rates of misses and of false alarms for fMRI detection of various conditions? Whatever they are, these error rates are only compounded when legal officials, most of whom know little neuroscience, need to draw conclusions from technical data. The release of noisy, unreliable neuroscientific evidence into the courtroom could actually serve to increase error rates in convictions, whereby judges and juries acquit the guilty and convict the innocent.

Will neuroscience bring more harm than good to criminal trials? Only time and careful analysis will tell. Still, some steps might help to minimize its destructive power and develop a constructive trajectory for its use.

One way to reduce the worst kinds of errors is to properly distribute the burden of proof or persuasion. If society is most concerned not to convict the innocent, then it can reduce that kind of error by placing a heavy burden of proof on prosecutors. The uncertainties in neuroscientific data will make it hard for prosecutors to use such data to prove beyond a reasonable doubt that the conditions of responsibility, including intention and sanity, are met. In contrast, if society is most concerned not to acquit and release the guilty and dangerous, then it can reduce that kind of error by shifting the burden of proof onto the defense. If the defense is required to prove, even to a preponderance of the evidence, that the defendant is insane in order to be found not guilty by reason of insanity, then it will be hard to carry that burden with uncertain evidence from neuroscience. It is, therefore, crucial for the law to develop appropriate rules governing the burden of proof to be able to handle the new evidence from neuroscience.

Finally, even if we tailor law to handle error asymmetries, we still face problems related to the admissibility of neuroscientific evidence, a domain in which procedural law might shape the way we do neuroscience. It is not clear when neuroscience findings should qualify as relevant, material, or competent, or reliable, as defined by the rules of evidence. It is also not obvious under what classification it should fall: real, demonstrative, documentary, or testimonial evidence? Finally, for evidence affirming responsibility, no such evidence can be admitted that violates the defendant's basic rights, as we noted above. Such questions of admissibility are generating increasing consideration (Tovino 2007).

What Do We Need from Neuroscience?

Chomsky (1975) once distinguished puzzles from mysteries. Puzzles are closed-ended problems to which solutions can be systematically approached and obtained. Mysteries are open-ended problems to which we are bewildered at the prospect of how to go about approaching a solution. Certainly the prospect of finding a simple "understanding" or "free will" center in the brain does seem doubtful to most scientists as well as philosophers. But the challenges we have charged to neuroscience—to make accurate probabilistic inferences about whether a brain is adequately equipped to deploy coordinated, goal-oriented plans of action, to reasonably anticipate consequences of these plans, and to be amenable to veto power by other brain processes—become a smaller puzzle every day. Extending our earlier analogy: Chemists perhaps cannot determine if a cake was baked with love, but they can determine if it was baked with cyanide, which in turn provides circumstantial evidence against the love hypothesis. Likewise, although neuroscience cannot locate responsibility in the brain, perhaps it can identify maladies that provide at least circumstantial evidence against guilt or liability. Several pivotal advancements lend support to our optimism.

Immersive Technology

Our findings can be only as rich as the environments in which we test them. But how could we possibly test complex, ecological environments in a crowded fMRI chamber? One exciting possibility lies in digital immersive virtual environment technology (IVET).

Digital IVET typically powers an interface among individuals and a computer-generated, three-dimensional world. The interface can take the form of a pair of stereoscopic display goggles and headphones. The resolution can approximate perfect photorealism, and environments can be as interactive as designers choose. In fMRI, users could traverse this environment with a simple joystick.

Armed with this technology, researchers could test models of cognition in environments that are as ecologically rich as the physical and social environments in which our cognitive mechanisms evolved. For instance, researchers seeking to understand intention formation may assess not just intentions to press a button but intentions to defend against a looming attacker. These different plans of action may or may not be formed in the same area of the brain, but advanced imaging technology combined with IVET can help us find out. IVET can enrich our ability to map sophisticated models of cognition onto the functional organization of the brain.

Advances in Temporal Resolution

A notorious drawback of research in fMRI scanning technology is its meager temporal resolution. A tremendous amount of activity can occur in the brain in a matter of seconds. The most cutting-edge fMRI scanners peak at a resolution of about 2000 ms—the length of one scan. The brain's blood oxygen level depletion response has an even longer duration. These two constraints make it difficult to know precisely when a predicted neural signal has occurred. Event-related designs can limit these problems to some extent, but these designs are expensive and taxing. Another solution is to supplement fMRI with higher temporal-resolution measures, such as event-related potentials. Synchronization between these technologies will provide the needed leverage to precisely localize brain events in both time and space. This triangulation tactic will enable neuroscientists to draw stronger inferences about causality between brain events, as well as between the brain and the body.

It's Not All about fMRI: Diffusion Tensor Imaging

A third technology with high hopes of building more sophisticated models of cognition is diffusion tensor imaging (DTI). DTI is a relatively new *in vivo* MRI technique used to measure the integrity, coherence, and directionality of white-matter fibers, which connect distal structures in the brain. The technique relies on the diffusion of water molecules within myelinated axons and measures the direction of the diffusion.

DTI can provide information about tissue microstructure and architecture for each voxel in the brain. It can also provide information related to the presence and coherence of the brain's white matter. Also, because the main direction of diffusion is linked to the orientation of structures in space, it allows for reconstruction of fiber pathways.

Information provided by DTI has recently been combined with cognitive–behavioral data and fMRI data to explore how the integrity and orientation of white-matter pathways relate to brain activation patterns and cognition (Baird et al. 2005). Knowledge about anatomical connections of distal cortical areas might even provide information about the temporal capacity of connecting fibers between activated foci from an fMRI experiment. This information can indirectly provide clues to the timing of the activation of each node in a cortical network. Whereas fMRI is limited to observations about localized brain activity, DTI can be particularly useful for exploring variations between cortical regions. Other techniques such as independent component analysis and dynamic causal modeling show similar prospects. A more complete understanding of functional connectivity could ultimately make possible better analysis of how brain abnormalities affect brain function and thus human behavior.

A Cautious Step Forward

As we brace for the future, the ideal test of the validity of neuroscience technology, it might be argued, is to predict in advance whether a person with observable abnormalities in legally relevant brain areas is at a specifiable risk of criminal behavior or can conform to the law. This inevitable goal may raise an entirely new set of moral and philosophical questions about how the law ought to regulate the behavior of innocent people. Therefore, this prospect should be approached by the scientific community with judicious reserve.

Neuroscience is much more limited in the kinds of conclusions it can support than the public, the legal system, and many neuroscientists would like to acknowledge. As we progress, many scientists and lawyers will undoubtedly make claims that are not warranted by the neuroscientific data. Like any new science, neuroscience is vulnerable to abuse. For these reasons, neuroscientists will, and ought to be, burdened with the responsibility not only of generating data but also of criticizing and thwarting those abuses. This dual role for neuroscientists is imperative if neuroscience is to have a positive effect on law.

Neuroscience has copious challenges to undertake before becoming a reliable benefit to courtroom procedures. As a case in point, this review has only touched on how neuroscience can inform determinations of intention and insanity, but a thorough understanding of the brain might also one day help us to inform legal determinations of the many other mental states relevant to criminal law, such as recklessness, negligence, duress, and automatism. There are also many areas within civil law procedures in which neuroscience will undoubtedly play an increasing role (Tovino 2007). Until such a thorough understanding is reached, stepwise advance in our theoretical models, experimental manipulations, and measurement technology should ultimately contribute to the overarching goal of bringing specificity to the problems that result from the application of neuroscience to questions of legal responsibility and exculpation.

Acknowledgments

We thank Jim Blascovich, Adina Roskies, Larry Crocker, Karl Doron, Emily Murphy, Suzanne Gazzaniga, Scott Grafton, Annie Wertz, Galia Aharoni, Matthew Green, Teneille Brown, Craig Bennett, and our reviewers for their invaluable feedback, as well as the MacArthur Foundation for its generous support.

Conflicts of Interest

The authors declare no conflicts of interest.

References

Aron, A. R., Behrens, T. E., Smith, S., Frank, M. J., & Poldrack, R. A. (2007). Triangulating a cognitive control network using diffusion-weighted magnetic resonance imaging (MRI) and functional MRI. *Journal of Neuroscience, 27*, 3743–3752.

Baird, A. A., Colvin, M. K., VanHorn, J. D., Inati, S., & Gazzaniga, M. S. (2005). Functional connectivity: integrating behavioral, diffusion tensor imaging and functional magnetic resonance imaging datasets. *Journal of Cognitive Neuroscience, 17*, 687–693.

Bandura, A. (1977). *Social Learning Theory*. Englewood Cliffs, NJ: Prentice Hall.

Blair, R. J., Jones, L., Clark, F., & Smith, M. (1995). Is the psychopath 'morally insane'? *Personality and Individual Differences, 19*, 741–752.

Blair, R. J., Jones, L., Clark, F., & Smith, M. (1997). The psychopathic individual: a lack of responsiveness to distress cues? *Psychophysiology, 34*, 192–198.

Brass, M., & Haggard, P. (2007). To do or not to do: the neural signature of self-control. *Journal of Neuroscience, 27*(34), 9141–9145.

Bratman, M. (1987). *Intention, Plans, and Practical Reason*. Cambridge, MA: Harvard University Press.

Castelli, F., Frith, C., Happé, F., & Frith, U. (2002). Autism, Asperger syndrome and brain mechanisms for the attribution of mental states to animated shapes. *Brain, 125*, 1839–1849.

Chomsky, N. (1975). *Reflections on Language*. New York, Pantheon.

Commonwealth v. Pirela, 929 A.2d 629 (Pa. 2007).

Cunnington, R., Windischberger, C., Deecke, L., & Moser, E. (2002). The preparation and execution of self-initiated and externally-triggered movement: a study of event-related fMRI. *Neuroimage, 15*(2), 373–385.

Desmurget, M., & Grafton, S. (2000). Forward modeling allows feedback control for fast reaching movements. *Trends in Cognitive Sciences, 4*, 423–431.

Dierks, T., Linden, D. E., Jandl, M., Formisano, E., Goebel, R., Lanfermann, H., et al. (1999). Activation of Heschl's gyrus during auditory hallucinations. *Neuron, 22*, 615–621.

Farrer, C., Franck, N., Paillard, J., & Jeannerod, M. (2003). The role of proprioception in action recognition. *Consciousness and Cognition, 12*, 609–619.

Farrer, C., Frey, S. H., Van Horn, J. D., Tunik, E., Turk, D., Inati, S. et al. (in press). The angular gyrus computes action awareness representations. *Cerebral Cortex*.

Fiddick, L., Spampinato, M. V., & Grafman, J. (2005). Social contracts and precautions activate different neurological systems: an fMRI investigation of deontic reasoning. *NeuroImage, 28*, 778–786.

Fine, C., & Kennett, J. (2004). Mental impairment, moral understanding and criminal responsibility: psychopathy and the purposes of punishment. *International Journal of Law and Psychiatry, 27*, 425–443.

Fischer, J. M., & Ravizza, M. (1998). *Responsibility and Control: A Theory of Moral Responsibility*. New York: Cambridge University Press.

Gazzaniga, M. S. (2005). *The Ethical Brain*. New York, Dana Press.

Gazzaniga, M. S., & Steven, M. S. (April 2005). Neuroscience and the law. *Scientific American Mind*, 42–49.

Grafton, S., Sinnott-Armstrong, W. P., Gazzaniga, S. I., & Gazzaniga, M. S. (December 2006/January 2007). Brain scans go legal. *Scientific American Mind*, 30–37.

Greene, J., & Haidt, J. (2002). How (and where) does moral judgment work? *Trends in Cognitive Science, 6*, 517–523.

Greene, J. D., Nystrom, L. E., Engell, A. D., Darley, J. M., & Cohen, J. D. (2004). The neural bases of cognitive conflict and control in moral judgment. *Neuron, 44*, 389–400.

Greene, J. D., Sommerville, R. B., Nystrom, L. E., Darley, J. M., & Cohen, J. D. (2001). An fMRI investigation of emotional engagement in moral judgment. *Science, 293*, 2105–2108.

Greene, J., & Cohen, J. (2004). For the law, neuroscience changes nothing and everything. *Philosophical Transactions of the Royal Society of London. Series B, Biological Sciences, 359*, 1775–1785. Also in S. Zeki & O. Goodenough, ed., *Law and the Brain*. New York: Oxford University Press.

Grèzes, J., & Decety, J. (2002). Does visual perception of object afford action? Evidence from a neuroimaging study. *Neuropsychologia, 40*, 212–222.

Halgren, E., & Marinkovic, K. (1996). General principles for the physiology of cognition as suggested by intracranial ERPs. In C. Ogura, Y. Koga & M. Shimokochi (Eds.), *Recent Advances in Event-Related Brain Potential Research* (pp. 1072–1084), Amsterdam, New York: Elsevier.

Haynes, J.-D., Sakai, K., Rees, G., Gilbert, S., Frith, C., & Passingham, E. E. (2007). Reading hidden intentions in the human brain. *Current Biology, 17*(4), 323–328.

Hoshi, E., Sawamura, H., & Tanji, J. (2005). Neurons in the rostral cingulate motor area monitor multiple phases of visuomotor behavior with modest parametric selectivity. *Journal of Neurophysiology, 94*, 640–656.

Hoshi, E., & Tanji, J. (2004). Differential roles of neuronal activity in the supplementary and presupplementary motor areas: from information retrieval to motor planning and execution. *Journal of Neurophysiology, 92*, 3482–3499.

Johansen-Berg, H., Behrens, T. E. J., Robson, M. D., Drobnjak, I., Rushworth, M. F. S., Brady, J. M., et al. (2004). Changes in connectivity profiles define functionally distinct regions in human medial frontal cortex. *Proceedings of the National Academy of Sciences USA, 101*, 13335–13340.

Kane, R. (1996). *The Significance of Free Will*. New York: Oxford University Press.

Kansas v. Wilburn, 822 P.2d 609, 615 (1991).

Kennett J., & Fine, C. (2008). Internalism and the evidence from psychopaths and "acquired sociopaths." In W.

Sinnott-Armstrong (ed.) *Moral Psychology, Volume 3: The Neuroscience of Morality* (pp. 173–190). Cambridge, MA: MIT Press.

Kiehl, K. (2008). Without morals: The cognitive neuroscience of criminal psychopaths. In W. Sinnott-Armstrong (ed.) *Moral Psychology, Volume 3: The Neuroscience of Morality* (pp. 119–149). Cambridge, MA: MIT Press.

Kilner, J. M., Vargas, C., Duval, S., Blakemore, S. J., & Sirigu, A. (2004). Motor activation prior to observation of a predicted movement. *Nature Neuroscience, 7*, 1299–1301.

Koenigs, M., Young, L., Adolphs, R., Tranel, D., Cushman, F., Hauser, M., et al. (2007). Damage to the prefrontal cortex increases utilitarian moral judgments. *Nature, 446*, 908–911.

Lau, H. C., Rogers, R. D., Haggard, P., & Passingham, R. E. (2004). Attention to intention. *Science, 303*, 1208–1210.

Levenston, G. K., Patrick, C. J., Bradley, M. M., & Lang, P. J. (2000). The psychopath as observer: emotion and attention in picture processing. *Journal of Abnormal Psychology, 109*, 373–385.

Libet, B. (2004). *Mind Time*. Cambridge, MA: Harvard University Press.

Mele, A. (2006). *Free Will and Luck*. New York: Oxford University Press.

M'Naghten's Case, 10 Clark, & F 200, 8 Reprint 718 (1843).

Model Penal code § 2.01 (1962).

Moll, J., Zahn, R., de Oliveira-Souza, R., Krueger, F., & Grafman, J. (October 2005). The neural basis of human moral cognition. *Nature Reviews Neuroscience, 6*, 799–809.

Moore, J. & Haggard, P. (in press). Awareness of action: Inference and prediction. *Consciousness and Cognition*.

Morse, S., & Hoffman, M. (2007). The uneasy entente between insanity and mens rea: beyond *Clark v. Arizona*. *University of Pennsylvania Law School. Scholarship at Penn Law*. Paper 143.

Nachev, P., Rees, G., Parton, A., Kennard, C., & Husain, M. (2005). Volition and conflict in human medial frontal cortex. *Current Biology, 15*, 122–128.

Nachev, P., Wydell, H., O'Neil, K., Husain, M., & Kennard, C. (2007). The role of pre-supplementary motor area in the control of action. *NeuroImage, 36*, T155–T163.

Pereboom, D. (2001). *Living Without Free Will*. Cambridge, UK: Cambridge University Press.

Perkins, R. N. (1969). *Perkins on Criminal Law* (2nd ed.). New York: Foundation Press.

Pinker, S. (2002). *The Blank Slate*. New York: Penguin Putnam, Inc.

Price, C. J., Mummery, C. J., Moore, C. J., Frakowiak, R. S. J., & Friston, K. J. (1999). Delineating necessary and sufficient neural systems with functional imaging studies of neuropsychological patients. *Journal of Cognitive Neuroscience, 11*, 371–382.

Raine, A. (1989a). Evoked potential models of psychopathy: a critical evaluation. *International Journal of Psychophysiology, 8*, 29–34.

Raine, A. (1989b). Evoked potentials and psychopathy. *International Journal of Psychophysiology, 8*, 1–16.

Robinson, P. H. 2 Criminal Law Defenses § 173 (West, 2007)

Roepstorff, A., & Frith, C. (2004). What's at the top in the top-down control of action? Script-sharing and "top-top" control of action in cognitive experiments. *Psychological Research, 68*, 189–198.

Roper v. Simmons, 543 U.S. 551, 125 S.Ct. 1183, 1200, 161 L.Ed.2d 1, 28 (Mo. 2005).

Sakai, K., Hikosaka, O., Miyauchi, S., Sasaki, N., Fujimaki, N., & Putz, B. (1999). Presupplementary motor area activation during sequence learning reflects visuo-motor association. *Journal of Neuroscience, 19*, 1–6.

Saxe, R. (2006). Uniquely human social cognition. *Current Opinion in Neurobiology, 16*, 235–239.

Saxe, R., & Wexler, A. (2005). Making sense of another mind: the role of the right temporo-parietal junction. *Neuropsychologia, 43*, 1391–1399.

Sinnott-Armstrong, W. (Ed.) (2008). *Moral Psychology, Volume 3: The Neuroscience of Morality*. Cambridge, MA: MIT Press.

Sirigu, A., Daprati, E., Sophie, C., Giraux, P., Nighoghossian, N., Posada, A., et al. (2004). Altered awareness of voluntary action after damage to the parietal cortex. *Nature Neuroscience, 7*, 80–84.

Sumner, P., Nachev, P., Morris, P., Peters, A. M., Jackson, S. R., Kennard, C., et al. (2007). Human medial frontal cortex mediates unconscious inhibition of voluntary action. *Neuron, 54*, 697–711.

Tovino, S. A. (2007). Functional neuroimaging and the law: trends and directions for future scholarship. *American Journal of Bioethics, 7*, 44–56.

U.S. v. Hinckley, 525 F. Supp. 1342 (D.D.C. 1981), clarified, 529 F. Supp. 520 (D.D.C. 1982), aff'd, 672 F.2d 115 (D.C. Cir. 1982).

van Inwagen, P. (1983). *An Essay on Free Will*. Oxford, UK: Oxford University Press.

Wegner, D. (2002). *The Illusion of Conscious Will*. Cambridge, MA: MIT Press.

Weichselbaum, S. (2004, May 1). Killer again beats death sentence. *Philadelphia Daily News*.

Wolbers, T., Schoell, E. D., Verleger, R., Kraft, S., McNamara, A., Jaskowski, P., et al. (2006). Changes in connectivity profiles as a mechanism for strategic control over interfering subliminal information. *Cerebral Cortex, 16*, 857–864.

Wolf, S. R. (1990). *Freedom Within Reason*. New York: Oxford University Press.

Young, L., Cushman, F., Hauser, M., & Saxe, R. (2007). The neural basis of the interaction between theory of mind and moral judgment. *Proceedings of the National Academy of Sciences USA, 104*, 8235–8240.

The Neural Basis of Moral Cognition
Sentiments, Concepts, and Values

JORGE MOLL,[a] RICARDO DE OLIVEIRA-SOUZA,[a,b] AND ROLAND ZAHN[c]

[a] *Cognitive and Behavioral Neuroscience Unit, LABS-D'Or Hospital Network, Rio de Janeiro, RJ, Brazil*

[b] *Gaffree e Guinle University Hospital, Rio de Janeiro, RJ, Brazil*

[c] *Neuroscience & Aphasia Research Unit (NARU), School of Psychological Sciences, The University of Manchester, Manchester, United Kingdom*

The human moral nature has perplexed laymen and academics for millennia. Recent developments in cognitive neuroscience are opening new venues for unveiling the complex psychological and neurobiological mechanisms underling human morality and its impairments. Here we review these lines of evidence and key topics of debate and explain why investigating the mechanisms of cognition–emotion interaction and of the neural bases of moral sentiments and values will be critical for our understanding of the human moral mind.

Key words: social cognition; motivation; moral judgment; emotion; cognitive control; values; sentiments; antisocial; psychopathy; social behavior

Introduction

Debates on the moral nature of man have occupied the center of discussions among theologians, philosophers, and laymen for millennia. This should not be surprising in view of the central role that morality plays in the constitution of human nature: people often risk material resources or even physical integrity to help or to punish perfect strangers based on a sense of fairness, concern for others, and observance of cultural norms (Goodenough & Prehn 2004; Zeki & Goodenough 2004). Strikingly, this inclination can go far beyond the interpersonal sphere, as humans often engage in costly behaviors to support abstract causes, beliefs, and ideologies. This "moral sensitivity" emerges from a sophisticated integration of cognitive, emotional, and motivational mechanisms (Moll, de Oliveira-Souza, Eslinger, et al. 2002), which are internalized through an active process of cultural learning during sensitive periods of individual development (Kagan 1984). Moral sensitivity relies on an array of complex motivations which enable social cohesion and reorganization. Puzzling as they might appear from biological and economical perspectives, such behaviors must have arisen from the human evolutionary process (Darwin 1871/1982), and evolutionary biology and psychology are quickly advancing towards new solutions (Milinski et al. 2002; Boyd et al. 2003; Fehr & Fischbacher 2003; Nowak & Sigmund 2005; Bowles 2006). How exactly nature implemented such mechanisms in our brains is a mystery that is beginning to be unveiled by modern neuroscience.

Defining morality is not a straightforward task, and any definition will suffer from shortcomings, especially when evaluated by scholars from different fields. "Moral" (derived from the Latin *moralis*) and "ethical" (from the Greek *êthikos*) originally referred to the consensus of manners and customs (MacIntyre 1985). Based on this rather broad notion, we have operationally adopted the definition of morality *as the sets of customs and values that are embraced by a cultural group to guide social conduct* (Moll, Zahn, et al. 2005). This working definition, we argue, has several advantages for a neuroscientific approach to moral cognition because: 1) it inherently allows for the existence cultural variability of values and norms; 2) it is compatible with the role of multiple psychological domains in moral cognition, including care, harm, fairness, disgust, and authority (Haidt & Graham 2007); and 3) it emphasizes the fact that morality, biologically speaking, is fundamentally tied to evaluation, and thus relies on *motivations*, which, importantly 4) emerged from our evolutionary history, probably by way of gene-culture

---

Address for correspondence: Jorge Moll, Cognitive and Behavioral Neuroscience Unit, LABS-D'Or Hospital Network, Rio de Janeiro, RJ, Brazil, 22281-080. Voice: +55-21-2538-3641.
mollj@neuroscience-rio.org

coevolution, enabling sophisticated forms of cooperation and reciprocity (Nowak & Sigmund 2005).

This definition of the scope of moral neuroscience, however, raises a central question: what distinguishes moral cognition from other forms of socially relevant abilities? Most instances of social behavior (i.e., behaviors that involve interactions with other people) are morally relevant because they have effects on others and are thus liable to be evaluated as "right" or "wrong." Therefore, one may argue that, on the outside, any kind of social behavior is also moral in nature and that the neural and cognitive mechanisms guiding moral and social behavior should therefore be identical. From the perspective of the specific motivations behind social behavior, however, moral choices can indeed be distinguished from nonmoral choices. Therefore, we propose that while moral cognition draws upon general social cognitive and motivational abilities, its most distinctive feature is the ability to altruistically motivate social behavior. As we argue here, these altruistic or "moral motivations" depend on the representation of complex moral sentiments and values.

From an agent's perspective, truly moral *choices* reside on doing something "right" (bearing consequence to either other people or to norms and values which are embraced by a social group) when more immediate selfish motives would tell the agent to do otherwise. Similarly, a moral agent will suffer when carrying out a moral violation (according to internalized moral standards).

Adopting a motivational perspective on moral behavior, we suggest the following four broad categories:

1. Self-serving actions that do not affect others
2. Self-serving actions that negatively affect others ("selfishness")
3. Actions that are beneficial to others, with a high probability of reciprocation ("reciprocal altruism")
4. Actions that are beneficial to others, with no direct personal benefits (material or reputation gains) and no expected reciprocation ("genuine altruism"). This includes altruistic helping as well as costly punishment of norm violators ("altruistic punishment").

The ordinary behaviors of social mammals, in general, fall into classes 1–3. In contrast, genuine altruism is primary a human attribute (Nowak & Sigmund 2005). (We here use the more generic term "genuine altruism" without discriminating between "pure altruism" and "warm glow"-based altruism, a topic of active debate that lies beyond the scope of this article.)

Although genuine altruism is costly to the individual and is less likely with increasing cost, it benefits the survival of a social group and therefore may have conveyed evolutionary advantages (Fehr & Fischbacher 2003). Altruistic choices underlie prosocial acts, such as costly helping, as well as costly punishment, in which one sacrifices one's own resources to punish somebody who violates a social norm (Fehr & Fischbacher 2003). Understanding the nature of such inclinations is a challenging task, as these behaviors can be quite costly and do not confer clear material or survival advantages from the agent's perspective. While theoretical biology and experimental economics have strongly substantiated the validity of these "selfless" human behaviors (Trivers 1971; Maynard-Smith & Szathmary 1997; Milinski et al. 2002; Fehr & Fischbacher 2003; Fehr & Rockenbach 2004), the motivational sources of altruistic inclinations have only recently started to be unveiled by neuroscience. Specifically regarding human moral behavior, it is reasonable to assume that without the engagement of motivational mechanisms, purely rational moral prescriptions ("oughts") could not be translated into actual behaviors.

Moral motivations have been claimed by virtue ethicists since antiquity (Casebeer 2003). Aristotle stressed that living according to moral virtues leads to human flourishing (*eudaimonia*) (Aristotle 1926). This point of view was expanded by the 12th-century physician, philosopher, and rabbi Moses Maimonides (Maimonides 1912) through prescribing virtuous behavior as a way to preserve and restore mental health. Moral motivations lie at the core of moral values (i.e., "virtues"). Moral values, described by concepts such as "courage," contain the moral "ought" that can be tied to actions conforming or opposing them. According to the notion of values proposed by British philosophers during the 18th century, "moral sentiments" determine whether we perceive something as a virtue or a vice, guiding our approval or disapproval accordingly (Hume 1739/1984), a point of view which has gained recent support from moral psychology (Haidt 2001). Hume emphasized the inextricable relation of actions as the objects of moral sentiments. He stated that the moral evaluation of such actions depends on whether these are caused internally or by external force (Hume 1739/1984). When we are agents of social actions conforming to our values, we may feel pride, whereas when another person is perceived as the agent, we may feel gratitude. On the negative side, when we act counter to our values, we may feel guilt, and when another person acts in the same way towards us, we feel indignation or anger instead (Moll, de Oliveira-Souza, Zahn, et al. 2007). Furthermore, the anticipation of these moral

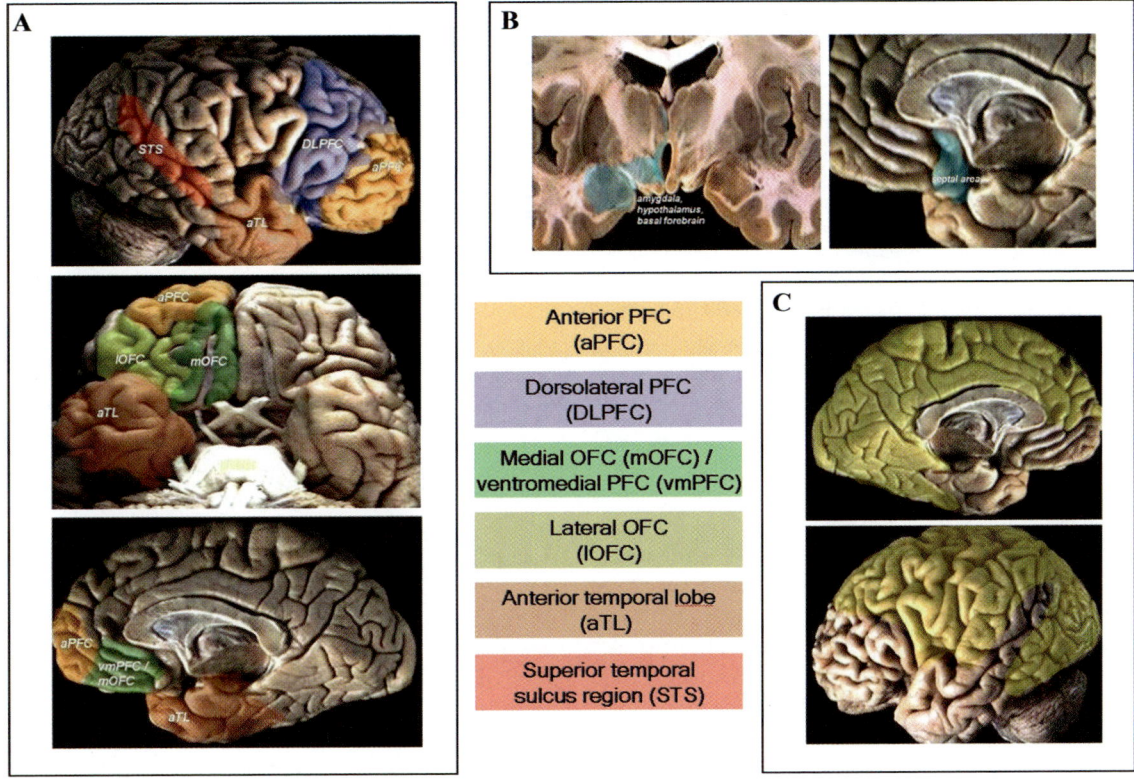

FIGURE 1. Brain regions implicated in moral cognition and behavior. Brain regions implicated in moral cognition and behavior in functional imaging and patient studies. **(A)** cortical regions (Stone et al. 2002; Moll et al. 2003; Eslinger et al. 2004) include the anterior prefrontal cortex (aPFC, mainly the frontopolar cortex), the medial and lateral orbitofrontal cortex (mOFC and lOFC), dorsolateral PFC (mostly the right hemisphere) and additional ventromedial sectors of the PFC (VMPFC), the anterior temporal lobes (aTL) (Luo et al. 2006), and the superior temporal sulcus region (STS). **(B)** subcortical structures (Weissenberger et al. 2001; Moll, de Oliveira-Souza, Eslinger, et al. 2002; Moll et al. 2003) include the amygdala, ventromedial hypothalamus, septal area and nuclei, basal forebrain (especially the ventral striatum-pallidum and extended amygdala), walls of the third ventricle, and rostral brain-stem tegmentum. **(C)** Brain regions that have not been consistently associated with moral cognition and behavior in patient studies include the parietal and occipital lobes, large areas of the frontal and temporal lobes, and the brain stem, basal ganglia, and additional subcortical structures.

sentiments in particular social situations often guides our behavior (Tangney et al. 2007).

Building on the first clues linking morality and brain function (Welt 1888; Macmillan 2000), modern neuroscience employed sophisticated cognitive probes along with structural and functional neuroimaging (Moll, Zahn, et al. 2005; Raine & Yang 2006) to address the neural underpinnings of moral judgments and moral emotions (de Oliveira-Souza & Moll 2000; Moll et al. 2001; Moll, de Oliveira-Souza, Bramati, et al. 2002; Moll, de Oliveira-Souza, Eslinger, et al. 2002; Heekeren, Wartenburger, et al. 2003; Eslinger et al. 2004; Greene et al. 2004; Koenigs et al. 2007), social concepts (Zahn et al. 2007), and attitudes (Cunningham et al. 2004; Luo et al. 2006). A picture that emerges from these recent studies is that there is large agreement about the brain regions supporting moral cognition, pointing to a reliable involvement of cortical (anterior and medial prefrontal and anterior temporal cortex) and subcortical-limbic (ventral striatum, hypothalamus, amygdala, basal forebrain) structures in morality (Moll, Zahn, et al. 2005) (Fig. 1). Key issues stand out as new sources of debate in moral cognition, however.

While it is common sense that both emotion and cognition play important roles in moral judgment, there is still much discussion on how they interact to produce moral thought and choices. According to one view, although emotion and cognition operate together to produce swift decision making, they are dependent on largely separable neural systems. This becomes evident in the context of difficult moral decisions associated with response conflict, leading to a competition between "emotional" (limbic) and "cognitive" brain regions (isocortical, especially the prefrontal cortex). In this situation, "prepotent" or automatic emotional responses must be suppressed by cognitive ("rational") top-down processes so that better decisions leading to overall "greater benefit" can be made. This view is in agreement with a large body of literature on the role of the prefrontal cortex in cognitive control and inhibitory function.

An alternative proposal, put forth here, emphasizes the idea that emotion and cognition are nondissociable elements underlying moral motivations, and that such motivations are represented within cortico-limbic neural assemblies. Conflicting moral decisions would not entail a conflict between emotion and cognition, but between two or more choices which rely on cortico-limbic assemblies encoding distinct motivationally salient goals. As such, a cognitive process that is devoid of motivational salience would never be able to overcome a motivationally laden choice—even if the "rational" option would be saving dozens of lives and the "emotional" one would be eating a piece of chocolate cake. As we will propose, moral sentiments and values are key players in moral cognition and decision making by providing these complex motivations.

While this neurocognitive framework of moral motivations as guided by moral values and sentiments is in agreement with the available evidence from patient lesion studies and functional imaging, it still remains in large part hypothetical and can only serve as a model to guide future experiments aiming to address two key questions: 1) how isocortical prefrontal and limbic regions interact in moral cognition; and 2) to what degree moral *reasoning* and *sentiments*, which may be distinguished subjectively, rely on distinct brain systems. Here, we briefly review the evidence on the neural bases of moral cognition, with a special focus on new evidence on the neural representation of moral motivations and their relationships to moral knowledge.

Lesion and Functional Imaging Evidence on the Neural Bases of Morality

Since the initial demonstrations that the moral faculties of the mind could be impaired by brain damage (Welt 1888; Macmillan 2000), systematic studies of acquired personality changes due to brain lesion, mostly to the frontal lobes, have strongly lent support to the notion that selective neurological impairments could lead to disturbances of moral cognition while leaving other cognitive domains relatively intact (Eslinger & Damasio 1985; Saver & Damasio 1991; Tranel et al. 2002). Damage to the ventromedial (VMPFC) and frontopolar sectors (FPC) of the prefrontal cortex (PFC) at an early age may lead to even more severe impairments in moral behavior, suggesting that moral development can be arrested by early PFC damage (Eslinger et al. 1992; Anderson et al. 1999). Given the similarities with developmental psychopathy (Cleckley 1976; Hare 2003), such impairments in social conduct were dubbed "acquired sociopathy" (Saver & Damasio 1991), though the complex constellation of behavioral abnormalities observed in developmental psychopathy can rarely, if at all, be produced by acquired brain lesions. Accordingly, a review of lesion studies of patients with acquired sociopathy and preserved general cognitive abilities showed that current models of normal social conduct have privileged the PFC at the expense of other brain regions (Moll et al. 2003).

However, damage to non-PFC brain regions can lead to impairments of moral behavior, including unprovoked physical assaults, paraphilias, inappropriate sexual advances, and teasing behavior (Moll et al. 2003). Evidence from studies on patients with neurodegenerative disorders, such as fronto-temporal dementia, shows that temporal lobe structures also play important roles in moral cognition and behavior. The anterior temporal isocortex stands among the most affected regions in cases of semantic dementia and has been directly implicated in the genesis of inappropriate social behaviors (Bozeat et al. 2000; Mendez et al. 2000). Abnormalities compatible with dysfunction of abstract conceptual knowledge in this brain region have also been described in psychopathy (Kiehl et al. 2004). Another sector of the temporal cortex, the posterior superior temporal sulcus region (STS) is critical for decoding social cues, including inferences on agency and intentionality, as part of an extended circuitry involved in "theory of mind" and social perception (Allison et al. 2000; Decety & Jackson 2004). In line with the role of an extended network of brain regions in the implementation and regulation of moral cognition and conduct, lesions to limbic and paralimbic structures can impair basic motivational mechanisms, including feeding, sex, social attachment, and aggression, which can result in severe impairments of moral conduct (Daigneault et al. 1999; Weissenberger et al. 2001; Burns & Swerdlow 2003).

During the past few years, a number of functional magnetic resonance imaging (fMRI) studies in normal volunteers have contributed to our understanding of the moral brain. In an early experiment of the neural basis of moral judgment, normal volunteers were scanned during the auditory presentation of short statements and instructed to silently make categorical judgments (right versus wrong) on each (de Oliveira-Souza & Moll 2000; Moll et al. 2001). Some statements had an explicit moral content (*The judge condemned an innocent man*), while others were factual statements without moral content (*Telephones never ring*). When the moral condition was contrasted to the factual one, the medial frontal gyrus and medial and lateral sectors of the FPC—cortical regions which are especially evolved in humans as compared to other primates (Allman et al. 2002)—were strongly activated. Robust effects were also observed in the right anterior temporal lobe (aTL) and the left angular gyrus/STS region. These effects could not be explained on the basis of overall degree of emotionality of stimuli.

Greene and colleagues (2001) addressed another important aspect of the moral domain, also by using fMRI. Normal subjects were exposed to moral and nonmoral dilemmas that were structurally more complex than the simple statements described above, which were associated with a higher load of reasoning and conflict. Moral dilemmas were divided into moral–personal (the agent personally inflicts an injury to another person to avoid a worse disaster, such as pushing an innocent person to death on the tracks of a runaway trolley in order to stop it and save five other individuals who would be killed otherwise) and moral–impersonal ones (the agent acts in an "impersonal" way, such as by pressing a button which will divert the trolley, thereby killing one innocent person instead of five others). The moral–personal condition evoked similar activations in the FPC and angular gyrus, as compared to Oliveira-Souza and Moll's study (de Oliveira-Souza & Moll 2000; Moll et al. 2001). Further studies followed, which addressed the contribution of general emotional arousal, bodily harm, response times, semantic content, cognitive load, conflict, intention, consequences, and emotional regulation (Berthoz et al. 2002; Moll, de Oliveira-Souza, Bramati, et al. 2002; Moll, de Oliveira-Souza, Eslinger, et al. 2002; Heekeren et al. 2003; Greene et al. 2004; Heekeren et al. 2005; Harenski & Hamann 2006; Schaich Borg et al. 2006). Collectively, these studies have confirmed the role of lateral and medial sectors of the orbitofrontal cortex (OFC), FPC, STS, and aTL in various aspects of moral judgment and moral sentiments.

The studies on moral judgment raised an important question: to what degree are these brain regions recruited by requirements of the task (semantic judgments, preference judgments, emotional judgments) and to what extent by the moral *contents* of moral scenarios (presence of written or visual stimuli having moral salience, i.e., stimuli associated with moral values, rights, responsibilities, moral sentiments, etc.)? This issue was addressed in another fMRI study by passively exposing participants to pictures which varied in their moral content and emotional salience (Moll, de Oliveira-Souza, Eslinger, et al. 2002). Activation of the anterior insula, amygdala, and subcortical structures were observed for both moral and nonmoral unpleasant stimuli. The FPC, medial OFC, and posterior STS region, however, were selectively activated by moral appraisals. The engagement of the same brain networks by moral appraisals independently of task demands originated the idea of *moral sensitivity* as a mechanism by which moral significance is automatically attributed to ordinary events (Moll, de Oliveira-Souza, Eslinger, et al. 2002). Moral sensitivity allows humans to quickly apprehend the moral implications of a social situation depending on context, agency, and consequences of one's choices. Such mechanism crucially depends on moral sentiments (Moll, Oliveira-Souza, Zahn, et al. 2007). Moral sentiments (Hume 1739/1984; Smith 1759/1966) are culturally ubiquitous (Fessler 1999; Ehrlich 2000), being intrinsically linked to daily social interactions. Anticipated or actual violations of one's own principles and beliefs automatically trigger aversive feelings such as guilt and shame (Eisenberg 2000). Contrariwise, standing up for one's core values may trigger positive feelings such as pride and awe. Moral sentiments are thus strong motivators for compliance with cultural norms and values. In this sense, cultural norms can become intrinsically motivating (Moll, Zahn, et al. 2005) (FIG. 2).

The Roles of Reason and Feeling in Moral Cognition

In Renaissance philosophical psychology emotive functions of the "sensitive soul" resided in the heart, while cognition and voluntary motion had their seat in the brain (Park 2000). While today such beliefs might sound amusing, it should be noted that modern science has tacitly retained the same dualistic principle when dealing with the relationships between mental processes and regional brain function. Different qualities of introspective experience, in this instance feeling and reasoning, are often assumed to "reside" in different anatomical loci (MacLean 1973), with feelings occupying the limbic system and reasoning the isocortex (especially the PFC).

Although there is now little question of the importance of reasoning and feeling in human morality

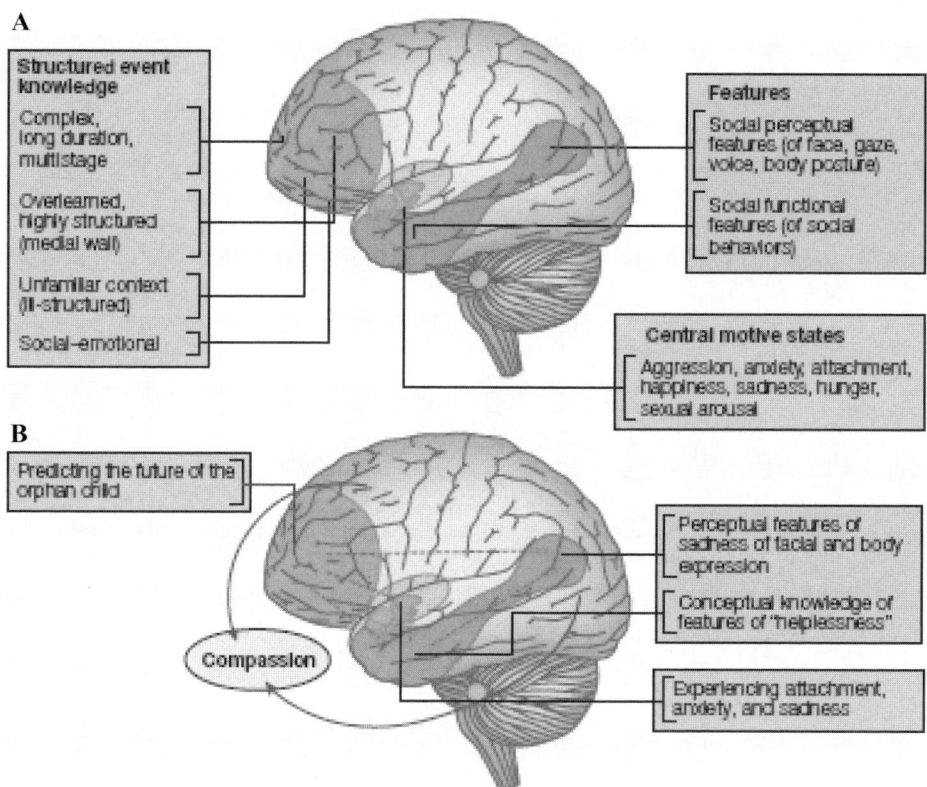

FIGURE 2. The event-feature-emotion model of moral cognition. **(A)** Three main components postulated by the event-feature-emotion complex (EFEC) framework. The EFEC framework postulates that moral cognitive and behavioral phenomena arise from the binding of three main components: structured event knowledge (provided by context-dependent representations within prefrontal subregions), social perceptual and functional features (stored in the posterior and anterior sectors of the temporal cortex), and central motive or basic emotional states (such as aggressiveness, sadness, attachment, or sexual arousal, represented within limbic and paralimbic regions). **(B)** Emergent representations predicted by the EFEC model. Relevant types of moral cognition phenomena that can be understood on the basis of the EFEC framework include moral sentiments, moral values, and long-term goals. The elements from the three main components of the EFEC framework interact to produce the moral sentiment *compassion*. The PFC provides contextual event representations (e.g. the girl is an orphan and the odds for adoption are low), the STS and anterior temporal cortex region contribute social perceptual (sad facial expression of a child) and functional (the concept of "helplessness") features, and limbic-paralimbic regions underlie central motive states (feeling sadness, anxiety, and attachment). These component representations give rise to a gestalt experience by way of temporal synchronization (W. Singer 2001). Reprinted with permission from Moll, Zahn, et al. (2005).

(Damasio 1994), the neural basis of these introspectively different ways of reaching moral decisions is hotly debated. One view is that reasoning ("cognition") and emotion rely on anatomically separable systems (cognition in the PFC and parietal areas, and emotion in limbic regions), and that cognition and emotion can be placed in conflict and compete with each other during choice behavior (McClure et al. in press). In the context of difficult moral choices, such as when one must decide whether it would be appropriate to push an innocent man to death on the tracks of a runaway trolley to save five other individuals, the emotional system would tell the decision maker "Don't do it!!" the prepotent response, whereas the cognitive system would recommend the "utilitarian" choice, the one that leads to the maximum overall benefit, the rational choice (Greene et al. 2004). According to this "dual-process theory," choosing to push the man means that cognitive brain areas were successful in overcoming or suppressing the emotional bias of not doing it. We have proposed an alternative view that moral reasoning and emotion depend on associatively linked representations within fronto-temporo-limbic networks (Moll, Zahn, et al. 2005). Whereas both views agree that limbic regions are primarily responsible for emotional states and that isocortical regions enable complex cognitive functions, they disagree on how information in limbic and isocortical systems interact to produce moral decisions. These contrasting views are described in the following section.

Control, Conflict, and the Cortex

The cognitive control approach is intuitive and builds on the classical distinction between reasoning and emotion. Reasoning is understood to be more explicit, effortful, and conscious and supports cost-benefit analyses (Miller & Cohen 2001). Emotion-based processes, on the other hand, are thought to be automatic, "hot," quick, and prepotent and, to a great extent, operate unconsciously. Together with cognitive mechanisms, they help guide decisions toward the appropriate behavioral choices. Reasoning is based on cognitive operations residing in isocortical regions (mainly the PFC), whereas emotions are produced by limbic regions.

Cognition and emotion, this view poses, rely on broadly separable brain systems, and information processing taking place in these two systems may be in direct opposition. According to the cognitive control view, cognitive and emotional systems can compete for behavioral output when prepotent responses arising from "emotional brain regions" favor one type of outcome while "cognitive brain regions" point to another outcome. When faced with difficult choices—say, staying in shape or eating fudge, or admitting a mistake instead of getting away without being caught—we vividly experience a feeling of conflict. Indulging in the fudge or failing to admit a mistake can thus be seen as a failure of this control mechanism over emotions. Neural theories on the workings of the frontal lobes have largely embraced this view. In fact, it has been consistently demonstrated that PFC lesions indeed lead to poor choices and impaired decision making (Grafman 1995). This led to the concept of the "central executive," an overarching controller of our behaviors, which is able to supervise and steer our choices according to performance criteria (Shallice & Burgess 1996).

Executive abilities subserved by the PFC have been variously described as tapping on diverse cognitive functions such as behavioral inhibition, selective attention, working memory, and cognitive control (Miller & Cohen 2001). PFC function is thought to be particularly important for novel situations, mainly when multiple behavioral options are present at the same time. According to this view, the PFC exerts top-down control over other brain processes. In the field of moral cognition and decision making, this approach is represented by the cognitive conflict and control model of moral cognition (Greene et al. 2004). Greene and colleagues (Greene et al. 2004; Greene et al. 2001) proposed a division between cognitive and emotional brain regions. Cognitive regions, in this model, would include the dorsolateral prefrontal cortex (DLPFC) and FPC and some posterior cortical areas. These areas are believed to exert inhibitory influence or control over emotional regions. Rational judgments in morally conflicting settings would therefore result from successful inhibition of emotional responses, whereas emotion-based choices (when a more "rationally appropriate" option is available) would represent a failure of this suppression mechanism.

Cortico-Limbic Integration

As discussed above, there are situations in which spontaneously evoked emotions and automatic intuitive mechanisms are insufficient to deal with contextual demands to guide appropriate behavioral choices. In the moral domain, these demands are typical of situations involving moral dilemmas. A moral dilemma is a problem which entails dissonant choices of roughly comparable motivational strength, giving rise to a slow and effortful process often referred to as *moral calculus* (Gottfried 1999; Moll et al. 2003). These processes presuppose the expression of the inner conflict between predicted outcomes of one's choices and how they relate to personal preferences and values. Higher order cognitive abilities, such as planning, executive flexibility, and strategy application, become decisive in these contexts. However the neural representations underlying these cognitive processes must work in the service of actions which are essentially motivationally salient. The cortico-limbic integration model of moral cognition (Moll, Zahn, et al. 2005), in contrast to the cognitive control approach, proposes that competing representations of behavioral choices cannot be split into cognitive and emotional ones. Instead, the competition will occur among *cognitive-emotional* alternatives— for example, should I opt for killing one innocent to save five other lives and forever suffer the angst of being a murderer, or opt for abstaining to do so and be responsible for causing the death of five people, thus committing a terrible act of omission? Should I indulge in tax evasion and thus be able to send my kid to a good school? In our view, rational or purely cognitive choices cannot be considered as *real* choices because they lack motivational power.

According to this view, all morally relevant experiences are considered to be essentially cognitive–emotional association complexes. Instead of competing with each other, cognition and emotion are continuously integrated during moral decision making. This view is in agreement with the finding that the PFC-mediated mechanisms are spontaneously engaged *whether or not* decisions or behavioral outputs are required in moral scenarios, suggesting that the PFC not only processes information stored elsewhere in the brain but is involved in representing aspects of morally salient contexts. Accordingly, certain PFC functions—for example, planning and representation of future outcomes—are believed to be central for enabling the experience of certain moral sentiments, such as anticipatory guilt for example. These sentiments require anticipation and evaluation of possible future consequences of one's choices and social acts. Following this model, emotional states would not compete with cognitive or rational information; cognitive representations are part of the subjective experience of complex feelings and provide essential ingredients for their emergence. In line with this proposal, recent studies on cognitive appraisals show that the PFC is involved both in up-regulation and down-regulation of emotional experience (Ochsner et al. 2004; Harenski & Hamann 2006; Kim & Hamann 2007). PFC–limbic networks would thus help in attaching value to whichever behavioral options are contemplated during decision making. Physiologically, interactions among cortical and subcortical-limbic brain regions in moral cognition are still not well understood but may result from temporal binding of neural activity across PFC–temporo-limbic networks (W. Singer 2001; Moll, Zahn, et al. 2005).

Recently published patient lesion studies have stirred up the debate about the roles of reason and emotion in moral cognition. These studies, carried out by Koenigs and colleagues (2007) and by Ciaramelli and colleagues (2007), employed classical trolley-type dilemmas (Thomson 1985) to investigate patterns of moral judgments in patients with bilateral damage to the VMPFC. They demonstrated that these patients endorsed "utilitarian" decisions in high-conflict scenarios—highly emotionally aversive choices that would nonetheless lead to greater aggregate welfare (e.g., more lives saved)—much more often than control subjects did. The increased preference of VMPFC patients for utilitarian choices could be interpreted according to different functional–anatomic hypotheses. One possibility would be that making more "rational," utilitarian choices in difficult dilemmas might have resulted from a general emotional blunting and reduced autonomic signaling arising from VMPFC damage—an interpretation that would fit with the somatic-marker hypothesis (Damasio et al. 1990). This possibility, however, is not supported by the results of another study by Koenigs and Tranel (2007). In this study, the performance of VMPFC patients in the two-person Ultimatum game was investigated. In this "single-shot" game (participants interact only one time, anonymously), participants sometimes must choose between accepting an unfair but financially rewarding proposal (the economically "rational" choice), or rejecting it to punish the unfair player (the "emotional" choice). VMPFC patients opted more often than controls for rejecting unfair offers (i.e., they were more "emotional"). Therefore, while VMPFC patients made more utilitarian ("rational") choices in trolley-type dilemmas, they opted more often for costly punishing ("emotional") responses). Thus, the choice patterns observed in these morally salient experimental settings can neither be explained by a single mechanism of overall emotional blunting (Damasio et al. 1990), nor by the dual-process proposal, in which cognition and emotion processes compete for behavioral output in conflicting situations (Greene et al. 2004; Greene 2007).

An alternative explanation would be the occurrence of a dissociation *within* the moral sentiment domain, with a more selective impairment of prosocial sentiments, such as guilt and compassion (Moll & de Oliveira-Souza 2007a, 2007b; Moll, de Oliveira-Souza, Garrido, et al. 2007). It is likely that distinct brain regions have differential roles in enabling different moral sentiments. The VMPFC, in particular, may be more critical for experience of prosocial sentiments associated with affiliative components (i.e., guilt, compassion, interpersonal attachment), whereas the DLPFC and lateral OFC/perirhinal cortex are more relevant for socially aversive sentiments (such as indignation and contempt) (Moll, de Oliveira-Souza, et al. 2005). The "cold-blooded" utilitarian choices (Ciaramelli et al. 2007; Koenigs et al. 2007) and preserved or increased punishment of others in the ultimatum game (Koenigs & Tranel 2007) observed in VMPFC patients may reflect an impairment in prosocial sentiments. Furthermore, the finding of decreased punishment of noncooperators following transient disruption of right DLPFC function by low-frequency, repetitive transcranial magnetic stimulation, demonstrated in a recent study by Knoch and others (2006), is compatible with a decrease in aggressive inclinations.

In summary, these data are in agreement with the notion that neither is moral reasoning only cortical and conscious nor is feeling only limbic and implicit. Though some brain regions are intrinsically tied to motivational/regulatory mechanisms and others are less so, this does not imply clear boundaries or competition between cognition and emotion. Instead, competition between behavioral options will only occur when choices are endowed with emotional salience.

The Neural Basis of Moral Motivations

The question of how unique our moral instinct is has been discussed for a long time (Smith 1759/1966; Darwin 1871/1982). There is a growing awareness, however, that the primitive affective–motivational building blocks of morality find clear parallels in other social species. These mechanisms can be operationally organized into two broad classes: one linked to approach and affiliation and the other linked to aversion and rejection. While attachment promotes care, cooperation, and reciprocity toward in-group members, aversion fosters blame, prejudice, and group dissolution (de Waal 1998; Schulkin 2000; Moll et al. 2003). As we aim to show here, such primitive social–motivational dispositions find a close correspondence to the prosocial and social–aversive counterparts at work in sophisticated psychological spheres of human moral cognition. These are manifested as moral sentiments and values, which embody motivational elements of social attachment/aversion and culturally shaped social knowledge (Schulkin 2004; Moll, Zahn, et al. 2005).

Here we briefly review the evidence on phylogenetically old mechanisms underlying prosocial motivations and social aversion. We argue that sophisticated forms of human prosocial (e.g., cooperation, altruism, and empathy) and socially aversive (e.g., moral outrage and prejudice) inclinations are deeply entrenched with motivational–emotional neuro-endocrine mechanisms underlying primitive social instincts. It follows that the experience of moral sentiments and values essentially emerges from interlocking cognitive–motivational systems integrating and reshaping social instincts into uniquely human neural and psychological dimensions.

Social Attachment and Prosocial Motivations

Attachment provides the basic ingredient for interindividual bonding and affiliative behaviors, such as mother–offspring ties. This depends on subcortical and limbic structures, including the ventral striatum, septal nuclei, amygdala, and hypothalamus (Insel & Fernald 2004; Keverne & Curley 2004). A broad array of neuropeptides in addition to monoaminergic neurotransmitters (serotonin, dopamine) and the opioid system (Depue & Morrone-Strupinsky 2005) contributes to attachment behaviors in animals. Neuropeptides which have a role in rewarding and/or affiliative states in animals include vasopressin, oxytocin, cocaine- and amphetamine-regulated transcript peptide, and neuropeptide Y. Distinct peptides can promote prosocial behaviors in different ways: for example, neuropeptide Y acts on the ventral striatum and perifornical region and has both anxiety-relieving properties and rewarding effects, while oxytocin facilitates social bonds and mediates animal contact and comfort (Insel & Young 2001). Serotonin has also been shown to promote constructive social interactions by decreasing aggression (S. N. Young & Leyton 2002) and might also be involved in regulating oxytocin expression.

Recent evidence has started to demonstrate the role of attachment-related neural mechanisms in humans. Structures of the brain reward system, that is the midbrain ventral tegmental area and ventral striatum, along with basal forebrain structures, were engaged when humans looked at their own babies or at their romantic partners (Bartels & Zeki 2004; Aron et al. 2005). Other studies have provided causal evidence for the effects of oxytocin on human social behavior. In a sequential economic game involving trust, oxytocin levels were found to be higher in subjects who received a monetary transfer signaling an intention to trust, in comparison to an unintentional monetary transfer of the same amount from another player (Zak et al. 2004). Higher oxytocin levels were associated with increased likelihood of reciprocation. Decreasing social anxiety or fear might also be an important effect of oxytocin, a hypothesis that was strengthened by a recent pharmacological fMRI study. In this study, oxytocin was shown to decrease amygdala activation to fearful stimuli (Kirsch et al. 2005). In another study, intranasal administration of oxytocin induced more cooperation in an anonymous economic game by boosting interpersonal trust (Kosfeld et al. 2005). In this game, the first player chooses to transfer an amount of money (if any) to another player. The amount is multiplied, and the second player may choose how much she/he will transfer back to the first player (reciprocation). Exogenous oxytocin administration was associated with increased amount transfers in the trust game by first movers.

It is possible that these primitive neuro-humoral attachment mechanisms, which appear to be relatively preserved across mammalian species, are relevant to the more sophisticated sphere of human morality. Because similar mechanisms can be adapted by evolution to serve novel *functions* across phylogenesis, we speculate that our proclivity to develop complex cultural constructs such as moral values may partially spring from integration of more "primitive" motivational systems with sophisticated cortical representations. In line with this hypothesis, a recent fMRI experiment provided evidence for a direct link between altruistic decision making in cultural settings and the functions of the brain reward and social attachment systems. In this study, subjects were scanned using fMRI while they made real-life anonymous decisions about whether to donate to or to oppose a number of charities (Moll et al. 2006). Decisions, depending on trial type, could be either financially costly or noncostly to the participant. In other trials, participants were able to receive "pure" monetary rewards (without consequences for the charities). The charities were associated with causes with important societal implications, such as abortion, children's rights, nuclear energy, war, and euthanasia. Both pure monetary rewards and decisions to donate activated the mesolimbic reward system, in agreement with the warm-glow hypothesis—it feels good to be good (Andreoni 1990).

Interestingly, in comparison to the pure monetary reward condition, decisions to donate selectively activated subgenual-septal area, which is intimately related to social attachment in other species (Freedman et al. 2000; L. J. Young & Wang 2004). When participants disliked the charities (e.g., many of them refused to make decisions that would benefit the National Rifle Association), the lateral OFC, an area more readily activated by experience of anger and disgust, was engaged. Furthermore, when decisions were costly to the participant—both costly donation and costly opposition—more anterior areas of the PFC were activated: the FPC and anterior OFC. This can be interpreted as a result of weighing the costs and benefits of decisions and anticipating the consequences of one's decisions to oneself and to the charities (Moll et al. 2006). Noteworthy, during costly donations these PFC areas showed increased functional connectivity with the subgenual-septal area (Moll et al. 2006 unpublished results). This indicates that moral motivations depend on the coactivation of limbic systems involved in affiliative rewards and of the more recently evolved anterior PFC, which work cooperatively (instead of competitively) during decision making. Finally, these findings extended the role of fronto-limbic networks in social cooperation from interpersonal economic interactions, as addressed by a number of previous studies (Sanfey et al. 2003; de Quervain et al. 2004; T. Singer et al. 2004; Delgado et al. 2005; King-Casas et al. 2005), to the realm of decisions based on internalized values and preferences shaped by culture (FIG. 3).

Social Aversion and Moralistic Aggression

Interindividual aggression typically occurs in disputes concerning sex, territory, power, and food resources. Primates possess highly structured dominance hierarchies regulating access to food resources, mating, and other social privileges (Byrne & Whiten 1988; de Waal 1998). Social status marks one as a "good" or "poor" partner for future interactions. In humans, aggressiveness is underlined by feelings of anger, frustration, and, arguably, disgust and contempt.

Neural and humoral systems underlying such behaviors have been studied in several species. There is extensive evidence pointing to the role of dopaminergic and serotonergic pathways. In primates, both dopamine and serotonin have modulatory effects on social interactions, depending on social status (Edwards & Kravitz 1997; Morgan et al. 2002; Muehlenbein et al. 2004). Although enhanced dopaminergic and serotonergic action have been related to increased dominance, these neurochemical systems probably exert partially separable effects. Increased serotonergic activity leads to a decrease of harm avoidance and hostility and an increase in dominance in social encounters in humans (Brody et al. 2000). It has been suggested that part of this effect may be mediated by regulation of oxytocin release, linked to social contact, or through the cortico-tropin-releasing hormone, linked to social withdrawal (Brody et al. 2000). In humans, D2-class receptor dopaminergic antagonism leads to a selective disruption in anger recognition, in line with the importance of dopamine mediating aggression in social-agonistic encounters (Lawrence et al. 2002).

In addition to anger, disgust also plays a central role in social aversion. Interestingly, proto-forms of disgust found in nonhumans are linked to essentially nonsocial functions: distaste and nausea from exposure to potentially toxic or contaminated foods and odors have a clear adaptive function (Darwin 1872/1965; Rozin & Haidt 1993; Rozin 1999). In humans, in contrast, disgust and its close relative, contempt, have clearly extended to the interpersonal realm. Different from anger, disgust and contempt are slower to fade away, tend to "stick" or become a property of the object, and intensely devalue it (Rozin et al. 1999; Haidt 2003). Thus, in the same way that neural systems underlying primitive forms of pleasure and social bonding operate in complex social situations associated with human cooperation, neural systems underlying aversive responses related to physical properties and odors of foods seem to have been adapted to sustain social disapproval and "moralistic" aggression (Arsenio & Lemerise 2004). Thus, while morality often promotes cooperation and helping, it can also motivate people to punish other individuals and social groups (Moll et al. 2003; Jones 2007).

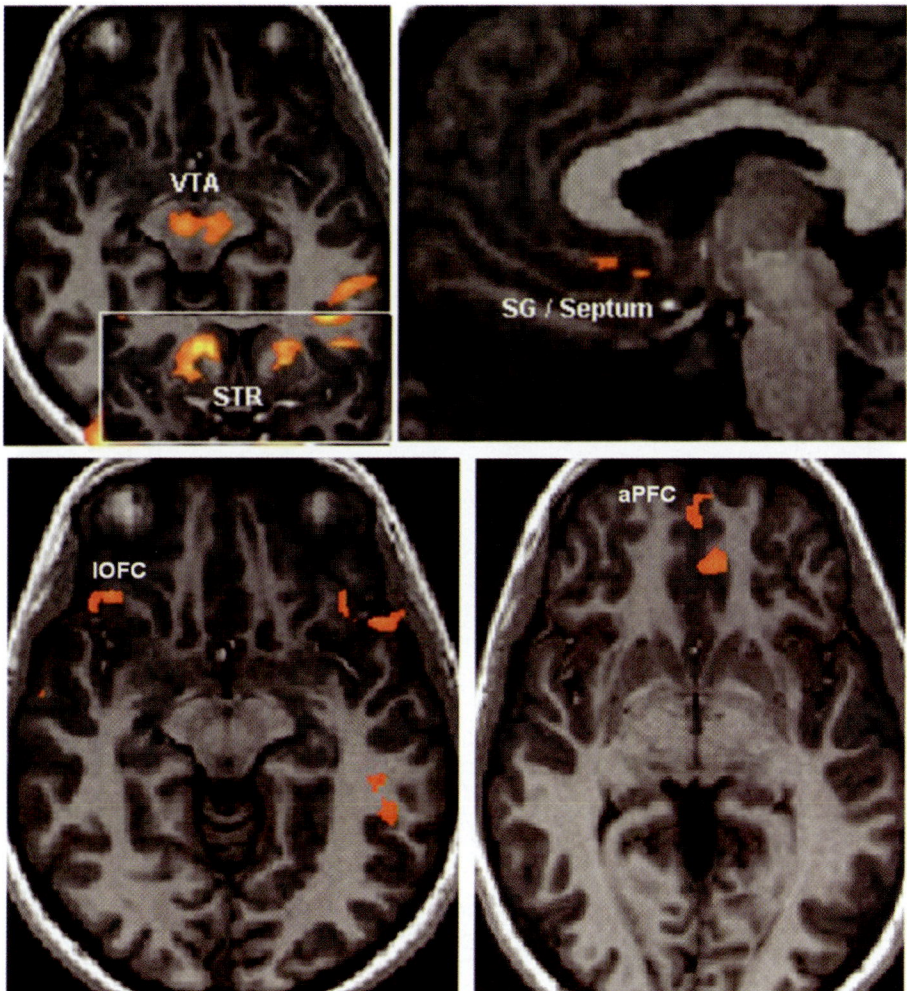

FIGURE 3. Brain regions involved in donation and opposition to charities. Brain regions showing increased activation in a functional magnetic resonance imaging (fMRI) study of charitable donations to societal causes (such as abortion, children's rights, nuclear energy, war, and euthanasia). Both pure monetary rewards (an experimental control condition) and decisions to donate (with or without personal financial costs) activated the mesolimbic reward system, including the ventral tegmental area (VTA, shown on a transversal cut across the midbrain) and the ventral and dorsal sectors striatum (STR) (figure inset depicting a coronal cut across the striatum). The subgenual-septal area (SG-septum), however, was selectively activated by decisions to donate, as compared to pure monetary rewards (both by costly and noncostly decisions, conjunction analysis; right side). The lateral orbitofrontal cortex (lOFC) was activated by decisions to oppose charities (transversal cut). This activation extended to the anterior insula and to the inferior dorsolateral prefrontal cortex (DLPFC) and was present both for costly and noncostly decisions (conjunction analysis). Ventral anterior sectors of the medial prefrontal cortex (aPFC) were activated when volunteers made costly decisions, that is, when they voluntarily chose to sacrifice their own monetary resources either to donate to a charity or to oppose it (conjunction analysis). Modified with permission from Moll et al. (2006).

Moral values powerfully incite people to challenge others' beliefs and ideologies (Allport 1954; Vogel 2004). Previous research has consistently implicated a number of brain regions and circuits in social aversion, including brain-stem regions, the amygdala, basal forebrain, and hypothalamic nuclei, pirifom and cingulate cortex, and temporal and frontal connections (Mega et al. 1997; Volavka 1999; Calder et al. 2001; Moll, de Oliveira-Souza, et al. 2005). Particularly, the lateral OFC and neighboring agranular insula have been implicated in interpersonal aversive mechanisms (Bechara et al. 2000; Kringelbach 2005), including punishment of noncooperators in economic interactions (Sanfey et al. 2003; de Quervain et al. 2004), anger responses (Blair et al. 1999; Bechara et al. 2000) and racial bias (Cunningham et al. 2004). Another fMRI study directly showed that brain regions involved in basic forms of disgust and moral disgust are largely shared (Moll, de Oliveira-Souza, et al. 2005). Accordingly, in the donation study described above, decisions to oppose charities, whether personally costly or not, were associated with activity in the lateral OFC and anterior insula, confirming the role of these regions in mediating aversive experiences in sophisticated cultural settings (Moll et al. 2006) (FIG. 3).

Morality and Human Attachment: The Extended Attachment Proposal

In this section we describe a recently developed hypothesis that focuses on the construct of an extended form of attachment as an important ingredient of human morality. Before proceeding, we would like to emphasize that this proposal is still, to a great degree, speculative. We believe, however, that it has the potential to aid the investigation of complex aspects of human social inclinations and behaviors in cultural settings, both by theoretical reframing and by guiding the development of novel experimental approaches. We suggest that extended attachment is rooted in a unique proclivity of humans to develop affiliative links to culturally shaped elements. More specifically, we postulate that ancient mechanisms supporting basic forms of attachment in other species, such as pair bonding (Insel & Young 2001), evolved to enable the unique human ability to attach to culturally shaped associations of symbols with abstract meaning. This form of attachment might have played a major role in cooperation and indirect reciprocity during evolution, promoting altruistic behaviors within sociocultural groups and facilitating out-group moralistic aggression. The fundamental aspect underlying extended attachment is based on a functional reorganization of basic mechanisms of social attachment, present in many social species, into their human counterparts. The neural architecture underlying this ability putatively involves the connection of limbic/brain-stem regions involved in basic mechanisms of interindividual bonding and attachment to phylogenetically recent association cortical systems. The specific mechanisms of cortico-limbic integration are articulated in our model of moral cognition (Moll, Zahn, et al. 2005). We speculate that this kind of integration may play a central role in the unique human ability to attach motivational significance to abstract ideas, cultural symbols, and beliefs, supporting the high level of cooperation among nonkin typically observed in human societies. Recent studies have started to provide support for this hypothesis (Moll et al. 2006; Krueger et al., 2007; Moll, de Oliveira-Souza, Garrido, et al. 2007).

The inclination to form affective bonds is one major driving force behind the behavior of social mammals. This motivation is manifested through the affiliative bonds that develop between mother and child from an early age, present in virtually all classes of mammals (Insel et al. 1998; Insel & Young 2001). In humans, mother–infant attachment provides a mold for the interpersonal affective bonds that the individual establishes in life (Bretherton 1997; Insel 1997). For our current purposes, "proximate" or "basic" attachment is operationally defined as a collection of motivated behaviors that bolsters the formation of three basic types of bonding (Insel 1997): parent–infant, filial, and pair bonding. Attachment provides a basic motivational ingredient for interindividual bonding and affiliative behaviors. In addition, a large body of research in social psychology indicates that interpersonal attachment may be associated with the experience of belongingness (Baumeister 2005), emotional empathy (Fultz et al. 1986; Batson et al. 1991), and, as some recent evidence from our laboratory suggests, with the prosocial moral sentiments of guilt and compassion (Moll Oliveira-Souza, Zahn, et al. 2007). Attachment-driven motivations and sentiments, we argue, are important for the reparation of broken social links and for the promotion of helping behaviors, and at the same time help restrain self-serving behaviors (Smith 1759/1966; Haidt 2003). Although attachment is typically established among humans or between a human and another living being (e.g., a pet, a Yayá orchid), in special circumstances it may extend to an inanimate surrogate of a living being (e.g., to a ring that belonged to your grandfather) (Harlow & Suomi 1970). Attachment also implies a special emotional stance in relation to the object of attachment, which may be reciprocated or not. Rupture of attachment bonds lead to frustration, despondency, and grief (Clayton et al. 1968). Humans are thus biologically endowed with the inclination to become emotionally attached to abstract concepts and values which can be denoted by symbols. The meaning of these symbols is highly arbitrary and fully comprehensible only to those individuals who belong to the particular group within which they have matured (Robb 1998).

In the field of developmental psychology, the work of Bowlby on child attachment has been highly influential (Bretherton 1997). Severe psychopathology is often associated with chronic childhood maltreatment, leading to pathological social fear and avoidance, aggressiveness, and other manifestations of poor psychological and emotional development. These developmental problems have been framed within the rubric of the "attachment disorders." Clinico-anatomic observations indicate that abnormalities in attachment result from disruption of discrete brain structures and pathways in the VMPFC, subgenual-septal-preoptic-anterior hypothalamic continuum, and ventral strio-pallidal and brain-stem nuclei (Insel & Young 2001; Moll et al. 2003). Researchers have seldom referred to attachment when describing the manifestations of impaired social behaviors in humans, however (with the notable exception of "separation anxiety" by child psychologists; Bowlby 1960; Bretherton 1997). Interestingly, patients fulfilling the clinical picture of "acquired sociopathy" have been variously described as "detached," "cold," and "aloof" (Damasio et al. 1990; Eslinger et al. 1992; Moll, Zahn, et al. 2005). For example, EVR, the patient who rekindled the modern interest in the cerebral correlates of human social behavior (Eslinger & Damasio 1985) became detached from his closest relatives and peers after an injury of the VMPFC. Patients like EVR, who also suffered bilateral VMPFC damage, have a disproportional impairment of prosocial moral sentiments (Koenigs et al. 2007; Moll & De Oliveira-Souza, Zahn, 2007), for which the basic drive for attachment is crucial (Moll, Oliveira-Souza, Zahn, et al. 2007).

The aforementioned observations indicate that basic forms of attachment can be impaired by lesions of the basal forebrain and connected structures. The basal forebrain is a general term for a collection of fiber pathways and nuclei that compound a longitudinal *continuum* that extends from the anterior frontal and temporal lobes to the upper brain-stem below the plane that cuts through the anterior and posterior commissures. The complex anatomy of this region has been subjected to several studies in the past years, and some neural systems with possible functional significance have been identified. The main anatomical structures that make up the basal forebrain continuum are i) the primary and accessory olfactory tracts and their central projections (Okuda et al. 2003), ii) the collection of nuclei that make up the amygdaloid complex, iii) the septal area and nuclei, iv) the preoptic and anterior hypothalamus, v) the pathways that traverse this region and interconnect them, and vi) the basal nuclei of Meynert, the extended amygdala, and the ventral (i.e., subcommissural) strio-pallidum. While these structures are not exclusively linked to attachment, they are necessary for establishing interpersonal bonds and for the experience of attachment. One major challenge for future studies is to define the part played by discrete circuits within these systems in the promotion of specific aspects of attachment and bonding.

As reviewed above, psychological, neurobiological, and evolutionary lines of evidence support the notion of a basic form of attachment shared by humans and other mammals. We now turn to the proposal that an extended form of attachment may have coevolved with, and at times acted as a driving force for, the capacity for artwork and symbolic thinking, which reached a critical point in the cultural explosion of the Upper Paleolithic around 100,000 years ago. This stage marks one of the major recent transitions in human evolution (Maynard-Smith & Szathmary 1997). Anthropological evidence suggests that humans invested significant amounts of time and energy—as they still do—in cultural and symbolic activities that did not provide immediate survival benefits. Those included carefully designed and executed symbolic burials, crafting adornments, taking part in communal rituals, and painting cave walls (Ehrlich 2000). Extended attachment may be a key ingredient that allowed our ancestors to develop emotional bonds to cultural artifacts and ideas, promoting social coherence in collective hunting, building shelter, rituals, and other kinds of social exchanges going beyond simple interpersonal reciprocity. Imprinting values to abstract symbols, practices, and beliefs rendered humans capable of developing and internalizing values and virtues, helping self-evaluations of performance in social groups of ever-growing complexities.

Affiliation to culture-specific shared values, agreed upon by members of the group, may have served as "commitment devices" (Frank 1988) for all individuals and rendered humans less dependent on the more unstable relationships based of social status, which govern reciprocal mechanisms of cooperation and punishment among individuals. It is possible that this mechanism might also have promoted intergroup competition. In this sense, extended attachment would not only drive intragroup altruism and cooperation, but also help demarcate out-group boundaries, enhancing group distinctiveness and promoting aggression towards outgroups—a haunting feature which has permeated human evolution (Bowles & Gintis 2004; Bowles 2006).

Although preliminary, recent imaging studies in humans have revealed that brain structures involved in attachment—such as the subgenual cortex, septal area, and neighboring basal forebrain structures—are engaged not only when humans are presented to beloved ones (such as mothers to their babies or romantic partners to each other) in experimental settings (Bartels and Zeki 2004; Aron et al. 2005), but also that these brain regions are activated by donation to abstract societal causes (Moll et al. 2006) and when individuals engage in "unconditional cooperation," but not during "strategic cooperation," in economic games (Krueger et al. 2007). We are currently testing the extended attachment hypothesis using novel behavioral and fMRI paradigms.

The Neural Basis of Moral Knowledge

As outlined in the Introduction, moral cognition can be clearly separated from social cognition when specifically moral (altruistic) motivations are distinguished from selfish motivations of social behavior. In the previous section we described a theoretical view according to which moral motivations play important roles in moral cognition. These moral motivations are hypothesized to be composed of basic attachment and aversion represented in mesolimbic and basal forebrain regions integrated with cortical representations to form complex moral sentiments and moral values. Although there is now cumulating evidence on the neural basis of moral sentiments, no direct evidence is available on the representation of moral values. Moral or social values consist of abstract conceptual knowledge linked to emotional states and social actions (Schwartz 1992). Therefore, the basis of moral values can only be established after identifying the basis of abstract moral knowledge. Following our previous argument, moral knowledge when stripped from its motivations will be part of general social knowledge. According to this view, what distinguishes moral from social values is not the knowledge of values but the motivation that drives us to strive to act towards them.

The neural representation of general social knowledge, however, is as poorly understood as is the representation of moral knowledge. Wood and Grafman (2003) proposed that social knowledge generally arises from knowledge of the sequences of social events and actions represented in the VMPFC. Other researchers, however, have stressed that when abstracted from the sequential context of action, social knowledge remains largely intact in patients with VMPFC damage (Eslinger & Damasio 1985).

Recently, we demonstrated that abstract conceptual social knowledge, which is independent of the sequential context of actions and emotions, is represented in the superior aTL (Zahn et al. 2007) (FIG. 4). Abstract conceptual social knowledge allows us to define the meaning of overarching social and/or moral values (e.g., intelligence, ambition, honor, politeness). Preserved aTL representations of this kind of knowledge may help explain the observation of intact abstract conceptual social knowledge and normal performance on tasks which probe social knowledge in patients with VMPFC damage when there is no requirement of flexibly accessing the full range of complex and far-reaching sequential unfoldings of one's actions as is necessary during real-life social behavior (Eslinger & Damasio 1985; Saver & Damasio 1991).

This separation of stable abstract conceptual representations in the aTL that can be flexibly embedded within different contexts of action implementation and emotional qualities, as encoded in fronto-limbic circuits, could account for our ability to adapt social and moral values to a wide range of interpersonal and cultural settings. This independence of stable abstract conceptual and flexible context-dependent action–emotion representations could account for our ability to communicate about the sense of concepts, such as "politeness," in diverse cultural settings, despite a great variability of the exact actions and emotional flavors in specific contexts. A polite greeting in Japan might be to bow one's head, in Germany to shake hands, and in the United States to say: "How are you?" Nevertheless, we are able to interpret each of these behaviors as "polite." Conversely, the same social action (e.g., a woman proposing to her boyfriend on a vacation) can be associated with different conceptual interpretations (e.g., "individualism," "boldness," or "desperation") depending on the sequential and cultural context. This flexibility of associative links between social concepts and actions also enables us to flexibly interpret social behavior because different associative links between social concepts and action contexts influence the emotional quality associated with the concept or action. A marriage proposal associated with boldness and individualism is more likely to lead to pride on the side of the agent, given that the person strives to act according to these values. This relinking of social actions and conceptual interpretations is successfully used to change emotional and moral evaluations of one's social behavior during the cognitive therapy of affective disorders (Beck et al. 1979).

Further studies are needed to test the interplay of these different representations which endow us with the remarkable ability to dynamically rearrange social concepts, actions, and emotional flavors to produce the rich variety of personal, moral, and social values which subtly steer our social lives.

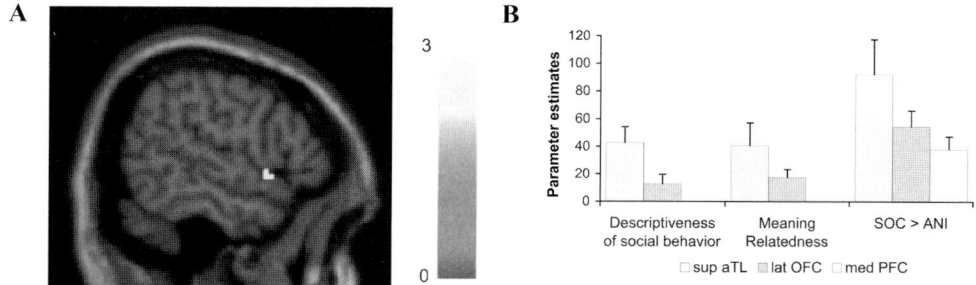

FIGURE 4. Abstract conceptual social knowledge and the anterior temporal lobe. In this functional magnetic resonance imaging (fMRI) study, word pairs were visually presented and subjects had to judge their relatedness in meaning. There were no differences between positive (e.g., "honor-brave") and negative (e.g., "tactless-impolite") social concepts within the anterior temporal lobe (aTL), so that in subsequent analyses we compared both conditions against a condition using animal function concepts (e.g., "nutritious-useful"). In addition to the subtraction analysis, an independent parametric regression analysis was employed within the social concept condition to determine whether the detected domain-specific superior aTL region indeed represents social conceptual knowledge. In order to test this we hypothesized that this region should change activity with meaning relatedness of social concept pairs and would increase activity with increasing richness of social conceptual detail. Both parameters were derived from normative studies on these concepts in which we had participants rate how closely two concepts were related in meaning (meaning relatedness) and how detailed each concept described social behavior (descriptiveness of social behavior). **(A)** Regions in which activity was higher for social than for animal concepts and which were independently correlated with descriptiveness of social behavior and meaning relatedness: conjunction null analysis for all of these three effects revealed a selective right *superior anterior* temporal region on a whole brain basis (BA38). **(B)** Parameter estimates and standard errors for descriptiveness of social behavior, meaning relatedness, and domain-specificity (Social > Animal) at right superior aTL, orbitofrontal, and medial prefrontal peak coordinates show that the frontal regions are not influenced by the measure of richness of social conceptual detail (descriptiveness of social behavior), whereas activity in the superior aTL is increased by increasingly descriptive social concepts. Reprinted with permission from Zahn et al. (2007).

Conclusions and Future Directions

As pointed out by Darwin (1871/1982) and Adam Smith (1759/1966) among others, moral sentiments are central for the regulation of social behaviors, enforcing the observance of social norms according to internalized values. Clinical and experimental studies have started to provide evidence on the influence of cultural and biological factors on human morality. The identification of neural components and their relationships to psychological processes underlying moral cognition is providing critical knowledge for our understanding of the strengths and weaknesses of our moral nature. We have argued that deeply entrenched neurohumoral mechanisms, which are largely shared with other social species, provide the motivational force underlying human moral sentiments and are uniquely combined with cognitive abilities only recently developed in our species, such as conceptual abstraction and elaborate representation of future consequences of actions. Thus, these motivational systems are not merely evolutionary remnants that must be tempered and modulated by "rational" cortical systems. Instead, social attachment and aversion are crucial motivators of moral actions and are inextricably linked to moral evaluations and judgments. These motivations are deeply influenced by social learning and by individual biological differences.

We have discussed evidence on a stable network of brain regions identified during functional imaging of moral cognition irrespective of task constraints. First evidence on distinct functional roles of components of this network, such as the specific role of the superior aTL in representations of abstract social conceptual knowledge and the role of the subgenual-septal and anterior PFC regions in altruistic decisions, have been articulated. We have also presented tentative evidence on categorical differences in patterns of activations for different moral sentiments, especially when prosocial and other critical sentiments are compared. These results raise hopes that the endeavor of elucidating functional subdivisions within the complex neural system which mediates moral cognition is worth pursuing.

Carefully designed neuroimaging and electrophysiological experiments and studies in patients with brain lesions are needed to further disentangle the localization of different cognitive components that make up moral sentiments and values and how these components are dynamically bound together. In order to study the neural basis of introspective entities such as moral sentiments, we will need to go beyond standard approaches of assuming that each person has a comparable response to the same stimulus. Instead, we need to assess how participants subjectively experience social stimuli and to employ analyses that effectively reflect individual assessments. This will allow researchers to directly probe whether brain regions underlying different types of subjective experience, moral reasoning, and moral sentiments are identical or different. Such experiments can only be successful if other experimental factors are carefully controlled.

Many assumptions of our hypotheses about moral cognition are built on collateral evidence from studies identifying the localization of other cognitive functions, such as sequence representation of events and actions, which we hypothesize to be a cognitive component of moral cognition. Two problems arise with this type of inference; 1) the postulate of such a cognitive component for moral cognition, even if reasonable, remains to be demonstrated experimentally; 2) the postulate that activation of the same brain region in two different imaging studies using different tasks points to a shared cognitive component between the two tasks may prove to be premature. This is because the resolution of functional imaging techniques, together with poor spatial reliability and individual variability of functional and structural anatomy, does not allow us to rule out further functional specializations of neuronal groups within those regions. Therefore, in order to test hypotheses about functional specializations we need to directly demonstrate the change in regional brain activity induced by varying loads of a hypothesized cognitive component during the moral cognitive task for which we claim the cognitive component to be relevant. For example, a direct demonstration of stronger activity within anterior PFC regions with increasing requirements of representation of future outcomes during the experience of moral sentiments would provide strong evidence for the assumption that anterior PFC activity observed for moral sentiments is indeed attributable to that cognitive component. Further, by demonstrating that lesions within this region in patients lead to impairments on the future outcome representation component of moral sentiments, but leaves other components of the sentiment relatively intact, would then provide strong evidence in favor of the claimed neurocognitive component.

The complexity and entanglement of cognitive components that make up moral cognition provide a challenge to future experimental designs in this field. However, we believe we have not only demonstrated, that the potential benefits of unveiling the secrets of this unique system should drive future pursuit of moral cognitive neuroscience, but also have provided a grain of empirical optimism fueled by the first successes recently made towards this end.

Acknowledgments

Jorge Moll is indebted to Fernanda Tovar-Moll and Pedro A. Andreiuolo for their support in various stages of this work. Ricardo de Oliveira-Souza is indebted to Omar da Rosa Santos for his continuous support and selfless benevolence.

Conflict of Interest

The authors declare no conflicts of interest.

References

Allison, T., Puce, A., & McCarthy, G. (2000). Social perception from visual cues: role of the STS region. *Trends Cogn. Sci.*, *4*(7), 267–278.

Allman, J., Hakeem, A., & Watson, K. (2002). Two phylogenetic specializations in the human brain. *Neuroscientist*, *8*(4), 335–346.

Allport, G. W. (1954). *The nature of prejudice*. Boston: Beacon Press.

Anderson, S. W., Bechara, A., Damasion, H., Tranel, D., & Damasio, A. R. (1999). Impairment of social and moral behavior related to early damage in human prefrontal cortex. *Nat. Neurosci.*, *2*(11), 1032–1037.

Andreoni, J. (1990). Impure altruism and donations to public good: A theory of warm glow giving. *The Economic Journal*, *100*(401), 464–477.

Aristotle. (1926). *The Nicomachean ethics*. London, New York: William Heinemann, G. P. Putnam's Sons.

Aron, A., Fisher, H., Mashek, D., Strong, G., Li, H.-F., et al. (2005). Reward, motivation, and emotion systems associated with early-stage intense romantic love. *J. Neurophysiol.*, *94*(1), 327–337.

Arsenio, W. F., & Lemerise, E. A. (2004). Aggression and moral development: Integrating social information processing and moral domain models. *Child Dev.*, *75*(4), 987–1002.

Bartels, A., & Zeki, S. (2004). The neural correlates of maternal and romantic love. *Neuroimage*, *21*(3), 1155–1166.

Batson, C. D., Batson, J. G., Slingsby, J. K., Harrell, K. L., Peekna, H. M., et al. (1991). Empathic joy and the empathy-altruism hypothesis. *J. Pers. Soc. Psychol.*, *61*(3), 413–426.

Baumeister, R. F. (2005). *The cultural animal*. New York: Oxford University Press.

Bechara, A., Tranel, D., & Damasio, H. (2000). Characterization of the decision-making deficit of patients with ventromedial prefrontal cortex lesions. *Brain*, *123*(Pt 11), 2189–2202.

Beck, A. T., Rush, A. J., Shaw, B. F., & Emery, A. (1979). *Cognitive therapy of depression*. New York: Guilford Press.

Berthoz, S., Armony, J. L., Blair, R. J. R., & Dolan, R. J. (2002). An fMRI study of intentional and unintentional (embarrassing) violations of social norms. *Brain, 125*(8), 1696–1708.

Blair, R. J., Morris, J. S., Frith, C. D., Perret, D. I., Dolan, R. J., et al. (1999). Dissociable neural responses to facial expressions of sadness and anger. *Brain, 122*(Pt 5), 883–893.

Bowlby, J. (1960). Separation anxiety. *Int. J. Psychoanal., 41*, 89–113.

Bowles, S. (2006). Group competition, reproductive leveling, and the evolution of human altruism. *Science, 314*(5805), 1569–1572.

Bowles, S., & Gintis, H. (2004). The evolution of strong reciprocity: cooperation in heterogeneous populations. *Theor. Popul. Biol., 65*(1), 17–28.

Boyd, R., Gintis, H., Bowles, S., & Richerson, P. J. (2003). The evolution of altruistic punishment. *Proc. Natl. Acad. Sci. U.S.A., 100*, 3531–3535.

Bozeat, S., Gregory, C. A., Ralph, M. A. L., & Hodges, J. R. (2000). Which neuropsychiatric and behavioural features distinguish frontal and temporal variants of frontotemporal dementia from Alzheimer's disease? *J. Neurol. Neurosurg. Psychiatry, 69*(2), 178–186.

Bretherton, I. (1997). Bowlby's legacy to developmental psychology. *Child Psychiatry Hum. Dev., 28*(1), 33–43.

Brody, A. L., Saxena, S., Fairbanks, L. A., Alborzian, S., Demaree, H. A., et al. (2000). Personality changes in adult subjects with major depressive disorder or obsessive-compulsive disorder treated with paroxetine. *J. Clin. Psychiatry, 61*(5), 349–355.

Burns, J. M., & Swerdlow, R. H. (2003). Right orbitofrontal tumor with pedophilia symptom and constructional apraxia sign. *Arch. Neurol., 60*(3), 437–440.

Byrne, R. W., & Whiten, A. (1988). *Machiavellian intelligence: Social expertise and the evolution of intellect in monkeys, apes and humans*. Oxford, UK: Oxford University Press.

Calder, A. J., Lawrence, A. D., & Young, A. W. (2001). Neuropsychology of fear and loathing. *Nat. Rev. Neurosci., 2*(5), 352–363.

Casebeer, W. D. (2003). Moral cognition and its neural constituents. *Nat. Rev. Neurosci., 4*(10), 840–846.

Ciaramelli, E., Muccioli, M., Làdavas, E., & di Pellegrino, G. (2007). Selective deficit in personal moral judgment following damage to ventromedial prefrontal cortex. *Soc. Cogn. Affect. Neurosci., 2*(2), 84–92.

Clayton, P. J., Desmarais, L., & Winokur, G. (1968). A study of normal bereavement. *Am. J. Psychiatry, 125*, 64–74.

Cleckley, H. M. (1976). *The mask of sanity*. St. Louis, MO: Mosby.

Cunningham, W. A., Raye, C. L., & Johnson, M. K. (2004). Implicit and explicit evaluation: fMRI correlates of valence, emotional intensity, and control in the processing of attitudes. *J. Cogn. Neurosci., 16*(10), 1717–1729.

Daigneault, S., Braun, C. M., & Montes, J. L. (1999). [Hypothalamic hamartoma: detailed presentation of a case]. *Encephale, 25*(4), 338–344.

Damasio, A. R. (1994). Descartes' error and the future of human life. *Sci. Am., 271*(4), 144.

Damasio, A. R., Tranel, D., & Damasio, H. (1990). Individuals with sociopathic behavior caused by frontal damage fail to respond autonomically to social stimuli. *Behav. Brain Res., 41*(2), 81–94.

Darwin, C. (1871/1982). *The descent of man and selection in relation to sex*. Princeton, NJ: Princeton University Press.

Darwin, C. (1872/1965). *The expression of emotions in man and animals*. Chicago: University of Chicago Press.

de Oliveira-Souza, R., & Moll, J. (2000). The moral brain: A functional MRI study of moral judgment. *Neurology, 54*, A104.

de Quervain, D. J., Fischbacher, U., Treger, V., Schellhammer, M., Schnyder, U., et al. (2004). The neural basis of altruistic punishment. *Science, 305*(5688), 1254–1258.

de Waal, F. (1998). *Chimpanzee politics power and sex among apes*. Baltimore: Johns Hopkins University Press.

Decety, J., & Jackson, P. L. (2004). The functional architecture of human empathy. *Behav. Cogn. Neurosci. Rev., 3*, 71–100.

Delgado, M. R., Frank, R. H., & Phelps, E. A. (2005). Perceptions of moral character modulate the neural systems of reward during the trust game. *Nat. Neurosci., 8*(11), 1611–1618.

Depue, R. A., & Morrone-Strupinsky, J. V. (2005). A neurobehavioral model of affiliative bonding: Implications for conceptualizing a human trait of affiliation. *Behav. Brain Sci., 28*(3), 313–350.

Edwards, D. H., & Kravitz, E. A. (1997). Serotonin, social status and aggression. *Curr. Opin. Neurobiol., 7*(6), 812–819.

Ehrlich, P. R. (2000). *Human natures: Genes, cultures, and the human prospect*. Washington, DC: Island Press.

Eisenberg, N. (2000). Emotion, regulation, and moral development. *Annu. Rev. Psychol., 51*, 665–697.

Eslinger, P. J., & Damasio, A. R. (1985). Severe disturbance of higher cognition after bilateral frontal lobe ablation: Patient EVR. *Neurology, 35*(12), 1731–1741.

Eslinger, P. J., Flaherty-Craig, C. V., & Benton, A. L. (2004). Developmental outcomes after early prefrontal cortex damage. *Brain Cogn., 55*(1), 84–103.

Eslinger, P. J., Grattan, L. M., Damasio, H., & Damasio, A. R. (1992). Developmental consequences of childhood frontal lobe damage. *Arch. Neurol., 49*(7), 764–769.

Fehr, E., & Fischbacher, U. (2003). The nature of human altruism. *Nature, 425*(6960), 785–791.

Fehr, E., & Rockenbach, B. (2004). Human altruism: economic, neural, and evolutionary perspectives. *Curr. Opin. Neurobiol., 14*(6), 784–790.

Fessler, D. (1999). Toward an understanding of the universality of second order emotions. In A. Hinton (Ed.), *Beyond nature or nurture: Biocultural approaches to the emotions* (pp. 75–116). New York: Cambridge University Press.

Frank, R. H. (1988). *Passions within reason: The strategic role of the emotions*. New York: W. W. Norton & Co Ltd.

Freedman, L. J., Insel, T. R., & Smith, Y. (2000). Subcortical projections of area 25 (subgenual cortex) of the macaque monkey. *J. Comp. Neurol., 421*(2), 172–188.

Fultz, J., Batson, C. D., Fortenbach, V. A., McCarthy, P. M., Varney, L. L., et al. (1986). Social evaluation and the empathy-altruism hypothesis. *J. Pers. Soc. Psychol., 50*(4), 761–769.

Goodenough, O. R., & Prehn, K. (2004). A neuroscientific approach to normative judgment in law and justice. *Philos. Trans. R. Soc. Lond. B Biol. Sci., 359*(1451), 1709–1726.

Gottfried, K. (1999). Moral calculus and the bomb. *Nature, 401*(6749), 117.

Grafman, J. (1995). Similarities and distinctions among current models of prefrontal cortical functions. *Ann. N Y Acad. Sci., 769,* 337–368.

Greene, J. D. (2007). Why are VMPFC patients more utilitarian? A dual-process theory of moral judgment explains. *Trends Cogn. Sci., 11*(8), 322–323. author reply 323–324.

Greene, J. D., Nystrom, L. E., Engell, A. D., Darley, J. M., & Cohen, J. D. (2004). The neural bases of cognitive conflict and control in moral judgment. *Neuron, 44*(2), 389–400.

Greene, J. D., Sommerville, R. B., Nystrom, L. E., Darley, T. M., & Cohen, J. D. (2001). An fMRI investigation of emotional engagement in moral judgment. *Science, 293*(5537), 2105–2108.

Haidt, J. (2001). The emotional dog and its rational tail: A social intuitionist approach to moral judgment. *Psychological Review, 108*(4), 814–834.

Haidt, J. (2003). The moral emotions. In R. J. Davidson, K. R. Scherer, & H. H. Goldsmith (Eds.), *Handbook of affective sciences* (pp. 852–870). Oxford, UK: Oxford University Press.

Haidt, J., & Graham, J. (2007). When morality opposes justice: conservatives have moral intuitions that liberals may not recognize. *Soc. Justice Res., 20*(1), 98–116.

Hare, R. D. (2003). *The Hare Psychopathy Checklist-Revised.* Toronto, Canada: Multi-Health Systems.

Harenski, C. L., & Hamann, S. (2006). Neural correlates of regulating negative emotions related to moral violations. *Neuroimage, 30*(1), 313–324.

Harlow, H. F., & Suomi, S. J. (1970). Nature of love-simplified. *Am. Psychol., 25,* 161–168.

Heekeren, H. R., Wartenburger, I., Schmidt, H., Prehn, K., Schwintowski, H. P., et al. (2005). Influence of bodily harm on neural correlates of semantic and moral decision-making. *Neuroimage, 24*(3), 887–897.

Heekeren, H. R., Wartenburger, I., Schmidt, H., Schwintowski, H. P., & Villringer, A. (2003). An fMRI study of simple ethical decision-making. *Neuroreport, 14*(9), 1215–1219.

Hume, D. (1739/1984). *A treatise of human nature.* New York: Penguin Classics.

Insel, T. R. (1997). A neurobiological basis of social attachment. *Am. J. Psychiatry, 154*(6), 726–735.

Insel, T. R., & Fernald, R. D. (2004). How the brain processes social information: searching for the social brain. *Annu. Rev. Neurosci., 27,* 697–722.

Insel, T. R., Winslow, J. T., Wang, Z., & Young, L. J (1998). Oxytocin, vasopressin, and the neuroendocrine basis of pair bond formation. *Adv. Exp. Med. Biol., 449,* 215–224.

Insel, T. R., & Young, L. J. (2001). The neurobiology of attachment. *Nat. Rev. Neurosci., 2*(2), 129–136.

Jones, D. (2007). Moral psychology: The depths of disgust. *Nature, 447*(7146), 768–771.

Kagan, J. (1984). *The nature of the child.* New York: Basic Books.

Keverne, E. B., & Curley, J. P. (2004). Vasopressin, oxytocin and social behaviour. *Curr. Opin. Neurobiol., 14*(6), 777–783.

Kiehl, K. A., Smith, A. M., Mendrek, A., Forster, B., & Hare, R. D. (2004). Temporal lobe abnormalities in semantic processing by criminal psychopaths as revealed by functional magnetic resonance imaging. *Psychiatry Res., 130*(3), 297–312.

Kim, S. H., & Hamann, S. (2007). Neural correlates of positive and negative emotion regulation. *J. Cogn. Neurosci., 19*(5), 776–798.

King-Casas, B., Tomlin, D., Anen, C., Camerer, C. F., Quartz, S. R., et al. (2005). Getting to know you: Reputation and trust in a two-person economic exchange. *Science, 308*(5718), 78–83.

Kirsch, P., Esslinger, C., Chen, Q., Mier, D., Lis, S., et al. (2005). Oxytocin modulates neural circuitry for social cognition and fear in humans. *J. Neurosci., 25*(49), 11489–11493.

Knoch, D., Pascual-Leone, A., Meyer, K., Treyer, V., & Fehr, E. (2006). Diminishing reciprocal fairness by disrupting the right prefrontal cortex. *Science, 314*(5800), 829–832.

Koenigs, M., & Tranel, D. (2007). Irrational economic decision-making after ventromedial prefrontal damage: evidence from the Ultimatum Game. *J. Neurosci., 27*(4), 951–956.

Koenigs, M., Young, L., Adolphs, R., Tranel, D., Cushman, F., et al. (2007). Damage to the prefrontal cortex increases utilitarian moral judgements. *Nature, 446*(7138), 908–911.

Kosfeld, M., Heinrichs, M., Zak, P. J., Fischbacher, U., & Fehr, E. (2005). Oxytocin increases trust in humans. *Nature, 435*(7042), 673–676.

Kringelbach, M. L. (2005). The human orbitofrontal cortex: linking reward to hedonic experience. *Nat. Rev. Neurosci., 6*(9), 691–702.

Krueger, F., McCabe, K., Moll, J., Kriegeskorte, N., Zahn, R., et al. (2007). Neural correlates of trust. *Proc. Natl. Acad. Sci., 104,* 20084–20089.

Lawrence, A. D., Calder, A. J., McGowan, S. W., & Grasby, P. M. (2002). Selective disruption of the recognition of facial expressions of anger. *Neuroreport, 13*(6), 881–884.

Luo, Q., Nakic, M., Wheatley, T., Richell, R., Martin, A., et al. (2006). The neural basis of implicit moral attitude—an IAT study using event-related fMRI. *Neuroimage, 30*(4), 1449–1457.

MacIntyre, A. (1985). *After virtue.* London: Duckworth.

MacLean, P. (1973). *A triune concept of the brain and behaviour: Hincks memorial lecture.* Oxford, UK: University of Toronto Press.

Macmillan, M. (2000). *An odd kind of fame: Stories of Phineas Gage.* Cambridge, MA: MIT Press.

Maimonides, M. (1912). *The eight chapters of Maimonides on ethics: Shemonah perakim. A psychological and ethical treatise.* New York: Columbia University Press.

Maynard-Smith, J., & Szathmary, E. (1997). *The major transitions in evolution.* New York: Oxford University Press.

McClure, S. M., Botvinick, M. M., Yeung, J. D., & Cohen, J. D. (in press). Conflict monitoring in cognition-emotion competition. In J. J. Gross (Ed.), *Handbook of emotion regulation.* New York: Guilford Press.

Mega, M., Cummings, J., Salloway, S., & Malloy, P. (1997). The limbic system: An anatomic, phylogenetic, and clinical perspective. *J. Neuropsychiatry Clin. Neurosci.*, *9*(3), 315–330.

Mendez, M. F., Chow, T., Ringman, J., Twitchell, G., & Hinkin, C. H. (2000). Pedophilia and Temporal Lobe Disturbances. *J. Neuropsychiatry Clin. Neurosci.*, *12*(1), 71–76.

Milinski, M., Semmann, D., & Krambeck, H.-J. (2002). Reputation helps solve the "tragedy of the commons." *Nature*, *415*(6870), 424–426.

Miller, E. K., & Cohen, J. D. (2001). An integrative theory of prefrontal cortex function. *Annu. Rev. Neurosci.*, *24*, 167–202.

Moll, J., & de Oliveira-Souza, R. (2007). Moral judgments, emotions and the utilitarian brain. *Trends Cogn. Sci.*

Moll, J., & de Oliveira-Souza, R. (2007). Response to Greene: Moral sentiments and reason: Friends or foes? *Trends Cogn. Sci.*, *11*(8), 323–324.

Moll, J., de Oliveira-Souza, R., Bramati, I. E., & Grafman, J. (2002). Functional networks in emotional moral and nonmoral social judgments. *Neuroimage*, *16*(3 Pt 1), 696–703.

Moll, J., de Oliveira-Souza, R., Eslinger, P. J., Gramati, I. E., & Mourão-Miranda, J. (2002). The neural correlates of moral sensitivity: a functional magnetic resonance imaging investigation of basic and moral emotions. *J. Neurosci.*, *22*(7), 2730–2736.

Moll, J., de Oliveira-Souza, R., & Eslinger, P. J. (2003). Morals and the human brain: A working model. *Neuroreport*, *14*(3), 299–305.

Moll, J., de Oliveira-Souza, R., Garrido, G. J., Bramati, I. E., Caparelli-Daquer, E. M. A., et al. (2007). The self as a moral agent: Linking the neural bases of social agency and moral sensitivity. *Social Neuroscience*, *2*, 336–352.

Moll, J., de Oliveira-Souza, R., Moll, F. T., Ignacio, F. A., Bramati, I. E., et al. (2005). The moral affiliations of disgust: A functional MRI study. *Cogn. Behav. Neurol.*, *18*(1), 68–78.

Moll, J., de Oliveira-Souza, R., Zahn, R., & Grafman, J. (2007). The cognitive neuroscience of moral emotions. In W. Sinnott-Armstrong (Ed.), *Moral psychology, Volume 3: Morals and the brain*. Cambridge, MA: MIT Press.

Moll, J., Eslinger, P. J., & de Oliveira-Souza, R. (2001). Frontopolar and anterior temporal cortex activation in a moral judgment task: Preliminary functional MRI results in normal subjects. *Arq Neuropsiquiatr*, *59*(3-B), 657–664.

Moll, J., Krueger, F., Zahn, R., Pardini, M., de Oliveira-Souza, R., et al. (2006). Human fronto-mesolimbic networks guide decisions about charitable donation. *Proc. Natl. Acad. Sci.*, *103*(42), 15623–15628.

Moll, J., Zahn, R., de Oliveira-Souza, R., Krueger, F., & Grafman, J. (2005). Opinion: The neural basis of human moral cognition. *Nat. Rev. Neurosci.*, *6*(10), 799–809.

Morgan, D., Grant, K. A., Gage, H. D., Mach, R. H., & Kaplan, J. R. (2002). Social dominance in monkeys: Dopamine D2 receptors and cocaine self-administration. *Nat. Neurosci.*, *5*(2), 169–174.

Muehlenbein, M. P., Watts, D. P., & Whitten, P. L. (2004). Dominance rank and fecal testosterone levels in adult male chimpanzees (Pan troglodytes schweinfurthii) at Ngogo, Kibale National Park, Uganda. *Am. J. Primatol.*, *64*(1), 71–82.

Nowak, M. A., & Sigmund, K. (2005). Evolution of indirect reciprocity. *Nature*, *437*(7063), 1291–1298.

Ochsner, K. N., Ray, R. D., Cooper, J. C., Robertson, E. R., Chopra, S., et al. (2004). For better or for worse: Neural systems supporting the cognitive down- and up-regulation of negative emotion. *Neuroimage*, *23*(2), 483–499.

Okuda, J., Fujii, T., Ohtake, H., Tsukura, T., Tanji, K., et al. (2003). Thinking of the future and past: The roles of the frontal pole and the medial temporal lobes. *Neuroimage*, *19*(4), 1369–1380.

Park, K. (2000). The organic soul. In C. B. Schmitt & Q. Skinner (Eds.), *The Cambridge history of renaissance philosophy* (pp. 464–484). Cambridge, UK: Cambridge University Press.

Raine, A., & Yang, Y. (2006). The neuroanatomical bases of psychopathy: A review of brain imaging findings. In C. J. Patrick (Ed.), *Handbook of psychopathy* (pp. 278–312). New York: Guilford Press.

Robb, J. E. (1998). The archaeology of symbols. *Ann. Rev. Anthropol.*, *27*, 329–346.

Rozin, P. (1999). The process of moralization. *Psychological Science*, *10*, 218–221.

Rozin, P., & Haidt, J. (1993). Disgust. In M. Lewis & J.M. Haviland (Eds.), *Handbook of emotions*. New York: Guilford Press.

Rozin, P., Lowery, L., Imada, S., & Haidt, J. (1999). The CAD triad hypothesis: A mapping between three moral emotions (contempt, anger, disgust) and three moral codes (community, autonomy, divinity). *J. Pers. Soc. Psychol.*, *76*(4), 574–586.

Sanfey, A. G., Rilling, J. K., Aronson, J. A., Nystrom, L. E., & Cohen, J. D. (2003). The neural basis of economic decision-making in the ultimatum game. *Science*, *300*(5626), 1755–1758.

Saver, J. L., & Damasio, A. R. (1991). Preserved access and processing of social knowledge in a patient with acquired sociopathy due to ventromedial frontal damage. *Neuropsychologia*, *29*(12), 1241–1249.

Schaich Borg, J., Hynes, C., Van Horn, J., Grafton, S., & Sinnott-Armstrong, W. (2006). Consequences, action, and intention as factors in moral judgments: An fMRI investigation. *J. Cogn. Neurosci.*, *18*(5), 803–817.

Schulkin, J. (2000). *Roots of social sensitivity and neural function*. Cambridge, MA: MIT Press.

Schulkin, J. (2004). *Bodily sensibility: Intelligent action*. New York: Oxford University Press.

Schwartz, S. H. (1992). Universals in the content and structure of values – theoretical advances and empirical tests in 20 countries. *Advances in Experimental Social Psychology*, *25*, 1–65.

Shallice, T., & Burgess, P. (1996). The domain of supervisory processes and temporal organization of behaviour. *Philos. Trans. R Soc. Lond. B Biol. Sci.*, *351*(1346), 1405–1411. discussion 1411–1412.

Singer, T., Kiebel, S. J., Winston, J. S., Dolan, R., & Frith, G. (2004). Brain responses to the acquired moral status of faces. *Neuron*, *41*, 653–662.

Singer, W. (2001). Consciousness and the binding problem. *Ann. N Y Acad. Sci.*, *929*, 123–146.

Smith, A. (1759/1966). *The theory of moral sentiments*. New York: Kelly.

Stone, V. E., Cosmides, L., Tooby, J., Kroll, N., & Knight, R. T. (2002). Selective impairment of reasoning about social exchange in a patient with bilateral limbic system damage. *Proc. Natl. Acad. Sci.*, *99*(17), 11531–11536.

Tangney, J. P., Stuewig, J., & Mashek, D. J. (2007). Moral emotions and moral behavior. *Annu. Rev. Psychol.*, *58*, 345–372.

Thomson, J. (1985). The Trolley Problem. *Yale Law Journal*, *94*, 1395–1415.

Tranel, D., Bechara, A., & Denburg, N. L. (2002). Asymmetric functional roles of right and left ventromedial prefrontal cortices in social conduct, decision-making, and emotional processing. *Cortex*, *38*(4), 589–612.

Trivers, R. L. (1971). The evolution of reciprocal altruism. *The Quarterly Review of Biology*, *46*, 35–57.

Vogel, G. (2004). Behavioral evolution. The evolution of the golden rule. *Science*, *303*(5661), 1128–1131.

Volavka, J. (1999). The neurobiology of violence: An update. *J. Neuropsychiatry Clin. Neurosci.*, *11*(3), 307–314.

Weissenberger, A. A., Dell, M. L., Liow, K., Theodore, W., Frattali, C. M., et al. (2001). Aggression and psychiatric comorbidity in children with hypothalamic hamartomas and their unaffected siblings. *J. Am. Acad. Child Adolesc. Psychiatry*, *40*(6), 696–703.

Welt, L. (1888). Ueber Charakterveraenderungen des Menschen. *Dtsch. Arch. Klin. Med.*, *42*, 339–390.

Wood, J. N., & Grafman, J. (2003). Human prefrontal cortex: processing and representational perspectives. *Nat. Rev. Neurosci.*, *4*(2), 139–147.

Young, L. J., & Wang, Z. (2004). The neurobiology of pair bonding. *Nat. Neurosci.*, *7*(10), 1048–1054.

Young, S. N., & Leyton, M. (2002). The role of serotonin in human mood and social interaction. Insight from altered tryptophan levels. *Pharmacol. Biochem. Behav.*, *71*(4), 857–865.

Zahn, R., Moll, J., Krueger, F., Huey, E. P., & Garrido, G. (2007). Social concepts are represented in the superior anterior temporal cortex. *Proc. Natl. Acad. Sci.*, *104*(15), 6430–6435.

Zak, P. J., Kurzban, R., & Matzner, W. T. (2004). The neurobiology of trust. *Ann. N Y Acad. Sci.*, *1032*, 224–227.

Zeki, S., & Goodenough, O. (2004). Law and the brain: Introduction. *Philos. Trans. R Soc. Lond. B Biol. Sci.*, *359*(1451), 1661–1665.

Intention, Choice, and the Medial Frontal Cortex

MATTHEW F.S. RUSHWORTH[a,b]

[a]*Department of Experimental Psychology, University of Oxford, South Parks Road, Oxford, United Kingdom*

[b]*Centre for Functional Magnetic Resonance Imaging of the Brain (FMRIB), John Radcliffe Hospital, University of Oxford, Oxford, United Kingdom*

The medial frontal cortex (MFC) has been identified with voluntary action selection. Recent evidence suggests that there are three principal ways in which the MFC is an essential part of the neural circuit for voluntary action selection. First, the MFC represents the reinforcement values of actions and is concerned with the updating of those action values. Because it is particularly concerned with the rate at which action values should be updated, it mediates the influence that the past reinforcement history has over the next choice that is made and it may determine the learning rate. The MFC's representation of action value does not just reflect the potential reward associations of an action but instead represents both the reward and effort costs that are intrinsic to the action. Second, the MFC is important when an exploratory action is generated in order to obtain more information about action values and the environment. Third, the MFC is critical when conflicting information in the immediate environment instructs more than one possible response. In such situations the MFC exerts an influence over how actions will be chosen by other motor regions of the brain.

Key words: action value; medial frontal cortex (MFC); supplementary eye field (SEF); voluntary action selection

Introduction

The cortex on the medial frontal surface of the brain consists of several component regions but is often referred to collectively as the medial frontal cortex (MFC). For some time we have known that it plays a critical role in the transformation of an intention into an action. Patients with lesions of the MFC make few spontaneous movements and say little—they are described as mute and akinetic (Devinsky et al. 1995; Laplane et al. 1977). Such effects are reported after lesions to more than one MFC subdivision and have meant that the MFC has been linked to volition and is sometimes thought to be necessary for the exercise of free will.

There is a widely held view that actions are selected by an animal or a person for one of two reasons (Passingham 1993). On the one hand an animal might make an action because of the appearance of a stimulus that is associated with the action. If we consider the example of someone driving a car, then the decision about which pedal to press may be a consequence of the driver seeing a red or a green traffic light signal. The red light is associated with one action, pressing down on the brake, while the green light is associated with quite another. The action that is selected is instructed by the presentation of the cue.

We know that in such situations action selection depends on several areas on the lateral surface of the frontal lobe (Koechlin & Summerfield 2007; Passingham 1993; Petrides 2005; Wise & Murray 2000). The lateral prefrontal cortex identifies stimuli that are relevant for behavior. In the macaque the activity of lateral prefrontal neurons reflects which stimuli will be used to guide behavior (Everling et al. 2002; Rainer et al. 1998), and lesions of ventrolateral prefrontal cortex impair the ability to identify behaviorally relevant stimuli unless they are immediately adjacent to the focus of action (Rushworth et al. 2005). Functional magnetic resonance imaging (fMRI) experiments suggest a similar area in the human brain has a similar function; activation changes reflect the selection of task-relevant information (Brass & von Cramon 2004). The activity of neurons in lateral prefrontal cortex and

Address for correspondence: M.F.S. Rushworth, Department of Experimental Psychology, University of Oxford, South Parks Road, Oxford, OX1 3UD, England, UK.
matthew.rushworth@psy.ox.ac.uk

particularly in the dorsal premotor cortex (PMd) reflect the actual stimulus–action association (Boussaoud & Wise 1993a; Boussaoud & Wise 1993b; Muhammad et al. 2006; Wallis & Miller 2003a; Wallis & Miller 2003b). Again, fMRI studies and investigations of the effect of disrupting PMd with transcranial magnetic stimulation (TMS) confirm that human PMd has a similar role (Amiez et al. 2006b; Boorman et al. 2007; Koechlin et al. 2003; O'Shea et al. 2007; O'Shea et al. in press)

In other situations, however, cues in the environment do not provide clear instructions about which action to make. Instead, in some situations, people and animals appear to act voluntarily and to decide for themselves what to do. It is in these situations that the MFC seems most important. In some cases there may be no obvious cue instructing action. In other cases it seems intuitively appealing to think that subjects have acted voluntarily because the instructing stimuli are ambiguous; there may be more than one stimulus, and they may instruct contradictory ways of responding or unexpected ways of responding. Recent research suggests that each MFC subdivision makes distinct contributions to the decision to act in such situations.

Voluntary Action and the Prospect of Reinforcement

Many of the choices organisms make are guided by an assessment of the expected value of the outcome that it is hoped will follow the action. As a general rule, whenever confronted by more than one possible course of action, an organism's goal is to pursue the option which results in the greatest utility—the option with the greatest value to the organism given its current motivational state and other constraining factors. Action selection is therefore thought to be based on the utility associated with each alternative. Once the action has been selected the outcome is received. Reinforcement learning theory describes how the valuation of the chosen action is revised in the light of any discrepancy between the expected and actual outcome (Sutton & Barto 1998). Thus decision making depends on two interdependent processes of value-based selection and value revision during learning. The anterior cingulate cortex (ACC) division of the MFC is central to both of these processes. The important region is centered on the dorsal bank of the sulcus of the ACC just anterior to a region called the rostral cingulate motor area (CMAr). Microstimulation in CMAr elicits limb movements, and tracer injections label motor regions of the spinal cord, (Dum & Strick 1996; Luppino et al. 1991). Although the more anterior parts of the ACC are almost certainly interconnected with CMAr, they are not directly connected to the spinal cord, and so they are likely to be less directly concerned with movement execution.

Some of the clearest evidence that ACC is involved in both value-guided action selection and in value revision comes from the work of K. Matsumoto, M. Matsumoto, and colleagues (Matsumoto et al. 2003; Matsumoto et al. 2007). In one experiment Matsumoto and colleagues (2003) trained macaques to select one of two responses to one of two stimuli during blocks of trials in which reward or no-reward was expected. The activity of most of a group of neurons in the MFC centered on the ACC sulcus encoded little information about the instructing cues, but many neurons encoded whether or not a reward was to be expected on a given trial, the type of action required, or both information about action selection and the expected reward. By contrast, neurons in the lateral prefrontal cortex were more likely to code information about the identity of the visual stimuli.

Not only do the neurons encode information pertinent to the guidance of action selection, but their activity is modulated when it is necessary to revise the estimate of the value of the outcome associated with an action. For some time it has been known that ACC neurons are active when monkeys make errors and fail to obtain anticipated rewards (Niki & Watanabe 1979; Shima & Tanji 1998). It is now clear that it is not just the occurrence of an error that is being detected but the need for revision of the action's value that appears to be represented in the activity of ACC neurons. Matsumoto and colleagues (2007) trained macaques to select one of two movements on the basis of presentations of a secondary reinforcer. Some neurons ("positive feedback"–preferring neurons) were responsive when the secondary reinforcer was presented, while others were more active when the secondary reinforcer was absent and another stimulus with no reinforcement association was presented ("negative feedback"–preferring neurons) (FIG. 1). Importantly, however, neurons in both classes were more active on the first trial of a new learning problem. The neurons became relatively inactive once the monkey had worked out which response was associated with delivery of the secondary reinforcer and therefore had the higher value.

Matsumoto and colleagues argued that the neurons were encoding action-value prediction errors. When monkeys obtained feedback on the first trial of a new problem they would either experience the actual outcome, positive feedback, as better than expected,

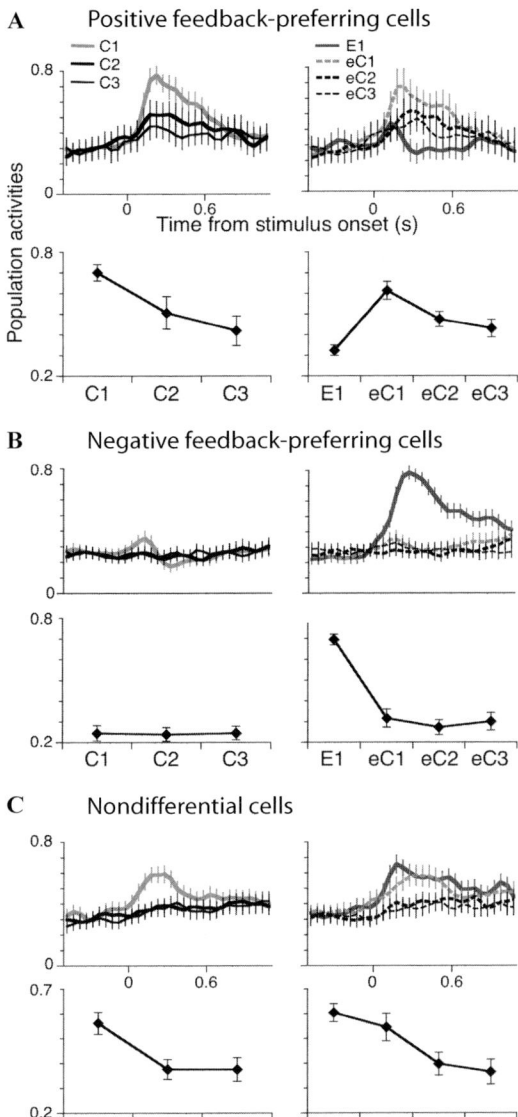

a positive prediction error, or if the feedback was negative, as worse than predicted and therefore as a negative prediction error. Once the monkey had worked out which response was associated with the positive feedback, however, there would be little discrepancy between the expected and the actual outcome. In some neurons activity encoded positive prediction errors, while in others it encoded negative prediction errors. A third class of neuron encoded both positive and negative prediction errors. What was important for these neurons was not so much whether the feedback indicated that the action's value estimate needed to be revised up or down but just simply the fact that it needed to be revised. By contrast, neurons in the lateral prefrontal cortex were less selective for particular types of prediction error and more likely to also be active in relation to other changes, for example, changes in visual stimulus identity.

A similar conclusion, that the ACC does not just detect errors but rather represents the discrepancy between predicted and actual outcomes and therefore the need to revise action values, was reached by another group of investigators. Amiez and colleagues (2005; Procyk et al. in press) also recorded from the macaque ACC. Although they focused on error trials, they examined ACC activity when the monkey had different levels of reward expectation. The responses of ACC neurons reflected not only the occurrence of the error but also the prior reward expectation.

In summary the anatomy of the macaque ACC suggests both that it is informed when actions are selected by other premotor areas and that it is in a position to influence action selection processes in those areas. The neurophysiology of the macaque ACC suggests that it represents the reinforcement values of the actions that are selected and that it is especially important when the values of those actions must be revised.

FIGURE 1. Changes of activity in the population of MFC neurons centered on the ACC sulcus during the course of correct-action learning: Averaged responses of 16 positive feedback–preferring cells (**A**), 32 negative feedback–preferring cells (**B**), and 34 nondifferential cells (**C**). Bin width in upper graphs in each section, 50 ms. The activity of each cell was normalized by its peak activity and then averaged across cells. Each graph shows activity across three trials of a typical problem set. On the first trial animals did not know which was the correct action to choose. On half of trials the animals guessed correctly and chose the action associated with a positive secondary reinforcer (data from these trials are labeled C1). Usually the animals continued to choose correctly on the subsequent trials on these blocks (data from these trials are labeled C2 and C3). Data from these blocks are shown on the left of the figure. The right-hand side of the figure shows data from the other half of blocks on which the monkeys' first choices were incorrect (E1 trial). The monkeys usually corrected their choices on the subsequent three trials (labeled eC1, eC2, and eC3). Positive feedback–preferring neurons and non differential neurons were active in relation to the positive prediction error when the first choice was made correctly but subsequently decreased their activity once the correct choice was known. Negative feedback–preferring neurons and nondifferential neurons were active in relation to the negative prediction error when the first choice was made incorrectly but subsequently decreased their activity once the correct choice was known. (Reprinted with permission from Matsumoto et al., *Nature Neuroscience*, 2007.)

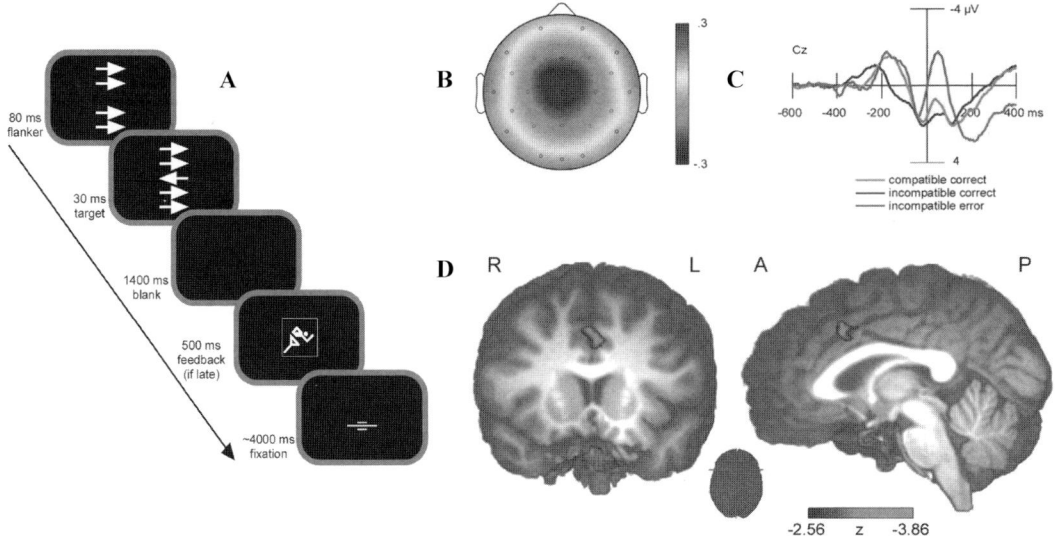

FIGURE 2. (A) Sequence of stimulus events in the speeded flanker task. Participants viewed four task-irrelevant flanker arrows, followed by a central arrow that indicated the response direction and pointed to the same or opposite direction as flanker arrows. Compatible (same direction) and incompatible (opposite direction) trials appeared in randomized order and with the same probability. For trials in which subjects responded slower than a dynamically adapting individual response deadline, a symbolic feedback occurred urging the subject to speed up in consecutive trials. **(B)** Grand mean topography of an independent component identified with the error-related negativity (ERN) isolated from simultaneous recordings of the electroencephalogram (EEG) while concurrently recording fMRI data (after root-mean-square normalization and in arbitrary units). **(C)** Grand average (13 subjects) independent component activation event–related potentials for the vertex electrode (Cz), time-locked to response-onset times (negativity plotted upwards) on correctly performed compatible trials (green), correctly performed incompatible trials (blue), and incompatible error trials (red). The ERN can be seen just after response onset on the error trials. **(D)** fMRI signal in the cingulate sulcus (x, y, z)_0, 17, 42; z__3.86) correlated with single-trial amplitudes of the ERN related independent component from the EEG signal solely in the RCZ along the banks of the cingulate sulcus [center of gravity at coordinates (x, y, z)_0, 17, 42; z__3.86]. The left part shows the coronal view; the right part shows the sagittal view on the right hemisphere. The red lines on the middle top view inset indicate slice sections (R, Right; L, left; A, anterior; P, posterior). Adapted from Debener et al. (*Journal of Neuroscience*, 2005) with permission.

The Encoding of Errors and Other Outcomes in the Human ACC

It is sometimes argued that the anatomy and function of ACC and prefrontal cortex (PFC) regions may have changed considerably during primate speciation (Nimchinsky et al. 1999), but there is evidence that the human ACC has a similar role in representing the outcomes of actions, particularly when there is a need to revise the valuation of an action. An event-related potential (ERP), often referred to as the error-related negativity (ERN), can be recorded from scalp electrodes placed over the frontal midline when human subjects make mistakes and select the wrong action (Falkenstein et al. 1991; Gehring et al. 1993). Debener and colleagues (2005) have recorded the ERN while simultaneously recording the blood oxygenation level dependent (BOLD) signal while subjects performed a "flanker" task as quickly as possible.

In the flanker test, subjects have to make one of two movements depending on the direction of a centrally presented arrow. The central arrow is flanked by pictures of other arrows that the subject is told are irrelevant and can be ignored. Reaction times (RTs) are slower and responses are more often incorrect when the flanking arrows point in a direction that is incongruent with that indicated by the central arrow. Debener and colleagues looked for brain regions in which the BOLD signal was related to trial-by-trial differences in the ERN; they argued that the ERN originates from the ACC because the ACC BOLD signal on error trials was correlated with the size of the ERN (FIG. 2). Several other fMRI studies concur in reporting BOLD signal increases in the ACC when errors are made under a variety of circumstances (Garavan et al. 2003; Holroyd et al. 2004; Magno et al. 2006; Ullsperger et al. 2007; Ullsperger & von Cramon 2001; Ullsperger & von Cramon 2003) sometimes even when subjects

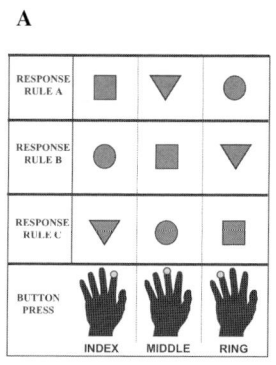 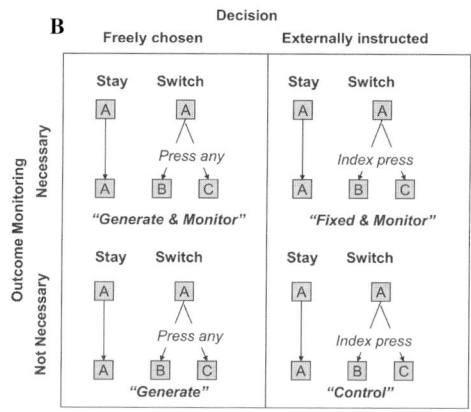

FIGURE 3. (A) Representation of the three response rules linking stimulus shapes to finger press actions during the task. **(B)** The four conditions constituted a factorial design. The first factor was the type of decision that was made by the subjects when they selected a candidate action after the cue informing them that the rule had changed. In the "generate and monitor" and the "generate" conditions, the subjects' had a free choice, but in the "fixed and monitor" and control conditions the subjectsdecision was externally determined. The second factor concerned the need to monitor the outcome of the decision. In the "generate and monitor" and the "fixed and monitor" conditions it was necessary to monitor the outcome of the decision, but the need to monitor outcomes was reduced in the "generate" and "control" conditions. Both factors were determinants of ACC activity (FIG. 4). (Reprinted with permission from Walton et al., *Nature Neuroscience*, 2004.)

are not aware that a mistake has been made or even when there is no strategic intention to correct errors (Fiehler et al. 2004; Hester et al. 2005; Klein et al. 2007).

In this task there was not the same opportunity for the human subjects to revise their estimates of the actions' values in quite such a straightforward way as the monkeys had done in the experiment conducted by Matsumoto and colleagues (2007); the subjects were told which way to respond at the beginning of the experiment, and the rules did not change during task performance. Subjects did, however, appear to revise their estimate of the value of responding quickly after an incorrect response was made. Not only did they slow down their speed of responding in both the flanker task and in a related antisaccade task after making a mistake, but the size of both the ERN and the ACC BOLD signal recorded on the error trial was correlated with the degree of slowing on the subsequent trial (Debener et al. 2005; Klein et al. 2007).

The ACC has been shown to be active when there are errors in a number of situations, but in many cases the errors that occur are inadvertent slips made under time pressure as in the study conducted by Debener and colleagues. Moreover in many experiments there is an asymmetry inasmuch as subjects can find out that, unexpectedly, they have responded incorrectly, but they rarely find they have responded correctly unexpectedly. In other words, unlike in the paradigm Matsumoto and colleagues (2007) taught to monkeys, positive prediction errors are not as likely as negative prediction errors.

Walton and colleagues (2004), however, devised a task in which human subjects revised the way that they selected actions in response to both positive and negative feedback. They taught human subjects to make one of three different possible actions in response to the presentation of three differently shaped visual stimuli. The stimuli were linked to the actions according to three different sets of rules (FIG. 3A). According to one set of rules, stimuli A, B, and C were mapped onto actions 1, 2, and 3, respectively, while according to the alternative rule sets they were mapped onto actions 3, 1, and 2, respectively, or actions 2, 3, and 1, respectively. In other words, the value of each action depended on the context provided by the stimulus on that trial and by the rule set currently in effect.

In some conditions cues told subjects which rule set was currently in effect (standard condition [S]). In another condition (generate and monitor [G&M] condition, experiment 2, FIG. 3B), there was no explicit instruction telling subjects which rule set to follow, only a cue telling them that the rule had changed in some way. In this condition subjects had to try making an exploratory action and then they had to monitor the feedback that followed in order to work out the current rule set. In this condition the ACC was found to be active (FIG. 4A, B). Moreover, on average, the ACC was active as long as the subject had to update the estimate of the action value in the context of each stimu-

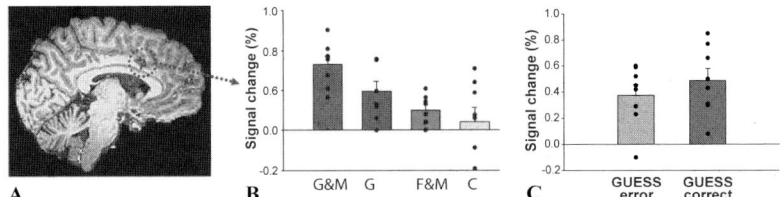

FIGURE 4. Monitoring the outcome of actions in order to establish the correct task set. **(A)** The region of significant ACC activation. The activation was actually derived by comparing the G&M and F&M conditions. **(B)** Percentage signal change in the region shown in part a in four conditions. In the "generate and monitor" (G&M) condition subjects had a free decision about which exploratory action to select and they had to monitor the outcome of that decision. In the "fixed and monitor" (F&M) condition subjects were instructed to always attempt the same action when the task sets changed. The F&M condition retained the element of outcome monitoring, but the initial choice of which action to make was not voluntary. In the "generate" condition, (G), the element of free decision making was retained, but the element of outcome monitoring was reduced by telling subjects that whatever exploratory action was generated it would be correct. In the fourth "control" condition (C) of the factorial design, choices were externally determined rather than free and the need for outcome monitoring was reduced—subjects were told which action to make and the instruction was always correct. ACC activation was a function of both the experimentally manipulated factors; it was determined by both the type of action (freely chosen exploratory action versus externally determined action, G&M and G versus F&M and C) and by the need for monitoring the outcome of the decision (G&M and F&M versus G and C). **(C)** Activations in the G condition were not specific to trials on which subjects made mistakes; there was a similar degree of signal change even on the trials on which subjects guessed correctly. Adapted from Walton et al., (2004) (*Nature Neuroscience*, 2004) with permission.

lus regardless of whether the feedback was positive or negative (FIG. 4C) as would have been predicted by the results of the single neuron recording study conducted by Matsumoto and colleagues (2007).

In summary it is clear that the human ACC, just like monkey ACC, is active when errors are made. ERN measurements demonstrate that similar activity occurs not just when we make mistakes but when we see other people make mistakes (Van Schie et al. 2004). Error detection is essential for ensuring that further mistakes do not occur when subsequent responses are made (Holroyd et al. 2005). ACC activity may precede the overt occurrence of a potential error, and some recent results suggest that it may even have a role in forestalling the occurrence of a mistake when the current response is made (Magno et al. 2006). There is now increasing agreement that error-related activity has a role to play in learning (Holroyd & Coles 2002; Mars et al. 2005). While early accounts of the ACC role in learning emphasized its importance for detecting mistakes and negative prediction errors, it is now apparent that the ACC is equally important when action values must be revised upwards as well as downwards.

Detecting Errors versus Representing Reinforcement History

The experiments of Matsumoto, Amiez, and colleagues (Amiez et al. 2005; Matsumoto et al. 2007) demonstrate ACC activity when the unexpected presence or absence of reinforcing feedback indicates there is a need to revise the estimate of an action's value. The value of an action does not, however, depend solely on the most recent outcome but on the extended history of reinforcement that is associated with it. A recent investigation of the effect of ACC lesions in the macaque suggests that the ACC mediates the influence that the reinforcement history will have on subsequent choices (Kennerley et al. 2006). Kennerley and colleagues (2006) taught macaques to either pull or turn the same lever to obtain food rewards. In one experiment the reward was associated with only one action at a time but which action was correct changed periodically. Which action was made by the animal was normally a function of the reinforcement each had produced over the course of about five trials (FIG. 5A, B). After an ACC lesion, however, choices were only influenced by the most recent action outcome rather than the more extended history of reinforcement associated with the action.

The deficit in the response reversal task reported by Kennerley and colleagues (2006) cannot be interpreted as simply a failure to change responses when errors occurred because there was no difference between the performance levels of ACC and control groups on the trial that immediately followed errors. This is apparent in FIGURE 5 (C, D) which shows performance on the first trial after an error (error+1 trial) on the left

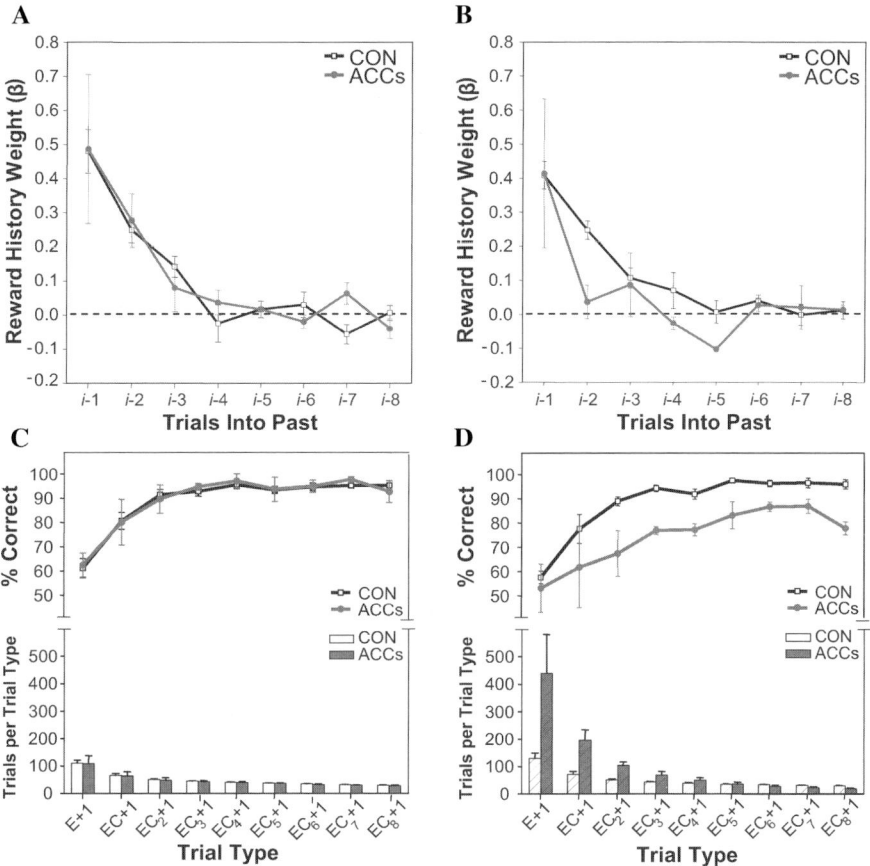

FIGURE 5. Estimates of the influence of previous reward history on current choice in control animals and animals with ACC sulcus lesions. Performance in the preoperative period **(A)** and postoperative period **(B)** is shown. Each point represents a group's mean regression coefficient value (± SEM) derived from multiple logistic regression analyses of choice on the current trial (i) against the outcomes (rewarded or unrewarded) on the previous eight trials for each animal. The height of the line can be read as an index of the influence of a previous outcome on the next choice that is made. The influence of the previous trial's outcome (i–1) is shown on the left-hand side of each figure, the influence of the outcome two trials back (i–2) is shown next, and so on up until the trial that occurred eight trials previously (i–8). Control and ACC_S lesion data are shown by the black and grey lines, respectively. While the choices of controls were influenced by outcomes that had occurred several trials previously, the choices of animals with ACC sulcus lesions were only influenced by the most recent outcome. **(C, D)** Sustaining rewarded behavior following an error. Pre- (a) and postoperative (b) performances are shown on separate figures. Each line graph shows the mean percentage of trials of each type that were correct (±SEM) for each group. Control and ACC lesion data are shown by the black and grey lines, respectively. The trial types are plotted across the x-axis and start on the left with the trial immediately following an error (E + 1). The next data point corresponds to the trial after one error and then a correct response (EC + 1), the one after corresponds to the trial after one error and then two correct responses (EC + 2), and so on. Moving from the left to the right of each panel corresponds to the animal acquiring more instances of positive reinforcement, after making the correct action, subsequent to an earlier error. The histogram in the bottom part of each graph indicates the number of instances of each trial type (±SEM). White and grey bars indicate the control and ACC_S lesion data respectively, while hatched bars indicate data from the postoperative session. Adapted from Kennerley et al. (*Nature Neuroscience*, 2006) with permission.

hand side of the figure. Performance is relatively poor even in control animals. Even after the experience of many thousands of trials of a task, macaques do not naturally treat reinforcement absence as an unambiguous instruction to one action or another in quite the same way as they treat sensory cues which have been linked with actions through conditional associations. The probability of making the correct action increases gradually as controls have more opportunity to revise the estimate of the correct action's value. The next point, to the right on the graph, represents performance on the error+2 trial; this is the trial that follows the error+1 trial if the choice on the error+1 trial is correct. The error+3 trial is the trial that follows the error+2 trial if, in turn, that is performed correctly. Moving across the figure from left to right it is clear that in the control animals the probability of making the next action correctly increases with an accumulating history of positive reinforcement in association with that action. The probability of making the correct response does not increase as rapidly with the accumulating history of reinforcement for that action in the ACC lesion animals.

The role of the ACC in error monitoring has received considerable attention, and correct and incorrect actions may be easily categorized in the laboratory by reference to the researchers' preprogrammed and fixed experimental contingencies. It can, however, be more difficult to draw a defining line between the two types of outcome in naturalistic settings. For a foraging animal, the natural environment is more uncertain and variable than the laboratory, and both positive and negative outcomes can be a source of information about the value of actions. If an outcome is only probabilistically associated with reward then what is important is not whether a given action on a given occasion failed to lead to reward, an occurrence normally referred to as an error, but whether the action is, on average, more profitable than an alternative. In summary, although the ACC may register when an error occurs (Amiez et al. 2005; Niki & Watanabe 1979; Shima & Tanji 1998), its function may not be error detection per se but instead may represent aspects of a more extended choice–outcome history, based on both positive and negative feedback, which can be used to guide future decisions.

The activity of single neurons in the macaque ACC also reflects more information than just whether or not the last trial terminated in the receipt of reward. ACC neurons also encode aspects of the history of reinforcement associated with a choice option. Amiez and colleagues (2006a), for example, have shown that ACC neuron activity encodes the *average* value of the rewards associated with a choice option. Amiez and colleagues (2006a) taught macaques to choose between two options that were associated with different rates of differently sized rewards. For example one option was associated with 1.2 ml of juice with a probability of 0.7 and 0.4 ml juice with a probability of 0.3. After experiencing the varying reward over the course over several trials it should be possible to learn that the option's average value was therefore 0.96 ml. Other options were consistently associated with either just 1.2 ml or just 0.4 ml rewards. The average value of the probabilistic option, 0.96 ml, was 70% of the difference in value between the certain 0.4 ml option and the certain 1.2 ml options. Correspondingly the increase in activity in many ACC neurons, on presentation of the probabilistic option, was 70% of that recorded when animals were presented with the certain 1.2 ml option as opposed to the certain 0.4 ml option (Fig. 6). Encoding of the average value of an option was not seen in all the brain areas investigated with this paradigm. Procyk and colleagues (in press) have reported that, by contrast, neurons in the orbitofrontal cortex (OFC) fire at similar rates when choosing the probabilistic option and the certain 1.2 ml option. Such a pattern of activity would be expected if the OFC were encoding the predicted or preferred reward outcome.

Not only do ACC neurons represent reinforcement history parameters such as the average value of a choice option, but the activity of neurons in monosynaptically interconnected regions of the posterior cingulate cortex also reflects variance in the reward rate (McCoy & Platt 2005). McCoy and Platt (2005) taught macaques a saccadic choice paradigm. They showed that the saccadic choices of macaques are best accounted for by both the size of rewards previously associated with each option and the variation in reward size, in other words the degree to which the reward sizes deviated from the mean value. Posterior cingulate neurons were more active when the target of the saccade in the receptive field was associated with greater variation in reward size. It should be mentioned, however, that in this study reward variance was also related to preference; both macaques that were studied preferred the riskier options.

Dynamic Changes in the Values of Choices

Outside of the laboratory, in many foraging situations, the value of an action will not be static but will vary depending on which actions have already been selected. To return to the example of the monkey foraging in the wild, the value of a course of action, such

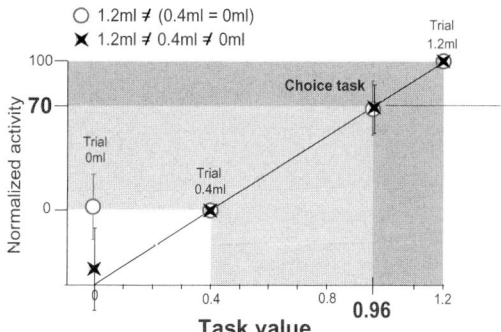

FIGURE 6. Activity of ACC neurons in the macaque to the presentation of stimuli with different associated probabilities of reward of different sizes. The right-hand side of the figure shows the neurons' activity in response to a stimulus consistently associated with 1.2 ml juice reward while the left-hand side of the figure shows the neurons' activity in response to the stimulus consistently associated with 0.4 ml juice reward. The activity recorded in each of these situations has been normalized so that the response to the 0.4 ml and the 1.2 ml rewards has become 0 and 100 on the y-axis. When the animals were given a choice between options with only probabilistic associations with reward (one option was associated with a 1.2 ml juice reward with a probability of 0.7 and 0.4 ml with a probability of 0.3, while the other stimulus was associated with a 0.4 ml juice reward with a probability of 0.7 and 1.2 ml with a probability of 0.3), the animals tended to choose the stimulus associated with the higher average reward of 0.96 ml (0.7 × 1.2 ml + 0.3 × 0.4 ml). The average expected reward of 0.96 ml occurs at the 70% point in between the reference reward expectations for the consistently rewarded stimuli. Notably, on such choice trials, ACC neural activity was also at 70% of the normalized maximum activity. The ACC neurons encode the average reward value associated with the choice of a particular option. By contrast, in the same situation when animals chose the preferred option, OFC activity was at its maximal rate. OFC neurons therefore may be encoding the predicted or preferred outcome instead of the average reward value. Consistent with the notion that the ACC may be concerned with exploring the value of options, it should also be noted that the ACC neurons encoded aspects of the animals' choices even while the animal was learning which option was the better one. By contrast the distinctive pattern of OFC activity was only seen once the animal had established a preference for one option rather than another. Adapted, with permission, from Amiez et al. (*Cerebral Cortex*, 2006) and Procyk et al. (*Attention and Performance*, XXII).

as foraging for fruit in a particular tree, will decrease if the course of action is repeated. Even if fruit is initially abundant in a given tree it will become depleted as it is consumed by the monkey. Although in the long term the tree's fruit will eventually be renewed as a result of growth, in the short term it may be better for the monkey to switch to an alternative tree even if the alternative is associated with less fruit. According to the marginal value theorem (Charnov 1976) the monkey should switch to the alternative tree once when the rate of payoff in the first tree falls below that associated with the alternative.

The dynamic foraging situation can be modeled in the laboratory using matching tasks similar to those first devised by Herrnstein et al. (1997) and used more recently with macaques by Sugrue and colleagues (2004). In a second experiment into the effect of ACC lesions Kennerley et al., (2006) programmed the two joystick movements to deliver reward with two different and independent probabilities. On any given trial the program could assign a reward to either the pull action, the turn action, both actions, or neither action. The monkey, however, had only one chance to make a response on each trial. If the monkey chose an action to which reward had been allocated then it received that reward. If a reward was assigned to an action but the action was not chosen then the "unharvested" reward was left assigned to the same action on the following trial. Reward was assigned to the other action with the same probability as usual.

In such situations the optimal strategy is not simply to choose the more profitable action on every trial but to switch between the more and less profitable actions. This is because the probability of the reward being associated with the less profitable action gradually increases on every consecutive trial that that action is not chosen; any unharvested reward that is allocated to the less profitable action when the more profitable action is selected will still be available on the next trial. After several trials the probability of reward associated with the normally less profitable action will exceed the average probability of reward associated with the better action. As in the natural foraging situation, neither one action nor the other is categorically correct or incorrect, although one is, on average, more likely to yield reward. Again, as in the natural setting, the probability of reward associated with each action is actually dependent on which responses the macaque has already made. Rewards are obtained at the highest rate if the fraction of responses of a given type is equal to the fraction of total rewards that can be earned by making that response. This is equivalent to the animal distributing its choices so that the average rate of reward associated with each option is equated. In summary, good performance on the matching task depends not just on error detection, but also on the possession of an estimate of the average reward rate associated with each option.

The number of trials taken before animals began to obtain rewards at 97% of the optimum rate was recorded for different matching problems involving re-

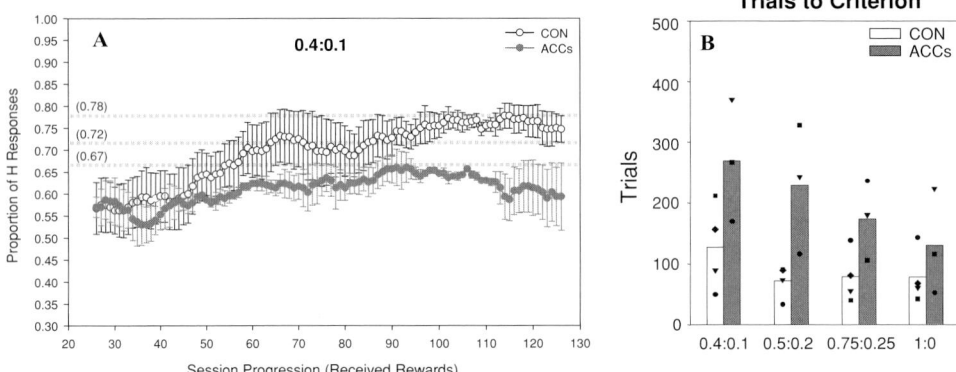

FIGURE 7. **(A)** Group response ratio plot in a matching task in which the probabilities of reward associated with the two actions were 0.4 and 0.1. The ratio of responses associated with the higher average reinforcement rate, as opposed to the lower average reinforcement rate, is shown. The ratio was calculated by smoothing behavioral performance across bins of 50 trials. In order to better compare performance of individuals the data are plotted as a function of collected rewards, as opposed to as a function of trials, on the abscissa. Dashed yellow lines denote 95%, 97%, and 99% optimum response thresholds for maximizing expected total reward income. **(B)** Summary of postoperative performance in the matching task in terms of the number of trials required to exceed the optimum response ratio threshold for four different pairs of action reward probabilities. Control and ACC lesion data are shown by white and grey bars respectively. Adapted from Kennerley et al. (*Nature Neuroscience*, 2006) with permission.

ward delivery of various rates. The yellow rectangle in FIGURE 7 demarcates the range of response ratios at which rewards are being received at 97% of the optimum rate in a matching problem in which the reward probabilities associated with the better and the worse action were 0.4 and 0.1, respectively. Animals with ACC lesions took significantly more trials to approach response ratios close to the optimum (FIG. 7A). The impairment was clear when the rewards were probabilistically associated with both responses (left-hand side of FIG. 7B) but not when one response was always rewarded and the other response never rewarded (1:0 condition, right-hand side of FIG. 7B). Such a pattern of results would be expected if the ACC is not simply monitoring each action to see whether it leads to an error but if it is part of a system for representing the value of each action on the basis of its integrated reward history. In order to work out which action is the more profitable in the matching task it is necessary to integrate the outcomes received for each action over time and simply switching whenever there is an error may not lead to the best allocation of responses.

How Far Back in Time Does the Effective Reinforcement History Extend?

If the ACC mediates the influence that the reinforcement history has over the next choice that is made, then the next question that should be asked is obviously from how far back in the past should an influence be exerted? In other words, what is the length of the effective reinforcement history that should influence voluntary choices? If it is not just whether or not the last trial resulted in an error that should determine the next choice, then how many previous outcomes should have a bearing?

Although the question may seem simple it has proved difficult to answer. Moreover any answer has profound implications for understanding one of the basic issues in cognitive science, namely how fast we should learn and how fast old memories should be overwritten by new memories (Courville et al. 2006; Dickinson & Mackintosh 1978; Doya 2002; Kakade & Dayan 2002; Pearce & Hall 1980). When the effective reinforcement history extends far into the past then learning is slow because the influence of the most recent outcomes will be counterbalanced by the influence of the historical outcomes. When the reinforcement history is short then the learning is fast because each new outcome has a major bearing on what choice is made next.

It is also useful to remember that the learning rate is one of the terms in the influential reinforcement learning model (Sutton & Barto 1998).

$$V_{t+1} = V_t + \delta\alpha$$

The prediction error, δ, which represents the difference between expected and actual reinforcement, has already been discussed above as encoding the required degree of action-value revision, from the old value V_t to the new value V_{t+1}. The new updated action value, V_{t+1}, however, does not depend only on the prediction error in isolation but on the product of the learning rate, α, and the prediction error δ. Often cognitive neuroscientists simply fit the learning rate in their models to that which is observed (e.g., Barraclough et al. 2004; Samejima et al. 2005) but if it were possible to predict what determines the effective length of the reinforcement history then it would also be possible to predict the learning rate.

The study by Kennerley and colleagues (2006) shows that the outcomes obtained up to five trials before a decision have a bearing on which choice control animals made even if they did not influence the choices of animals with ACC lesions (FIG. 5). Other studies, however, have come up with very different estimates of how many previous outcomes should influence the next choice. Sugrue and colleagues (2004) looked at saccadic choices made by monkeys in which rewards were allocated on the basis of matching schedules similar to those explained above. The estimate they derive in their study suggests that the outcomes of actions made even 25 trials ago still exerted some influence over the monkeys' choices.

There is also evidence that outcomes received several trials ago still influence the activity of ACC neurons. Seo and Lee (2007) taught macaques to choose between making a saccade to one of two locations in order to receive reward. The computer program that presented the saccade task also chose a target on each trial, and a reward was given if the computer's choice matched that made by the monkey. The task is sometimes referred to as a "matching pennies game" because rewards are won when the monkey chooses the same option as the computer program. Seo and Lee examined whether the activity of ACC neurons reflected information about the history of the monkey's past choices, the history of the computer's past choices, or the history of reinforcement (FIG. 8). On any given trial, ACC neuron activity reflected not just the choice the animal was making, but in addition activity in approximately 54% of neurons reflected whether or not a reward had been delivered in the last trial. In approximately 14% of neurons activity also reflected whether or not a reward had been delivered three trials earlier. In addition to encoding information about the presence or absence of reward delivery, the ACC neurons encoded other aspects of the choices and the actions from the previous three trials. The neurons' activity also reflected the prediction errors associated with recent choices made and the sum of the values of the actions that could have been chosen on recent trials.

Behrens and colleagues (2007) have recently argued that an organism should set its learning rates so that it maximizes its power to make the best choices. They argued that the learning-rate, α, should depend on the levels of uncertainty in the estimate of the action's value and that, in turn, such uncertainty is determined by the statistics of the reward environment. If the reward environment is *volatile* and fast changing then historical outcomes have less bearing on what it is best to choose next while recent experience is a better predictor. Such an approach would predict the different reinforcement history lengths reported by Kennerley and colleagues (2006) and by Sugrue and colleagues (2004) because the environment was more volatile in the first situation.

The volatility of the reward environment appears to influence the learning rate via the ACC. Behrens and colleagues used fMRI to record the BOLD signal while human subjects performed a probability tracking task. The probability that a secondary reinforcer was associated with one of two choice options was changed throughout the course of the experiment so that the reward environment changed from being stable to volatile or, in some subjects, from volatile to stable. The subjects' learning rates were faster at the end of the volatile period than at the end of the stable period and in fact the observed learning rates corresponded to rates predicted by an optimal Bayesian learning model. The volatility of the reinforcement environment also significantly modulated the ACC BOLD signal as each choice outcome was witnessed (FIG. 9). Subjects' estimates of the volatility of the reward environment are related to their estimates of the variance in the reward rate and so Behrens' findings are consistent with the evidence for the encoding of reward variance in interconnected posterior cingulate regions reported by McCoy and Platt (2005).

It is important to emphasize that the Markovian approach adopted in the proposal made by Behrens and colleagues (2007) suggests that it is not necessary for the chooser to store explicit and separate representations of each outcome in the effective reinforcement history. There is no need to remember details of each outcome obtained on previous trials. Instead representations of only a limited number of summary parameters are needed in order to make the next choice. If there is access to an estimate of the option's previous value estimate, the prediction error, and the volatility, then the degree to which the option's value should be revised in the light of the most recent prediction error is known.

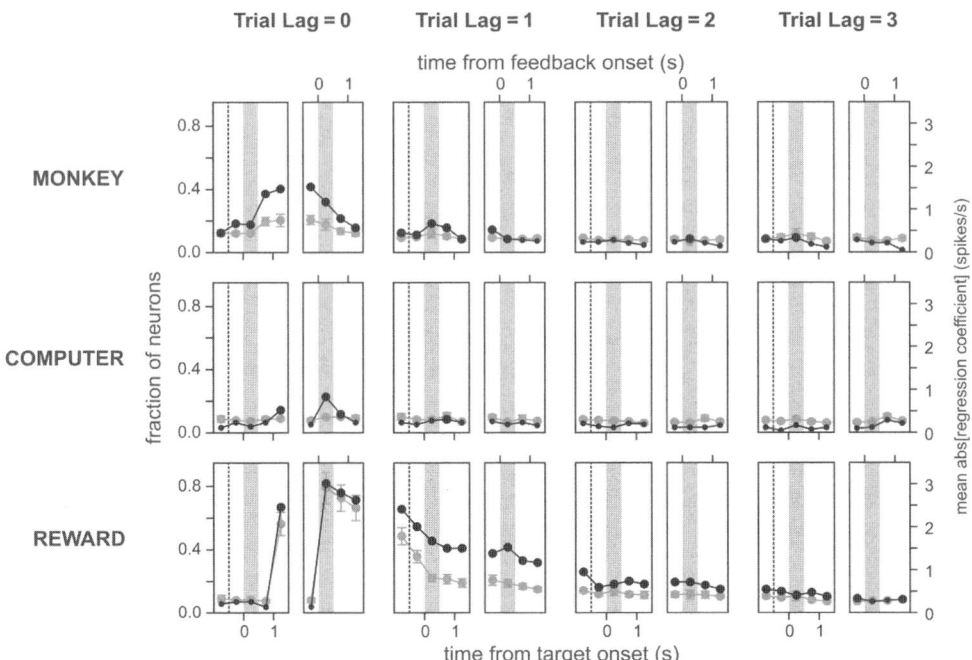

FIGURE 8. Time course of activity in the recorded population of ACC sulcus neurons related to the history of choices made by the animal (top), the history of choices made by the computer program (middle), and reward (bottom). In each row the first graph on the left illustrates the degree to which neural activity on the current trial encodes each choice parameter in the current trial (trial lag = 0), while the next graph illustrates the degree to which activity in the current trial also encodes the same choice variable in the previous trial (trial lag = 1). The third and fourth graphs on each row show how neural activity on the current trial encodes the same variables but in relation to events that occurred two (trial lag = 2) and three trials (trial lage = 3) ago. Black symbols (left axis) indicate the percentage of neurons that displayed significant modulations in their activity according to each variable (t test, $P < 0.05$). Gray symbols (right axis) indicate the average magnitude of the regression coefficients related to each variable. These values were estimated separately for different time bins using a series of multiple linear regression models. Large black symbols indicate that the percentage of neurons was significantly higher than the significance level used in the regression analysis (binomial test, $P < 0.05$). The dotted vertical lines in the left panels correspond to the onset of fore-period, and the gray background the delay (left panels) or feedback (right panels) period. Adapted, with permission, from Seo and Lee (*Journal of Neuroscience*, 2007).

The volatility parameter on each choice determines the degree to which the new action-value estimate is weighted toward the previous action-value estimate as opposed the most recent prediction error. The new action-value estimate then optimally summarizes the reinforcement history into a single value so that the next choice can be made.

Expected Costs as Well as Benefits Determine Which Choices Will Be Made

So far it has been suggested that choices should be made on the basis of which action is associated with the better outcome, and it has been argued that the ACC region of the MFC is a critical component of the brain circuit for representing action values and choices. Unfortunately, as most of us know only too well, many choices do not involve only a single option that is more advantageous in every respect than the alternatives. Each course of action, instead, can be perceived as having both advantages and disadvantages or both benefits and costs. For example one action may lead to a larger reward than another, but it may do so only after more effort has been invested. To return to the previous example of a monkey foraging in the wild, it may be the case that one type of tree has larger fruit than another type; but if the larger fruits are only to be obtained after climbing higher and after expending more effort then it may be better to opt for the more easily obtained smaller fruit. In choosing which one of two food items should be sought an animal may decide that it is worth investing more effort in order to obtain the larger food reward in some situations but not in others.

The effort that a course of action entails is known to be an important factor in determining whether it will

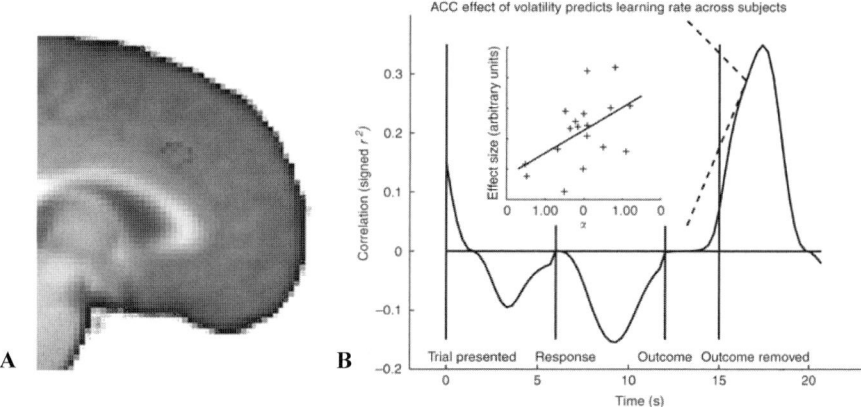

FIGURE 9. **(A)** Sagittal slice through z-statistic maps relating to the effect of volatility on the monitoring of outcomes in a decision-making task. A region in the ACC sulcus was the only one to survive thresholding at $z = 3.5$ and the only region of greater than 50 voxels to survive thresholding at $z = 3.1$ (shown). **(B)** Volatility-related activity in the ACC explains between-subject variation in overall learning rates. The figure shows a timeseries of correlations (signed r^2) between the effect size in the ACC and the mean learning rate fitted to subject behavior over both phases of the experiment. Subjects showing a greater effect of volatility in the ACC in the outcome-monitoring period are likely to display a higher average learning rate in the behavioral data. Insert shows the scatter plot at the time of the peak effect of volatility in the ACC ($r^2 = 0.27$, $P < 0.01$ [F test], max $r^2 = 0.32$). (Reprinted with permission from Behrens et al., *Nature Neuroscience*, 2007.)

be chosen by animals in natural environments. This is not surprising if the larger food item entails greater handling costs before it can be consumed (Stephens & Krebs 1986) or if more energy has first to be spent in reaching its location (Charnov 1976). In the laboratory, animals choose between foraging modes not just on the basis of the rates at which rewards are encountered but also on the basis of the metabolic costs associated with each action (Bautista et al. 2001). When choosing between two levers rats consider the number of times that the lever must be pressed before reward is delivered as well as the size of the reward (Walton et al. 2006b). A similar influence of expected effort also influences the choices that monkeys make in a related paradigm (Walton et al. 2006b). In summary, the costs as well as the potential benefits of a course of action should influence the choice that is made. Although, economists and behavioral ecologists have been interested in the effect of different costs, including delay, effort, and risk, on decision making in humans and animals (Bautista et al. 2001; Kacelnik & Bateson 1997; Long & Platt 2005; Stevens et al. 2005a; Stevens et al. 2005b), the neural mechanisms that mediate the effect of such costs on choice have only recent begun to be elucidated. Once again, however, recent research suggests that the ACC plays a critical role, especially when the cost to be considered is the effort that the action entails.

Effort-based cost–benefit decision making has been investigated in the rat (Mingote et al. 2005; Salamone et al. 2003; Salamone et al. 1994). In one paradigm, first used by Salamone and colleagues, the rats are given a choice between two options defined by the two arms of a T-maze. During preliminary training rats learn that each arm is consistently associated with either a "high reward" or a "low reward" (e.g., four versus two food pellets). As well as being associated with consistently different levels of reward, the two maze arms are also consistently associated with the requirement to invest different amounts of effort; the high-reward maze arm also contains a barrier that the rat must climb before it can reach the food pellets. A series of experiments have shown that the Cg1 and Cg2 fields of the rat ACC are critical for integrating the costs and benefits of each action when choices are made (Floresco & Ghods-Sharifi 2007; Rudebeck et al. 2006; Schweimer & Hauber 2005; Walton et al. 2003; Walton et al. 2002; Walton et al. 2005). After several days' experience climbing the 30 cm barrier in the preoperative period most rats were fairly consistent in choosing the high-reward option even though it was associated with the expenditure of greater effort. After large medial frontal lesions, including Cg1 and Cg2 cortex, as well as prelimbic cortex, rats consistently chose the low-reward option (Walton et al. 2002). Similar effects were seen after circumscribed lesions of Cg1 and Cg2 but not when the lesions were restricted to the prelimbic cortex (Walton et al. 2003). The impairments could not be attributed to a simple loss of spatial or reward memory or an inability to climb because rats reverted to choosing the high-reward option when a second barrier was placed in the low-reward arm of the T-maze. When there is a barrier in each arm of the T-maze there is no need to integrate both the costs and the benefits associated with each option before coming to a decision because the costs of each option are equal and the choice is simply determined by reward size. In the case of large lesions that included the prelimbic cortex as well as the ACC, the rats returned to choosing the low-reward option when the barrier was removed from that arm of the T-maze.

The Influence of Effort and Other Costs on Decision Making

There are different types of costs that should be considered before pursuing a course of action, such as the effort that will be required, the expected delay until receipt of the reward, and the risk and probability of obtaining the reward after the action has been completed. There is increasing evidence that different costs are treated in different ways by the brain. Not only does it seem that the ACC has a central role in mediating effort-based cost–benefit decision making, but it also seems that its role is quite specific to the consideration of only certain types of decision costs.

In addition to the recent work on effort-based decision making there has also been particular interest in delay-based decision making. In the paradigms used to investigate delay-based decision making there may be no need to invest more effort in order to obtain the larger food reward but instead the larger reward may only be obtained after a longer delay. Typically researchers have examined animals' choices when low-reward and high-reward options are available immediately and after a delay, respectively (Cardinal et al. 2001; Cardinal et al. 2004; Cheung & Cardinal 2005; Kheramin et al. 2002; Mobini et al. 2002; Winstanley et al. 2004). In some cases animals refrain from the temptation of choosing an option that leads immediately to reward, albeit a small reward, and choose to wait a longer delay for the larger reward. Choosing to wait through the delay is promoted by the presence of a conditioned stimulus that evokes the expectation of the large reward at the end of the delay period (Cardinal 2006b; Cardinal et al. 2002; Schoenbaum & Roesch 2005).

Several studies attest to the biological separation of delay and effort cost mechanisms by demonstrating that they are subject to different evolutionary forces. Stevens and colleagues have reported that cotton-top tamarins (*Saguinus oedipus*) and common marmosets (*Callithrix jacchus*) are, respectively, more inclined to tolerate high effort costs incurred in traveling further to a larger food amount, or high delay costs in order to obtain larger food amounts (Long & Platt 2005; Stevens et al. 2005a; Stevens et al. 2005b). The different predispositions of the two species may be due to their natural feeding ecology; while tamarins range over larger distances in pursuit of insects, marmosets wait patiently for tree exudates within a limited area.

Rudebeck and colleagues (2006) have directly contrasted effort-based and delay-based decision making in the rat. They trained two sets of rats on two versions of the cost/benefit T-maze task. In one version of the task the cost was the effort entailed in climbing over the barrier to obtain the high reward. In the other version of the task the cost comprised waiting for 15 seconds in the high-reward arm before the high reward was delivered. Either OFC or ACC lesions were made in separate groups of animals trained on each task and, in each case, performance was compared with a sham-operated control group trained at the same time on the same task. After OFC lesions, rats continued to choose the high-effort/high-reward option but became significantly more likely to choose the short-delay/low-reward option in the delay-cost paradigm. Rats with ACC lesions still chose the delayed high-reward option but, as in previous experiments when response effort was a factor, chose the low-effort, low-reward option. While OFC lesions significantly affected performance on the delay task but not the effort task, ACC lesions caused the opposite pattern of disruption (FIG. 10). Because the deficits are different and specific, neither can be explained as just the consequence of a poorer representation of reward. Instead, any account of OFC and ACC decision-making impairments must also make reference to the representation of the options' costs.

The results suggest that the ACC and OFC are involved in the *integration* of the costs and benefits associated with possible options when choices are made. This was demonstrated by showing that neither the ACC nor OFC deficits were significant once the costs associated with each option were equated. Imposing a delay in both maze arms or requiring barrier climbing in both maze arms in the delay and effort tasks, respectively, meant that the better option was simply a function of reward size and there was no need to integrate both benefit and costs before making a decision.

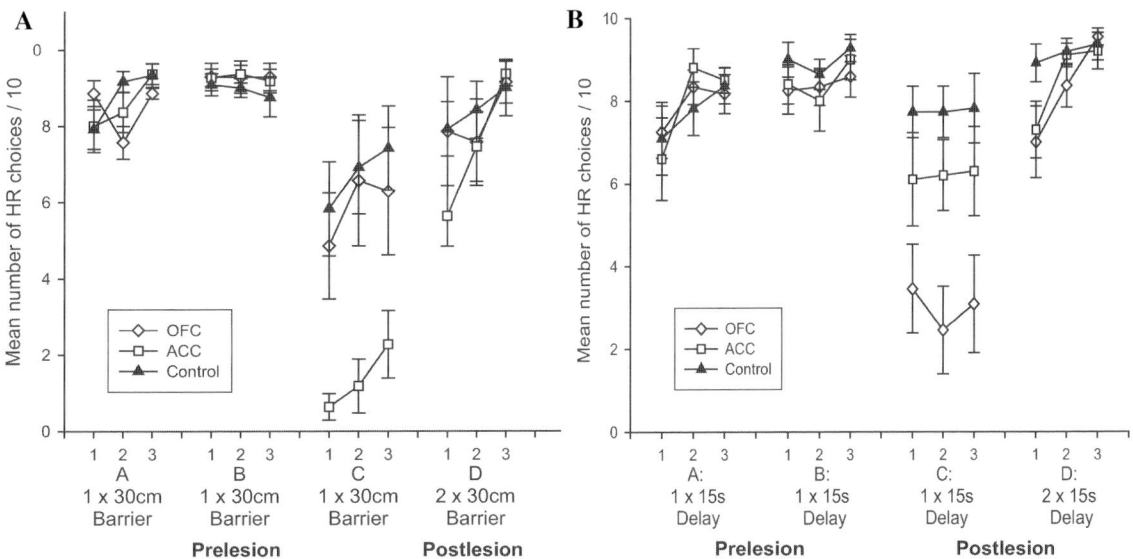

FIGURE 10. (**A**) Rats were trained to choose one of two arms of a T-maze, each of which was baited with food pellets. Choosing one arm of the maze, the high-reward arm (HR responses plotted on the ordinate), was consistently associated with more food rewards. In addition to the larger reward, however, the same arm of the maze was also associated with a greater cost—the animal had to climb a barrier before it could consume the food reward. Although rats normally chose the high-reward but high-cost option (left and center panels A and B), they stopped doing so after a lesion was made in the Cg1 and Cg2 fields of the ACC (panel C). When a second barrier was placed into what had been the low-cost arm, there was no longer a need to integrate both the costs and benefits associated with each option before a choice was made; because the costs associated with each T-maze option were equated, the choice could simply be based on the difference in expected reward. Under such conditions the choices of the ACC lesion group returned to normal (right panel D). (**B**) The ACC appears to be specifically concerned with effort costs. The same lesion did not alter the way in which rats made choices in which the cost was the delay before food was delivered. The opposite pattern of impairment was seen after OFC lesions (again preoperative data are shown in Panels A and B, postoperative data are shown in C, and data from an equal delay condition are shown in D). OFC lesions did not change effort-based decision making but it did affect delay-based decision making. (Reprinted with permission from Rudebeck et al., *Nature Neuroscience*, 2007.)

Such manipulations led to amelioration of both the ACC and OFC deficits (FIG. 10).

Despite the superficial similarity of decisions about delay and effort it is clear that overcoming impulsivity or apathy when choosing are quite distinct processes. There has been some confusion in the literature regarding whether frontal lesions impair cost–benefit decision making. That the two types of cost–benefit decisions are different can explain why it has been difficult to determine whether frontal lobe lesions consistently cause impaired decision making and the choosing of the easier option rather than the ultimately more rewarding outcome. The results of Rudebeck's study demonstrate, first, that it is essential to consider the type of cost—effort or delay—that is pertinent to the decisions that are examined. Second, the results suggest that different frontal regions—the ACC and the OFC—are differentially concerned with the two types of cost.

Contradictory tendencies toward impulsivity and apathy have been reported in patients with frontal lobe lesions and frontotemporal dementia (Levy & Dubois 2006; Rosen et al. 2005; van Reekum et al. 2005), and it is possible that the two types of decision bias are associated with dysfunction in two different circuits centered on the OFC and ACC respectively (Cummings 1993). It is certainly clear that degeneration of a relatively anterior part of the ACC, anterior to the genu of the corpus callosum, is correlated with apathy, a failure to exert effort, but not disinhibition in patients with fronto-temporal dementia (Rosen et al. 2005).

The distinction between the two patterns of impairment may reflect the fact that deciding how much effort to invest and how long to wait may depend on two very distinct types of psychological process. Deciding how much effort to expend may be related to considerations of the opportunity costs of not responding (Niv et al. 2005; Niv et al. 2007; Niv et al. 2006) and energy expenditure (Bautista et al. 2001; Walton et al. 2006a), whereas deciding how long to wait for an outcome may be inextricably linked to associative learning mechanisms and the representation of reward expectancies

(Cardinal 2006a; Kacelnik 2003; Kacelnik & Bateson 1997; Schoenbaum & Roesch 2005).

The OFC may be pre-eminent in delay-based decision making because of its importance for stimulus-related associative learning and for representing reward expectancies (Rushworth et al. 2007a; Schoenbaum & Roesch 2005). A rat will only choose the delayed, high-reward option if it is able to maintain a representation of the expected reward at the end of the delay period, but such representations are degraded after OFC lesions. This has been most directly demonstrated by using a reward devaluation paradigm in which the value of the food reward is reduced by association with illness induced by lithium chloride injection. While a normal rat will approach the foodwell where a reinforcer is delivered less frequently after devaluation, this is not the case after an OFC lesion (Pickens et al. 2003). In the normal rat behavior is guided by the revised valuation assigned to the reward, but that does not happen after OFC removal. Neurons encoding reward expectation are found not just in the OFC but also in the basolateral amygdala. The degree of activity in the basolateral amygdala related to reward expectation is, however, reduced after an OFC lesion (Saddoris et al. 2005; Schoenbaum et al. 2003). The delayed, high-reward option may no longer seem the most valuable when the rat is weighing up the costs and benefits associated with each option after an OFC lesion.

The involvement of the ACC in effort-based decision making may be linked to its importance in representing arousal states (Critchley et al. 2003) which could provide a proximate indicator of energy expenditure and therefore be critical for making a decision about whether or not it is worth working hard for a given reward. The ACC is interconnected with areas associated with autonomic control such as the hypothalamus and periaqueductal grey (Floyd et al. 2000; Gabbott et al. 2005). Recording studies conducted in the macaque ACC have identified neurons that encode the number of actions still to be made, in other words the amount of remaining work, before a reward is expected (Shidara & Richmond 2002).

Climbing the barrier in the effort task entailed little delay and the pursuit of either option required animals to maintain representations of the expected rewards over similar time periods. Instead, deciding whether to climb the barrier required consideration of a cost–effort–intrinsic to the action itself. The ACC may update or represent the value of the action itself. Such a representation would reflect not just the action's association with reward but also the intrinsic costs entailed by the action (Rushworth et al. 2007a).

In such a representation, because it is the value of the action rather than the expected outcome that is represented, reward devaluation would not have an immediate impact, at least not before the animal had the opportunity to experience the reward in the context of a choice. Instead, if the animal only possessed such a representation, the action would be taken until it was devalued in the combined representation of the recent outcome history. The ACC may contribute to the action-value "caching" system proposed by Daw and colleagues (2005). The computationally simple caching system involves the association of reward with an action or other event through reinforcement learning. Through such an association the action itself comes to have a value that need not immediately reflect a change in the value of the outcome, such as its devaluation through association with illness or satiety. The cached action value may also incorporate information about the effort costs that are intrinsic to the action (Rushworth et al. 2007b).

Voluntary Action and the Balancing of Exploitation with Exploration in the ACC

ACC activity is not just related to the receipt of informative feedback that can be used to revise action-value estimates. It is also driven by whether or not subjects are in an exploratory mode and trying to find out more about how best to respond in a potentially new situation. The fMRI investigation conducted by Walton and colleagues (2004) into the monitoring of feedback during task switching also examined the degree to which subjects were actively generating exploratory actions in order to obtain reinforcement feedback. In addition to asking subjects to guess which might be the correct response when the task rules changed Walton and colleagues (2004) also asked their subjects to perform another condition in which they were instructed to always attempt a particular response whenever they were warned that a rule change had occurred (FIGS. 3 and 4). In this "fixed" condition subjects did not have to generate an intention of their own in order to explore the value of the different possible actions in different contexts even though they still monitored the action's outcome. The ACC signal was significantly lower. In a second experiment (FIG. 4) Walton and colleagues (2004) compared the importance of having to generate one's own choice and the importance of feedback monitoring; both were important determinants of ACC activity. Forstmann and colleagues (2006) have also reported fMRI data that underline the central

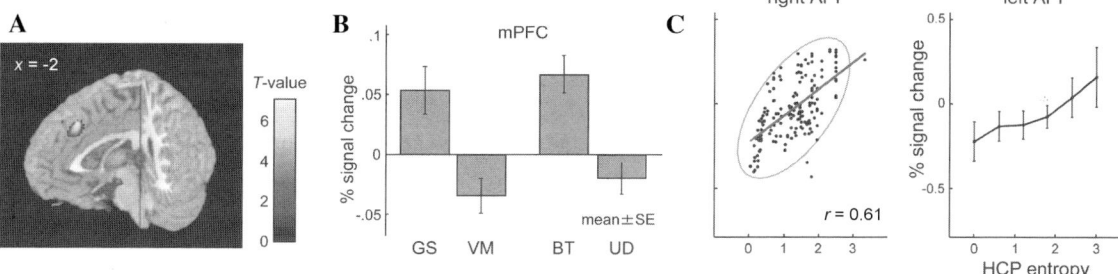

FIGURE 11. (A) MFC activity was significantly correlated with the "back track probability," an index of the subjects' likely need to revise their estimate of their position in the maze. (B) The left-hand bars show the relative percent change of BOLD signal in MFC when subjects attempted to estimate their position in the maze by monitoring the outcome of their own exploratory actions (GS, goal search condition) and when they followed cues that guided them through the maze (VM, visuomotor condition). The right-hand bars show the percent change of BOLD signal for two types of trials in the GS task. A major revision of the position estimate was required on back track (BT) trials but not update trials (UD). The error bars indicate the standard error. (C) Activity in lateral prefrontal cortex, as opposed to the MFC, changes in relation to quite distinct cognitive processes. The percentage BOLD signal change relative to the mean activity in the GS task in the anterior and lateral prefrontal cortex was associated with "hidden current position" (HCP) entropy—an index of the subjects' uncertainty about their position in the maze. The error bars indicate the standard deviations. Adapted from Yoshida and Ishii (*Neuron*, 2006) with permission.

importance of the ACC to the generation of one's own choice of task set.

In the situations investigated by Walton and Forstmann and colleagues a cue told subjects *when* to generate an exploratory action even if it did not instruct them which action to make. In many environments, however, there may be no explicit indication of when contingencies are changing and that exploratory actions should be attempted. In such a situation, particularly in an uncertain environment, there is a tension between the balancing of exploitation of knowledge about the high value of one action with the exploration of the value of alternatives. It seems intuitive that an action with a high value should be made whenever there is an opportunity, but if the same action is made on every occasion then the actor forgoes the opportunity to explore and the possibility of finding out that another action has an even higher value. Ways of attempting to address the exploration–exploitation dilemma in the context of reinforcement learning theory are beginning to provide a formal way to describe a core aspect of voluntary behavior (Ishii et al. 2002).

Other experiments underline the central importance of the ACC to the generation of exploratory behavior. In a recent experiment Yoshida and Ishii (2006) gave their human subjects the opportunity to move around a virtual maze and then scanned with fMRI while the subjects explored the same maze. The fMRI experiment was broken down into trials on each of which the subject had to get to a goal position from a new and unknown starting position. In one condition subjects had to work out by trial and error where they were in the maze and how they might best approach the goal, while in another they simply followed a series of instructions. The conditions were referred to as the goal search and visuomotor control conditions, respectively. Yoshida and Ishii (2006) reported greater ACC activity in the first condition when the subjects were generating exploratory actions (FIG. 11A, B). Using an incremental Bayes belief update analysis of each subject's behavior and the information available to them, Yoshida and Ishii derived estimates of belief about current maze position and estimates of when an observation would have been discrepant with a previously held belief. On such "back track" trials subjects had to revise their belief about their position, and ACC activity was again prominent.

Single-neuron recording studies confirm the central importance of the ACC in exploratory behavior. Procyk and colleagues (Procyk et al. in press; Procyk et al. 2000) have recorded activity in the ACC while macaques learned, by trial and error, the correct order in which to touch three targets in order to obtain a food reward. ACC neurons were more active when the macaques were searching for the correct order in which to respond, but they became less active once the correct order had been learned and the macaque merely had to repeat it in order to obtain the next reward.

One possibility is that the ACC controls the *balance* between exploitative and exploratory behaviors (Aston-Jones & Cohen 2005). Aston-Jones and Cohen argue that the ACC, and perhaps some other areas in the frontal cortex such as the OFC, may influence the activity of noradrenergic neurons in the locus coeruleus (LC). LC neurons exhibit phasic and tonic modes of activity associated with the outcomes of decisions when animals are engaged in exploitative behaviors and exploratory behaviors respectively (Usher et al. 1999). According to this account changes in noradrenergic activity mediate the ACC's influence over a widely distributed set of brain regions when an animal is engaged in exploratory behavior.

Neural Circuits for Voluntary Action: Distinct Roles for ACC and Lateral Prefrontal Cortex in Generating Exploratory Actions

The ACC is not alone among cortical areas in being active during exploratory behavior, but it may have a critical role in the generation of each exploratory action and in the revision of the estimate of the action's value once feedback is obtained. There is evidence implicating adjacent, more dorsal medial frontal areas such as the presupplementary motor area (pre-SMA) and both the dorsolateral prefrontal cortex (DLPFC) and the frontopolar cortex in exploratory behavior. These different brain regions are known to be interconnected (Bates & Goldman-Rakic 1993; Lu et al. 1994; Petrides & Pandya 2007), so it is plausible that they might work together in order to facilitate exploratory behavior, but the special contribution of each remains unclear.

DLPFC neurons in the macaque are also active when monkeys are searching for the correct way in which to respond (Procyk et al. in press; Procyk & Goldman-Rakic 2006). Both TMS and fMRI studies implicate human DLPFC in the generation of intentions and choices; DLPFC TMS interferes with the speed with which unconstrained choices are made (Hadland et al. 2001), while DLPFC BOLD signals change when subjects decide when to respond (Lau et al. 2004). Yoshida and Ishii (2006) also reported an increase in activity in DLPFC when their human subjects were exploring the maze rather than following instructions. One possibility is that DLPFC continuously represents the alternative possible courses of action. More potential courses of action will have to be represented when the subject is most uncertain about which particular course should be pursued. Yoshida and Ishii (2006) were able to use their Bayesian incremental belief updating approach in their maze learning task to calculate the subjects' most likely estimates of their position in the maze on each trial and the probability distribution over the estimates. The probability distribution over the estimates corresponds to the subjects' conditional uncertainty about their positions in the maze given the observations that they have been able to make up to that time. When this is high, subjects will have to consider the largest possible number of positions, and they will have to represent the largest number of different possible courses of action. It was found that BOLD changes in anterior DLPFC and frontopolar regions increased with increasing uncertainty in the maze position estimate (FIG. 11C).

Remarkably we also know something of the activity of individual DLPFC neurons in a similar situation. The neuron-recording studies conducted in macaques confirm that DLPFC holds information about possible courses of action even before the monkey embarks on the course of action. In addition the studies confirm that DLPFC activity reflects certainty in a particular course of action being the correct one to pursue. Evidence that different possible courses of action are represented in DLPFC comes from studies conducted by Mushiake, Saito, and colleagues who taught monkeys to pronate or supinate the wrist of each arm in order to move a cursor through a maze presented on a computer monitor (Mushiake et al. 2006; Saito et al. 2005). Stimuli of different colors presented at different locations within the maze at the start of each trial informed the monkey about the start and end positions for a particular trial. DLPFC activity encoded not just the initial cursor movement that the monkey was first going to effect but also the final intended goal position for the cursor and the intervening cursor positions.

Evidence that DLPFC neuron activity reflects the individual's certainty about a course of action comes from a study conducted by Averbeck and colleagues, who taught monkeys to make eight series of three saccades to three positions in a nine-point grid (Averbeck & Lee 2007; Averbeck et al. 2006). Saccades were only allowed between adjacent grid positions. At the start of a block of trials the monkey knew that it had to start the first saccade at the center point of the grid, but it did not know which three positions were then to be targets for each saccade. The correct sequence was only gradually established by trial and error. Averbeck and colleagues recorded from ensembles of several DLPFC neurons at a time and reported different patterns of activity depending on the sequence to be performed. The activity patterns of the neuronal ensembles were distinctive once good performance of the sequences was well established. Each distinctive activity pattern, however, only emerged gradually during the course of learning each sequence. Moreover, the emergence of the distinctive pattern paralleled the animal's apparent certainty, as indexed by errors, as to which was the correct sequence to perform.

Like ACC neurons, DLPFC neurons may also contribute to the monitoring of the success of actions. Mansouri and colleagues have reported DLPFC neuron activity that encoded reinforcing feedback in a task-switching paradigm (Mansouri et al. 2006). Barraclough, Seo, and Lee taught their monkeys to perform a saccade choice task in which unpredictable rather than repetitive behavior was rewarded (Barraclough et al. 2004; Lee et al. 2005; Seo et al. 2007). DLPFC neuron activity encoded not just which action the animal made on any trial but also which actions had been made previously and the recent history of reward delivery. Seo et al. (2007) argued that the sustained signal encoding which action had been made provided an "eligibility trace" necessary for the association of the action with a reinforcer delivered only some time later.

Both Yoshida and Ishii (2006) and Daw and colleagues (Daw et al. 2006) have particularly emphasized the activation of the frontopolar cortex when human subjects are engaged in exploratory behavior. Daw and colleagues (2006) also used fMRI to record activity from human subjects while they chose between gambling on one of four options with gradually shifting values. They classified decisions as exploitative when subjects chose the option observed to have the highest value and exploratory when they chose differently. While the exploitative choices were associated with the activation of the ventromedial frontal cortex, the exploratory choices were again associated with both MFC activity centered on the ACC and frontopolar activity. One possibility is that the frontopolar cortex is not directly concerned with the generation of the exploratory action or the monitoring of its consequence but instead that it is holding information about the value of an alternative option or options to the one currently being chosen but which might be chosen again in the future. It would be important to hold information about alternative options; if the value of the alternative option turned out to be less than that of the explored and chosen option, then it would be important to be able to make a comparison and to revert back to the previous option. Koechlin and colleagues have provided evidence that the frontopolar cortex holds information about tasks that subjects have performed recently and may have to perform again later on in an experiment, and so it is possible that it also holds information about alternative option values (Koechlin et al. 2003; Koechlin & Summerfield 2007).

In summary, a distributed network of frontal brain regions is active when monkeys and people explore a situation or environment or make exploratory actions in the course of learning. While lateral and polar prefrontal areas represent possible alternative courses of actions, the ACC is active when each exploratory action is generated and when the value of the courses of action must be revised.

Conflict and Voluntary Action Selection

So far this review of voluntary action and the MFC has focused on situations in which action selection is based not on an instruction or cue but instead on the action's expected value or an exploratory attempt to find out more about an action's value. There has, however, also been considerable interest in the possibility that the MFC is important when cues and affordances in the immediate environment prompt the selection of more than one action and there is "conflict" between the different possible actions that might be made (Botvinick et al. 2001; Botvinick et al. 2004). The idea of conflict has an immediate relevance to any discussion of voluntary action because it is in just such conflict situations, where there appears to be more than one way to respond, that volition is most in evidence. In addition the notion of an MFC role in conflict has prompted the development of a rich computational theory that has guided interpretation of many fMRI and EEG studies (Botvinick et al. 2001; Botvinick et al. 2004; Brown & Braver 2005; Yeung et al. 2004; Yeung et al. 2006).

A number of influential fMRI studies of conflict have focused on the ACC region of the MFC and the role that it may have in the initial *detection* of response conflict (Botvinick et al. 2004; Ridderinkhof et al. 2004). The approach has been criticized partly on the basis of some animal studies in which ACC lesions did not appear to cause straightforward conflict-detection deficits (Rushworth et al. 2003) and in which ACC neuron activity did not appear to be modulated in a variety of paradigms thought to induce response conflict (Ito et al. 2003; Nakamura et al. 2005). On the other hand, some caution is warranted in interpreting the data from animal studies in which the subjects may have had unusually extensive experience of performance in high-conflict situations. There are also several investigations of the effects of human ACC lesions, but in these cases it is necessary to be cautious about the precise location of the lesions within the ACC. One investigation of the effects of lesions in human patients focused on a very ventral and anterior region of the ACC. In fact the lesion was ventral and anterior to the typical location of conflict related activity in fMRI studies, but surprisingly the study reported a change in conflict-task performance (di Pellegrino et al. 2007).

Other human patient lesion studies, however, have reported no change in conflict detection (Fellows & Farah 2005; Swick & Turken 2002).

Despite the uncertainty about the role of the ACC in response conflict detection, it is clear that some part of the MFC—perhaps even the pre-SMA and an adjacent region called the supplementary eye field (SEF)—that is more concerned with the control of eye movements than arm movements is more active in situations of response conflict (Dux et al. 2006; Garavan et al. 2003; Nachev et al. 2005; Rushworth et al. 2004; Ullsperger & von Cramon 2001) and when subjects first start selecting actions according to a new set of rules associated with a new task or when they switch between tasks (Crone et al. 2006; Dosenbach et al. 2006; Rushworth et al. 2002).

In the macaque the activity of single neurons in the pre-SMA and SEF is modulated by the context (conflict or nonconflict), in which an action is selected. Importantly, however, SEF and pre-SMA neurons also encode information about action selection while they do not seem to have properties consistent with a simple role in conflict *detection* (Isoda & Hikosaka 2007; Nakamura et al. 2005; Stuphorn et al. 2000). Nakamura and colleagues (2005) taught macaques a "spatial incompatibility task" in which saccadic eye movements were made to the left or to the right in response to red and green cues, respectively. Because the cue itself could appear on either the left or the right, it drew each animal's attention to the same location and predisposed them to make a saccade in that direction. Conflict, indexed by increased RT, occurred when the cue color was associated with the making of a response in a direction opposite to the cue position. The SEF role in response selection was indicated by the fact that the majority of SEF neurons responded more when saccades were made in a preferred direction than in the opposite direction. The firing rates of many neurons also reflected whether it was a conflict or nonconflict trial. There was, however, little evidence for the existence of neurons that responded only to conflict in isolation from response selection, as would predicted by a simple conflict monitoring account.

Even if the SEF and pre-SMA do not detect conflict, they may be part of a system that changes the way in which actions are selected or inhibited depending on the current task and context. Stuphorn and Schall (2006) used microstimulation to alter MFC activity while macaques were performing a saccadic stop-signal RT task. In this paradigm monkeys are cued to make a saccade, but on some trials an additional cue instructs them to withhold the planned saccade. In many instances SEF microstimulation led to a greater probability of countermanding the saccade when the stop signal was presented even though it had no impact on performance on the other control trials. Such context-specific effects suggest the SEF may be changing the way in which actions are selected when conflicting information in the immediate environment affords different ways of responding.

It might be argued that the stop-signal paradigm used by Stuphorn and Schall does not really examine the processing of choosing between alternative actions but rather simply the inhibition of a given action. Isoda and Hikosaka (2007), however, have reported related effects in an action-selection paradigm that was investigated while recording and microstimulating neurons in the pre-SMA. They trained macaques to make saccades to yellow or purple squares shown on the left or right of a central fixation point (FIG. 12). The fixation point turned either yellow or purple and instructed the monkeys to make a saccade to the similarly colored peripheral square. Animals' RTs decreased when the central cue color remained the same over the course of several trials but increased on trials when the color switched. Again Isoda and Hikosaka found that pre-SMA neurons often coded for one direction of response or the other, but in addition the activity of a number of pre-SMA neurons changed on switch trials. Although pre-SMA microstimulation was found to affect RT on both switch and nonswitch trials, it only affected the likelihood of making the correct action on switch trials.

Perhaps the most direct evidence that the MFC exerts an influence, in conflict situations, over action selection comes from a recent study conducted by Taylor and colleagues (2007) in which the human MFC was stimulated with TMS at the same time that ERPs were recorded from the primary motor cortex. The subjects in the experiment performed a flanker task similar to the one used by Debener and colleagues (2005, described above) while TMS was administered and ERPs were recorded. In brief, the subjects responded by making left- or right-hand actions in response to central arrows pointing in left or right directions. Peripheral arrows either pointed in a congruent or incongruent direction on nonconflict and conflict trials, respectively. Taylor and colleagues focused on a particular ERP called the lateralized readiness potential (LRP), which represents the degree to which the motor cortex in the hemisphere contralateral to the correct response hand is more active than the motor cortex in the hemisphere contralateral to the incorrect response hand. As in previous studies Taylor and colleagues found that the motor cortex contralateral to the incorrect hand was more active on conflict trials than

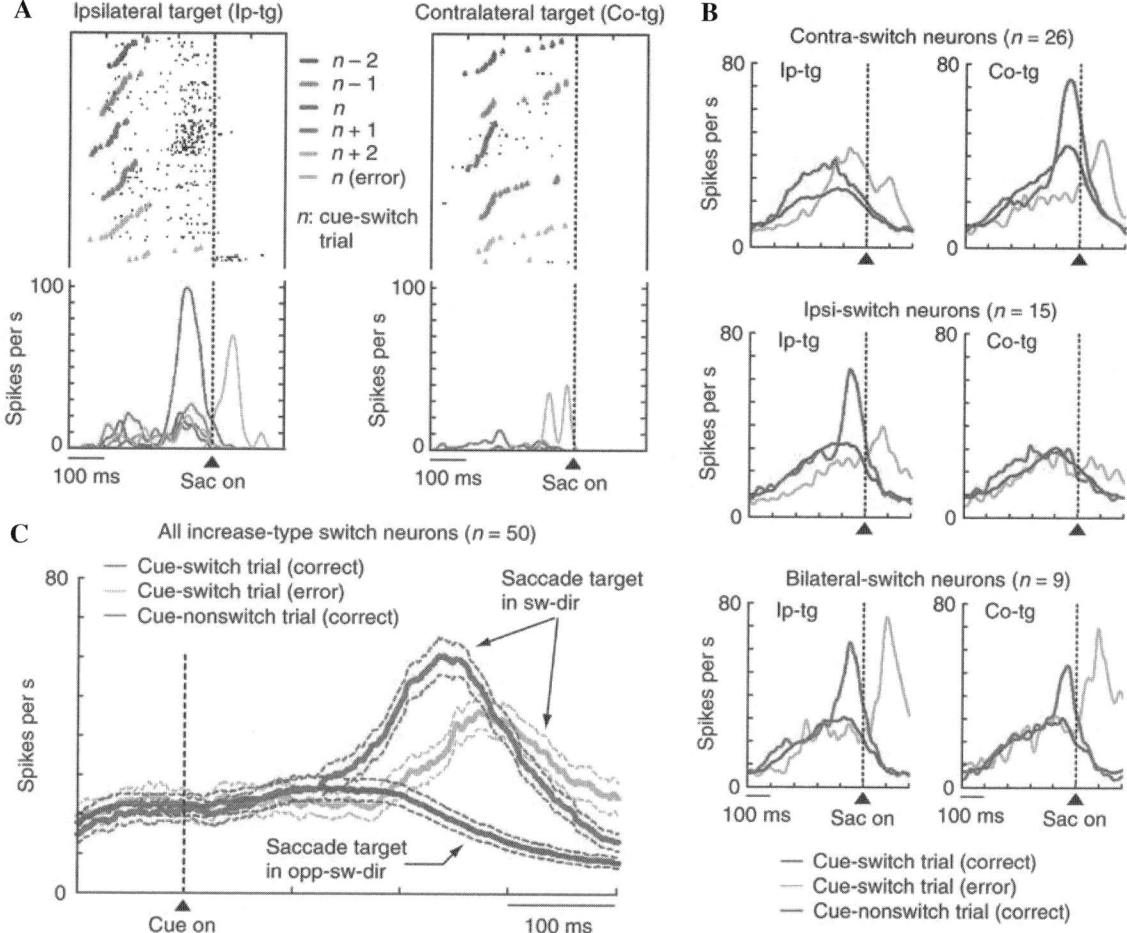

FIGURE 12. Switch-selective activity of pre-SMA neurons. **(A)** Activity of a single "ipsi-switch" neuron—a neuron with greater activity when saccades were made to the same side as the hemisphere in which recordings were made. Rastergrams and spike density functions (SDFs) are sorted according to the trial position in each block (n represents the cue-switch trials) and aligned with saccade onset. In rastergrams, black dots indicate the time of individual action potentials and colored triangles indicate the time of cue onset; trials are arranged in order of saccadic RTs. Activity in switch-error trials is shown in gray. **(B)** Ensemble average SDFs for contra-switch neurons (top), ipsi-switch neurons (middle), and bilateral-switch neurons (bottom) shown separately for the correct cue-switch trials (red), correct cue-nonswitch trials (blue), and switch error trials (gray). All SDFs are aligned with saccade onset. **(C)** Ensemble SDFs (mean ± SD) for all increase-type switch neurons. SDFs are aligned with cue onset. Note that the direction of the saccade target for the cue-switch trials is opposite that for the cue-nonswitch trials. Reprinted with permission from Isoda and Hikosaka (*Nature Neuroscience*, 2007).

on nonconflict trials consistent with the activation of the incorrect action representation. MFC TMS exacerbated this effect and particularly affected the LRP on conflict trials (FIG. 13). In other words, the experiment confirms that, as in the MFC microstimulation experiments of Stuphorn and Schall (2006) and Isoda and Hikosaka (2007), the control over action exerted by the MFC is context dependent. In addition the results provide information about the mechanism by which the MFC affects action selection in conflict situations; they suggest that MFC activity changes lead to changes in action selection–related activity in other motor regions of the brain. In the absence of normal MFC activity, for example on TMS trials, the representation of the wrong action is not suppressed relative to the representation of the correct action.

Taylor and colleagues were not able to measure whether MFC TMS particularly disrupted the facilitation of the correct action or whether it particularly disrupted the inhibition of the incorrect action. Isoda and Hikosaka (2007) were able to show that the pre-SMA is concerned both with inhibition of the in-

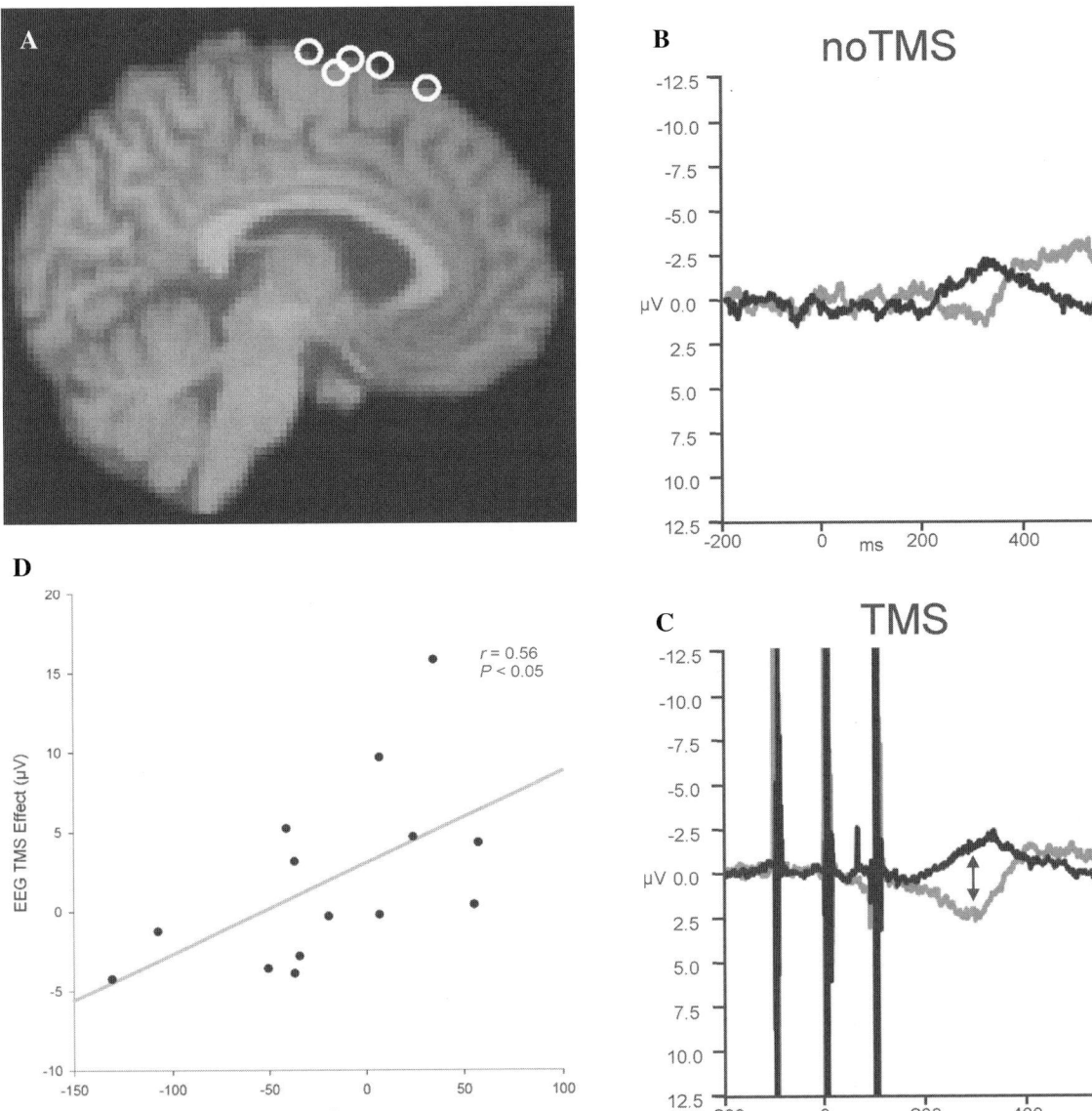

FIGURE 13. **(A)** Left dMFC TMS site. The circles represent the MNI coordinates at which TMS was applied over left dMFC in a subset of the subjects from Experiment 1 (mean $x=-5$, $y=7$, $z=73$). The circles are superimposed over the brain of an example subject that had also been registered into MNI space. The site is just left of the midline and over tissue normally assigned to the pre-SMA. **(B)** On noTMS congruent trials (black) there was a clear negative deflection in the LRP (negative is plotted upwards for the LRP) indicative of the preparation of correct responses, peaking at approximately 300 ms. On incongruent trials (grey) the waveform was, instead, displaced in the positive direction, associated with the preparation of the wrong response. The negative deflection associated with the correct response was delayed. **(C)** When dMFC TMS was applied there was a significant increase in the difference between the waveforms recorded on congruent and incongruent trials starting at 180 ms. This was due to dMFC TMS causing a positive deflection in the LRP on incongruent trials. **(D)** Positive correlation between dMFC TMS effects on behavior and the LRP. The effect of dMFC on conflict resolution was calculated for both behavior and the LRP as $TMS_{incongruent-congruent} - noTMS_{incongruent-congruent}$. Subjects who showed the strongest effects of TMS on the behavioral measure of conflict also showed the strongest effects on the LRP measure of conflict. Adapted from Taylor et al. (*Journal of Neuroscience*, 2007) with permission.

correct action and facilitation of the correct action. Moreover, they were able to show that neurons that are more concerned with inhibition of the incorrect action tended to be active at an earlier time prior to neurons concerned with the facilitation of the correct action. Isoda and Hikosaka came to these conclusions by examining the activity of neurons that had had increased firing rates on switch trials in a second paradigm in which a single colored square was presented to the left or right of a central fixation point. The monkeys made a "go" response and saccaded to the peripheral square when the central cue changed to the same color, but they made a "no-go" response and refrained from responding when the central and peripheral colors differed. Facilitation and inhibition neurons were identified by the fact that they were more active on go and no-go trials, respectively. Significant increases in activity were seen first in the inhibition neurons and only later in those concerned with facilitation. "Dual" neurons that were active on both go and no-go trials were active at an intermediate time.

A number of lines of evidence demonstrate the MFC's importance in another aspect of voluntary action selection: when there is conflict between different possible actions. While particular attention has been devoted to the possibility that the MFC detects conflict between competing action representations, there is clear evidence that some MFC regions, particular the pre-SMA and SEF, have a role in the *resolution* of conflict.

Conclusions

Cognitive neuroscientists have been interested in the mechanisms that underlie voluntary action and have paid special attention to situations in which subjects either have a free choice about which action to make and no instruction is given or in which different instructions provide conflicting information about what to do. The MFC plays a critical role in these situations for three reasons. First, the MFC, particularly the ACC, is concerned with the representation and updating of action values. It may have a particular role in determining the rate at which action values are updated. The ACC action-value representation may incorporate the effort costs that are intrinsic to an action as well as the action's potential reward benefit. Second, the MFC may be important when exploratory actions are generated in order to establish more about the potential value of actions. Finally, the MFC, perhaps particularly dorsal MFC areas such as the pre-SMA and SEF, has a role in inhibiting and facilitating the selection of undesired and desired actions, respectively, when the environment provides conflicting information about which action should be made.

Conflict of Interest

The author declares no conflicts of interest.

References

Amiez, C., Joseph, J. P., & Procyk, E. (2005). Anterior cingulate error-related activity is modulated by predicted reward. *Eur J Neurosci, 21*, 3447–3452.

Amiez, C., Joseph, J. P., & Procyk, E. (2006a). Reward encoding in the monkey anterior cingulate cortex. *Cereb Cortex, 16*, 1040–1055.

Amiez, C., Kostopoulos, P., Champod, A. S., & Petrides, M. (2006b). Local morphology predicts functional organization of the dorsal premotor region in the human brain. *J Neurosci, 26*, 2724–2731.

Aston-Jones, G., & Cohen, J. D. (2005). An integrative theory of locus coeruleus-norepinephrine function: adaptive gain and optimal performance. *Annu Rev Neurosci, 28*, 403–450.

Averbeck, B. B., & Lee, D. (2007). Prefrontal neural correlates of memory for sequences. *J Neurosci, 27*, 2204–2211.

Averbeck, B. B., Sohn, J. W., & Lee, D. (2006). Activity in prefrontal cortex during dynamic selection of action sequences. *Nat Neurosci, 9*, 276–282.

Barraclough, D. J., Conroy, M. L., & Lee, D. (2004). Prefrontal cortex and decision making in a mixed-strategy game. *Nat Neurosci, 7*, 404–410.

Bates, J. F., & Goldman-Rakic, P. S. (1993). Prefrontal connections of medial motor areas in the rhesus monkey. *J Comp Neurol, 335*, 1–18.

Bautista, L. M., Tinbergen, J., & Kacelnik, A. (2001). To walk or to fly? How birds choose among foraging modes. *Proc Natl Acad Sci U S A, 98*, 1089–1094.

Behrens, T. E., Woolrich, M. W., Walton, M. E., & Rushworth, M. F. (2007). Learning the value of information in an uncertain world. *Nat Neurosci, 10*, 1214–1221.

Boorman, E., O'Shea, J., Sebastian, C., Rushworth, M. F. S., & Johansen-Berg, H. (2007). Individual differences in white-matter microstructure reflect variation in functional connectivity during choice. *Curr Biol, 17*, 1426–1431.

Botvinick, M. M., Braver, T. S., Barch, D. M., Carter, C. S., & Cohen, J. D. (2001). Conflict monitoring and cognitive control. *Psychol Rev, 108*, 624–652.

Botvinick, M. M., Cohen, J. D., & Carter, C. S. (2004). Conflict monitoring and anterior cingulate cortex: an update. *Trends Cogn Sci, 8*, 539–546.

Boussaoud, D., & Wise, S. P. (1993a). Primate frontal cortex: effects of stimulus and movement. *Exp Brain Res, 95*, 28–40.

Boussaoud, D., & Wise, S. P. (1993b). Primate frontal cortex: neuronal activity following attentional versus intentional cues. *Exp Brain Res, 95*, 15–27.

Brass, M., & von Cramon, D. Y. (2004). Selection for cognitive control: a functional magnetic resonance imaging study

on the selection of task-relevant information. *J Neurosci, 24*, 8847–8852.
Brown, J. W., & Braver, T. S. (2005). Learned predictions of error likelihood in the anterior cingulate cortex. *Science, 307*, 1118–1121.
Cardinal, R. N. (2006a). Neural systems implicated in delayed and probabilistic reinforcement. *Neural Netw, 19*, 1277–1301.
Cardinal, R. N. (2006b). Neural systems implicated in delayed and probabilistic reinforcement. *Neural Netw, 19*, 1277–1301.
Cardinal, R. N., Parkinson, J. A., Hall, J., & Everitt, B. J. (2002). Emotion and motivation: the role of the amygdala, ventral striatum, and prefrontal cortex. *Neurosci Biobehav Rev, 26*, 321–352.
Cardinal, R. N., Pennicott, D. R., Sugathapala, C. L., Robbins, T. W., & Everitt, B. J. (2001). Impulsive choice induced in rats by lesions of the nucleus accumbens core. *Science, 292*, 2499–2501.
Cardinal, R. N., Winstanley, C. A., Robbins, T. W., & Everitt, B. J. (2004). Limbic corticostriatal systems and delayed reinforcement. *Ann N Y Acad Sci, 1021*, 33–50.
Charnov, E. (1976). Optimal foraging: the marginal value theorem. *Theoretical and Population Biology, 9*, 129–136.
Cheung, T. H., & Cardinal, R. N. (2005). Hippocampal lesions facilitate instrumental learning with delayed reinforcement but induce impulsive choice in rats. *BMC Neurosci, 6*, 36.
Courville, A. C., Daw, N. D., & Touretzky, D. S. (2006). Bayesian theories of conditioning in a changing world. *Trends Cogn Sci, 10*, 294–300.
Critchley, H. D., Mathias, C. J., Josephs, O., O'Doherty, J., Zanini, S., et al. (2003). Human cingulate cortex and autonomic control: converging neuroimaging and clinical evidence. *Brain, 126*, 2139–2152.
Crone, E. A., Wendelken, C., Donohue, S. E., & Bunge, S. A. (2006). Neural evidence for dissociable components of task-switching. *Cereb Cortex, 16*, 475–486.
Cummings, J. L. (1993). Frontal-subcortical circuits and human behavior. *Arch Neurol, 50*, 873–880.
Daw, N. D., Niv, Y., & Dayan, P. (2005). Uncertainty-based competition between prefrontal and dorsolateral striatal systems for behavioral control. *Nat Neurosci, 8*, 1704–1711.
Daw, N. D., O'Doherty, J. P., Dayan, P., Seymour, B., & Dolan, R. J. (2006). Cortical substrates for exploratory decisions in humans. *Nature, 441*, 876–879.
Debener, S., Ullsperger, M., Siegel, M., Fiehler, K., von Cramon, D. Y., & Engel, A. K. (2005). Trial-by-trial coupling of concurrent electroencephalogram and functional magnetic resonance imaging identifies the dynamics of performance monitoring. *J Neurosci, 25*, 11730–11737.
Devinsky, O., Morrell, M. J., & Vogt, B. A. (1995). Contributions of anterior cingulate to behaviour. *Brain, 118*, 279–306.
di Pellegrino, G., Ciaramelli, E., & Ladavas, E. (2007). The regulation of cognitive control following rostral anterior cingulate cortex lesion in humans. *J Cogn Neurosci, 19*, 275–286.
Dickinson, A., & Mackintosh, N. J. (1978). Classical conditioning in animals. *Annu Rev Psychol, 29*, 587–612.
Dosenbach, N. U., Visscher, K. M., Palmer, E. D., Miezin, F. M., Wenger, K. K., et al. (2006). A core system for the implementation of task sets. *Neuron, 50*, 799–812.

Doya, K. (2002). Metalearning and neuromodulation. *Neural Netw, 15*, 495–506.
Dum, R. P., & Strick, P. L. (1996). Spinal cord terminations of the medial wall motor areas in macaque monkeys. *J Neurosci, 16*, 6513–6525.
Dux, P. E., Ivanoff, J., Asplund, C. L., & Marois, R. (2006). Isolation of a central bottleneck of information processing with time-resolved FMRI. *Neuron, 52*, 1109–1120.
Everling, S., Tinsley, C. J., Gaffan, D., & Duncan, J. (2002). Filtering of neural signals by focused attention in the monkey prefrontal cortex. *Nat Neurosci, 5*, 671–676.
Falkenstein, M., Hohnsbein, J., Hoorman, J., & Blanke, L. (1991). Effects of crossmodal divided attention on late ERP components. II. Error processing in choice reaction tasks. *Electroencephalography and Clinical Neurophysiology, 78*, 447–455.
Fellows, L. K., & Farah, M. J. (2005). Is anterior cingulate cortex necessary for cognitive control? *Brain, 128*, 788–796.
Fiehler, K., Ullsperger, M., & von Cramon, D. Y. (2004). Neural correlates of error detection and error correction: is there a common neuroanatomical substrate? *Eur J Neurosci, 19*, 3081–3087.
Floresco, S. B., & Ghods-Sharifi, S. (2007). Amygdala-prefrontal cortical circuitry regulates effort-based decision making. *Cereb Cortex, 17*, 251–260.
Floyd, N. S., Price, J. L., Ferry, A. T., Keay, K. A., & Bandler, R. (2000). Orbitomedial prefrontal cortical projections to distinct longitudinal columns of the periaqueductal gray in the rat. *J Comp Neurol, 422*, 556–578.
Forstmann, B. U., Brass, M., Koch, I., & von Cramon, D. Y. (2006). Voluntary selection of task sets revealed by functional magnetic resonance imaging. *J Cogn Neurosci, 18*, 388–398.
Gabbott, P. L., Warner, T. A., Jays, P. R., Salway, P., & Busby, S. J. (2005). Prefrontal cortex in the rat: projections to subcortical autonomic, motor, and limbic centers. *J Comp Neurol, 492*, 145–177.
Garavan, H., Ross, T. J., Kaufman, J., & Stein, E. A. (2003). A midline dissociation between error-processing and response-conflict monitoring. *Neuroimage, 20*, 1132–1139.
Gehring, W. J., Goss, B., Coles, M. G. H., Meyer, D. E., & Donchin, E. (1993). A neural system for error detection and compensation. *Psychol Sci, 4*, 385–390.
Hadland, K. A., Rushworth, M. F. S., Passingham, R. E., Jahanshahi, M., & Rothwell, J. C. (2001). Interference with performance of a response selection task that has no working memory component: an rTMS comparison of the dorsolateral prefrontal and medial frontal cortex. *J Cogn Neurosci, 13*, 1097–1108.
Herrnstein, R., Rachlin, H., & Laibson, D. (1997). *The Matching Law: Papers in Psychology and Economics*. Cambridge, Massachusetts, London, England: Harvard University Press.
Hester, R., Foxe, J. J., Molholm, S., Shpaner, M., & Garavan, H. (2005). Neural mechanisms involved in error processing: a comparison of errors made with and without awareness. *Neuroimage, 27*, 602–608.
Holroyd, C. B., & Coles, M. G. (2002). The neural basis of human error processing: reinforcement learning, dopamine, and the error-related negativity. *Psychol Rev, 109*, 679–709.
Holroyd, C. B., Nieuwenhuis, S., Yeung, N., Nystrom, L., Mars, R. B., et al. (2004). Dorsal anterior cingulate cortex shows

fMRI response to internal and external error signals. *Nat Neurosci, 7*, 497–498.

Holroyd, C. B., Yeung, N., Coles, M. G., & Cohen, J. D. (2005). A mechanism for error detection in speeded response time tasks. *J Exp Psychol Gen, 134*, 163–191.

Ishii, S., Yoshida, W., & Yoshimoto, J. (2002). Control of exploitation-exploration meta-parameter in reinforcement learning. *Neural Netw, 15*, 665–687.

Isoda, M., & Hikosaka, O. (2007). Switching from automatic to controlled action by monkey medial frontal cortex. *Nat Neurosci, 10*, 240–248.

Ito, S., Stuphorn, V., Brown, J. W., & Schall, J. D. (2003). Performance monitoring by the anterior cingulate cortex during saccade countermanding. *Science, 302*, 120–122.

Kacelnik, A. (2003). The evolution of patience. In G. Loewenstein, D. Read, & R. Baumeister, (Eds.), *Time and decision: economic and psychological perspectives on intertemporal choice* (pp. 115–138). New York: Russell Sage Foundation.

Kacelnik, A., & Bateson, M. (1997). Risk-sensitivity: crossroads for theories of decision making. *Trends Cogn Sci, 1*, 304–309.

Kakade, S., & Dayan, P. (2002). Acquisition and extinction in autoshaping. *Psychol Rev, 109*, 533–544.

Kennerley, S. W., Walton, M. E., Behrens, T. E., Buckley, M. J., & Rushworth, M. F. (2006). Optimal decision making and the anterior cingulate cortex. *Nat Neurosci, 9*, 940–947.

Kheramin, S., Body, S., Mobini, S., Ho, M. Y., Velazquez-Martinez, D. N., et al. (2002). Effects of quinolinic acid-induced lesions of the orbital prefrontal cortex on intertemporal choice: a quantitative analysis. *Psychopharmacology (Berl), 165*, 9–17.

Klein, T. A., Endrass, T., Kathmann, N., Neumann, J., von Cramon, D. Y., & Ullsperger, M. (2007). Neural correlates of error awareness. *Neuroimage, 34*, 1774–1781.

Koechlin, E., Ody, C., & Kouneiher, F. (2003). The architecture of cognitive control in the human prefrontal cortex. *Science, 302*, 1181–1185.

Koechlin, E., & Summerfield, C. (2007). An information theoretical approach to prefrontal executive function. *Trends Cogn Sci, 11*, 229–235.

Laplane, D., Talairach, J., Meininger, V., Bancaud, J., & Orgogozo, J. M. (1977). Clinical consequences of corticectomies involving the supplementary motor area in man. *J Neurol Sci, 34*, 301–314.

Lau, H. C., Rogers, R. D., Haggard, P., & Passingham, R. E. (2004). Attention to intention. *Science, 303*, 1208–1210.

Lee, D., McGreevy, B. P., & Barraclough, D. J. (2005). Learning and decision making in monkeys during a rock-paper-scissors game. *Brain Res Cogn Brain Res, 25*, 416–430.

Levy, R., & Dubois, B. (2006). Apathy and the functional anatomy of the prefrontal cortex-Basal Ganglia circuits. *Cereb Cortex, 16*, 916–928.

Long, A., & Platt, M. (2005). Decision making: the virtue of patience in primates. *Curr Biol, 15*, R874–876.

Lu, M. -T., Preston, J. B., & Strick, P. L. (1994). Interconnections between the prefrontal cortex and the premotor areas in the frontal lobe. *J Comp Neurol, 341*, 375–392.

Luppino, G., Matelli, M., Camarda, R. M., Gallese, V., & Rizzolatti, G. (1991). Multiple representations of body movements in mesial area 6 and the adjacent cingulate cortex: an intracortical microstimulation study in the macaque monkey. *J Comp Neurol, 311*, 463–482.

Magno, E., Foxe, J. J., Molholm, S., Robertson, I. H., & Garavan, H. (2006). The anterior cingulate and error avoidance. *J Neurosci, 26*, 4769–4773.

Mansouri, F. A., Matsumoto, K., & Tanaka, K. (2006). Prefrontal cell activities related to monkeys' success and failure in adapting to rule changes in a Wisconsin Card Sorting Test analog. *J Neurosci, 26*, 2745–2756.

Mars, R. B., Coles, M. G., Grol, M. J., Holroyd, C. B., Nieuwenhuis, S., et al. (2005). Neural dynamics of error processing in medial frontal cortex. *Neuroimage, 28*, 1007–1013.

Matsumoto, K., Suzuki, W., & Tanaka, K. (2003). Neuronal correlates of goal-based motor selection in the prefrontal cortex. *Science, 301*, 229–232.

Matsumoto, M., Matsumoto, K., Abe, H., & Tanaka, K. (2007). Medial prefrontal cell activity signaling prediction errors of action values. *Nat Neurosci, 10*, 647–656.

McCoy, A. N., & Platt, M. L. (2005). Risk-sensitive neurons in macaque posterior cingulate cortex. *Nat Neurosci, 8*, 1220–1227.

Mingote, S., Weber, S. M., Ishiwari, K., Correa, M., & Salamone, J. D. (2005). Ratio and time requirements on operant schedules: effort-related effects of nucleus accumbens dopamine depletions. *Eur J Neurosci, 21*, 1749–1757.

Mobini, S., Body, S., Ho, M. Y., Bradshaw, C. M., Szabadi, E., et al. (2002). Effects of lesions of the orbitofrontal cortex on sensitivity to delayed and probabilistic reinforcement. *Psychopharmacology (Berl), 160*, 290–298.

Muhammad, R., Wallis, J. D., & Miller, E. K. (2006). A Comparison of Abstract Rules in the Prefrontal Cortex, Premotor Cortex, Inferior Temporal Cortex, and Striatum. *J Cogn Neurosci, 18*, 974–989.

Mushiake, H., Saito, N., Sakamoto, K., Itoyama, Y., & Tanji, J. (2006). Activity in the lateral prefrontal cortex reflects multiple steps of future events in action plans. *Neuron, 50*, 631–641.

Nachev, P., Rees, G., Parton, A., Kennard, C., & Husain, M. (2005). Volition and conflict in human medial frontal cortex. *Curr Biol, 15*, 122–128.

Nakamura, K., Roesch, M. R., & Olson, C. R. (2005). Neuronal activity in macaque SEF and ACC during performance of tasks involving conflict. *J Neurophysiol, 93*, 884–908.

Niki, H., & Watanabe, M. (1979). Prefrontal and cingulate unit activity during timing behaviour in the macaque. *Brain Res, 171*, 213–224.

Nimchinsky, E. A., Gilissen, E., Allman, J. M., Perl, D. P., Erwin, J. M., & Hof, P. R. (1999). A neuronal morphologic type unique to humans and great apes. *Proc Natl Acad Sci U S A, 96*, 5268–5273.

Niv, Y., Daw, N. D., & Dayan, P. (2005). How fast to work: Response vigor, motivation and tonic dopamine. In Y. Weiss, B. Scholkopf, & J. Platt, (Eds.), *Advances in neural information processing systems* (pp. 1019–1026). MIT Press.

Niv, Y., Daw, N. D., Joel, D., & Dayan, P. (2007). Tonic dopamine: opportunity costs and the control of response vigor. *Psychopharmacology (Berl), 191*, 507–520.

Niv, Y., Joel, D., & Dayan, P. (2006). A normative perspective on motivation. *Trends Cogn Sci, 10*, 375–381.

O'Shea, J., Johansen-Berg, H., Trief, D., Gobel, S., & Rushworth, M. F. (2007). Functionally specific reorganization in human premotor cortex. *Neuron, 54*, 479–490.

O'Shea, J., Sebastian, C., Boorman, E., Johansen-Berg, H., & Rushworth, M. (in press). Functional specificity of premotor-motor cortical interactions during action selection. *Eur J Neurosci, 26*, 2085–2095.

Passingham, R. E. (1993). *The frontal lobes and voluntary action.* Oxford: Oxford University Press.

Pearce, J. M., & Hall, G. (1980). A model for Pavlovian learning: variations in the effectiveness of conditioned but not of unconditioned stimuli. *Psychol Rev, 87*, 532–552.

Petrides, M. (2005). Lateral prefrontal cortex: architectonic and functional organization. *Philos Trans R Soc Lond B Biol Sci, 360*, 781–795.

Petrides, M., & Pandya, D. (2007). Efferent association pathways from the rostral prefrontal cortex in the macaque monkey. *J Neurosci, 27*, 11573–11586.

Pickens, C. L., Saddoris, M. P., Setlow, B., Gallagher, M., Holland, P. C., & Schoenbaum, G. (2003). Different roles for orbitofrontal cortex and basolateral amygdala in a reinforcer devaluation task. *J Neurosci, 23*, 11078–11084.

Procyk, E., Amiez, C., Quilodran, R., & Joseph, J. P. (2007). Modulations of prefrontal activity related to cognitive control and performance monitoring. In Y. Rossetti, P. Haggard, & M Kawato (Eds.), *Attention and performance XXII: Sensorimotor foundations of higher cognition* (pp. 235–250). Oxford: Oxford University Press.

Procyk, E., & Goldman-Rakic, P. S. (2006). Modulation of dorsolateral prefrontal delay activity during self-organized behavior. *J Neurosci, 26*, 11313–11323.

Procyk, E., Tanaka, Y. L., & Joseph, J. P. (2000). Anterior cingulate activity during routine and non-routine sequential behaviors in macaques. *Nat Neurosci, 3*, 502–508.

Rainer, G., Asaad, W. F., & Miller, E. K. (1998). Selective representation of relevant information by neurons in the primate prefrontal cortex. *Nature, 393*, 577–579.

Ridderinkhof, K. R., Ullsperger, M., Crone, E. A., & Nieuwenhuis, S. (2004). The role of the medial frontal cortex in cognitive control. *Science, 306*, 443–447.

Rosen, H. J., Allison, S. C., Schauer, G. F., Gorno-Tempini, M. L., Weiner, M. W., & Miller, B. L. (2005). Neuroanatomical correlates of behavioural disorders in dementia. *Brain, 128*, 2612–2625.

Rudebeck, P. H., Walton, M. E., Smyth, A. N., Bannerman, D. M., & Rushworth, M. F. (2006). Separate neural pathways process different decision costs. *Nat Neurosci, 9*, 1161–1168.

Rushworth, M. F., Behrens, T. E., Rudebeck, P. H., & Walton, M. E. (2007a). Contrasting roles for cingulate and orbitofrontal cortex in decisions and social behaviour. *Trends Cogn Sci, 11*, 168–176.

Rushworth, M. F., Buckley, M. J., Behrens, T. E., Walton, M. E., & Bannerman, D. M. (2007b). Functional organization of the medial frontal cortex. *Curr Opin Neurobiol, 17*, 220–227.

Rushworth, M. F., Buckley, M. J., Gough, P. M., Alexander, I. H., Kyriazis, D., et al. (2005). Attentional selection and action selection in the ventral and orbital prefrontal cortex. *J Neurosci, 25*, 11628–11636.

Rushworth, M. F. S., Hadland, K. A., Gaffan, D., & Passingham, R. E. (2003). The effect of cingulate cortex lesions on task switching and working memory. *J Cogn Neurosci, 15*, 338–353.

Rushworth, M. F. S., Hadland, K. A., Paus, T., & Sipila, P. K. (2002). Role of the human medial frontal cortex in task switching: a combined fMRI and TMS study. *J Neurophysiol, 87*, 2577–2592.

Rushworth, M. F. S., Walton, M. E., Kennerley, S. W., & Bannerman, D. M. (2004). Action sets and decisions in the medial frontal cortex. *Trends Cogn Sci, 8*, 410–417.

Saddoris, M. P., Gallagher, M., & Schoenbaum, G. (2005). Rapid associative encoding in basolateral amygdala depends on connections with orbitofrontal cortex. *Neuron, 46*, 321–331.

Saito, N., Mushiake, H., Sakamoto, K., Itoyama, Y., & Tanji, J. (2005). Representation of immediate and final behavioral goals in the monkey prefrontal cortex during an instructed delay period. *Cereb Cortex, 15*, 1535–1546.

Salamone, J. D., Correa, M., Mingote, S., & Weber, S. M. (2003). Nucleus accumbens dopamine and the regulation of effort in food-seeking behavior: implications for studies of natural motivation, psychiatry, and drug abuse. *J Pharmacol Exp Ther, 305*, 1–8.

Salamone, J. D., Cousins, M. S., & Bucher, S. (1994). Anhedonia or anergia? Effects of haloperidol and nucleus accumbens dopamine depletion on instrumental response selection in a T-maze cost/benefit procedure. *Behav Brain Res, 65*, 221–229.

Samejima, K., Ueda, Y., Doya, K., & Kimura, M. (2005). Representation of action-specific reward values in the striatum. *Science, 310*, 1337–1340.

Schoenbaum, G., & Roesch, M. (2005). Orbitofrontal cortex, associative learning, and expectancies. *Neuron, 47*, 633–636.

Schoenbaum, G., Setlow, B., Saddoris, M. P., & Gallagher, M. (2003). Encoding predicted outcome and acquired value in orbitofrontal cortex during cue sampling depends upon input from basolateral amygdala. *Neuron, 39*, 855–867.

Schweimer, J., & Hauber, W. (2005). Involvement of the rat anterior cingulate cortex in control of instrumental responses guided by reward expectancy. *Learn Mem, 12*, 334–342.

Seo, H., Barraclough, D. J., & Lee, D. (2007). Dynamic signals related to choices and outcomes in the dorsolateral prefrontal cortex. *Cereb Cortex., 17* (Suppl I), i110–i117.

Seo, H., & Lee, D. (2007). Temporal filtering of reward signals in the dorsal anterior cingulate cortex during a mixed-strategy game. *J Neurosci, 27*, 8366–8377.

Shidara, M., & Richmond, B. J. (2002). Anterior cingulate: single neuronal signals related to degree of reward expectancy. *Science, 296*, 1709–1711.

Shima, K., & Tanji, J. (1998). Role for cingulate motor area cells in voluntary movement selection based on reward. *Science, 282*, 1335–1338.

Stephens, D. W., & Krebs, J. R. (1986). *Foraging Theory.* Princeton, NJ: Princeton University Press.

Stevens, J. R., Hallinan, E. V., & Hauser, M. D. (2005a). The ecology and evolution of patience in two New World monkeys. *Biol Lett, 1*, 223–226.

Stevens, J. R., Rosati, A. G., Ross, K. R., & Hauser, M. D. (2005b). Will travel for food: spatial discounting in two new world monkeys. *Curr Biol, 15*, 1855–1860.

Stuphorn, V., & Schall, J. D. (2006). Executive control of countermanding saccades by the supplementary eye field. *Nat Neurosci, 9*, 925–931.

Stuphorn, V., Taylor, T. L., & Schall, J. D. (2000). Performance monitoring by the supplementary eye field. *Nature, 408*, 857–860.

Sugrue, L. P., Corrado, G. S., & Newsome, W. T. (2004). Matching behavior and the representation of value in the parietal cortex. *Science, 304*, 1782–1787.

Sutton, R., & Barto, A. G. (1998). *Reinforcement Learning*. Cambridge, Massachusetts: MIT Press.

Swick, D., & Turken, A. U. (2002). Dissociation between conflict detection and error monitoring in the human anterior cingulate cortex. *Proc Natl Acad Sci U S A, 99*, 16354–16359.

Taylor, P. C., Nobre, A. C., & Rushworth, M. F. S. (2007). Subsecond changes in top-down control exerted by human medial frontal cortex during conflict and action selection: a combined TMS-EEG study. *J Neurosci, 27*, 11343–11353.

Ullsperger, M., Nittono, H., & von Cramon, D. Y. (2007). When goals are missed: dealing with self-generated and externally induced failure. *Neuroimage, 35*, 1356–1364.

Ullsperger, M., & von Cramon, D. Y. (2001). Subprocesses of performance monitoring: a dissociation of error processing and response competition revealed by event-related fMRI and ERPs. *Neuroimage, 14*, 1387–1401.

Ullsperger, M., & von Cramon, D. Y. (2003). Error monitoring using external feedback: specific roles of the habenular complex, the reward system, and the cingulate motor area revealed by functional magnetic resonance imaging. *J Neurosci, 23*, 4308–4314.

Usher, M., Cohen, J. D., Servan-Schreiber, D., Rajkowska, J., & Aston-Jones, G. (1999). The role of the locus coeruleus in the regulation of cognitive performance. *Science, 283*, 549–554.

van Reekum, R., Stuss, D. T., & Ostrander, L. (2005). Apathy: why care? *J Neuropsychiatry Clin Neurosci, 17*, 7–19.

Van Schie, H. T., Mars, R. B., Coles, M. G., & Bekkering, H. (2004). Modulation of activity in medial frontal and motor cortices during error observation. *Nat Neurosci, 7*, 549–554.

Wallis, J. D., & Miller, E. K. (2003a). From rule to response: neuronal processes in the premotor and prefrontal cortex. *J Neurophysiol, 90*, 1790–1806.

Wallis, J. D., & Miller, E. K. (2003b). Neuronal activity in primate dorsolateral and orbital prefrontal cortex during performance of a reward preference task. *Eur J Neurosci, 18*, 2069–2081.

Walton, M. E., Bannerman, D. M., Alterescu, K., & Rushworth, M. F. S. (2003). Functional specialization within medial frontal cortex of the anterior cingulate for evaluating effort-related decisions. *J Neurosci, 23*, 6475–6479.

Walton, M. E., Bannerman, D. M., & Rushworth, M. F. S. (2002). The role of rat medial frontal cortex in effort-based decision making. *J Neurosci, 22*, 10996–11003.

Walton, M. E., Croxson, P. L., Rushworth, M. F. S., & Bannerman, D. M. (2005). The mesocortical dopamine projection to anterior cingulate cortex plays no role in guiding effort-related decisions. *Behav Neurosci, 119*, 323–328.

Walton, M. E., Devlin, J. T., & Rushworth, M. F. S. (2004). Interactions between decision making and performance monitoring within prefrontal cortex. *Nat Neurosci, 7*, 1259–1265.

Walton, M. E., Kennerley, S. W., Bannerman, D. M., Phillips, P., & Rushworth, M. F. (2006a). Weighing up the benefits of work: behavioral and neural analyses of effort-related decision making. *Neural Netw, 19*, 1302–1314.

Walton, M. E., Kennerley, S. W., Bannerman, D. M., Phillips, P. E., & Rushworth, M. F. (2006b). Weighing up the benefits of work: Behavioral and neural analyses of effort-related decision making. *Neural Netw, 19*, 1302–1314.

Winstanley, C. A., Theobald, D. E., Cardinal, R. N., & Robbins, T. W. (2004). Contrasting roles of basolateral amygdala and orbitofrontal cortex in impulsive choice. *J Neurosci, 24*, 4718–4722.

Wise, S. P., & Murray, E. A. (2000). Arbitrary associations between antecedents and actions. *Trends Neurosci, 23*, 271–276.

Yeung, N., Cohen, J. D., & Botvinick, M. M. (2004). The neural basis of error detection: conflict monitoring and the error-related negativity. *Psychol Rev, 111*, 931–959.

Yeung, N., Nystrom, L. E., Aronson, J. A., & Cohen, J. D. (2006). Between-task competition and cognitive control in task switching. *J Neurosci, 26*, 1429–1438.

Yoshida, W., & Ishii, S. (2006). Resolution of uncertainty in prefrontal cortex. *Neuron, 50*, 781–789.

Evaluating Faces on Trustworthiness

An Extension of Systems for Recognition of Emotions Signaling Approach/Avoidance Behaviors

ALEXANDER TODOROV

Department of Psychology and Center for the Study of Brain, Mind and Behavior, Princeton University, Princeton, New Jersey, USA

People routinely make various trait judgments from facial appearance, and such judgments affect important social outcomes. These judgments are highly correlated with each other, reflecting the fact that valence evaluation permeates trait judgments from faces. Trustworthiness judgments best approximate this evaluation, consistent with evidence about the involvement of the amygdala in the implicit evaluation of face trustworthiness. Based on computer modeling and behavioral experiments, I argue that face evaluation is an extension of functionally adaptive systems for understanding the communicative meaning of emotional expressions. Specifically, in the absence of diagnostic emotional cues, trustworthiness judgments are an attempt to infer behavioral intentions signaling approach/avoidance behaviors. Correspondingly, these judgments are derived from facial features that resemble emotional expressions signaling such behaviors: happiness and anger for the positive and negative ends of the trustworthiness continuum, respectively. The emotion overgeneralization hypothesis can explain highly efficient but not necessarily accurate trait judgments from faces, a pattern that appears puzzling from an evolutionary point of view and also generates novel predictions about brain responses to faces. Specifically, this hypothesis predicts a nonlinear response in the amygdala to face trustworthiness, confirmed in functional magnetic resonance imaging (fMRI) studies, and dissociations between processing of facial identity and face evaluation, confirmed in studies with developmental prosopagnosics. I conclude with some methodological implications for the study of face evaluation, focusing on the advantages of formally modeling representation of faces on social dimensions.

Key words: social cognition; face perception; trustworthiness

Introduction

References to the belief that the nature of the mind and human personality can be inferred from facial appearance can be dated back to ancient Greece, Persia, Rome, and China (McNeill 1998). At the end of 18th century, Johann Kaspar Lavater, a Swiss pastor, wrote "Essays on physiognomy, designed to promote the knowledge and love of mankind," in which he described how to read a person's character from their face. The book caused a craze in Europe. It underwent more than 150 editions until 1940. As Darwin noted in his autobiography, he was almost denied the chance to take the historic *Beagle* voyage because of this book. The captain of the ship, a fan of Lavater, did not believe that a person with such a nose would possess "sufficient energy and determination" for the voyage (Darwin 1887/1950, p. 36). In the 19th century, the pseudo-science of physiognomy reached its apogee. Cesare Lombroso, who provided his "scientific" testimony at several trials, argued that "each type of crime is committed by men with particular physiognomic characteristics." For example, "thieves are notable for their expressive faces and manual dexterity, small wandering eyes that are often oblique in form, thick and close eyebrows, distorted or squashed noses, thin beards and hair, and sloping foreheads" (Lombroso 1876/2006, p. 51).

Although nowadays such notions strike most of us as ludicrous, there is abundant research in social psychology about the effects of facial appearance on social outcomes (e.g., Blair et al. 2004; Eberhardt et al. 2006; Hamermesh & Biddle 1994; Hassin & Trope 2000; Little et al. 2007; Langlois et al. 2000; Montepare & Zebrowitz 1998; Mueller & Mazur 1996; Zebrowitz 1999). Most of this work has been on the effects of attractiveness (e.g., Langlois et al. 2000), but specific

---

Address for correspondence: Alexander Todorov, Department of Psychology, Green Hall, Princeton University, Princeton, NJ 08544-1010. Voice: +609-258-7463; fax: +609-258-1113.

atodorov@princeton.edu

trait impressions also impact social outcomes. For example, inferences of competence, based solely on facial appearance, predict the outcomes of political elections (Ballew & Todorov 2007; Hall et al. in press; Todorov et al. 2005), and inferences of dominance predict military rank attainment (Mazur et al. 1984; Mueller & Mazur 1996).

In this article, I argue that evaluation of emotionally neutral faces is an extension of functionally adaptive systems for understanding the communicative meaning of emotional expressions and explore the implications of this hypothesis for brain responses to faces. I review evidence that a) trait judgments from faces, in particular judgments of trustworthiness, are highly efficient (Section I); b) trustworthiness judgments approximate the valence evaluation of faces that underlies multiple social judgments (Section II); c) the amygdala plays a key role in the automatic evaluation of faces on trustworthiness (Section III); and d) exaggerating the facial features that make a neutral face look trustworthy produces expressions of happiness, whereas exaggerating the facial features that make a face look untrustworthy produces expressions of anger (Section IV).

The emotion overgeneralization hypothesis can explain highly efficient but not necessarily accurate trait judgments from faces, a pattern that appears puzzling from an evolutionary point of view (Section V) and also generates novel predictions about brain responses to faces. Specifically, this hypothesis predicts a nonlinear response in the amygdala to face trustworthiness, a prediction confirmed in two functional magnetic resonance imaging (fMRI) studies (Section VI). Second, the hypothesis predicts that it should be possible to observe dissociations between processing of facial identity and face evaluation, a prediction confirmed in studies with developmental prosopagnosics who are unable to process facial identity but are able to make trustworthiness judgments (Section VII). I conclude with some methodological implications for the study of face evaluation, focusing on the advantages of formally modeling representation of faces on social dimensions (Section VIII).

I. The Efficiency of Trait Judgments from Faces

What is the minimal time exposure to a face sufficient for people to form a person impression? We studied five trait judgments from emotionally neutral faces: likeability, trustworthiness, competence, aggressiveness, and attractiveness (Willis & Todorov 2006). Prior studies have shown that judgments of physical attractiveness can be made after extremely brief presentations of faces (Locher et al. 1993; Olson & Marshuetz 2005). However, attractiveness is a property of facial appearance, and it is not clear whether these findings generalize to specific trait judgments such as trustworthiness and competence.

We included attractiveness judgments as a benchmark against which to compare the efficiency of other judgments. Faces were presented for 100, 500, or 1000 ms and participants were asked to make one of the five judgments. For all five judgments, judgments made after 100 ms exposure to faces closely agreed with control judgments made in the absence of time constraints. More importantly, this agreement did not improve with additional time exposure, suggesting that 100 ms exposure is sufficient for people to form a reliable person impression. Additional time exposure had the effect of increasing confidence in judgments.

The findings did not change when the analysis controlled for the shared variance of trait judgments with attractiveness. Importantly, the agreement for judgments of trustworthiness was as high as the agreement for judgments of attractiveness. The response times for these two judgments were also almost identical and faster than the response times for judgments of competence, likeability, and aggressiveness, suggesting that people are particularly efficient at making trustworthiness judgments.

In a series of subsequent studies focusing on judgments of trustworthiness (Todorov & Pakrashi, under review), we tested whether exposure times shorter than 100 ms are sufficient for these judgments. In fact, in three experiments we found that even after 33 ms exposure, judgments were better than chance in discriminating trustworthy-looking from untrustworthy-looking faces. In one of the experiments, we used 8 different presentation times ranging from subliminal presentation of faces (17 ms) to unlimited viewing time. As shown in FIGURE 1, judgments changed systematically as a function of time exposure. These judgments were almost perfectly described by a sigmoid function of time exposure, accounting for 95% of the variance. Participants were unable to discriminate between trustworthy-looking and untrustworthy-looking faces after subliminal exposure but were able to discriminate after 33 ms exposure. With the increase in exposure from 33 to 100 ms, the correlation between judgments made after limited exposure and control judgments made in the absence of time constraints increased dramatically. This correlation improved relatively little with the increase in exposure from 100 to 167 ms, and additional increases in time exposure did not improve the correlation at all.

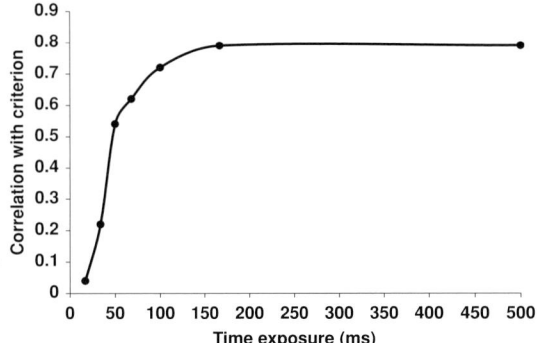

FIGURE 1. Correlation of judgments of trustworthiness made after limited time exposure to emotionally neutral faces and control judgments made in the absence of time constraints as a function of exposure time. Faces were presented for 17, 33, 50, 67, 100, 167, and 500 ms. Correlations at the level of mean trustworthiness judgment averaged across participants.

Bar and colleagues (2006) obtained similar findings for judgments of perceived threat in emotionally neutral faces. Judgments made after 39 ms (but not judgments made after 26 ms) correlated highly with judgments made after 1700 ms. As in our studies, participants were not able to make trait judgments after subliminal exposure to faces but were able to make these judgments after presentation times that are at the subjective threshold of visual awareness of faces (Pessoa et al. 2006a; Pessoa et al. 2006b).

Bar and colleagues also showed that after rapid exposures, threat judgments were predicted by judgments of low spatial frequency (LSF) face images but not by judgments of high spatial frequency (HSF) face images. This finding is interesting because it suggests that such judgments may be computed via fast coarse magnocellular pathways, guaranteeing a processing advantage for these judgments. Low frequency information may be carried through either superior colliculus/pulvinar subcortical pathways (Hamm et al. 2003; Vuilleumier 2005) or cortical pathways (Bar 2003; Pessoa 2005; Pessoa et al. 2002). In the case of emotional expressions, there is evidence that their perception depends on LSF information (Schyns & Oliva 1999), and functional neuroimaging studies suggest that the amygdala is particularly sensitive to this information in the discrimination of fearful from neutral faces (Vuilleumier et al. 2003; Winston et al. 2003). In one of our experiments, described in Section VI, we tested whether the amygdala response to face trustworthiness is modulated by spatial frequency information (Said et al., under review).

To summarize, person impressions are formed after face exposures shorter than 100 ms. Such exposure times are not sufficient for saccadic eye movements and, thus, do not allow for visual exploration of the face. In other words, trait impressions formed after rapid face presentations are "single glance" impressions.

II. What Do Judgments of Trustworthiness Measure?

As the first three panels of FIGURE 2 show, judgments of trustworthiness are highly correlated with other trait judgments. For example, for a set of standardized neutral faces (Lundqvist et al. 1998), trustworthiness judgments correlate 0.75 with judgments of attractiveness, −0.76 with judgments of aggressiveness, and 0.63 with judgments of intelligence. In fact, it is very difficult to find a trait judgment that is not correlated with trustworthiness. These high correlations suggest that trustworthiness judgments from faces may reflect the general evaluation of the face or, at least, approximate this evaluation rather well. Such valence evaluation permeates social judgments (Kim & Rosenberg 1980; Rosenberg et al. 1968; cf. Osgood et al. 1957) and is one of the organizing principles of person impressions (Wyer & Srull 1989).

A series of data-driven behavioral studies confirmed the hypothesis that trustworthiness judgments approximate the valence evaluation of faces (Oosterhof & Todorov, under review). First, we identified trait dimensions that are spontaneously used to characterize faces. Second, for each of these trait dimensions, a group of participants rated emotionally neutral faces. Third, the mean trait judgments were submitted to a principal component analysis. The first principal component accounted for 63% of the variance. All positive judgments (trustworthy, emotionally stable, responsible, sociable, caring, attractive, intelligent, and confident) had positive loadings. and all negative judgments (weird, mean, aggressive, unhappy, and dominant) had negative loadings on this component. Most important, judgments of trustworthiness had the highest loading (.94), suggesting that these judgments best approximate the valence dimension of face evaluation. This was the case even when we excluded trustworthiness judgments from the principal component analysis. The correlation between the first principal component (the evaluation factor) obtained from all trait judgments except trustworthiness and trustworthiness judgments was .94 (FIG. 2D), indicating that a single trustworthiness judgment was sufficient to summarize the evaluative information present in all other trait judgments.

Thus, it appears that in situations where no context is provided, trustworthiness judgments from faces

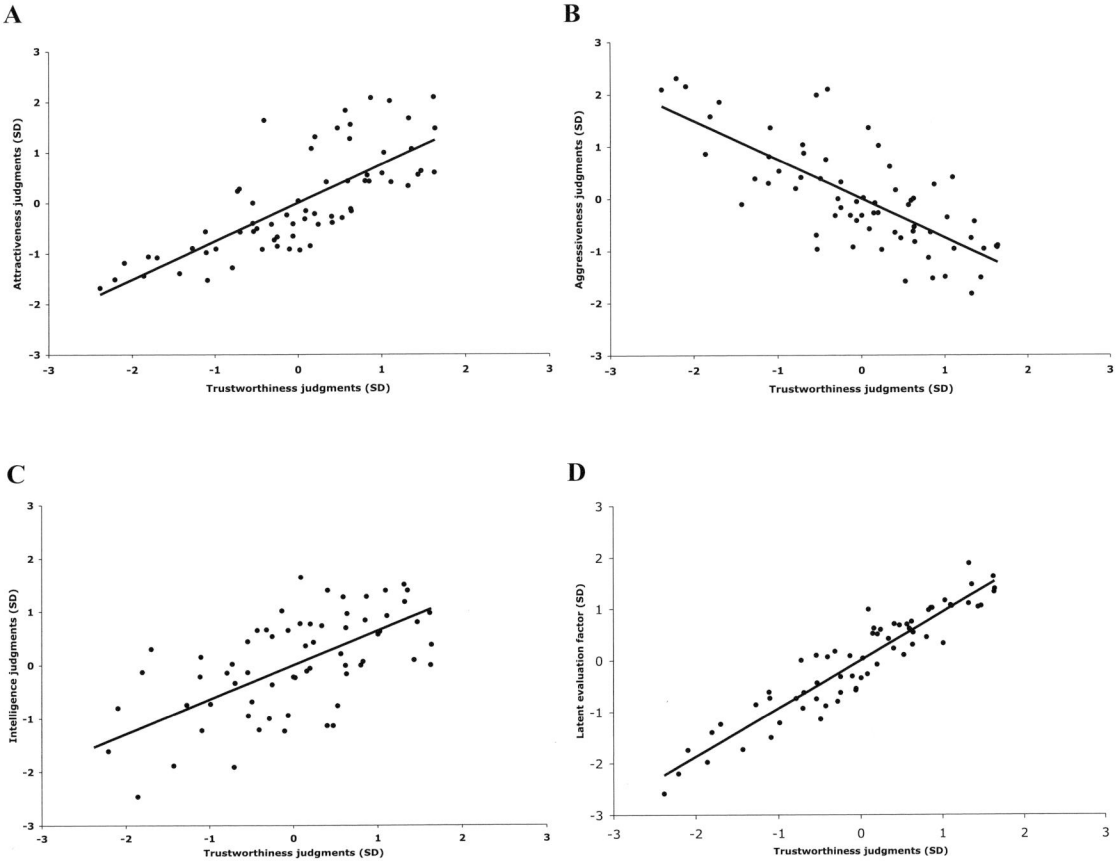

FIGURE 2. Scatter plots of judgments of trustworthiness from emotionally neutral faces and **(A)** judgments of attractiveness, **(B)** judgments of aggressiveness, **(C)** judgments of intelligence, and **(D)** a latent evaluation factor, which is a linear combination of judgments on 12 traits used to spontaneously categorize faces. Each point represents a face. The judgments are plotted in standardized scores. The line represents the best linear fit.

reflect inferences about the positivity/negativity of the face. If the valence evaluation of a stimulus is directly linked to automatic approach/avoidance responses (Chen & Bargh 1999), then judgments of trustworthiness may serve precisely this function in social interactions: determining whether to approach or avoid a stranger. In fact, Fenske and colleagues (2005) showed that momentary associations of motor approach/avoidance responses with faces affected subsequent trustworthiness judgments of these faces. Faces for which participants had to withhold a response were rated as less trustworthy than faces for which they did not have to withhold a response.

Adolphs and colleagues (1998) asked patients with bilateral amygdala–damage to make trustworthiness and approachability judgments ("how much would they want to walk up to that person and strike up a conversation") from faces. The results were identical for these two judgments, and the correlation between the mean control judgments was 0.89. Relative to three comparison groups (normal controls, brain-damaged patients with no damage in the amygdala, and patients with unilateral amygdala-damage), the bilateral amygdala damage patients judged untrustworthy-looking faces as trustworthy and "unapproachable" faces as approachable. This is consistent with experimental primate research showing that bilateral amygdala lesions lead to uninhibited approach behaviors in social interactions (Amaral 2002; Emery et al. 2001).

To summarize, the functional role of face evaluation is to prepare one's behavior in relation to the other person. When clear emotional cues broadcasting the intentions of the other person are absent, judgments of trustworthiness are tantamount to an approach/avoidance decision.

III. The Neural Underpinnings of Judgments of Trustworthiness

Three studies have implicated the amygdala in the computation of trustworthiness judgments (Adolphs et al. 1998; Engell et al. 2007; Winston et al. 2002). The amygdala is involved in multiple psychological functions (Phelps & LeDoux 2005) from learning of fear responses and consolidation of emotional memories (McGaugh 2004) to implicit evaluation of stimuli (Davis & Whalen 2001; Sander et al. 2003; Vuilleumier 2005; Whalen 1998). The findings suggesting that the amygdala plays a key role in the evaluation of face trustworthiness are consistent with the latter role.

As described above, patients with bilateral amygdala damage show a bias to perceive untrustworthy faces as trustworthy (Adolphs et al. 1998). Two subsequent functional neuroimaging studies (Engell et al. 2007; Winston et al. 2002) confirmed the involvement of the amygdala in face evaluation on trustworthiness and, further, showed that faces are spontaneously evaluated on this dimension. Winston and colleagues (2002) asked participants to make explicit trustworthiness judgments and implicit (with respect to trustworthiness) age judgments of unfamiliar faces. Independent of the task, the amygdala activity increased as the subjective *untrustworthiness* of the faces increased. The judgments of trustworthiness were collected after the imaging experiment and the brain responses were modeled as a function of these judgments.

We used a different implicit task and replicated the Winston et al. findings (Engell et al. 2007). In our experiment, participants were ostensibly engaged in a memory task. They were presented with blocks of faces and asked to indicate whether a test face was presented in the preceding block or not. Judgments of trustworthiness or person evaluation were never mentioned during the course of the experiment. Although the task did not demand face evaluation, the amygdala response to faces increased as the untrustworthiness of the faces increased (FIG. 3).

In the same study, we also tested whether the amygdala response is driven by face properties that signal untrustworthiness across individuals or by an individual's idiosyncratic perceptions of untrustworthiness. Although people agree when making trait judgments from faces, there is a large individual variation. For example, for the set of faces that we used, the average correlation between individual judgments and the mean judgments of the other individuals (consensus judgments) was 0.52. We collected trustworthiness judgments from a large sample of participants who did not participate in the fMRI study and used the mean judgments to predict the individual's amygdala response to the faces. These consensus judgments predicted the amygdala's response better than the individual's own judgments collected after the fMRI session. There was little residual variance explained by individual judgments in the amygdala's response after removing their shared variance with consensus judgments. Because consensus judgments reflect properties of the face rather than idiosyncratic perceptions of the judge (e.g., Hönekopp 2006), we argued that the amygdala response is driven in a bottom-up fashion by structural properties of the face that convey cues for untrustworthiness. This finding suggests that a more powerful approach to modeling the amygdala's response to face trustworthiness is to use formal models for representing face trustworthiness rather than rely on individual judgments, an approach that is outlined in the next section.

IV. The Origins of Face Evaluation

Secord (1958) suggested that one of the mechanisms for forming person impressions is "temporal extension"—misattributing a momentary state of the person to an enduring attribute. This hypothesis implies that person impressions may be grounded in momentary emotional expressions, and three empirical studies provide support for this idea. Knutson (1996) showed that emotional expressions were associated with trait judgments of dominance and affiliation. For example, faces expressing anger were rated as more dominant. Two subsequent studies replicated these findings (Hess et al. 2000; Montepare & Dobish 2003). Montepare and Dobish also showed that emotion ratings of neutral faces correlated with trait ratings of these faces.

Emotional expressions, among other things, broadcast behavioral intentions (e.g., Adams & Kleck 2005; Fridlund 1994). Expressions of anger communicate that the person should be avoided, and expressions of happiness communicate that the person can be approached. For example, recent studies show that angry faces trigger automatic avoidance responses (Adams et al. 2006; Marsh et al. 2005). If face evaluation reflects inferences of behavioral intentions related to one's approach/avoidance behavior, as argued in Section II, it may be derived from emotional expressions that signal approach/avoidance behaviors. Specifically, faces that are evaluated negatively may contain subtle features that resemble angry expressions and faces that are evaluated positively may contain subtle features that resemble happy expressions.

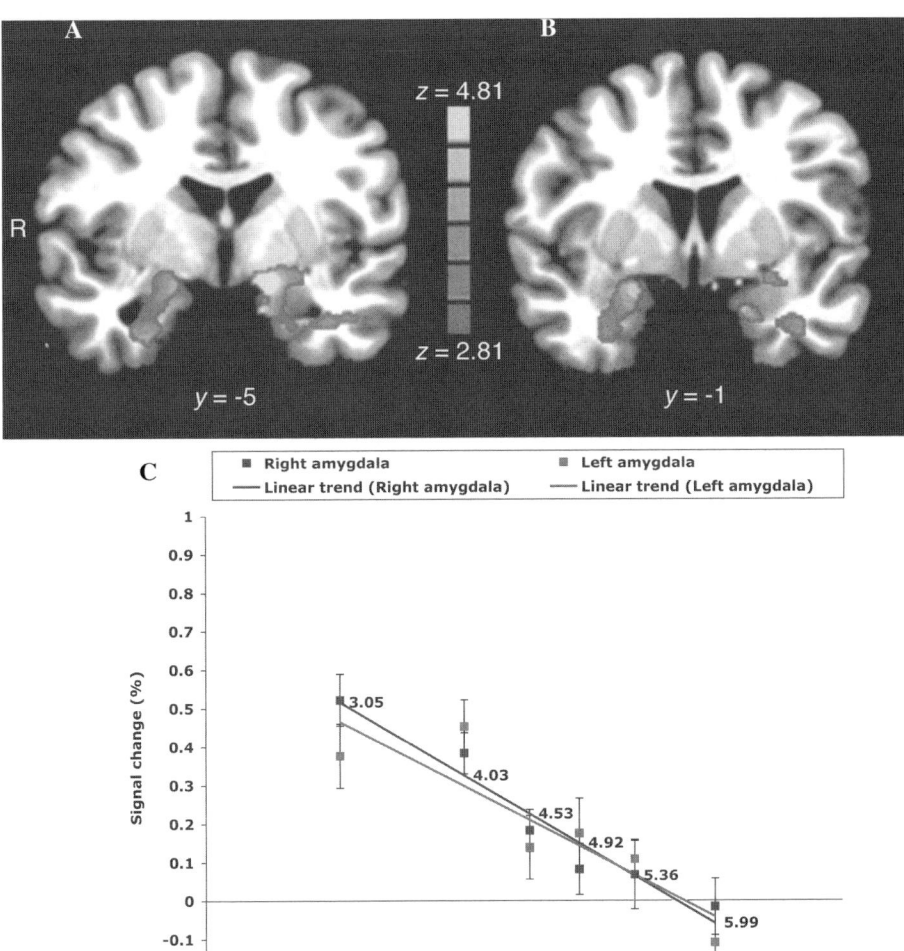

FIGURE 3. Amygdala response as a linear function of face trustworthiness. Activity is overlaid on slices of a standardized brain containing the peak response for **(A)** the left amygdala and for **(B)** the right amygdala. **(C)** Blood oxygenated level-dependent response (% signal change) in voxels in the amygdala showing a significant linear trend as a function of face trustworthiness. To extract percent signal change, faces were divided into 6 categories according to their perceived trustworthiness. For example, the mean for the least trustworthy faces was 3.05 ($SD = 0.45$) and the mean for the most trustworthy faces was 5.99 ($SD = 0.21$) on a scale ranging from 1 (untrustworthy) to 9 (trustworthy).

To test the hypothesis that face evaluation is an overextension of the mechanisms for understanding the communicative meaning of emotional expressions, we combined behavioral studies and computer modeling (Oosterhof & Todorov, under review). First, we built and validated a computer model for representing face trustworthiness. Second, using this model, we exaggerated the features that make a face look trustworthy or untrustworthy and tested how the perceptions of the face change as a function of these features.

We used a data-driven statistical model based on 3D laser scans of faces, in which faces are represented as points in a multidimensional space (Blanz & Vetter 1999; Singular Inversions 2006). We worked with 50 dimensions (50 independent principal components) representing 3D face shape. Using the model, we randomly generated 200 emotionally neutral faces with the constraint that the faces were Caucasian to avoid the influence of ethnic stereotypes on judgments. We asked participants to judge these faces on trustworthiness and used the mean judgments to find a vector (representing a weighted combination of the principal components) in the 50-dimensional face space whose direction is optimal in changing trustworthiness (FIG. 4A).

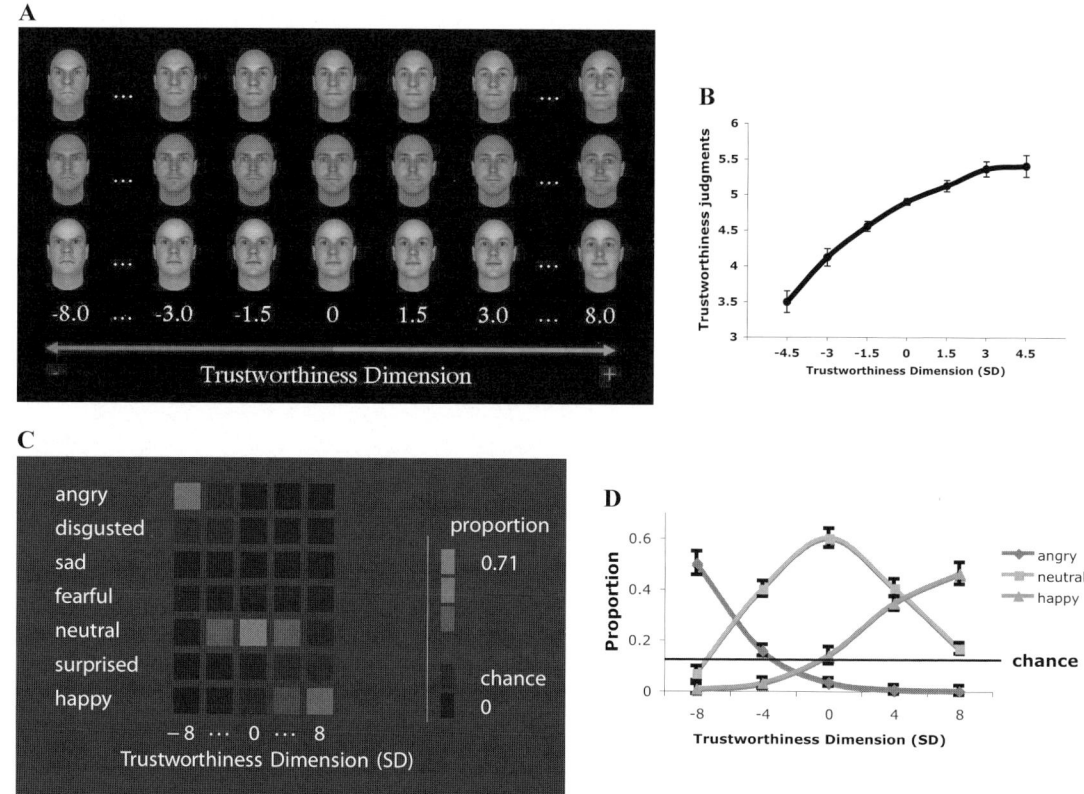

FIGURE 4. (A) Examples of faces with exaggerated trustworthiness features. The faces in the center column were randomly generated and then their features were exaggerated to decrease (left three columns) and increase (right three columns) their perceived trustworthiness. These changes were implemented in a computer model based on trustworthiness judgments of neutral faces. **(B)** Trustworthiness judgments of faces generated by the computer model. The judgments were made on a 9-point scale, ranging from 1 (not at all trustworthy) to 9 (extremely trustworthy). **(C)** Intensity color plot showing the emotion categorization of faces as a function of their trustworthiness. **(D)** Categorization of faces as angry, happy, and neutral as a function of their trustworthiness. The x-axis in the figures represents the extent of exaggeration of facial features in standard deviation units. Error bars show within-subjects standard error of the mean.

To validate that the model successfully manipulates face trustworthiness, we randomly generated neutral faces and produced untrustworthy and trustworthy versions for each face. Then, we asked participants to judge these faces on trustworthiness. As shown in FIGURE 4B, trustworthiness judgments of faces tracked the trustworthiness predicted by the model, although people were more sensitive to changes in trustworthiness at the low end of the spectrum than at the high end. A quadratic monotonic function accounted for 99% of the variance of the mean judgments. That is, although the physical distance between any two categories of faces was the same (1.5 SD), people were better at discriminating faces at the negative end of the trustworthiness dimension.

If face evaluation builds on the mechanisms underlying perception of emotional expressions, then exaggerating facial features that increase or decrease perceived trustworthiness should produce faces with emotional expressions (FIG. 4A). In other words, "neutral" expressions should contain subtle features that resemble emotional expressions and that people interpret to signify personality dispositions. To test this hypothesis, we presented participants with extreme trustworthy and untrustworthy versions of randomly generated neutral faces and asked them to classify the faces as neutral or as expressing one of the six basic emotions (FIG. 4C). The only responses above the chance level were for the categories of neutral, angry, and happy. The original faces (0 SD) were classified as neutral (FIG. 4D). As the facial features become more exaggerated, the neutral categorization approached chance, and this was particularly clear on the negative end of the continuum. As the facial features become more exaggerated in the negative direction (−8 SD), the faces were mostly classified as angry, whereas the trustworthy facial features become more exaggerated in the positive direction (+8 SD), the faces were mostly classified as happy.

To summarize, although the model for representing face trustworthiness was a) based on judgments of faces with neutral expressions and b) data driven without a priori assumptions about which facial parts are important for trustworthiness judgments, exaggerating the features specific for trustworthiness produced faces with emotional expressions. These findings suggest that face evaluation is an overextension of the ability to read emotional expressions. That is, trustworthiness judgments are an attempt to infer behavioral intentions and are derived from facial features that resemble emotional expressions signaling approach/avoidance behaviors. For the positive end of the trustworthiness continuum, these are expressions of happiness. For the negative end of the continuum, these are expressions of anger.

The emotion overgeneralization hypothesis can account for rapid, efficient trait judgments from faces that are not necessarily accurate, a pattern that appears puzzling from an evolutionary point of view (Section V). This hypothesis also generates novel predictions about brain responses to faces, namely the amygdala response to face trustworthiness should change as a nonlinear function (Section VI) and it should be possible to observe dissociations between processing of facial identity and face evaluation (Section VII).

V. Implications for the Accuracy of Trait Judgments from Faces

Granted the notoriety of physiognomy, is there evidence that judgments of trustworthiness from still images of faces are accurate? Berry (1990) found that judgments of honesty from faces correlated with self-reports and judgments of acquaintances. In the one study measuring the trustworthiness of actual behavior, judgments of honesty from faces accounted for 4% of the variance of behavior (Bond et al. 1994). Bond and colleagues (1994) found that participants who were rated as dishonest based on their photos were more likely to express willingness to participate in experiments that involved deceiving another participant. There are multiple possible pathways of developing behavioral patterns that confirm social expectations, and these can account for such correlations (Zebrowitz 1999). For example, according to a self-fulfilling prophecy perspective, a person with an untrustworthy appearance who is consistently treated as an untrustworthy individual may develop corresponding behavioral responses. Of course, the opposite prediction can also be made, namely that people may work hard to overcome stereotypes triggered by their appearance, and there is evidence for this self-defeating prophecy effect (Collins & Zebrowitz 1995; Zebrowitz et al. 1998a; Zebrowitz et al. 1998b).

In the one longitudinal study on the accuracy of trustworthiness judgments, Zebrowitz and colleagues (1996) failed to find correspondence between judgments of honesty from faces and clinical assessments of honesty. Additional analyses showed positive correlations for men with a stable appearance of honesty across the life span, but negative correlations for women with a stable appearance. It is interesting to note that some evolutionary theories predict negative correlations (Bond & Robinson 1988). Starting from the argument that deception confers an adaptive advantage, they argue that people with nondeceptive (trustworthy) faces can learn to be more successful liars and, correspondingly, can develop deceptive personality traits as a result of positive reinforcement of their deceptive behaviors.

From the point of view of the emotion overgeneralization hypothesis, it is not necessary to have a reliable relationship between trustworthiness judgments from faces and measures of personality. To the extent that these judgments are a measure of reading emotional cues in "neutral" faces that are misattributed to stable personality dispositions, one should not expect that they are accurate.

Finally, if one assumes that personality dispositions are combinations of emotion tendencies (e.g., Plutchik 1980), it should be possible to find positive correlations between facial appearance and personality dispositions. At the end of 19th century, Theodor Piderit, a German physician who rejected Lavater's physiognomy, argued that because emotional expressions involve exercising of facial muscles, frequent exercise of these muscles could leave its permanent trace on the face (cited in Fridlund 1994, p. 11). One hundred years later, Malatesta and colleagues (1987) found some support for this hypothesis. They showed that posed neutral expressions of a sample of elderly subjects were perceived as conveying specific emotions and that these perceptions correlated with self-reports of the frequency of experiencing the emotions. For example, people who looked angry when posing for neutral photos also reported high frequency of experiencing anger.

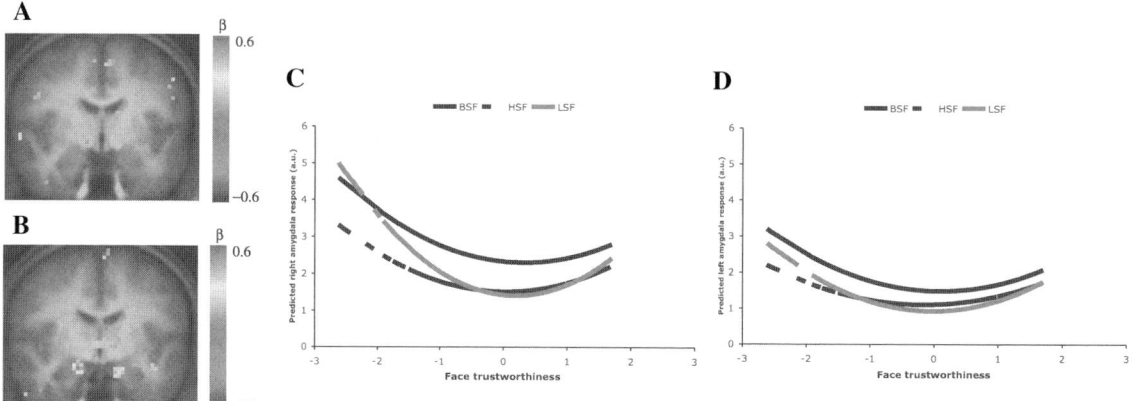

FIGURE 5. Amygdala response as a function of face trustworthiness. **(A)** Clusters in both amygdalae (y = 6) showing a linear response to trustworthiness. The blue shading indicates more activity as trustworthiness decreases. **(B)** Clusters (y = 8) showing significant quadratic effects of trustworthiness. Predicted quadratic response in clusters in the **(C)** right and **(D)** left amygdala as a function of face trustworthiness and spatial frequency. The curves were generated by extracting the mean parameter estimates of zero-order (presence of a face), linear, and quadratic effects from each spatial frequency category within the functionally defined region of interest.

VI. Implications for the Amygdala Response to Face Trustworthiness

In the first two functional neuroimaging studies on the evaluation of face trustworthiness (Engell et al. 2007; Winston et al. 2002), the amygdala response was modeled as a linear function of trustworthiness. As described above, in both studies, this response increased as the untrustworthiness of the faces increased. However, a number of functional neuroimaging studies have found a stronger amygdala response to happy than to neutral faces (e.g., Breiter et al. 1996; Pessoa, Japee, Sturman, et al. 2006; Winston et al. 2003; Yang et al. 2002). These findings, coupled with our findings that trustworthy faces have features resembling expressions of happiness, suggest that trustworthy faces can evoke a stronger amygdala response than faces in the middle of the trustworthiness dimension. That is, one should observe a nonlinear response to face trustworthiness with elevated responses to both extremely trustworthy and untrustworthy faces. Modeling the amygdala response as a linear function of face trustworthiness would miss this effect. Thus, the first implication of the emotion overgeneralization hypothesis for the amygdala's response is that this response should be a nonmonotonic function of face trustworthiness given sufficient range of trustworthiness.

In general, there is substantial evidence for the attention-grabbing power of negative information (e.g., Fiske 1980; Skowronski & Carlston 1989; Pratto & John 1991). In our own studies, as described above (FIG. 4B), we found that people are more sensitive to differences at the negative than at the positive end of the trustworthiness dimension (Oosterhof & Todorov, under review). From an evolutionary point of view, it is more important to detect untrustworthy than trustworthy individuals (cf., Cosmides & Tooby 1992), and our findings are consistent with this view. The second implication of the emotion overgeneralization hypothesis is that the amygdala's response should be more sensitive to differences at the negative than at the positive end of the trustworthiness dimension.

To test these predictions, we modeled the amygdala response as a quadratic function of face trustworthiness in two fMRI studies (Said et al. under review; Todorov et al. under review). In the first study, we found that the quadratic function provided a better fit of the amygdala response than the linear function in both left and right amygdala (FIG. 5). The amygdala response was stronger to both trustworthy and untrustworthy faces than to faces in the middle of the trustworthiness dimension. However, consistent with the previous findings of linear amygdala response to trustworthiness (Engell et al. 2007; Winston et al. 2002), the amygdala response was more sensitive to differences at the negative than at the positive end of the trustworthiness dimension (FIG. 5C & D).

In this study, we also tested whether the amygdala response was better predicted by LSF face images than by HSF images. We found that both LSF and HSF faces provided sufficient information to differentiate faces on trustworthiness and that this was the case for the behavioral and the functional neuroimaging data. Trustworthiness judgments from both the HSF and the LSF images correlated with judgments from unfiltered (broad spatial frequency faces) images. In addition, as shown in FIGURE 5C, D, the amygdala response for these images was similar, although at the negative end of the trustworthiness dimension, the slope was steeper for LSF images. One possible reason for the discrepancy with the behavioral findings of Bar et al. (2006), described in Section I, is that we used a longer presentation time in our experiment (200 ms as compared to 38 ms). In other words, it is likely that the advantage in processing of LSF images can only be seen after rapid exposure to faces. Our findings suggest that the amygdala response to face trustworthiness is robust with respect to the informational input for exposures as short as 200 ms.

In our second fMRI study (Todorov et al. under review), we used faces generated by a computer model for representing trustworthiness. The development of this model preceded the work of Oosterhof and Todorov (under review), which was described in Section IV. As it turned out, the two models converged on very similar representations of trustworthiness. We asked participants to judge computer-generated faces on trustworthiness and then regressed the mean judgments on facial features that can be controlled (e.g., moving up or down the inner part of the brow ridge) in the program for face manipulation (*FaceGen 3.1*, Singular Inversions 2006). Based on the four features that showed the highest correlation with the judgments and also had low correlations among them, we built a regression model for predicting face trustworthiness. Then we generated novel faces and manipulated the four features in both directions of increasing and decreasing face trustworthiness. The trustworthiness scores predicted by the regression model were used as regressors in the fMRI analysis.

As in Said and colleagues (under review), we found a cluster of voxels in the left amygdala that showed a non monotonic quadratic response to face trustworthiness (FIG. 6). However, this was limited to the left amygdala. A cluster of voxels in the right amygdala, which showed the same response in Engell and colleagues (2007), showed a significant linear trend. As the untrustworthiness of the faces increased, so did the right amygdala response. The findings suggest that the right amygdala may exhibit a more linear response than the left amygdala. In Engell et al., the linear trend was stronger for the right than the left amygdala, and in Said et al. (FIG. 5C & D), the slope of the response to untrustworthy faces was steeper in the right than in the left amygdala. Possible laterality differences should be addressed in future studies.

In the two studies described above, we found that the amygdala response to face trustworthiness may be better described as a quadratic rather than as a linear function of trustworthiness and that this response is more sensitive to differences at the negative than at the positive end of the trustworthiness dimension. It is interesting to note in the context of the latter finding that the relatively poor discrimination between trustworthy-looking and untrustworthy-looking faces in bilateral amygdala damage patients is due to a bias to perceive untrustworthy faces as trustworthy (Adolphs et al. 1998; see also Section VII). This also seems to be the case for people with Asperger syndrome (Adolphs et al. 2001; White et al. 2006).

The findings from patient studies and functional neuroimaging studies suggest that the amygdala is better tuned to detecting differences in the negative valence than in the positive valence of faces. This can also explain the linear trends observed in the prior studies. A linear trend can provide a reasonable fit of data that are better described by a quadratic function with a steeper slope at the negative than at the positive end of the trustworthiness dimension. This question is revisited in the section on methodological implications.

VII. Implications for Models of Face Perception

Models of face perception posit different neural pathways for processing of relatively invariant facial features essential for recognizing identity and gender and changeable facial features essential for recognizing emotions and gaze direction (Bruce & Young 1986; Haxby et al. 2000; Perrett et al. 1992; but see Calder & Young 2005 for an alternative view). Trait judgments from faces do not fit neatly in this categorization. The current findings suggest that face evaluation is subserved by the mechanisms underlying perception of emotional expressions. Thus, it should be possible to observe dissociations between processing of face evaluation and facial identity. For example, given that there are prosopagnosics who can recognize emotional expressions but not identity (Bentin et al. 2007; Damasio et al. 1990; Duchaine et al. 2003; Humphreys et al. in press; Tranel et al. 1988), there should be prosopagnosics who can make normal trustworthiness judgments.

In fact, data from four individuals with developmental prosopagnosia, a condition characterized by face recognition deficits due to a failure to develop face recognition mechanisms (Behrmann & Avidan 2005;

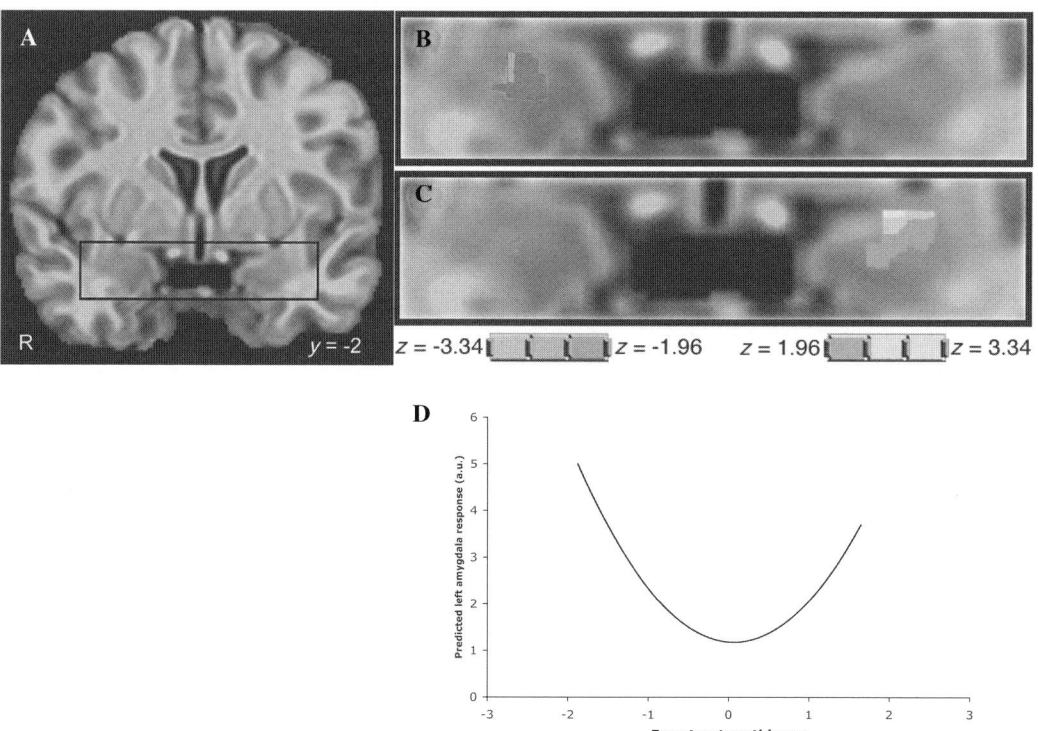

FIGURE 6. Amygdala response as a function of face trustworthiness. **(A)** Amygdala region of a standardized brain. **(B)** A cluster in the right amygdala showing a significant linear response. This cluster showed the same linear response in Engell et al. (2007). **(C)** A cluster in the left amygdala showing a significant quadratic response. **(D)** Predicted quadratic response in the left amygdala cluster as a function of face trustworthiness. The curve was generated by extracting the mean parameter estimates of zero-order (presence of a face), linear, and quadratic effects within the functionally defined region of interest.

Duchaine & Nakayama 2006a), confirmed this prediction (Todorov & Duchaine, under review). Although all four prosopagnosics had a normal performance on tests of low-level vision (Riddoch & Humphreys 1993), they had severe impairments in both long-term memory for faces and perception of facial identity. On five different measures—two measuring face memory problems and three measuring identity perception problems—each prosopagnosic individual was more than 2 standard deviations below the mean control performance (Duchaine & Nakayama 2006b; Yovel & Duchaine 2006). For example, as a group, they were 6.7 SD below the control mean on a recognition test of famous faces and 3.1 SD below the mean on a recognition test of newly learned faces (Bentin et al. 2007; Duchaine & Nakayama 2006b). On a task requiring the sorting of morphed faces in terms of similarity to a target face (Duchaine et al. in press), they were 3.3 SD below the control mean.

We asked the prosopagnosics to make trustworthiness judgments of three different sets of faces. The first set of faces was used to test patients with bilateral amygdala damage (Adolphs et al. 1998). As shown in FIGURE 7A, all four prosopagnosics showed normal performance on this set of faces. To compare their judgments with the judgments of the bilateral amygdala-damage patients studied by Adolphs and colleagues, we split the faces into the 50 most and the 50 least trustworthy faces. As described earlier, these patients show a bias to perceive untrustworthy-looking faces as trustworthy. Relative to our controls, their judgments of untrustworthy faces were 2.8 SD above the control mean. In contrast, the prosopagnosics' judgments of untrustworthy faces were within 1 SD of the control mean. For both groups, the judgments of trustworthy faces were within 1 SD of the control mean (FIG. 7B). Given that there are patients with bilateral amygdala damage who process the identity of faces normally (Adolphs et al. 1995), the results suggest a possible double dissociation between encoding identity and face evaluation. This is not surprising in light of the findings that these judgments reflect the detection of facial cues that resemble expressions of anger and happiness.

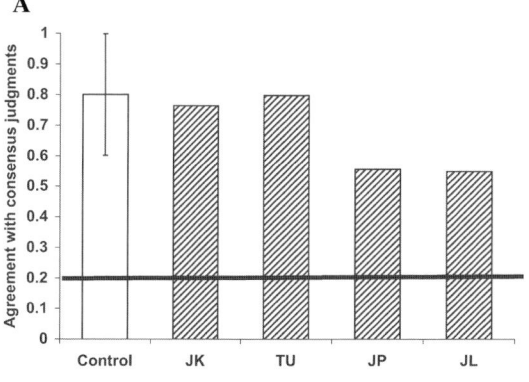

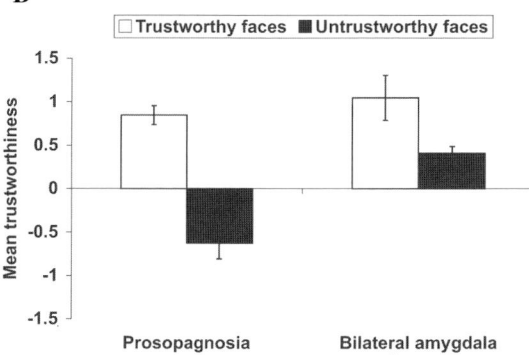

FIGURE 7. (A) Agreement between prosopagnosics' judgments and control judgments of trustworthiness of faces. The agreement is measured in Fisher z transformations of the raw correlations between individual judgments and the mean judgments of control participants. The error bar shows 1 standard deviation. Scores above the thick black line indicate significant correlations. **(B)** Mean perceived trustworthiness of faces categorized as trustworthy and untrustworthy for four patients with bilateral amygdala damage and four developmental prosopagnosics. The trustworthiness was measured on a scale from −3 (untrustworthy) to +3 (trustworthy). The error bars show standard error of the mean.

The faces in the first set varied on a number of dimensions including hair, expression, gaze, and age. It is possible that the prosopagnosics' normal performance on trustworthiness judgments can be accounted for by reliance on these cues. To rule out this explanation, we used two sets of standardized faces. In both sets, the faces had direct gaze, neutral expression, and a similar age. In the final set, the hair and facial blemishes of all faces were removed, and the faces were presented as grayscale images. Thus, the face sets consisted of increasingly homogeneous face images in order to force reliance on facial structure and complexion. For both sets of faces, two of the prosopagnosics showed typical trustworthiness judgments that agreed with control judgments. The judgments of the other two weakly agreed with control judgments, but even their judgments were within the normal range of control performance. The prosopagnosics with worse performance on the trustworthiness tests were not more severely impaired with the facial identity tests than the prosopagnosics with normal performance.

The findings suggest that the mechanisms underlying face evaluation are separable from the mechanisms underlying processing of facial identity. We tested developmental prosopagnosics, but these findings should be extended to individuals with acquired prosopagnosia and defined brain lesions in inferotemporal cortex.

VIII. Methodological Implications

The most important methodological implication of our findings is the value of using data-driven formal models for representing the variation of faces on social dimensions. First, by exaggerating the facial features that define the variation of a face on a specific dimension, one can discover the cues in the face that are critical for judgments on this dimension. We applied this technique to judgments of trustworthiness, but it can be applied to any other judgment. Second, from an experimental point of view, these models allow the researcher to have precise control over the facial stimuli and to generate an unlimited number of faces. This can lead to new discoveries and potential theory advancement, as well as facilitate comparisons across different studies. I illustrate the value of using models for face representation with three examples.

First, as described in Section IV (FIG. 4B), we found that participants were more sensitive to changes at the negative than at the positive end of the trustworthiness dimension, controlling for the distance between faces on the trustworthiness dimension. A computer model provides the means for objective scaling of differences on a specific dimension and, consequently, precise modeling of how judgments change as a function of this distance. Without a model for representing face trustworthiness, we would not have been able to discover that judgments are more sensitive to changes at the negative end of the trustworthiness dimension.

Second, the finding that the amygdala response was more sensitive to differences at the negative than at the positive end of the trustwothiness dimension (Said et al. under review; Todorov et al. under review) can partially explain the linear trends observed in the prior studies (Engell et al. 2007; Winston et al. 2002). However, one variable that is critical about the observed amygdala response and that can vary across studies is the range of face trustworthiness. Comparing behavioral ratings of faces across studies to test for differences in this range is not sufficient because people can shift their standard of judgment as a function of the specific set of faces (Biernat et al. 1991; Parducci 1965). In other words, two face sets may have the same behavioral ratings in two different studies but if judged within the same study may be very different. In fact, in a behavioral study conducted after the fMRI studies, we found that the faces used by Said and colleagues had a higher range of positivity than the faces used by Engell and colleagues (2007). Such variables external to the experiment may lead to different neural responses further complicating comparisons across studies. Having a formal model for representing face variations on the dimension of interest can solve this problem, because different face sets can be objectively scaled in terms of the model representation.

Third, as described in Section III, trait judgments from faces are highly correlated with each other. This makes it very difficult to disentangle the specific contributions of different judgments to neural responses. For example, Winston and colleagues (2007) recently found a nonlinear amygdala response to facial attractiveness. However, given that trustworthiness and attractiveness judgments are highly correlated (e.g., FIG. 2A), it is possible that this response was driven by the shared variance with perceptions of trustworthiness. The standard approach is to statistically control for the shared variance among different judgments, but this can reduce the statistical power of experiments and, in cases of specific trait judgments, it would be difficult to decide on an a priori basis what judgments should be controlled. The alternative is to experimentally rather than statistically unconfound contributions of different judgments. This can be easily achieved with formal models that can produce an unlimited number of faces varying on specific dimensions. Further, this would be a shift from exploratory correlational approaches (e.g., Engell et al. 2007) to theory validation approaches.

In our research, we focused on the spontaneous bottom-up valence evaluation of faces. This research should be extended to testing a) theory-driven multi-dimensional models of face evaluation using the same modeling tools and b) the role of top-down evaluation triggered by specific goals. For example, validated models of interpersonal perception posit two fundamental dimensions of dominance and affiliation (e.g., Wiggins et al. 1989). Similarly, models of perception of social groups posit two dimensions of competence and warmth that mapped into assessments of group status and group competition (Fiske et al. 2007).

Whether these dimensions obtained from behavioral studies have specific neural correlates is an open empirical question.

Finally, it would be important to integrate the present research with research on social categorization. Social category information such as age, gender, and race is rapidly extracted from facial information (e.g., Cloutier et al. 2005; Ito, in press; Ito et al. 2004; Ito & Urland 2003; Mason et al. 2006) and many models of person perception make a fundamental distinction between social category and individuating information (Bodenhausen & Macrae 1998; Brewer 1988; Fiske & Neuberg 1990; but see Kunda 1999). Social category information can be easily manipulated in models of face representation allowing for the identification of the relative contributions of social category and individuating (e.g., variations on trustworthiness) information to both behavioral and neural responses.

Conclusions

Evaluation permeates social judgments, and its functional role is to prepare the individual for an appropriate action. Evaluating emotionally neutral faces on trustworthiness approximates the basic valence evaluation of faces and involves the amygdala. I argue that this evaluation is grounded in the mechanisms for perception of emotional expressions. Trustworthiness judgments from faces reflect inferences of behavioral intentions that signal approach/avoidance behaviors. Specifically, these judgments are based on facial features that resemble emotional expressions—happiness and anger—that ordinarily signal approach and avoidance behaviors, respectively. This emotion overgeneralization hypothesis can account for the persistence and subjectively compelling character of trait impressions from faces, as well as for rapid, efficient judgments that are not necessarily accurate. Finally, this hypothesis makes novel predictions about brain responses to faces that were confirmed in fMRI studies and studies with prosopagnosics.

We are in the beginning of the study of the neural underpinnings of face evaluation. Although I focused on findings about the role of the amygdala in face evaluation, clearly there are multiple regions involved in this evaluation. This chapter outlines a set of tools that can be used to characterize the neural systems underlying face evaluation. We should be able to build formal representational models of any specific trait dimension (e.g., competence), decompose the face variation on this dimension to facial properties such as features resembling emotional expressions and masculine

/feminine face shape, and characterize the neural systems involved in the evaluation on this dimension.

Acknowledgments

This research was supported by National Science Foundation Grant BCS-0446846. I thank Ralph Adolphs for providing the stimuli used to test patients with bilateral amygdala damage and the raw data for my reanalysis and Sean Baron, Jason Barton, Andy Engell, Susan Fiske, Crystal Hall, Todd Heatherton, Valerie Loehr, Chris Olivola, Nick Oosterhof, Chris Said, Sara Verosky, and an anonymous reviewer for their comments on previous versions of this chapter.

Conflict of Interest

The author declares no conflicts of interest.

References

Adams, R. B., Ambady, N., Macrae, N., & Kleck, R. E. (2006). Emotional expressions forecast approach-avoidance behavior. *Motivation & Emotion, 30*, 179–188.

Adams, R. B., & Kleck, R. E. (2005). Effects of direct and averted gaze on the perception of facially communicated emotion. *Emotion, 5*, 3–11.

Adolphs, R., Sears, L., & Piven, J. (2001). Abnormal processing of social information from faces in autism. *Journal of Cognitive Neuroscience, 13*, 232–240.

Adolphs, R., Tranel, D., & Damasio, A. R. (1998). The human amygdala in social judgment. *Nature, 393*, 470–474.

Adolphs, R., Tranel, D., Damasio, H., & Damasio, A. R. (1995). Fear and the human amygdala. *Journal of Neuroscience, 15*, 5879–5891.

Amaral, D. G. (2002). The primate amygdala and the neurobiology of social behavior: Implications for understanding social anxiety. *Biological Psychiatry, 51*, 11–17.

Ballew, C. C., & Todorov, A. (2007). Predicting political elections from rapid and unreflective face judgments. *Proceedings of the National Academy of Sciences of the USA, 104*, 17948–17953.

Bar, M. (2003). A cortical mechanism for triggering top-down facilitation in visual object recognition. *Journal of Cognitive Neuroscience, 15*, 600–609.

Bar, M., Neta, M., & Linz, H. (2006). Very first impressions. *Emotion, 6*, 269–278.

Behrmann, M., & Avidan, G. (2005). Congenital prosopagnosia: Face blind from birth. *Trends in Cognitive Sciences, 9*, 180–187.

Bentin, S., Degutis, J. M., D'Esposito, M., & Robertson, L. C. (2007). Too many trees to see the forest: Performance, event-related potential, and functional magnetic resonance imaging manifestations of integrative congenital prosopagnosia. *Journal of Cognitive Neuroscience, 19*, 132–146.

Berry, D. S. (1990). Taking people at face value: Evidence for the kernel of truth hypothesis. *Social Cognition, 8*, 343–361.

Biernat, M., Manis, M., & Nelson, T. E. (1991). Stereotypes and standards of judgment. *Journal of Personality and Social Psychology, 60*, 485–499.

Blair, I. V., Judd, C. M., & Chapleau, K. M. (2004). The influence of Afrocentric facial features in criminal sentencing. *Psychological Science, 15*, 674–679.

Blanz, V., & Vetter, T. (1999). A morphable model for the synthesis of 3D faces. In *Proceedings of the 26th Annual Conference on Computer Graphics and Interactive Techniques*, 187–194.

Bodenhausen, G. V., & Macrae, C. N. (1998). Stereotype Activation and Inhibition. In R. S. Wyer, Jr. (Ed.). *Stereotype Activation and Inhibition* (pp. 1–52). Mahwah, NJ: Lawrence Erlbaum.

Bond, C. F., Berry, D. S., & Omar, A. (1994). The kernel of truth in judgments of deceptiveness. *Basic and Applied Social Psychology, 15*, 523–534.

Bond, C. F., & Robinson, M. (1988). The evolution of deception. *Journal of Nonverbal Behavior, 12*, 295–307.

Breiter, H. C., Etcoff, N. L., Whalen, P. J., Kennedy, W. A., Rauch, S. L., Buckner, R. L., et al. (1996). Response and habituation of the human amygdala during visual processing of facial expression. *Neuron, 17*, 875–887.

Brewer, M. C. (1988). A dual process model of impression formation. In R. Wyer, & T. Scrull (Eds.). *Advances in Social Cognition* (Vol. 1 pp. 1–36). Hillsdale, NJ: Erlbaum.

Bruce, V., & Young, A. (1986). Understanding face recognition. *British Journal of Psychology, 77*, 305–327.

Calder, A. J., & Young, A. W. (2005). Understanding the recognition of facial identity and facial expression. *Nature Reviews Neuroscience, 6*, 641–651.

Chen, M., & Bargh, J. A. (1999). Consequences of automatic evaluation: Immediate behavioral predispositions to approach or avoid the stimulus. *Personality and Social Psychology Bulletin, 25*, 215–224.

Cloutier, J., Mason, M. F., Macrae, C. N. (2005). The perceptual determinants of person construal: Reopening the social-cognitive toolbox. *Journal of Personality and Social Psychology, 88*, 885–894.

Collins, M. A., & Zebrowitz, L. A. (1995). The contributions of appearance to occupational outcomes in civilian and military settings. *Journal of Applied Social Psychology, 25*, 129–163.

Cosmides, L., & Tooby, J. (1992). Cognitive adaptations for social exchange. In J. H. Barkow, L. Cosmides, & J. Tooby (Eds.), *The Adapted Mind: Evolutionary Psychology and the Generation of Culture* (pp. 163–228). London: Oxford University Press.

Damasio, A. R., Tranel, D., & Damasio, H. (1990). Face agnosia and the neural substrates of memory. *Annual Review of Neuroscience, 13*, 89–109.

Darwin, F. (Ed.) (1950). *Charles Darwin's Autobiography*. New York: Henry Schuman.

Davis, M., & Whalen, P. J. (2001). The amygdala: vigilance and emotion. *Molecular Psychiatry, 6*, 13–34.

Duchaine, B., & Nakayama, K. (2006a). Developmental prosopagnosia: A window to content-specific face processing. *Current Opinion in Neurobiology, 16*, 166–173.

Duchaine, B., & Nakayama, K. (2006b). The Cambridge Face Memory Test: Results for neurologically intact individuals and an investigation of its validity using inverted face stimuli and prosopagnosic participants. *Neuropsychologia*, *44*, 576–585.

Duchaine, B. C., Parker, H., & Nakayama, K. (2003). Normal emotion recognition in a developmental prosopagnosic. *Perception*, *32*, 827–838.

Duchaine, B., Yovel, G., & Nakayama, K. (in press). No global processing deficit in the Navon task in 14 developmental prosopagnosics. *Social, Cognitive, and Affective Neuroscience*.

Eberhardt, J. L., Davies, P. G., Purdie-Vaughns, V. J., & Johnson, S. L. (2006). Looking deathworthy: Perceived stereotypicality of Black defendants predicts capital-sentencing outcomes. *Psychological Science*, *17*, 383–386.

Emery, N. J., Capitanio, J. P., Mason, W. A., Machado, C. J., Mendoza, S. P., & Amaral, D. G. (2001). The effects of bilateral lesions of the amygdala on dyadic social interactions in rhesus monkeys (Macaca mulatta). *Behavioral Neuroscience*, *115*, 515–544.

Engell, A. D., Haxby, J. V., & Todorov, A. (2007). Implicit trustworthiness decisions: Automatic coding of face properties in human amygdala. *Journal of Cognitive Neuroscience*, *19*, 1508–1519.

Fenske, M. J., Raymond, J. E., Kessler, K., Westoby, N., & Tipper, S. P. (2005). Attentional inhibition has social-emotional consequences for unfamiliar faces. *Psychological Science*, *16*, 753–758.

Fiske, S. T. (1980). Attention and weight in person perception: The impact of negative and extreme behavior. *Journal of Personality and Social Psychology*, *38*, 889–906.

Fiske, S. T., Cuddy, A. J. C., & Glick, P. (2007). Universal dimensions of social cognition: warmth and competence. *Trends in Cognitive Sciences*, *11*, 77–83.

Fiske, S. T., & Neuberg, S. L. (1990). A continuum of impression formation, from category–based to individuating processes: Influences of information and motivation on attention and interpretation. *Advances in Experimental Social Psychology*, *23*, 1–73.

Fridlund, A. J. (1994). *Human Facial Expression: An Evolutionary View*. San Diego, CA: Academic Press.

Hall, C. C., Goren, A., Chaiken, S., & Todorov, A. (In press). Shallow cues with deep effects: Trait judgments from faces and voting decisions. In E. Borgida, J. L. Sullivan, & C. M. Federico (Eds.), *The Political Psychology of Democratic Citizenship*. Oxford University Press.

Hamermesh, D., & Biddle, J. (1994). Beauty and the labor market. *American Economic Review*, *84*, 1174–1194.

Hamm, A. O., Weike, A. I., Schupp, H. T., Treig, T., Dressel, A., & Kessler, C. (2003). Affective blindsight: intact fear conditioning to a visual cue in a cortically blind patient. *Brain*, *126*, 267–275.

Hassin, R., & Trope, Y. (2000). Facing faces: Studies on the cognitive aspects of physiognomy. *Journal of Personality and Social Psychology*, *78*, 837–852.

Haxby, J. V., Hoffman, E. A., & Gobbini, M. I. (2000). The distributed human neural system for face perception. *Trends in Cognitive Sciences*, *4*, 223–233.

Hess, U., Blairy, S., & Kleck, R. E. (2000). The influence of facial emotion displays, gender, and ethnicity on judgments of dominance and affiliation. *Journal of Nonverbal Behavior*, *24*, 265–283.

Hönekopp, J. (2006). Once more: Is beauty in the eye of the beholder? Relative contributions of private and shared taste to judgments of facial attractiveness. *Journal of Experimental Psychology: Human Perception and Performance*, *32*, 199–209.

Humphreys, K., Avidan, G., & Behrmann, M. (2007). A detailed investigation of facial expression processing in congenital prosopagnosia as compared to acquired prosopagnosia. *Experimental Brain Research*, *176*, 356–373.

Ito, T. A. (In press). Perceiving social category information from faces: Using ERPs to study person perception. In A. Todorov, S. T. Fiske, & D. Prentice (Eds.), *Social Neuroscience: Toward Understanding the Underpinnings of the Social Mind*. Oxford University Press.

Ito, T. A., Thompson, E., & Cacioppo, J. T. (2004). Tracking the timecourse of social perception: The effects of racial cues on event-related brain potentials. *Personality and Social Psychology Bulletin*, *30*, 1267–1280.

Ito, T. A., & Urland, G. R. (2003). Race and gender on the brain: Electrocortical measures of attention to race and gender of multiply categorizable individuals. *Journal of Personality and Social Psychology*, *85*, 616–626.

Kim, M. P., & Rosenberg, S. (1980). Comparison of two structural models of implicit personality theory. *Journal of Personality and Social Psychology*, *38*, 375–389.

Knutson, B. (1996). Facial expressions of emotion influence interpersonal trait inferences. *Journal of Nonverbal Behavior*, *20*, 165–181.

Kunda, Z. (1999). Parallel processing of stereotypes and behaviors. In S. Chaiken & Y. Trope (Eds). *Dual-Process Theories in Social Psychology* (pp. 314–322). New York: Guilford Press.

Langlois, J. H., Kalakanis, L., Rubenstein, A. J., Larson, A., Hallam, M., & Smoot, M. (2000). Maxims or myths of beauty? A meta-analytic and theoretical review. *Psychological Bulletin*, *126*, 390–423.

Little, A. C., Burriss, R. P., Jones, B. C., & Roberts, S. C. (2007). Facial appearance affects voting decisions. *Evolution and Human Behavior*, *28*, 18–27.

Locher, P., Unger, R., Sociedade, P., & Wahl, J. (1993). At first glance: Accessibility of the physical attractiveness stereotype. *Sex Roles*, *28*, 729–743.

Lombroso, C. (1876/2006). *Criminal Man*. Duke University Press.

Lundqvist, D., Flykt, A., & Öhman, A. (1998). *The Karolinska Directed Emotional Faces*. Psychology Section, Department of Clinical Neuroscience, Karolinska Institute, Stockholm, Sweden.

Malatesta, C. Z., Fiore, M. J., & Messina, J. J. (1987). Affect, personality, and facial expressive characteristics of older people. *Psychology and Aging*, *2*, 64–69.

Marsh, A. A., Ambady, N., & Kleck, R. E. (2005). The effects of fear and anger facial expressions on approach- and avoidance-related behaviors. *Emotion*, *5*, 119–124.

Mason, M. F., Cloutier, J., & Macrae, C. N. (2006). On construing others: Category and stereotype activation from facial cues. *Social-Cognition*, *24*, 540–562.

Mazur, A., Mazur, J., & Keating, C. (1984). Military rank attainment of a West Point class: Effects of cadets' physical features. *American Journal of Sociology*, *90*, 125–150.

McGaugh, J. L. (2004). The amygdala modulates the consolidation of memories of emotionally arousing experiences. *Annual Review of Neuroscience, 27*, 1–28.

McNeill, D. (1998). *The Face* (pp. 165–169). Boston: Little, Brown & Company.

Montepare, J. M., & Dobish, H. (2003). The contribution of emotion perceptions and their overgeneralizations to trait impressions. *Journal of Nonverbal Behavior, 27*, 237–254.

Montepare, J. M., & Zebrowitz, L. A. (1998). Person Perception comes of age: The salience and significance of age in social judgments. *Advances in Experimental Social Psychology, 30*, 93–161.

Mueller, U., & Mazur, A. (1996). Facial dominance of West Point cadets as a predictor of later military rank. *Social Forces, 74*, 823–850.

Olson, I. R., & Marshuetz, C. (2005). Facial attractiveness is appraised in a glance. *Emotion, 5*, 498–502.

Oosterhof, N. N., & Todorov, A. (under review). *The Functional Basis of Face Evaluation.*

Osgood, C. E., Suci, G. I., & Tennenbaum, P. H. (1957). *The Measurement of Meaning.* Urbana: University of Illinois Press.

Parducci, A. (1965). Category judgment: A range-frequency model. *Psychological Review, 72*, 407–418.

Perrett, D. I., Hietanen, J. K., Oram, M. W., & Benson, P. J. (1992). Organization and functions of cells responsive to faces in the temporal cortex. *Philosophical Transactions of the Royal Society of London. Series B, Biological Sciences, 335*, 23–30.

Pessoa, L. (2005). To what extent are visual emotional stimuli processed without attention and awareness? *Current Opinion in Neurobiology, 15*, 188–196.

Pessoa, L., Japee, S., Sturman, D., & Underleider, L. G. (2006a). Target visibility and visual awareness modulate amygdala responses to fearful faces. *Cerebral Cortex, 16*, 366–375.

Pessoa, L., Japee, S., & Underleider, L. G. (2006b). Visual awareness and the detection of fearful faces. *Emotion, 5*, 243–247.

Pessoa, L., McKenna, M., Gutierrez, E., & Ungerleider, L. G. (2002). Neural processing of emotional faces requires attention. *Proceedings of the National Academy of Sciences USA, 99*, 11458–11463.

Phelps, E. A., & LeDoux, J. E. (2005). Contributions of the amygdala to emotion processing: From animal models to human behavior. *Neuron, 48*, 175–187.

Plutchik, R. (1980). *Emotion: A Psychoevolutionary Synthesis.* New York: Harper & Row.

Pratto, F., & John, O. P. (1991). Automatic vigilance: The attention-grabbing power of negative social information. *Journal of Personality and Social Psychology, 61*, 380–391.

Riddoch, M. J., & Humpheys, G. W. (1993). *Birmingham Object Recognition Battery.* Hove, UK: Lawrence Erlbaum Associates.

Rosenberg, S., Nelson, C., & Vivekananthan, P. S. (1968). A multidimensional approach to the structure of personality impressions. *Journal of Personality and Social Psychology, 9*, 283–294.

Said, C. P., Baron, S., & Todorov, A. (under review). *Nonlinear Amygdala Response to Face Trustworthiness: Contributions of High and Low Spatial Frequency Information.*

Sander, D., Grafman, J., & Zalla, T. (2003). The human amygdala: An evolved system for relevance detection. *Reviews in the Neurosciences, 14*, 303–316.

Schyns, P. G., & Oliva, A. (1999). Dr. Angry and Mr. Smile: When categorization flexibly modifies the perception of faces in rapid visual presentations. *Cognition, 69*, 243–265.

Secord, P. F. (1958). Facial features and inference processes in interpersonal perception. In R. Tagiuri & L. Petrullo (Eds.), *Person Perception and Interpersonal Behavior* (pp. 300–315). Stanford, CA: Stanford University Press.

Singular Inversions (2006). *FaceGen 3.1 Ful l SDK Documentation.* http://facegen.com

Skowronski, J. J., & Carlston, D. E. (1989). Negativity and extremity biases in impression formation: A review of explanations. *Psychological Bulletin, 105*, 131–142.

Todorov, A., Pakrashi, M., Loehr, V. R., & Oosterhof, N. N. (under review). *Evaluating Faces on Trustworthiness: Automatic Assessment of Face Valence.*

Todorov, A., & Duchaine, B. (under review). *Recognizing Trustworthiness in Faces Without Recognizing Faces.*

Todorov, A., Mandisodza, A. N., Goren, A., & Hall, C. C. (2005). Inferences of competence from faces predict election outcomes. *Science, 308*, 1623–1626.

Todorov, A., & Pakrashi, M. (under review). *Trait Judgments From Faces: Rapid, Unreflective, and Robust.*

Tranel, D., Damasio, A. R., & Damasio, H. (1988). Intact recognition of facial expression, gender, and age in patients with impaired recognition of face identity. *Neurology, 38*, 690–696.

Vuilleumier, P. (2005). How brains beware: neural mechanisms of emotional attention. *Trends In Cognitive Sciences, 9*, 585–594.

Vuilleumier, P., Armony, J. L., Driver, J., & Dolan, R. J. (2003). Distinct spatial frequency sensitivities for processing faces and emotional expressions. *Nature Neuroscience, 6*, 624–631.

Whalen, P. J. (1998). Fear, vigilance, and ambiguity: Initial neuroimaging studies of the human amygdala. *Current Directions in Psychological Science, 7*, 177–188.

White, S., Hill, E., Winston, J., & Frith, U. (2006) An islet of social ability in Asperger Syndrome: Judging social attributes from faces. *Brain and Cognition, 61*, 69–77.

Willis, J., & Todorov, A. (2006). First impressions: Making up your mind after 100 ms exposure to a face. *Psychological Science, 17*, 592–598.

Winston, J., O'Doherty, J., & Dolan, R. J. (2003). Common and distinct neural responses during direct and incidental processing of multiple facial emotions. *NeuroImage, 20*, 84–97.

Winston, J., O'Doherty, J., Kilner, J. M., Perrett, D. I., & Dolan, R. J. (2007). Brain systems for assessing facial attractiveness, *Neuropsychologia, 45*, 195–206.

Winston, J., Strange, B., O'Doherty, J., & Dolan, R. J. (2002). Automatic and intentional brain responses during evaluation of trustworthiness of face. *Nature Neuroscience, 5*, 277–283.

Winston, J. S., Vuilleumier, P., & Dolan, R. J. (2003). Effects of low-spatial frequency components of fearful faces on fusiform cortex activity. *Current Biology, 13*, 1824–1829.

Wiggins, J. S., Philips, N., & Trapnell, P. (1989). Circular reasoning about interpersonal behavior: Evidence concerning some untested assumptions underlying diagnostic classification. *Journal of Personality and Social Psychology, 56*, 296–305.

Wyer, R. S., Jr., & Srull, T. K. (1989). *Memory and Cognition in Social Context*. Hillsdale, NJ: Erlbaum.

Yang, T. T., Menon, V., Eliez, S., Blasey, C., White, C. D. et al. (2002). Amygdalar activation associated with positive and negative facial expressions. *NeuroReport, 13*, 1737–1741.

Yovel, G., & Duchaine, B. (2006). Specialized face perception mechanisms extract both part and spacing information: Evidence from developmental prosopagnosia. *Journal of Cognitive Neuroscience, 18*, 580–593.

Zebrowitz, L. A. (1999). *Reading Faces: Window to the Soul?* Boulder, CO: Westview Press.

Zebrowitz, L. A., Andreoletti, C., Collins, M. A., Lee, S. Y., & Blumenthal, J. (1998a). Bright, bad, babyfaced boys: Appearance stereotypes do not always yield self-fulfilling prophecy effects. *Journal of Personality and Social Psychology, 75*, 1300–1320.

Zebrowitz, L. A., Collins, M. A., & Dutta, R. (1998b). The relationship between appearance personality across the life span. *Personality and Social Psychology Bulletin, 24*, 736–749.

Zebrowitz, L. A., Voinescu, L., & Collins, M. A. (1996). "Wide-eyed" and "crooked-faced": Determinants of perceived and real honesty across the life span. *Personality and Social Psychology Bulletin, 22*, 1258–1269.

Disorders of Consciousness

ADRIAN M. OWEN

MRC Cognition and Brain Sciences Unit, Cambridge, United Kingdom

The vegetative state and other so-called disorders of consciousness present some of the most significant practical and ethical challenges in modern medicine. It is extremely difficult to assess residual cognitive function in these patients because their movements may be minimal or inconsistent, or because no cognitive output may be possible. In recent years, behavioral and neuroimaging techniques developed within the cognitive neurosciences have provided a number of new approaches for investigating these disorders, leading to significant advances in current understanding. In several cases, residual cognitive function and even conscious awareness have been demonstrated in patients who are assumed to be vegetative yet retain cognitive abilities that have evaded detection using standard clinical methods. In this article, I review these data, focusing primarily on the vegetative and minimally conscious states.

Key words: vegetative state; fMRI; minimally conscious state; locked-in syndrome; coma; imaging; consciousness; awareness

Introduction

In recent years, improvements in intensive care have increased the number of patients who survive severe acute brain injuries. Although some of these patients go on to make a good recovery, many do not and remain in one of several states now known collectively as "disorders of consciousness" (Bernat 2006). These include the vegetative state, the minimally conscious state, the minimally conscious state, and coma. The assessment of such patients is extremely difficult and depends frequently on subjective interpretations of the observed spontaneous and volitional behavior. This difficulty is reflected in frequent misdiagnoses between these conditions and confusion about precise definitions (Andrews et al. 1996; Childs et al. 1993). For those patients who retain peripheral motor function, rigorous behavioral assessment supported by structural imaging and electrophysiology is usually sufficient to establish a patient's level of wakefulness and awareness. However, it is becoming increasingly apparent that, in some patients, damage to the peripheral motor system may prevent overt responses to command, even though the cognitive ability to perceive and understand such commands may remain intact.

Recent advances in functional neuroimaging suggest a novel solution to this problem; so-called activation studies can be used to assess cognitive functions in altered states of consciousness without the need for any overt response on the part of the patient. For example, this approach has been used to identify residual brain functions in patients who behaviorally meet all of the standard clinical criteria for the vegetative state yet retain cognitive abilities that have evaded detection using standard clinical methods. Similarly, in some patients diagnosed as minimally conscious, functional neuroimaging has been used to demonstrate residual cognitive capabilities even when there is no clear and consistent external behavioral evidence to support this conclusion. Such studies have led several leading groups in this area to suggest that the future integration of emerging functional neuroimaging techniques with existing clinical and behavioral methods of assessment will be essential for improving our ability to reduce diagnostic errors between these related conditions (Laureys et al. 2006; Schiff et al. 2006). Moreover, such efforts may provide important new prognostic indicators, helping to disentangle differences in outcome on the basis of a greater understanding of the underlying mechanisms responsible and thus improve therapeutic choices in these challenging populations (Laureys et al. 2006). Finally, the use of functional neuroimaging in this context will undoubtedly contribute to our understanding of concepts such as awareness, arousal, volition, and even consciousness itself.

Disorders of Consciousness: Descriptions and Definitions

Although the term "disorders of consciousness" provides a useful short hand for referring to a group

---

Address for correspondence: Adrian M. Owen Ph.D., MRC Cognition and Brain Sciences Unit, Cambridge, CB2 7EF, UK. Voice: +44 1223 355294 ext 511; fax: +44 1223 359062.

adrian.owen@mrc-cbu.cam.ac.uk

of related disorders, it is also problematic because it implies that they are all linked by disruption to some common, underlying, clearly defined system known as consciousness. Unfortunately, there is, as yet, no universally agreed definition of *consciousness*. Widely accepted definitions often refer to *awareness* of the self and the environment (Plum & Posner 1966); and, accordingly, patients with disorders of consciousness (e.g., the vegetative state) are often described as lacking awareness of self or environment. Such descriptions inevitably provoke further questions, including what constitutes *awareness* and what level of awareness is sufficient for a patient to be described as *consciously aware*. On the other hand, Koch (2007) recently stated that the distinction between consciousness and awareness is a largely one of social convention, there being no clear distinction between them. It is far beyond the remit of this article to provide even a brief summary of the consciousness literature. Indeed, the central problem in the investigation of disorders of consciousness is not in understanding the nature of consciousness itself, but rather in defining where the transition point lies between what most people would agree is an unconscious or unaware state and what most would agree is a conscious or aware state. This transition point is not always easily recognized in people with severe brain damage, particularly in patients whose neurological course (improvement or deterioration) is evolving slowly. Accordingly, for the purposes of this review, "consciousness," "awareness," and the combined term "conscious awareness," which is often heard in common parlance, will be used interchangeably.

The Vegetative State

The clinical features of the vegetative state were formally introduced into the literature by Jennett and Plum (1972) and later clarified and refined by the Multi-Society Task Force on Persistent Vegetative State (1994a, b) and the Royal College of Physicians (1996). Etiology is variable, although the condition may arise as a result of road traffic accident, stroke, hypoxia (oxygen deficiency), encephalitis, or viral infection. After stroke or hypoxia, the damage is usually cell death in the cortex, almost always associated with thalamic damage, although occasionally the cortex is relatively spared (Jennett 2002). After traumatic brain injury, the dominant lesion is diffuse damage to the subcortical white matter, often referred to as diffuse axonal injury (DAI), although the degree and extent of this damage is highly variable. A diagnosis of vegetative state is only made after repeated examinations that have yielded *no evidence whatsoever* of sustained, reproducible, purposeful, or voluntary behavioral response to visual, auditory, tactile, or noxious stimuli. There must also be no evidence of language comprehension or expression, although there is generally sufficiently preserved hypothalamic and brain-stem autonomic functions to permit survival with medical care. Unlike patients in coma, the vegetative state is characterized by cycles of eye closure and eye opening giving the appearance of a sleep/wake cycle. It is this waking pattern, combined with the wide range of reflexive responses that are often observed in vegetative patients, that can result in this activity being misinterpreted as evidence of volitional behavior and even the return of conscious awareness. However, although these patients will often appear to be awake and will make nonpurposeful movements, rigorous observation reveals no consistent activities that are voluntary or learned and no responses to command or mimicry (Jennett 2002). In short, these patients show no signs of being aware of themselves or of their environment (Schnakers et al. 2006; Tresch et al. 1991).

The term *persistent* vegetative state has been used arbitrarily to denote that the vegetative state has persisted for more than one month after brain injury. However, because it is often confused with the term *permanent* vegetative state its use in the first few months is now discouraged in favor of simply the vegetative state. The Multi-Society Task Force (1994a, b) on the vegetative state recommended that six months following a nontraumatic brain injury and twelve months following a traumatic brain injury the condition should be regarded as a permanent vegetative state. Although the chances of recovery at this stage are diminishingly small, some exceptional patients may begin to show signs of limited recovery even after very long delays.

Minimally Conscious State

The minimally conscious state is a relatively new diagnostic category (Giacino et al. 2002) and describes patients who show limited but clear evidence of awareness. Some vegetative patients pass through the minimally conscious state on the road to further recovery, while others remain minimally conscious indefinitely. Like vegetative patients, cycles of eye closure and eye opening give the appearance of a sleep/wake cycle and reflexive and nonpurposeful movements are commonly observed. However, unlike vegetative patients, at least one of the following behaviors must also be observed on a reproducible or sustained basis: simple command following (e.g., "move your right hand"), verbal or gestural yes/no responses, intelligible speech, nonreflexive purposeful movements. A patient is considered to have progressed beyond the minimally conscious state when there is consistent functional interactive communication and/or the functional use of more than one object. Because the minimally conscious state is characterized by *inconsistent* responses, such patients can be difficult to distinguish from vegetative patients, particularly in the initial stages. Given the strong relationship between the vegetative and minimally conscious states, similar pathophysiological changes are likely to underlie the two conditions (i.e., multifocal or diffuse cortical and/or thalamic damage or very severe DAI). However, the clear behavioral distinction between the two conditions suggests a difference in the extent of cortical dysfunction such that minimally conscious patients are likely to have resumed some associative cortical activity.

Locked-in Syndrome

Another group of patients who may be mistaken for vegetative are those in what has been termed the "locked-in syndrome" (Plum & Posner 1966). Patients who are locked in are unable to speak or move, although limited eye movements and blinks are usually possible. This condition arises when a lesion of the pons disrupts the descending motor pathways, leaving sensation and consciousness entirely intact, while disrupting almost all forms of motoric behavior.

Coma

In contrast to the vegetative state, coma is characterized by a complete absence of arousal (Laureys et al. 2004). Thus, comatose patients lie, completely unresponsive, with their eyes closed. Unlike the vegetative state, there are no periods of wakefulness. Stimulation does not lead to arousal, and it is widely assumed that such patients have no awareness of themselves or their surroundings. Reflexes frequently remain, but unlike in the vegetative and minimally conscious states, sleep/wake cycles are absent. Of those that survive, most comatose patients begin to recover within 2–4 weeks, although many will not recover beyond the vegetative or minimally conscious state. A comatose state may arise as a result of diffuse cortical or white-matter damage following neuronal or axonal injury, or from a focal brain-stem lesion affecting the pontomesencephalic tegmentum or paramedian thalami, bilaterally.

Functional Neuroimaging in Disorders of Consciousness

Until recently, the majority of neuroimaging studies in disorders of consciousness used either flurodeoxyglucose (FDG) positron emission tomography (PET), or single photon emission computed tomography (SPECT) to measure resting cerebral blood flow and glucose metabolism (e.g., Beuthien-Baumann et al. 2003; De Volder et al. 1990; Laureys et al. 1999a, b; Levy et al. 1987; Momose et al. 1989; Rudolf et al. 1999; Schiff et al. 2002; Tommasino et al. 1995). Typically, widespread reductions in metabolic activity of up to 50% have been reported in the vegetative state, although in a few cases normal cerebral metabolism (Schiff et al. 2002) and blood flow (Agardh et al. 1983) have been found in such patients. In some cases isolated islands of metabolism have been identified in circumscribed regions of cortex, suggesting the potential for cognitive processing in a subset of patients (Schiff et al. 2002). PET studies have shown significantly higher metabolic levels in the brains of patients diagnosed as locked-in syndrome compared to patients diagnosed as vegetative state (Levy et al. 1987). Indeed, several reports have suggested that no grey matter areas show metabolic signs of reduced function in acute or chronic locked-in patients compared to age-matched healthy controls (e.g., Laureys et al. 2004). In one recent and remarkable case of late recovery from minimally conscious state, longitudinal PET examinations revealed increases in resting metabolism coincident with marked clinical improvements in motor function (Voss et al. 2006). While metabolic studies are useful in this regard, they can only identify functionality at the most general level; that is, mapping cortical and subcortical regions that are *potentially* recruitable, rather than relating neural activity within such regions to specific cognitive processes. On the other hand, methods such as $H_2^{15}O$ PET and functional magnetic resonance imaging (fMRI) can be used to link distinct and specific physiological responses (changes in regional cerebral blood flow or changes in regional cerebral hemodynamics) to specific cognitive processes in the absence of any overt response (e.g., a motor action or a verbal response) on the part of the patient.

Early activation studies in patients with disorders of consciousness used $H_2^{15}O$ PET, in part because the technique was more widely available and in part because the multiple logistic difficulties of scanning critically ill patients in the strong magnetic field that is integral to fMRI studies had yet to be resolved. In the first of such studies, $H_2^{15}O$ PET was used to measure regional cerebral blood flow in a posttraumatic vegetative patient during an auditorily presented story told by his mother (de Jong et al. 1997). Compared to nonword sounds, activation was observed in the anterior cingulate and temporal cortices, possibly reflecting emotional processing of the contents, or tone, of the mother's speech. In another patient diagnosed as vegetative, Menon et al. (1998) used PET to study covert visual processing in response to familiar faces. When the patient was presented with pictures of the faces of family and close friends, robust activity was observed in the right fusiform gyrus, the so-called human face area. Importantly, both of these studies involved single, well-documented cases; in cohort PET studies of patients unequivocally meeting the clinical diagnosis of the vegetative state, normal brain activity in response to external stimulation has generally been the exception rather than the rule. For example, in one PET study of 15 vegetative patients, high-intensity noxious electrical stimulation activated midbrain, contralateral thalamus, and primary somatosensory cortex in every patient (Laureys et al. 2002). However, unlike control subjects, the patients did not activate secondary somatosensory, insular, posterior parietal, or anterior cingulate cortices.

$H_2^{15}O$ PET studies are limited by issues of radiation burden which may preclude essential longitudinal or follow-up studies in many patients or even a comprehensive examination of multiple cognitive processes within any one session. The power of PET studies to detect statistically significant responses is also low, and group studies are often needed to satisfy standard statistical criteria. Given the heterogeneous nature of disorders of consciousness and the clinical need to define individuals in terms of their individual diagnosis, residual functions, and potential for recovery, such limitations are of paramount importance in the evaluation of these patients.

A significant development in this rapidly evolving field has been the relative shift of emphasis from PET activation studies using $H_2^{15}O$ methodology, to fMRI. Not only is MRI more widely available than PET, it offers increased statistical power, improved spatial and temporal resolution, and has no associated radiation burden. Recently, Di and colleagues (2007) used event-related fMRI to measure brain activation in seven vegetative patients and four minimally conscious patients in response to the patient's own name spoken by a familiar voice. Two of the vegetative patients exhibited no significant activity at all, three patients exhibited activation in primary auditory areas, and two vegetative patients and four minimally patients exhibited activity in higher-order associative temporal-lobe areas. Although this result is encouraging (particularly because the two vegetative patients who showed the most widespread activation subsequently improved to the minimally conscious state in the following months), it lacks cognitive specificity; that is to say, responses to the patient's own name spoken by a familiar voice were compared only to responses to the attenuated noise of the MRI scanner. Therefore, the activation observed may have reflected a specific response to one's own name, but it is equally possible that it reflected a low-level orienting response to speech in general, an emotional response to the speaker (see Bekinschtein et al. 2004), or any one of a number of possible cognitive processes relating to the unmatched auditory stimuli. As a result, the interpretation hinges on a reverse inference, an unfortunately common practice in neuroimaging by which the engagement of a given cognitive process is inferred solely from the observed activation in a particular brain region (Poldrack 2006; Christoff & Owen 2006). Thus, in the study by Di and colleagues (2007), conclusions about higher-order cognitive processing were derived on the basis of activation in associative temporal-lobe areas, without any evidence that those processes are actually recruited by the task.

Staffen et al. (2006) have recently used event-related fMRI to compare sentences containing the patient's own name (e.g., "James, hello James"), spoken by a variety of unfamiliar voices, with sentences containing another first name, in a patient who had been vegetative for 10 months at the time of the scan. In this case, because identical speech stimuli were used which differed only with respect to the name itself, activations can be confidently attributed to cognitive processing that is specifically related to the patient's own name. Differential cortical processing was observed to the patient's own name in a region of the medial prefrontal cortex, similar to that observed in three healthy volunteers. These findings concur closely with a recent electrophysiological study that has shown differential P3 responses to patient's own names (compared to other names) in locked-in, minimally conscious, and some vegetative patients (Perrin et al. 2006). Selective cortical processing of one's own name (when it is compared directly with another name) requires the ability to perceive and access the meaning of words and may imply some level of comprehension on the part of this patient. However, as the authors point out (Staffen et al. 2006), a response to one's own name is one of the most basic forms of language, is elicited automatically (you cannot choose to *not* orient to your own name), and may not depend on the higher-level linguistic processes that are assumed to underpin comprehension.

A Hierarchical Approach to Studying Disorders of Consciousness

It has recently been argued that fMRI studies in patients in the vegetative state and other disorders of consciousness should be conducted hierarchically (Owen et al. 2005a, b) beginning with the simplest form of processing within a particular domain (e.g., auditory) and then progressing sequentially through more complex cognitive functions. Many patients with disorders of consciousness suffer serious damage to auditory and/or visual input systems, which may impede performance of any higher cognitive functions (e.g., voice discrimination), which place demands on these lower sensory systems (e.g., hearing). This is particularly crucial for functional neuroimaging studies in this patient group because, unlike the majority of studies in healthy volunteers, the participants are unlikely to be able to verify that stimuli have been perceived as they were intended by the experimenter. By way of example, a series of auditory paradigms were described that have all been successfully employed in functional neuroimaging studies of vegetative patients (Coleman et al. 2007). These paradigms increase in complexity systematically from basic acoustic processing to more complex aspects of language comprehension and semantics.

Acoustic Processing

At the most basic level, it is important to establish normal or near-normal sensory perception in any candidate patient for functional neuroimaging studies of higher cognitive functions (e.g., language processing). For the most part, functional neuroimaging is not necessary in this regard; that is to say, the measurement of auditory or visual evoked potentials are usually sufficient to establish that the respective neural pathways are intact. The integrity of the auditory neural axis can be assessed using a number of tests including the brain-stem auditory evoked response (BAER) and passive mismatch negativity (MMN). The MMN is widely thought to reflect a precognitive response generated from a comparison between the deviant input and a neural memory trace encoding the physical features of the repetitive sound (Naatanen 2003). The MMN has been successfully applied to the assessment of vegetative patients, although with considerable variability in results (Jones et al. 2000; Kotchoubey et al. 2001).

Speech Perception

Once basic neural responses to sounds have been established, it becomes possible to investigate whether the damaged brain is able to discriminate between different categories of sound. Speech perception in healthy volunteers has been widely investigated within the functional neuroimaging literature, and the findings have obvious clinical and therapeutic relevance for the investigation of preserved cognitive function in patients with disorders of consciousness. Most often, studies of speech perception involve volunteers being scanned during an experimental condition (e.g., while listening to binaurally presented spoken words) and an acoustic control condition (e.g., while listening to sounds that have the same duration, spectral profile, and amplitude envelope as the original speech, but are entirely unintelligible because all spectral detail has been replaced with noise, commonly referred to as signal correlated noise) or a silence condition (no auditory stimulus at all). For example, Mummery et al. (1999) scanned six neurologically normal volunteers while they listened to concrete nouns or signal correlated noise at a rate of 30 items per minute. The task instruction was to pay attention to the stimuli without responding. When speech was compared to signal correlated noise, they found a broad swathe of activation along both superior temporal gyri, extending ventrolaterally into the superior temporal sulcus (see FIG. 1A).

The same paradigm, or variants of it, has been applied recently to groups of patients meeting the clinical criteria for the vegetative state or the minimally conscious state (Owen et al. 2002, 2005b; Coleman et al. 2007). For example, Owen and colleagues (2002), described one case of a 30-year-old female bank manager who suffered severe head injuries during a road traffic accident involving a head-on collision with another vehicle. Over several weeks, the patient developed a withdrawal to pain but showed no consistent evidence of volitional activity and was diagnosed as vegetative. The decision to use an auditory speech task was made largely on the basis of the partially intact BAERs. The patient was scanned while being presented with spoken words, matched signal-correlated noise bursts, or silence. The comparison of noise bursts with rest revealed significant foci of activation bilaterally in the auditory region, confirming the BAER results suggesting that basic auditory processes were at least somewhat functional. More remarkably, the comparison of speech sounds with matched noise bursts revealed significant activity on the superior temporal plane bilaterally and posterior to auditory cortex, in the region of the planum temporale, in the left hemisphere only (see FIG. 1B). These findings correspond extremely closely with previous results in healthy volunteers (Mummery et al. 1999, see FIG. 1A), suggesting that this patient's brain processed speech in a way that was indistinguishable from controls. Similar findings were described in a second patient who also met the clinical criteria for the vegetative state (Owen et al. 2005b). In that study, a similar contrast between speech stimuli and signal-correlated noise yielded an almost identical pattern of activity in the vegetative patient and in a group of healthy volunteers (FIG. 1C).

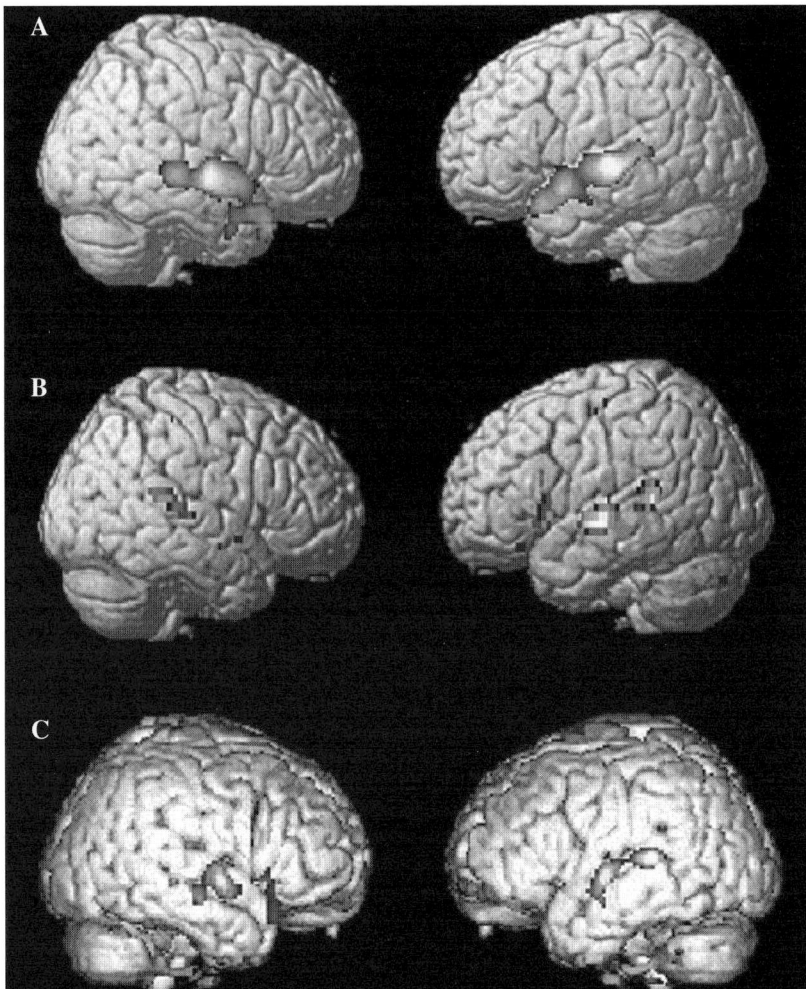

FIGURE 1. Brain activity when speech is compared with signal-correlated noise in healthy volunteers **(A)** and in two patients **(B, C)** meeting the clinical criteria for vegetative state. The speech-specific bilateral superior temporal-lobe activity observed in the two patients is similar to that observed in controls. Adapted from Owen et al. (2005a).

These preliminary findings in individual case studies have been extended recently using fMRI in a mixed group of 12 vegetative and minimally conscious patients (Coleman et al. 2007). Three of seven vegetative patients and two of five minimally conscious patients demonstrated some evidence of preserved speech processing, while four patients showed no significant activity at all, even when responses to any sound were compared to silence.

In short, simple perceptual tasks that compare speech with psycho-acoustically matched auditory stimuli can be used to demonstrate normal patterns of brain activity in some patients diagnosed with disorders of consciousness. Of course, recognizing speech as speech does not imply anything about comprehension; that is, whether the content of the speech is understood or not (consider the experience of listening to speech in a language of which you have no prior experience). To assess speech comprehension in disorders of consciousness it is necessary to employ more complex experiment designs that tap aspects of phonological processing.

Phonological Processing

Although the results from studies of speech processing in disorders of consciousness (e.g., Boly et al. 2004; Owen et al. 2002, 2005a, b; Coleman et al. 2007), have suggested that some level of covert linguistic functioning may be preserved, such tasks do not allow any conclusions to be drawn about comprehension; that is, whether speech is processed beyond the point at which it is identified as speech. One approach to this problem, which has met with some success, is to document responses to a set of stimuli of graded complexity. Davis and Johnsrude (2003) have developed such a task using graded intelligibility as a measure of speech comprehension. During the task, volunteers listen passively to sentences that have been distorted by adding noise such that they produce a range of six levels of intelligibility (as measured by subsequent word report scores). In a parallel fMRI study, intelligibility (operationalized as "the amount of a sentence that is understood") was found to correlate with activation in a region of the left anterior and superior temporal lobe; as intelligibility increased, so did signal intensity in this region (Davis & Johnsrude 2003). This increase was also significantly positively correlated with word report scores; signal intensity increasing linearly as the subjects reported more words as being understood correctly. These findings in healthy volunteers suggest that activity in the left anterior and superior temporal lobe reflects processing of the linguistic content of spoken sentences (words and meanings), rather than their more general acoustic properties.

This auditory comprehension paradigm has been adapted for use in patients with disorders of consciousness (Owen et al. 2005b). In one case, a 30-year-old male was diagnosed as vegetative following a basilar thrombosis and posterior circulation infarction. Four months after his brain injury, the auditory comprehension task described above was administered; the comparison of speech (collapsed across three levels of intelligibility) with a silence baseline condition revealed significant foci of activation over the left and right superior temporal planes confirming preliminary BAER and MMN findings suggesting that basic auditory processes were probably functional. Moreover, when low intelligibility sentences were compared with high intelligibility sentences in order to isolate any residual activity related specifically to the comprehension of spoken language, two peaks were observed in the superior and middle temporal gyri of the left hemisphere that were extremely similar to the pattern of results reported previously in healthy volunteers (Davis & Johnsrude 2003).

These results suggest that a test of graded intelligibility may be a useful indicator of some level of speech comprehension in patients with disorders of consciousness. Thus, while the left superior temporal sulcus responds to the presence of phonetic information in general, its anterior part (which was similarly activated in the patient and in healthy volunteers) appears to respond only when the stimuli become intelligible (Scott et al. 2000). However, whether the responses observed reflect speech comprehension per se (i.e., understanding the contents of spoken language) or a more basic response to the acoustic properties of intelligible speech that distinguish it from less intelligible speech can not be determined on the basis of these data alone.

Semantic Processing

Understanding natural speech is ordinarily so effortless that we often overlook the complex computations that are necessary to make sense of what someone is saying. Not only must we identify all the individual words on the basis of the acoustic input, we must also retrieve the meanings of these words and appropriately combine them to construct a representation of the whole sentence's meaning. When words have more than one meaning, contextual information must be used to identify the appropriate meaning. For example, given the sentence "The boy was frightened by the loud bark," the listener must work out that the ambiguous word "bark" refers to the sound made by a dog and not the outer covering of a tree. This process of selecting appropriate word meanings is important because the majority of English words have more than one meaning and are therefore ambiguous (Rodd et al. 2005). Selecting appropriate word meanings is likely to place a substantial load on the neural systems involved in computing sentence meanings.

Recently, an fMRI study in healthy volunteers has used semantic ambiguity to identify the brain regions that are specifically involved in speech comprehension and in particular in the processes of activating, selecting, and integrating contextually appropriate word meanings (Rodd et al. 2005). During the fMRI scan, the volunteers were played sentences containing two or more ambiguous words (e.g., "the *creak/creek* came from a *beam* in the *ceiling/sealing*") and well-matched, low-ambiguity sentences (e.g., "her secrets were written in her diary"). The ambiguous words were either homonyms (the two meanings have the same spelling and pronunciation; e.g., *beam*), or homophones (the two meanings that have the same pronunciation but different spellings; e.g., *creak/creek*). While the two types of sentences have similar acoustic, phonological, syntactic, and prosodic properties (and are rated as being equally natural), the high-ambiguity sentences require additional processing to identify and select contextually appropriate word meanings. Relative to low-ambiguity sentences, high-ambiguity stimuli produced increases in signal intensity in the left posterior inferior temporal cortex and inferior frontal gyri bilaterally (FIG. 2B).

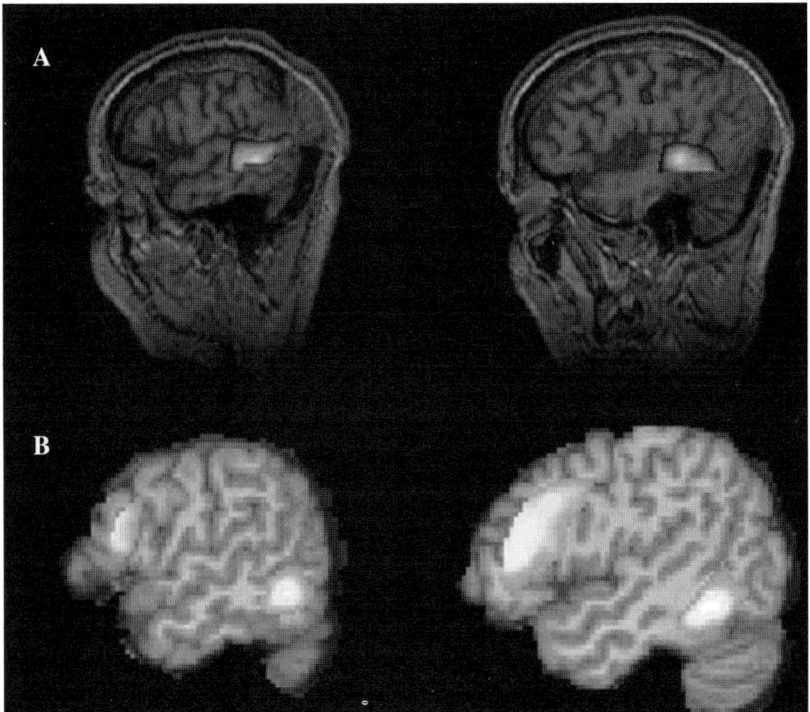

FIGURE 2. fMRI data for the ambiguous sentences versus unambiguous sentences comparison. Like healthy volunteers (**B**; adapted from Rodd et al. 2005), this patient (**A**) exhibited significant signal intensity changes in the left posterior inferior temporal cortex, suggesting that some of the processes involved in activating, selecting, and integrating contextually appropriate word meanings may be intact, despite the clinical diagnoses.

The results of this study demonstrate that a key aspect of spoken language comprehension—the resolution of semantic ambiguity—can be used to identify the brain regions involved in the semantic aspects of speech comprehension (e.g., activating, selecting, and integrating word meanings). Moreover, they support models of speech comprehension in which posterior inferior temporal regions are involved in semantic processing (Hickok & Poeppel 2000), and they demonstrate that the lateral inferior frontal gyrus, which has long been known to be important in syntactic processing of sentences and the semantic properties of single words, also plays an important role in processing the meanings of words in sentences.

Two recent studies have explored the utility of this approach in identifying residual comprehension in disorders of consciousness (Owen et al. 2005b; Coleman et al. 2007). In the more recent study, seven vegetative state and five minimally conscious patients were scanned during the semantic paradigm developed by Rodd et al. (2005). Two of the vegetative patients showed a significant response in the semantic ambiguity contrast, consistent with high-level comprehension of the semantic aspects of speech. These results provide compelling evidence for high-level residual linguistic processing in some patients meeting the clinical criteria for vegetative state and suggest that some of the processes involved in activating, selecting and integrating contextually appropriate word meanings may be intact, despite their clinical diagnoses.

Conscious Awareness

A question that is often asked, however, is whether the presence of normal brain activation in patients with disorders of consciousness (e.g., de Jong et al. 1997; Menon et al. 1998; Laureys et al. 2002; Owen et al. 2002; Boly et al. 2004; Owen et al. 2005a, b; Coleman et al. 2007), indicates a level of awareness, perhaps even similar to that which exists in healthy volunteers when performing the same tasks. Many types of stimuli, including faces, speech, and pain will elicit relatively automatic responses from the brain; that is to say, they will occur without the need for active intervention on the part of the participant (e.g., you can not choose to *not* recognize a face, or to *not* understand speech that is presented clearly in your native language). In addition, there is a wealth of data in healthy volunteers, from studies of implicit learning and the effects of priming (e.g., see Schacter 1994 for review), to studies of learning and speech perception during anesthesia (e.g., Bonebakker et al. 1996; Davis et al. 2007) that have demonstrated that many aspects of human cognition can go on in the absence of awareness. Even the semantic content of masked information can be primed to affect subsequent behavior without the explicit knowledge of the participant, suggesting that some aspects of semantic processing may occur without conscious awareness (Dehaene et al. 1998). By the same argument, normal neural responses in patients who are diagnosed with disorders of consciousness do not necessarily indicate that these patients have any conscious experience associated with processing those same types of stimuli. Thus, such patients may retain discreet islands of subconscious cognitive function, which exist in the absence of awareness.

The logic described above exposes a central conundrum in the study of conscious awareness and, in particular, how it relates to disorders of consciousness. As noted above, there is, as yet, no universally agreed definition of consciousness and even less so self-consciousness or sense of self/being (Laureys et al. 2007). Deeper philosophical considerations notwithstanding, the only reliable method that we have for determining if another being is consciously aware is to ask him/her. The answer may take the form of a spoken response or a nonverbal signal (which may be as simple as the blink of an eye, as documented cases of the locked-in syndrome have demonstrated), but it is this answer, and only this answer, that allows us to infer conscious awareness. In short, our ability to know unequivocally that another being is consciously aware is ultimately determined, not by whether they are aware or not, but by their ability to communicate that fact through a recognized behavioral response. But what if the ability to blink an eye or move a hand is lost, yet conscious awareness remains? Much of the debate about the vegetative state revolves around what behaviors reflect cortical activity and whether signs of activity in the cortex necessarily indicate conscious awareness. Yet the crux of the diagnosis is that the patient displays no evidence of awareness or self or surroundings. Thus, by definition, patients who are diagnosed as vegetative are not able to elicit any behavioral responses. Following the logic of this argument then, even if such a patient *were* consciously aware, he/she would have no means for conveying that information to the outside world.

A novel approach to this conundrum has recently been described, using fMRI, to demonstrate preserved conscious awareness in a patient fulfilling the criteria for a diagnosis of vegetative state (Owen et al. 2006). Between the time of the accident and the fMRI scan in early January 2006, the patient was assessed by a multidisciplinary team employing repeated standardized assessments consistent with the procedure described by Bates (2005). Throughout this period the patient's behavior was consistent with accepted guidelines defining the vegetative state. She would open her eyes spontaneously, exhibited sleep/wake cycles, and had preserved, but inconsistent, reflexive behavior (startle, noxious, threat, tactile, olfactory). No elaborated motor behaviors (regarded as voluntary or willed responses) were observed from the upper or lower limbs. There was no evidence of orientation, fixation greater than 5 seconds, or tracking to visual or auditory stimuli. No overt motor responses to command were observed.

Prior to the fMRI scan, the patient was instructed to perform two mental imagery tasks when cued by the instructions "imagine playing tennis" or "imagine visiting the rooms in your home." Importantly, these particular tasks were chosen, not because they involve a set of fundamental cognitive processes that are known to reflect conscious awareness, but because imagining playing tennis and imagining moving around the house elicit extremely reliable, robust, and statistically distinguishable patterns of activation in specific regions of the brain (Boly et al. 2007). For example, in a series of studies in healthy volunteers (Boly et al. 2007; Owen et al. 2006) imagining playing tennis has been shown to elicit activity in the supplementary motor area, a region known to be involved in imagining (as well as actually performing) coordinated movements, in each and every one of 34 participants scanned. In contrast, imagining moving from room to room in a house commonly activates the parahippocampal cortices, the posterior parietal lobe, and the lateral premotor cortices, all regions that have been shown to contribute to imaginary, or real, spatial navigation (FIG. 3A).

Given the reliability of these responses across individuals, activation in these regions in patients with disorders of consciousness can be used as a neural marker, confirming that the patient retains the ability to understand instructions, to carry out different mental tasks in response to those instructions, and, therefore, is able to exhibit willed, voluntary behavior in the absence of any overt action. Thus, they permit the identification of volitional brain activity (and thus of consciousness) at the single-subject level, without the need for any motor response (Boly et al. 2007).

During the periods that the vegetative patient was asked to imagine playing tennis, significant activity was observed in the supplementary motor area (Owen

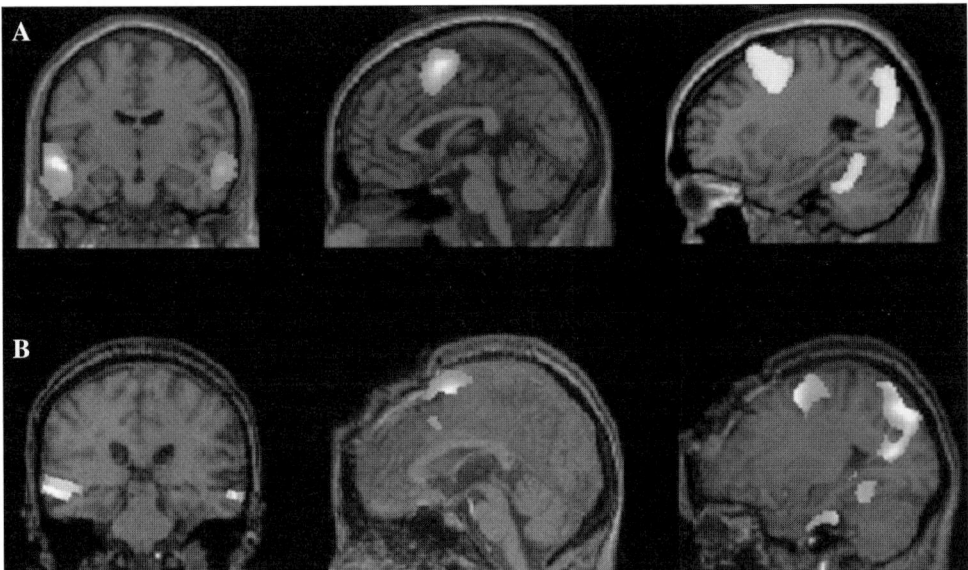

FIGURE 3. Indistinguishable fMRI activity in healthy controls **(A)** and in a vegetative patient **(B)** while listening to speech versus signal-correlated white noise (left column), while imagining playing tennis (middle column), or while imagining walking around the house (right column). Adapted from Owen et al. (2006).

et al. 2006; FIG. 3B). In contrast, when she was asked to imagine walking through her home, significant activity was observed in the parahippocampal gyrus, the posterior parietal cortex, and the lateral premotor cortex (FIG. 3B). Her neural responses were indistinguishable from those observed in healthy volunteers performing the same imagery tasks in the scanner (Boly et al. 2007; Owen et al. 2006; FIG. 4A). It was concluded that, despite fulfilling all the clinical criteria for a diagnosis of vegetative state, this patient retained the ability to understand spoken commands and to respond to them through her brain activity, rather than through speech or movement, confirming beyond any doubt that she was consciously aware of herself and her surroundings.

Of course, skeptics may argue that the words "tennis" and "house" could have automatically triggered the patterns of activation observed in the supplementary motor area, the parahippocampal gyrus, the posterior parietal lobe, and the lateral premotor cortex in this patient in the absence of conscious awareness. However, no data exist supporting the inference that such stimuli can unconsciously elicit sustained hemodynamic responses in these regions of the brain. Indeed, considerable data exist to suggest such words do not elicit the responses that were observed. For example, although it is well-documented that some words can, under certain circumstances, elicit wholly automatic neural responses in the absence of conscious awareness, such responses are typically transient (i.e., lasting for a few seconds) and, unsurprisingly, occur in regions of the brain that are associated with word processing. In the patient described by Owen et al. (2006, 2007a, b), the observed activity was not transient but persisted for the full 30 seconds of each imagery task, that is, far longer than would be expected, even given the hemodynamics of the fMRI response (FIG. 4B). In fact, these task-specific changes persisted until the patient was cued with another stimulus indicating that she should rest (Owen et al 2007b). Such responses are impossible to explain in terms of automatic brain processes. In addition, the activation observed in the patient was not in brain regions that are known to be involved in word processing, but rather in regions that are known to be involved in the two imagery tasks that she was asked to carry out. Again, sustained activity in these regions of the brain is impossible to explain in terms of unconscious responses to either single key words or to short sentences containing those words. In fact, in a supplementary study (Owen et al. 2007a), noninstructive sentences containing the same key words as those used with the patient (e.g., "The man enjoyed playing tennis") were shown to produce no sustained activity in any of these brain regions in healthy volunteers.

The most parsimonious explanation is, therefore, that this patient was consciously aware and actively following the instructions given to her, despite her diagnosis of vegetative state.

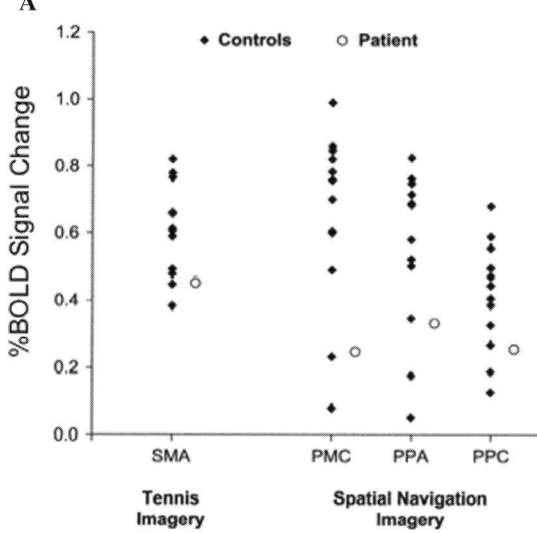

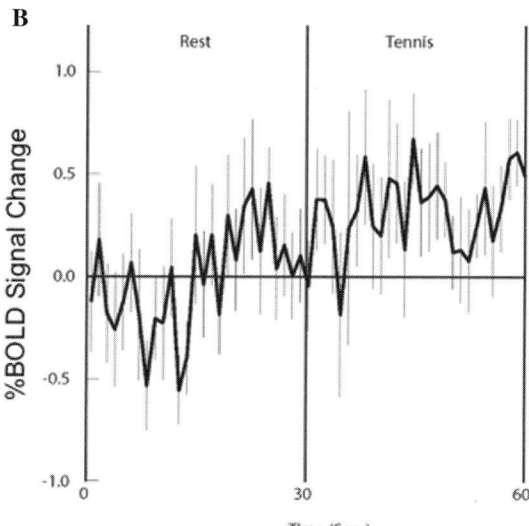

FIGURE 4. (A) Signal intensity changes in the vegetative patient described by Owen et al. (2006) plotted against 12 healthy volunteers while imagining playing tennis or while imagining moving around their own house. SMA, supplementary motor area; PMC, lateral premotor cortex; PPA, parahippocampal gyrus; PPC, posterior parietal cortex. Signal intensity changes for the patient are all within the normal range. **(B)** Mean signal intensity changes in the patient over two 30s epochs of the imaginary tennis playing task. A sustained 30s fMRI response in the supplementary motor cortex was observed when the vegetative patient was asked to imagine playing tennis relative to rest.

Limitations

This work raises a number of important issues regarding the use of fMRI in the assessment of patients with disorders of consciousness. First, although this technique provides a new means for detecting conscious awareness when standard clinical approaches are unable to provide that information, the method will not be applicable to all vegetative patients. For example, after 5 months (as was the case in the patient described by Owen et al. 2006, 2007a) the incidence of recovery of consciousness following a traumatic brain injury remains at nearly 20%, with a quarter of those recovering moving on to some level of social independence. Nontraumatic injuries are considered to have a much poorer prognosis. Similarly, the likelihood of recovery is much lower in patients who meet the diagnostic criteria for the permanent vegetative state. International guidelines, including those of the Royal College of Physicians in the U.K. and the Multi-Society Task Force, representing five major medical societies in the United States, suggest that a diagnosis of permanent vegetative state should not be made in cases of traumatic brain injury until 12 months postinjury and 6 months postinjury for cases of anoxic brain injury. In many of these cases, standard clinical techniques, including structural MRI, may be sufficient to rule out any potential for normal activation, without the need for fMRI.

More generally, the acquisition, analysis, and interpretation of fMRI data from patients with severe brain damage are also complex (Giacino et al. 2006). For example, the coupling of neuronal activity and local hemodynamics, essential for fMRI activation measurements, is likely to be different from that in healthy controls (Gsell et al. 2000; Hamzei et al. 2003; Rossini et al. 2004; Sakatani et al. 2003), making interpretation of such data sets extremely difficult. Notwithstanding this basic methodological concern, the choice of the study design is also crucial. For example, if brain-stem auditory evoked responses are abnormal, auditory stimuli may be inappropriate and alternatives (e.g., visual stimuli) should be considered. The investigation should also be complex enough that the cognitive processes of interest will be studied (i.e., preferably beyond stimulus perception), yet not so complex that the tasks could easily overload the cognitive capacities of a tired or inattentive patient. Many studies also suffer from the reverse inference problem described above (Christoff & Owen 2006; Poldrack 2006). For example, activity in the amygdala is not sufficient evidence for an emotional response unless well-documented studies in healthy volunteers have established previously that the task in question produces such a response, accompanied by an anatomically specific, robust, and reproducible activation pattern in this brain region. In vegetative state, minimally conscious state, and locked-in syndrome, episodes of low arousal and sleep are common and close patient monitoring—preferably through EEG recording—during activation scans is essential so that these periods can be avoided. Spontaneous movements during the scan itself may also compromise the interpretation of functional neuroimaging data, particularly with fMRI scans. Processing of functional neuroimaging data may also present challenging problems in this patient group. For example, the presence of gross hydrocephalus or focal pathology may complicate the fitting of functional imaging data to structural imaging data, and the normalization of these images through reference to a healthy brain. Under these circumstances, statistical assessment of activation patterns is complex and interpretation of activation foci with standard stereotaxic coordinates may be impossible.

Finally and most importantly, negative fMRI findings in patients with disorders of consciousness should never be used as evidence for impaired cognitive function or lack of awareness. For example, a patient may fall asleep during the scan or may not have properly heard or understood the task instructions, leading to so-called false negative results. False negative findings in functional neuroimaging studies are common, even in healthy volunteers. Whether this will ultimately limit the practical application that functional neuroimaging might have for distinguishing between those patients who are likely to recover and those who are not will only be determined when the technique has been applied to many more patients who have been followed longitudinally. Nevertheless, positive findings, when they occur and can be verified by careful statistical comparison with data from healthy volunteers, can be used to detect conscious awareness in patients, without the need for conventional methods of communication such as movement or speech.

Conclusions

In the last two decades, rapid technological developments in the field of neuroimaging have produced a cornucopia of new techniques for examining both the structure and function of the human brain *in vivo*. Detailed anatomical images, acquired through computerized tomography (CT) and magnetic resonance imaging (MRI), can now be combined with PET, fMRI, quantitative electroencephalography (EEG), and magnetoencephalography (MEG) to produce a cohesive picture of normal and abnormal brain function. As a result, functional neuroimaging has become the technique of choice for neuropsychologists, cognitive neuroscientists, and many others in the wider neuroscientific community with an interest in the relationship between brain and behavior. Until recently, these new methods of investigation have been used primarily as a correlational tool to map the cerebral changes that are associated with a particular cognitive process or function, be it an action, a reaction (e.g., to some kind of external stimulation), or a thought. But recent advances in imaging technology, and in particular the ability of fMRI to detect reliable neural responses in individual participants in real time, are beginning to reveal a participant's thoughts, actions, or intentions based solely on the pattern of activity that is observed in their brain. The case of the vegetative patient described above provides a clear example of such an application (Owen et al. 2006, 2007a). In the absence of any overt action on her part, the fact that she was consciously aware was evident only by examination of her time-locked and sustained fMRI responses following instructions to perform specific mental tasks. On this basis, it was possible to infer not only that she was thinking, but what she was thinking at any given point in time (within the constraints of the tasks given to her). Similarly, Boly et al. (2007) have demonstrated that when healthy volunteers are instructed to choose to imagine either playing tennis or navigating around their homes (without informing the investigators of their choice), it is possible to determine, with 100% accuracy, which task is being imagined by each and every participant based solely on their brain activity. Finally, in another recent fMRI study, participants were asked to freely decide which of two different tasks to perform and to covertly hold onto that intention during a variable delay (Haynes et al. 2007). During the delay, it was possible to decode from activity in the prefrontal cortex which of the two tasks the participants were covertly intending to perform.

Such feats of rudimentary "mind-reading" using fMRI pave the way for new and innovative applications of functional neuroimaging, both in basic neuroscience and in clinical practice. For example, the presence of reproducible and robust task-dependent fMRI responses to command without the need for any practice or training (Owen et al. 2006, 2007a) suggests a novel method by which both healthy participants and patients with disorders of consciousness may be able to communicate their thoughts to those around them by simply modulating their own neural activity. The use of functional neuroimaging in this context will clearly continue to present innumerable logistic, theoretical, and ethical problems. However, its clinical and scientific implications are so major that such efforts are clearly justified.

Acknowledgments

I thank M. Coleman, M. Davis, J. D. Pickard, J. Rodd, D. Menon, I. Johnsrude, M. Boly, S. Laureys, and the Cambridge Impaired Consciousness Research Group for their contributions to work discussed in this review.

Conflict of Interest

The author declares no conflicts of interest.

References

Agardh, C. D., Rosen, I., & Ryding, E. (1983). Persistent vegetative state with high cerebral blood flow following profound hypoglycemia. *Ann. Neurol.*, *14*(4), 482–486.

Andrews, K., Murphy, L., Munday, R., et al. (1996). Misdiagnosis of the vegetative state: retrospective study in a rehabilitation unit. *BMJ*, *313*, 13–16.

Bates, D. (2005). Incidence and prevalence of the vegetative and minimally conscious states. *Neuropsychol Rehabil*, *15*, 175.

Bekinschtein, T., Leiguarda, R., Armony, J., et al. (2004). Emotional processing in the minimally conscious state. *Journal of Neurosurgery, Neurology and Psychiatry*, *75*, 788.

Bernat, J. L. (2006). Chronic disorders of consciousness. *Lancet*, *367*, 1181–1192.

Beuthien-Baumann, B., Handrick, W., Schmidt, T., et al. (2003). Persistent vegetative state: evaluation of brain metabolism and brain perfusion with PET and SPECT. *Nucl Med Commun*, *24*(6), 643–639.

Boly, M., Faymonville, M. E., Peigneux, P., et al. (2004). Auditory processing in severely brain injured patients: differences between the minimally conscious state and the persistent vegetative state. *Arch Neurol*, *61*(2), 233–238.

Boly, M., Coleman, M. R., Davis, M. H., et al. (2007). When thoughts become action: an fMRI paradigm to study volitional brain activity in non-communicative brain injured patients. *Neuroimage*, *36*, 979–992.

Bonebakker, A., Bonke, B., Klein, J., Wolters, G., Stijnen, T., Passchier, J., et al. (1996). Information processing during general anaesthesia: Evidence for unconscious memory. In B. Bonke, J.G.W. Bovill, & N. Moerman (Eds.), *Memory and Awareness in Anaesthesia* (pp. 101–109). Lisse, Amsterdam: Swets and Zeitlinger.

Childs, N. L., Mercer, W. N., & Childs, H. W. (1993). Accuracy of diagnosis of persistent vegetative state. *Neurology*, *43*, 1465–1467.

Christoff, K., & Owen, A. M. (2006). Improving reverse neuroimaging inference: cognitive domain versus cognitive complexity. *Trends Cogn. Sci.*, *10*(8), 352–353.

Coleman, M. R., Rodd, J. M., Davis, M. H., et al. (2007). Do vegetative patients retain aspects of language Evidence from fMRI. *Brain*, *130*, 2494–2507.

Davis, M. H., Coleman, M. R., Absalom, A. R., Rodd, J. M., Johnsrude, I. S., Matta, B. F., et al. (2007). Dissociating speech perception and comprehension at reduced levels of awareness. *Proc Natl Acad Sci*, *104*(41), 16032–16037.

Davis, M. H., & Johnsrude, I. S. (2003). Hierarchical processing in spoken language comprehension. *J Neurosc Sci*, *23*(8), 3423–3431.

de Jong, B., Willemsen, A. T., & Paans, A. M. (1997). Regional cerebral blood flow changes related to affective speech presentation in persistent vegetative state. *Clin. Neurol. Neurosurg.*, *99*(3), 213–216.

De Volder, A. G., Goffinet, A. M., Bol, A., et al. (1990). Brain glucose metabolism in postanoxic syndrome. Positron emission tomographic study. *Arch. Neurol.*, *47*(2), 197–204.

Dehaene, S., Naccache, L., Le Clec'h, G., Koechlin, E., Mueller, M., Dehaene-Lambertz, G., et al. (1998). Imaging unconscious semantic priming. *Nature*, *395*, 597–600.

Di, H. B., Yu, S. M., Weng, X. C., et al. (2007). Cerebral response to patient's own name in the vegetative and minimally conscious states. *Neurology*, *68*, 895–899.

Giacino, J., Hirsch, J., Schiff, N., et al. (2006). Functional neuroimaging applications for assessment and rehabilitation planning in patients with disorders of consciousness. *Arch Phys Med Rehabil*, *87*, 67–76.

Gsell, W., De Sadeleer, C., Marchalant, Y., et al. (2000). The use of cerebral blood flow as an index of neuronal activity in functional neuroimaging: experimental and pathophysiological considerations. *J Chem Neuroanat*, *20*(3–4), 215–224.

Giacino, J. T., Ashwal, S., Childs, N., et al. (2002). The minimally conscious state: Definition and diagnostic criteria. *Neurology*, *58*(3), 349–353.

Hamzei, F., Knab, R., Weiller, C., et al. (2003). The influence of extra- and intracranial artery disease on the BOLD signal in FMRI. *Neuroimage*, *20*(2), 1393–1399.

Haynes, J. D., Sakai, K., Rees, G., et al. (2007). Hidden intentions in the human brain. *Curr. Biol.*, *10*, 1016.

Hickok, G., & Poeppel, D. (2000). Towards a functional neuroanatomy of speech perception. *Trends Cogn Sci*, *4*, 131–138.

Jennett, B. (2002). *The Vegetative State. Medical Facts, Ethical and Legal Dilemmas*. Cambridge: Cambridge University Press.

Jones, S. J., Vaz Pato, M., Sprague, L., Stokes, M., Munday, R., & Haque, N. (2000). Auditory evoked potentials to spectro-temporal modulation of complex tones in normal subjects and patients with severe brain injury. *Brain*, *123*, 1007–1016.

Koch, C. (2007). *The quest for consciousness: A neurobiological approach*. Englewood, CO: Roberts and Company.

Kotchoubey, B., Lang, S., Baales, R., Herb, E., Maurer, P., Mezger, G., et al. (2001). Brain potentials in human patients with extremely severe diffuse brain damage. *Neurosci Lett*, *301*, 37–40.

Jennett, B., & Plum, F. (1972). Persistent vegetative state after brain damage. *Lancet*, *1*, 734–737.

Laureys, S., Faymonville, M. E., Peigneux, P., et al. (2002). Cortical processing of noxious somatosensory stimuli in the persistent vegetative state. *Neuroimage*, *17*(2), 732–741.

Laureys, S., Giacino, J. T., Schiff, N. D., et al. (2006). How should functional imaging of patients with disorders of consciousness contribute to their clinical rehabilitation needs? *Curr Opin Neurol*, *19*(6), 520–527.

Laureys, S., Goldman, S., Phillips, C., et al. (1999a). Impaired effective cortical connectivity in vegetative state: preliminary investigation using PET. *Neuroimage*, *9*(4), 377–382.

Laureys, S., Lemaire, C., Maquet, P., et al. (1999b). Cerebral metabolism during vegetative state and after recovery to consciousness. *J. Neurol. Neurosurg. Psychiatry*, *67*, 121.

Laureys, S., Owen, A. M., & Schiff, N. (2004). Brain function in coma, vegetative state, and related disorders. *The Lancet Neurology*, *3*(9), 537–546.

Laureys, S., Perrin, F., & Brédart, S. (2007). Self-consciousness in non-communicative patients. *Conscious Cogn*. *16*, 722–741.

Levy, D. E., Sidtis, J. J., Rottenberg, D. A., et al. (1987). Differences in cerebral blood flow and glucose utilization in vegetative versus locked-in patients. *Ann. Neurol.*, *22*(6), 673–682.

Menon, D. K., Owen, A. M., Williams, E. J., et al. (1998). Cortical processing in persistent vegetative state. *Lancet*, *352*(9123), 200.

Momose, T., Matsui, T., & Kosaka, N. (1989). Effect of cervical spinal cord stimulation (cSCS) on cerebral glucose metabolism and blood flow in a vegetative patient assessed by positron emission tomography (PET) and single photon emission computed tomography (SPECT). *Radiat. Med.*, *7*(7), 243–246.

Multi-Society Task Force on PVS. (1994a). Medical aspects of the persistent vegetative state (first part). *N Eng J Med*, *330*, 1400–1508.

Multi-Society Task Force on PVS (1994b). Medical aspects of the persistent vegetative state (second part). *N Eng J Med*, *330*, 1572–1579.

Mummery, C. J., Ashburner, J., Scott, S. K., & Wise, R. J. S. (1999). Functional neuroimaging of speech perception in six normal and two aphasic subjects. *Journal of the Acoustical Society of America*, *106*, 449–456.

Naatanen, R. (2003). Mismatch negativity: clinical research and possible applications. *International Journal of Psychophysiology*, *48*, 179–188.

Owen, A. M., Menon, D. K., Johnsrude, I. S., Bor, D., Scott, S. K., Manly, T., et al. (2002). Detecting residual cognitive function in persistent vegetative state. *Neurocase*, *8*, 394–403.

Owen, A. M., Coleman, M. R., Menon, D. K., et al. (2005a). Using a heirarchical approach to investigate residual auditory cognition in persistent vegetative state. In S. Laureys (Ed.), *The Boundaries of Consciousness: Neurobiology and Neuropathology. Progress in Brain Research* (Vol. 150, pp. 461–476). London: Elsevier.

Owen, A. M., Coleman, M. R., Menon, D. K., et al. (2005b). Residual auditory function in persistent vegetative state: A combined PET and fMRI study. *Neuropsychological Rehabilitation*, *15*(3–4), 290–306.

Owen, A. M., Coleman, M. R., Davis, M. H., et al. (2006). Detecting awareness in the vegetative state. *Science*, *313*, 1402.

Owen, A. M., Coleman, M. R., Davis, M. H., et al. (2007a). Response to Comments on "Detecting awareness in the vegetative state". *Science*, *315*, 1221c.

Owen, A. M., Coleman, M. R., Davis, M. H., et al. (2007b). Using fMRI to detect awareness in the vegetative state. *Archives of Neurology*, *64*, 1098–1102.

Perrin, F., Schnakers, C., Schabus, M., et al. (2006). Brain response to one's own name in vegetative state, minimally conscious state, and locked-in syndrome. *Arch Neurol*, *63*, 562–569.

Plum, F., & Posner, J. B. (1966). *The Diagnosis of Stupor and Coma*. Philadelphia, PA: F.A. Davis Co.

Poldrack, R. A. (2006). Can cognitive processes be inferred from neuroimaging data? *Trends Cogn. Sci.*, *10*, 59–63.

Rossini, P. M., Altamura, C., Ferretti, A., et al. (2004). Does cerebrovascular disease affect the coupling between neuronal activity and local haemodynamics? *Brain*, *127*(Pt 1), 99–110.

Rudolf, J., Ghaemi, M., Haupt, W. F., et al. (1999). Cerebral glucose metabolism in acute and persistent vegetative state. *J. Neurosurg. Anesthesiol.*, *11*(1), 17–24.

Rodd, J. M., Davis, M. H., & Johnsrude, I. S. (2005). The neural mechanisms of speech comprehension: fMRI studies of semantic ambiguity. *Cereb. Cortex*, *15*, 1261.

Royal College of Physicians Working Group (1996). The permanent vegetative state. *Journal of the Royal College of Physicians of London*, *30*, 119–121.

Schacter, D. L. (1994). Priming and multiple memory systems: Perceptual mechanisms of implicit memory. In D.L. Schacter & E. Tulving (Eds.), *Memory Systems* (pp. 233–268). Cambridge, MA: MIT Press.

Sakatani, K., Murata, Y., Fukaya, C., et al. (2003). BOLD functional MRI may overlook activation areas in the damaged brain. *Acta Neurochir Suppl*, *87*, 59–62.

Schiff, N. D. (2006). Multimodal Neuroimaging Approaches to Disorders of Consciousness. *Journal of Head Trauma Rehabilitation*, *21*(5), 388–397.

Schiff, N. D., Ribary, U., Moreno, D. R., et al. (2002). Residual cerebral activity and behavioural fragments can remain in the persistently vegetative brain. *Brain*, *125*(Pt 6), 1210–1234.

Schnakers, C., Giacino, J., Kaknar, K., et al. (2006). Does the FOUR score correctly diagnose the vegetative and minimally conscious states? *Ann Neurol*, *60*, 744–745.

Scott, S. K., Blank, C., Rosen, S., & Wise, R. J. S. (2000). Identification of a pathway for intelligible speech in the left temporal lobe. *Brain*, *123*, 2400–2406.

Staffen, W., Kronbichler, M., Aichhorn, M., et al. (2006). Selective brain activity in response to one's own name in the persistent vegetative state. *J Neurol Neurosurg Psychiatry*, *77*, 1383–1384.

Tommasino, C., Grana, C., & Lucignani, G. (1995). Regional cerebral metabolism of glucose in comatose and vegetative state patients. *J. Neurosurg. Anesthesiol.*, *7*(2), 109–116.

Tresch, D. D., Sims, F. H., & Duthie, E. H. (1991). Clinical characteristics of patients in the persistent vegetative state. *Arch Intern Med*, *151*, 930–912.

Voss, H. U., Uluc, A. M., & Dyke, J. P. (2006). Possible axonal regrowth in late recovery from the minimally conscious state. *J Clin Invest*, *116*, 2005–2011.

The Neural Correlates of Consciousness
An Update

GIULIO TONONI[a] AND CHRISTOF KOCH[b]

[a]*Department of Psychiatry, University of Wisconsin, Madison, Wisconsin, USA*
[b]*Division of Biology and the Division of Engineering and Applied Science, California Institute of Technology, Pasadena, California, USA*

This review examines recent advances in the study of brain correlates of consciousness. First, we briefly discuss some useful distinctions between consciousness and other brain functions. We then examine what has been learned by studying global changes in the level of consciousness, such as sleep, anesthesia, and seizures. Next we consider some of the most common paradigms used to study the neural correlates for specific conscious percepts and examine what recent findings say about the role of different brain regions in giving rise to consciousness for that percept. Then we discuss dynamic aspects of neural activity, such as sustained versus phasic activity, feedforward versus reentrant activity, and the role of neural synchronization. Finally, we briefly consider how a theoretical analysis of the fundamental properties of consciousness can usefully complement neurobiological studies.

Key words: consciousness; brain; information

Introduction

There are several strategies by which scientists can approach the relationship between the brain and consciousness. One is to wait and hope that, once we know all there is to know about neuroanatomy and neurophysiology (or maybe when we can model in detail the working of the entire brain; Markram 2006), the answer will somehow pop out. A more practical approach is to use the tools of neuroscience that are available now to shed light on the neural structures and activity patterns that underlie consciousness. For example, one can examine how brain activity changes when, everything else being as equal as possible, a stimulus is experienced or not. In this way, one can attempt to identify, more and more precisely, the neural correlates of consciousness (NCC), defined as the *minimal neuronal mechanisms jointly sufficient for any one specific conscious percept* (Koch 2003). A complementary strategy is to consider conditions in which consciousness is globally diminished, such as deep sleep or anesthesia, and ask what has changed in the brain. Finally, another approach is to develop a theoretical framework that clarifies what consciousness is, how it can be generated by a physical system, and how it can be measured and then to test the predictions of the theory against data from neuroscience (Tononi 2004b).

This review focuses on recent advances in the study of the NCC. First, we briefly discuss some useful distinctions between consciousness and other brain functions. We then examine what has been learned about the NCC by studying global changes in the level of consciousness, such as sleep, anesthesia, and generalized seizures. Next, we consider some of the most common paradigms used to study the NCC for specific conscious percepts and examine what recent findings say about the role of different brain regions in giving rise to consciousness for that percept. Finally, we discuss the relation to the NCC of dynamic aspects of neural activity, such as sustained versus phasic activity, feedforward versus reentrant activity, and the role of neural synchronization. We end with a few remarks on the importance of a combined theoretical and neurobiological approach.

Consciousness and Other Brain Functions

Many suggestions have been ventured in the hope of alleviating the puzzle of subjective experience. Perhaps consciousness emerges somehow when an organism is

Address for correspondence: Christof Koch, Division of Biology and the Division of Engineering and Applied Science, 216-76, California Institute of Technology, Pasadena, CA 91125. Fax: +1-626-796-8876.
koch@klab.caltech.edu

immersed in some complex sensorimotor loop that includes the environment. Another common idea is that consciousness may somehow arise when one part of the brain, acting as the "subject" (typically the front), looks upon another part as its "object" (typically the back), and evaluates or reflects upon its activity. It is often thought that in the end consciousness may reduce to attention and its brain mechanisms, since we are usually conscious of what we attend. Much could be said about each of these suggestions. Here, we briefly consider some recent results (and some very old evidence) indicating that consciousness—in the sense of having an experience—does not require sensorimotor loops involving the body and the world, does not require self-reflection (or language), and does not reduce to attention.

Consciousness and Sensory Input/Motor Output

We are usually conscious of what goes on around us, and occasionally of what goes on within our body. So it is only natural to think that consciousness may be tightly linked to the ongoing interaction we maintain with the world and the body. However, there are many examples to the contrary. We are conscious of our thoughts, which do not seem to correspond to anything out there; we can also imagine things that are not out there. When we do so, sensory areas can be activated from the inside (Kosslyn et al. 2001), though there are some differences (Amedi et al. 2005). Also, stimulus-independent consciousness is associated with its own patterns of activation within cortex and thalamus (Mason et al. 2007). During dreams, we are virtually disconnected from the environment (Hobson et al. 2000)—hardly anything of what happens around us enters consciousness, and our muscles are paralyzed (except for eye muscles and diaphragm). Nevertheless, we are vividly conscious: all that seems to matter is that the thalamocortical system continues to function more or less as in wakefulness, as shown by unit recording, EEG, and neuroimaging studies performed during rapid eye movement (REM) sleep, when dreams are most intense (Maquet et al. 1996). Interestingly, certain regions of the thalamocortical systems, such as dorsolateral prefrontal cortex, are deactivated in REM sleep, which likely accounts for some peculiarities of dreaming experiences, such as the reduction of voluntary control.

Neurological evidence also indicates that neither sensory inputs nor motor outputs are needed to generate consciousness. For instance, retinally blind people can both imagine and dream visually if they become blind after 6–7 years of age or so (Hollins 1985; Buchel et al. 1998). Patients with the locked-in syndrome can be almost completely paralyzed, and yet they are just as conscious as healthy subjects (Laureys et al. 2005) and can compose eloquent accounts of their condition (Bauby 1997). A transient form of paralysis is one of the characteristic features of narcolepsy. Severe cataleptic attacks can last for minutes and leave the patient collapsed on the floor, utterly unable to move or to signal, but fully aware of her surroundings (Guilleminault 1976; Siegel 2000). Or consider the Californian drug addicts known as the *frozen addicts* who acquired some of the symptoms of severe, late-stage Parkinson's disease, fully conscious, yet unable to move or speak (Langston & Palfreman 1995). All six had previously taken synthetic heroin tainted with MPTP, which selectively and permanently destroyed dopamine-producing neurons in their basal ganglia. Thus, consciousness here and now seems to depend on what certain parts of the brain are doing, without requiring any obligatory interaction with the environment or the body.

Consciousness and Self-Reflection

Consciousness is usually evaluated by verbal reports, and questions about consciousness ("Did you see anything on the screen?") are answered by "looking inside" retrospectively and reporting what one has just experienced. So it is perhaps natural to suggest that consciousness may arise through the ability to reflect on our own perceptions: our brain would form a scene of what it sees, but we would become conscious of it—experience it subjectively—only when we, as a subject of experience, watch that scene from the inside. This suggestion is often framed in a neurobiological context by assuming that patterns of activity corresponding to "unconscious" or "subconscious" percepts form in posterior regions of the cerebral cortex involved in the categorization/association of sensory stimuli. These percepts then become conscious when mainly anterior prefrontal and cingulate regions involved in self-representations interact with posterior cortex, perhaps by reading in signals through forward connections and selectively amplifying them through back connections (more on this later).

There is of course no doubt that the brain categorizes its own patterns of activity in the sense that neurons respond mainly to the activity of other neurons, so the brain is constantly "looking at itself." However, this is not necessarily in terms of a "subject" (the front) looking at an "object" represented in sensory cortices (the back). Leaving aside the mystery of why reflecting on something should make it conscious, this scenario is made less plausible by a common observation: when we become absorbed in some intense perceptual task, for example watching an engrossing movie, playing a fast-paced video game, or rushing through the woods at high speed, we are vividly conscious—we are immersed in the rapid flow of experience—without any need for reflection or introspection. Often, we become so immersed in such flow that we may lose the sense of self, the inner voice. Perhaps the habit of thinking about consciousness has distracted the scholars who write upon such matters to devalue the unreflective nature of much of experience.

A recent neuroimaging study by Malach and collaborators (Hasson et al. 2004) throws some interesting light on these old observations. Subjects were scanned with fMRI in three conditions. In the slow categorization task, subjects were asked to categorize pictures into animal/no-animal categories. During the introspective task, subjects viewed the images and then introspected about their emotional response (strong/neutral). Finally, the fast categorization task was identical to the "slow" condition but at triple the stimulation rate. Thus, "slow" and "introspection" conditions were identical in terms of sensory stimuli and motor output but differed in the cognitive task. On the other hand, "slow" and "rapid" conditions were similar in the cognitive task but differed in the sensorimotor processing and attentional loads. Behavioral measurements confirmed that self-awareness was high during the introspection task, and virtually abolished during rapid categorization. The neuroimaging results were clear: during introspection there was an activation of prefrontal regions, whereas sensory cortex was strongly activated during rapid categorization. Crucially, during introspection self-related cortex was deactivated below the rest condition. This deactivation of prefrontal regions was thus the neural correlate of "losing oneself" in the task. To the extent that these prefrontal regions were indeed involved in self-representation, these findings suggest that their activation is not necessary for the emergence of perceptual consciousness, but only to reflect upon it and report it to others. Indeed, it appears that self-related activity is actually shut off during highly demanding sensory tasks.

Lesion studies also seem to support the notion that consciousness does not require prefrontal cortex and, by inference, the functions it performs. Though patients with widespread, bilateral damage to prefrontal cortex are rare, two recent clinical studies provide some intriguing evidence. A man who, at the age of 21, had fallen on an iron spike that completely penetrated through both of his frontal lobes, nevertheless went on to live a stable life—marrying and raising two children—in an appropriate professional and social setting. Although displaying many of the typical frontal lobe behavioral disturbances, he never complained of loss of sensory perception, nor did he show visual or other deficits (Mataro et al. 2001). Another case is that of a 27-year-old woman with massive bilateral prefrontal damage of unclear etiology (Markowitsch & Kessler 2000). While manifesting grossly deficient scores in frontal lobe sensitive tests, she showed no abnormal perceptual abilities (that is not to say that such patients do not suffer from subtle visual deficits; Barcelo et al. 2000).

Consciousness and Attention

Consciousness and attention have resisted clear and compelling definitions. Few would dispute that the relationship between the two is an intimate one. When subjects pay attention to an object, they become conscious of its various attributes; when the focus of attention shifts away, the object fades from consciousness. Indeed, more than a century of research efforts have quantified the ample benefits accrued to attended and consciously perceived events (Pashler 1998; Braun et al. 2001). This has prompted many to posit that the two processes are inextricably interwoven, if not identical (Posner 1994; Merikle & Joordens 1997; Chun & Wolfe 2000; O'Regan & Noe 2000). Others, however, going back to the 19th century, have argued that attention and consciousness are distinct phenomena, with distinct functions and neuronal mechanisms (Iwasaki 1993; Hardcastle 1997; Lamme 2003; Baars 2005; Block 2005; Dehaene et al. 2006; Koch & Tsuchiya 2007). Recent psychophysical and neurophysiological evidence argues in favor of a dissociation between selective attention and consciousness, suggesting that events or objects can be attended to without being consciously perceived. Conversely, an event or object can be consciously perceived in the near absence of top-down attentional processing.

Attention without Consciousness

Consider that subjects can attend to a location for many seconds and yet fail to see one or more attributes of an object at that location. In lateral masking (*visual crowding*), the orientation of a peripherally presented grating is hidden from conscious sight but remains sufficiently potent to induce an orientation-dependent aftereffect (He et al. 1996) Montaser-Kouhsari and Rajimehr (2004) showed that an aftereffect induced by an invisible illusory contour required focal attention, even though the object at the center of attention was invisible. Naccache and colleagues (2002) elicited priming for invisible words (suppressed by a combination of forward and backward masking) but only if the subject was attending to the invisible prime-target pair; without attention, the same word failed to elicit priming. That is, the subject needs to attend to the masked stimulus for priming to occur, but the actual stimulus is not seen (with an associated $d' = 0$). In another experiment, male/female nudes attracted attention and induced involuntary eye movements when they were rendered completely invisible by continuous flash suppression (Jiang et al. 2006). When subjects had to discriminate the location of the masked nude from the location of a masked shuffled nude, they were at chance; without the intraocular masking, the images are clearly visible. fMRI evidence confirms attentional modulation of invisible images in primary visual cortex (Bahrami et al. 2007). In conclusion, attentional selection does not necessarily engender phenomenal sensations, although it may often do so.

Consciousness in the Absence of Attention

When focusing intensely on one event, the world is not reduced to a tunnel, with everything outside the focus of attention gone: we are always aware of some aspects of the world surrounding us, such as its gist. Indeed, gist is immune from inattentional blindness (Mack & Rock 1998)—when a photograph covering the entire background is briefly and unexpectedly flashed onto the screen, subjects can accurately report a summary of its content. In the 30 ms necessary to apprehend the gist of a scene, top-down attention cannot play much of a role (because gist is a property associated with the entire image, any process that locally enhances features is going to be of limited use).

Or take the perception of a single object (say a bar) in an otherwise empty display, a nonecological but common arrangement in many animal and human experiments. Here, what function would top-down, selective attention need to perform without any competing item in or around fixation? Indeed, the most popular neuronal model of attention, *biased competition* (Desimone & Duncan 1995), predicts that in the absence of competition, no or little attentional enhancement occurs, yet we are perfectly aware of the object and its background.

In a dual-task paradigms, the subject's attention is drawn to a demanding central task, while at the same time a secondary stimulus is flashed somewhere in the periphery. Using the identical retinal layout, the subject either performs the central task, the peripheral task, or both simultaneously (Sperling & Dosher 1986; Braun & Sagi 1990; Braun & Julesz 1998). With focal attention busy at the center, the subject can still distinguish a natural scene containing an animal (or a vehicle) from one that does not include an animal (or a vehicle), while being unable to distinguish a red-green bisected disk from a green-red one (Li et al. 2002). Likewise, subjects can tell male from female faces or even distinguish a famous from a nonfamous face (Reddy et al. 2004; Reddy & Koch 2006) but are frustrated by tasks that are computationally much simpler (e.g., discriminating a rotated letter "L" from a rotated "T"). This is quite remarkable. Thus, while we cannot be sure that observers do not deploy some limited amount of top-down attention in these dual-task experiments that require training and concentration (i.e., high arousal), it remains true that subjects can perform certain discriminations but not others in the near absence of top-down attention. And they are not guessing. They can be quite confident of their choices and "see," albeit often indistinctly, what they can discriminate.

The existence of such dissociations—attention without consciousness and consciousness without attention—should not be surprising when considering their different functions. Attention is a set of mechanisms whereby the brain selects a subset of the incoming sensory information for higher level processing, while the nonattended portions of the input are analyzed at a lower band width. For example, in primates, about one million fibers leave each eye and carry on the order of one megabyte per second of raw information. One way to deal with this deluge of data is to select a small fraction and process this reduced input in real time, while the nonattended data suffer from benign neglect. Attention can be directed by bottom-up, exogenous cues or by top-down endogenous features and can be applied to a spatially restricted part of the image (focal, spotlight of attention), an attribute (e.g., all red objects), or to an entire object. By contrast, consciousness appears to be involved in providing a kind of "executive summary" of the current situation that is useful for decision making, planning, and learning (Baars).

Changes in the Level of Consciousness

In neurology, a distinction is traditionally made between the level of consciousness and the content of consciousness. When you fall asleep, for example, the level of consciousness decreases to the point that you become virtually unconscious—the degree to which you are conscious (of anything) becomes progressively less and less. The content of consciousness, instead, refers to the particular experience you're having at any given time, for the same level of consciousness. It is useful to maintain this distinction when considering the

NCC, and begin by considering changes in the level of consciousness.

Sleep

Sleep offers a commonplace, daily demonstration that the level of consciousness can change dramatically. In the laboratory, a subject is awakened during different stages of sleep and asked to report "anything that was going through your mind just before waking up." What is most noteworthy for the present purposes is that a number of awakenings from non-REM (NREM) sleep, especially early in the night when EEG slow waves are prevalent, can yield no report whatsoever. Thus, early slow-wave sleep is the only phase of adult life during which healthy human subjects may deny that they were experiencing anything at all. When present, reports from NREM sleep early in the night are often short and thought-like. However, especially later in the night, reports from NREM sleep can be longer, more hallucinatory and, generally speaking, more dream-like. On the other hand, awakenings during REM sleep almost always yield dreams—vivid conscious experiences, sometimes organized within a complex narrative structure (Hobson et al. 2000; Hobson & Pace-Schott 2002).

What are the processes underlying the fading of the level of consciousness during early slow-wave sleep? Though metabolic rates decrease in many cortical areas, especially frontal and parietal areas, the thalamocortical system is far from shutting down. Instead, triggered by a decrease in acetylcholine and other modulators, cortical and thalamic neurons undergo slow oscillations (1 Hz or less) between an up and a down state (Steriade et al. 2001). During the up state, cortical cells remain depolarized at waking levels for around a second and fire at waking rates, often in the gamma range (Destexhe et al. 2007). However, the up state of NREM sleep is not stable as in wakefulness and REM sleep, but it is inherently bistable. The longer neurons remain depolarized, the more likely they become to precipitate into a hyperpolarized down state—a complete cessation of synaptic activity that can last for a tenth of a second or more—after which they revert to another up state. The transition from up to down states appears to be due to depolarization-dependent potassium currents and to short-term synaptic depression, both of which increase with the amount of prior activation (Steriade 2003). The slow oscillation is found in virtually every cortical neuron and is synchronized across the cortical mantle by cortico-cortical connections, which is why the EEG records high-voltage, low-frequency waves.

An intriguing possibility is that changes in the level of consciousness during sleep may be related to the degree of bistability of thalamocortical networks (Tononi 2004b; Massimini et al. 2007). In a recent study, transcranial magnetic stimulation (TMS) was used in conjunction with high-density EEG to record cortical evoked responses to direct stimulation in waking and sleep (Massimini et al. 2005; Massimini et al. 2007). During wakefulness, TMS induced a sustained response made of rapidly changing patterns of activity that persisted until 300 ms and involved the sequential activation of specific brain areas, depending on the precise site of stimulation. During early NREM sleep, however, the brain response to TMS changed markedly. When applied to lateral cortical regions, the activity evoked by TMS remained localized to the site of stimulation, without activating connected brain regions, and lasted for less than 150 ms (Massimini et al. 2005). This finding indicates that during early NREM sleep, when the level of consciousness is reduced, effective connectivity among cortical regions breaks down, implying a corresponding breakdown of cortical integration. Computer simulations suggest that this breakdown of effective connectivity may be due to the induction of a local down state (Esser & Tononi, in preparation). When applied over centromedian parietal regions, each TMS pulse triggered a stereotypical response implying the induction of a global down state: a full-fledged, high-amplitude slow wave (Massimini et al. 2007) that closely resembled spontaneous ones and that traveled through much of the cortex (Massimini et al. 2004). Such stereotypical responses could be induced even when, for the preceding seconds, there were no slow waves in the spontaneous EEG, indicating that perturbations can reveal the potential bistability of a system irrespective of its observed state. Altogether, these TMS–EEG measurements suggest that the sleeping brain, despite being active and reactive, becomes inherently bistable: it either breaks down in causally independent modules or bursts into a global, stereotypical response. By contrast, during REM sleep late in the night, when dreams become long and vivid and consciousness returns to levels close to those of wakefulness, the responses to TMS also recover and come to resemble more closely those observed during wakefulness: evoked patterns of activity become more complex and spatially differentiated, although some late components are still missing (Massimini & Tononi, unpublished).

Anesthesia

The most common among exogenous manipulations of the level of consciousness is general anesthesia. Anesthetics come in two main classes: intravenous agents used for induction, such as propofol and ketamine, which are generally administered together with sedatives such as midazolam and dexmedetomidine; and inhaled agents, such as isoflurane, sevoflurane, and desflurane or the gases xenon and nitrous oxide. The doses of inhaled anesthetics are usually referred to their minimum alveolar concentration (MAC): a MAC value of 1 is the dose that prevents movement in 50% of subjects in response to a painful surgical stimulation. At low MAC values (0.1–0.2) anesthetics produce amnesia, first explicit and then implicit. Frequently there are distortions of time perception, such as slowing down and fragmentation, and a feeling of disconnection from the environment. Also, at low MAC values anesthetics produce increasing sleepiness and make arousal progressively more difficult, suggesting that to some extent they can mimic neurophysiological events underlying sleep. At around 0.3 MAC people experience a decrease in the level of consciousness, also described as a "shrinking" in the field of consciousness, as if they were kept on the verge of falling asleep. MAC-awake, usually around 0.3–0.4 MAC, is the point at which response to verbal command is lost in 50% of patients and is considered the point at which consciousness is lost (LOC). The transition to unconsciousness (LOC) appears to be rather brusque, not unlike the collapse of muscle tone that usually accompanies it, suggesting that neural processes underlying consciousness change in a nonlinear manner. At concentrations above LOC, movements are still possible, especially partially coordinated responses to painful stimuli, suggesting that some degree of "unconscious" processing is still possible. Complete unresponsiveness is usually obtained just above MAC of 1.0.

At the cellular level, many anesthetics have mixed effects, but the overall result is a decrease in neuronal excitability by either increasing inhibition or decreasing excitation. Most anesthetics act by enhancing GABA inhibition or by hyperpolarizing cells through an increase of potassium-leak currents. They can also interfere with glutamatergic transmission and antagonize acetylcholine at nicotinic receptors (Campagna et al. 2003; Franks 2006). But what are critical circuits mediating the LOC induced by anesthetics?

A considerable number of neuroimaging studies in humans have recently shed some light on this issue (Alkire & Miller 2005). The most consistent effects produced by most anesthetics at LOC is a reduction of thalamic metabolism and blood flow, suggesting the possibility that the thalamus may serve as a consciousness switch (Alkire et al. 2000). (Another common site of action of several anesthetics is the posterior cingulate/medial parietal cortical areas, as well as the medial basal forebrain). However, both PET and fMRI signals mostly reflect synaptic activity rather than cellular firing, and the thalamus receives a massive innervation from cortex. Moreover, the relative reduction in thalamic activity occurs on a background of a marked decrease in global metabolism (30–60%) that involves many cortical regions. Thus, thalamic activity as recorded by neuroimaging may represent an especially sensitive, localized readout of the extent of widespread cortical deactivation, rather than the final common pathway of unconsciousness (Ori et al. 1986). In fact, spontaneous thalamic firing in animal models of anesthesia is mostly driven by corticothalamic feedback (Vahle-Hinz et al. 2007), and the metabolic effects of enflurane on the thalamus can be abolished by an ipsilateral cortical ablation (Nakakimura et al. 1988), suggesting that the switch in thalamic unit activity is driven primarily through a reduction in afferent corticothalamic feedback more than by a direct effect of anesthesia on thalamic neurons. Recently, thalamic activity was recorded using depth electrodes in a patient undergoing anesthesia for the implant of a deep brain stimulator (Velly et al. 2007). With either propofol or sevoflurane, when the patient lost consciousness, the cortical EEG changed dramatically. However, there was little change in the thalamic EEG until almost 10 min later. This result implies that the deactivation of cortex alone is sufficient for loss of consciousness, and conversely that thalamic activity alone is insufficient to maintain it.

These findings do not imply that the thalamus is irrelevant, but rather suggest that its effects on consciousness are largely accounted for by its effects on cortical circuits, most notably by providing a tonic facilitatory action that can help to restore consciousness, or cause its collapse when it fails. A dramatic demonstration is provided by a recent study, where rats kept under anesthetic concentration of sevoflurane could be awakened by a minute injection of nicotinic agents in an intralaminar thalamic nucleus (Alkire et al. 2007). Conversely, GABA agonists infused into the same side caused an immediate loss of consciousness (Miller et al. 1989; Miller & Ferrendelli 1990) (though nicotinic antagonists did not).

Coma and Vegetative States

While consciousness may nearly fade during certain phases of sleep and be kept at very low levels for a prescribed period during general anesthesia, coma and vegetative states are characterized by a loss of consciousness that is hard or impossible to reverse. Coma—an enduring sleep-like state of immobility with eyes closed from which the patient cannot be aroused—represents the paradigmatic form of pathological loss of consciousness. Typically, coma is caused by a suppression of thalamocortical function by drugs, toxins, or internal metabolic derangements. Other causes of coma are head trauma, strokes, or hypoxia due to heart failure, which again cause widespread destruction of thalamocortical circuits. Smaller lesions of the reticular activating system can also cause unconsciousness, presumably by deactivating the thalamocortical system indirectly.

Patients who survive a coma may recover, while others enter the so-called vegetative state, in which eyes reopen, giving the appearance of wakefulness, but unresponsiveness persists. Soon, regular sleep/waking cycles follow. Respiration, other autonomic functions and brainstem functions are relatively preserved, and stereotypic, reflex-like responses can occur, including yawning and grunting, but no purposeful behavior. Patients may remain vegetative for a long time or may emerge to a "minimally conscious state." This is distinguished from the vegetative state by the occasional occurrence of some behaviors that do not appear to be purely reflexive, suggesting that some degree of consciousness may be present.

Post-mortem analysis in vegetative patients reveals that the brainstem and hypothalamus, and specifically the reticular activating system, are largely spared, which explains why patients look awake. Usually the vegetative state is due to widespread lesions of gray matter in neocortex and thalamus, to widespread white-matter damage and diffuse axonal injury, or to bilateral thalamic lesions, especially of the paramedian thalamic nuclei. It is not clear whether thalamic damage is largely a reflection of diffuse cortical damage (as in metabolic studies of anesthesia, changes in the thalamus are much more concentrated and therefore easier to document than changes in cortex) or whether even isolated thalamic damage can cause persistent unconsciousness. Matrix, calbindin-positive thalamic cells, which are most numerous within intralaminar nuclei, project diffusely to supragranular layers of cortex (Jones 1998) where they facilitate coherent high-frequency oscillations (Joliot et al. 1994). Such cells may be especially important in enabling effective interactions among many cortical regions: if their activating function is lost, patients may remain vegetative even though cortical tissue may be relatively intact. Indeed, Steven Laureys and colleagues showed that recovery from a vegetative state was associated with the restoration of functional connectivity between intralaminar thalamic nuclei and prefrontal and anterior cingulate cortices (Laureys et al. 2000a). A recent study by Niko Schiff and colleagues shows the role of the thalamus even more dramatically: bilateral deep brain electrical stimulation of the central thalamus restored a degree of behavioral responsiveness in a patient who had remained in a minimally conscious state for 6 years following brain trauma (Schiff et al. 2007).

In vegetative states, brain metabolism is globally reduced by 50 to 60%, most notably in regions such as the posterior cingulate cortex and the precuneus (Laureys et al. 2004; Schiff 2006a). These are also the areas that reactivate most reliably if a patient regains consciousness. A recent case study reported an extraordinary recovery of verbal communication and motor function in a patient who had remained in a minimally conscious state for 19 years (Voss et al. 2006). Diffusion tensor MRI showed increased fractional anisotropy (assumed to reflect myelinated fiber density) in posteromedial cortices, encompassing cuneus and precuneus. These same areas showed increased glucose metabolism as studied by PET scanning, likely reflecting the neuronal regrowth paralleling the patient's clinical recovery. This and other neuroimaging studies of vegetative or minimally conscious patients are demonstrating ever more clearly that a purely clinical diagnosis of persistent loss of consciousness may at times be dramatically inaccurate. It was already known that patients with locked-in syndromes due to pontine lesions that left them almost completely paralyzed may seem unresponsive, but if they preserve even a minimal ability to signal (typically by moving an eye or eyelid up or down) they can communicate a rich subjective experience. What about patients who show no voluntary movement at all? Several imaging studies have now shown that, even in completely unresponsive patients, as long as significant portions of the thalamocortical system are preserved, cognitive stimuli can induce patterns of activation similar to those seen in healthy subjects (Laureys et al. 2004; Schiff 2006b). As we have seen in a previous section, stimuli that are not perceived consciously can still activate appropriate brain areas. Thus, inferring the presence of consciousness may be unwarranted. However, in a recent, thought-provoking study, a clinically vegetative, seemingly unresponsive patient was put in the scanner and asked to imagine playing tennis or navigating through her room. Remarkably, the patient showed fMRI activation patterns of the appropriate cortical regions, exactly like healthy subjects. Obviously, these activations could not be due to unconscious processing of stimuli (Owen et al. 2006). Of note, this patient had widespread frontal lesions, while posterior cortex was largely preserved.

Seizures

The abnormal, hypersynchronous discharge of neurons is a frequent cause of short-lasting impairments of consciousness. Consciousness is lost or severely affected in so-called generalized seizures, such as absence and tonic-clonic seizures, and to a lesser extent in complex partial seizures. Absence seizures, which are more frequent in children, are momentary lapses of consciousness during which a child stops what she was doing and stares straight ahead blankly. Absence seizures are accompanied by spike-and-wave complexes at around 3 Hz in the EEG, reflecting cycles of synchronous firing and silence of large numbers of neurons. There is great variability in the degree of unresponsiveness both across subjects and, within the same subject, between seizures. Sometimes, simple behaviors such as repetitive tapping or counting can proceed unimpaired during the seizures, but more complex tasks come to a halt.

Generalized convulsive seizures usually comprise a tonic phase of muscle stiffening, followed by a clonic phase with jerking of the arms and legs. After the convulsion the person may be lethargic or in a state of confusion for minutes up to hours. During the tonic phase of a convulsive seizure neural activity is greatly increased, as indicated by high frequency activity in the EEG. The clonic phase is accompanied by synchronous spikes and waves in the EEG, corresponding to millions of neurons alternately firing in strong bursts and turning silent. Loss of consciousness during the tonic phase of generalized seizures is noteworthy because it occurs at times when neuronal activity is extremely high and synchronous.

Partial complex seizures often begin with strange abdominal sensations, fears, premonitions, or automatic gestures. The person progressively loses contact with the environment, exhibits a fixed stare, and is unable to respond adequately to questions or commands. Stereotyped, automatic movements are common. Complex partial seizures usually last from 15 sec to 3 min. Seizure activity is usually localized to the medial temporal lobe.

The diagnosis of seizures is made through clinical observation and EEG recordings. In absence and tonic-clonic seizures the scalp EEG shows diffuse abnormalities, suggesting a generalized involvement of brain networks, whereas in partial complex seizures the abnormalities are confined to a medial temporal focus on one side. However, neuroimaging studies using SPECT, PET, and fMRI, and depth EEG recordings in humans and animals have revealed that generalized seizures do not affect all brain areas indiscriminately, whereas complex partial seizures alter brain activity less focally than initially thought (Blumenfeld & Taylor 2003; Blumenfeld et al. 2003; Blumenfeld et al. 2004; Blumenfeld 2005). In fact, it now appears that all seizures causing an impairment of consciousness are associated with changes in activity in three sets of brain areas, namely: i) increased activity in the upper brainstem and medial thalamus; ii) decreased activity in the anterior and posterior cingulate, medial frontal cortex, and precuneus; iii) altered activity in the lateral and orbital frontal cortex and in the lateral parietal cortex. In tonic-clonic seizures, fronto-parietal association areas show increased activity, while the pattern is more complex and variable in absence seizures, though parietal areas are usually deactivated. Complex partial seizures show decreased activity in frontal and parietal association cortex, which is associated with the onset of slow waves similar to those of sleep or anesthesia (rather than to epileptiform discharges).

At this stage, it is not clear which of these three sets of areas, alone or in combination, are crucial for the loss of consciousness. However, two things are clear: first, the areas involved in the loss of consciousness associated with seizures correspond to those affected in sleep, anesthesia, and the vegetative state, pointing to a common substrate for the most common forms of loss of consciousness; and second, especially during the tonic phase of convulsive seizures, it would seem that consciousness is lost when neurons are excessively and synchronously active, rather than inactive.

Changes in the Content of Consciousness—Localizing the NCC

As we have seen, much can be learned by studying how brain activity changes with changes in the overall level of consciousness. A complementary approach is to examine how brain activity changes when a specific content of consciousness changes—for example, a visual stimulus becomes visible or invisible—while everything else, including the overall level of consciousness as well as the sensory input, remains as constant as possible. Recording spike trains from individual neurons or measuring hemodynamic signals while the subject is looking at a stimulus in an MR scanner allows researchers to investigate what kind of neuronal activity is correlated with the conscious perception of the stimulus rather than with the mere presentation of the stimulus. The goal is to follow the footprints of consciousness in the brain by ultimately identifying the neural correlates of consciousness (NCC)—the minimal neuronal mechanisms that are jointly sufficient for any one specific conscious percept (Crick & Koch 1995,

1998, 2003). Thus, every phenomenal, subjective state will have associated NCC: one for seeing a red patch, another one for seeing grandmother, yet a third one for hearing a siren, another one for feeling free to act one way or another and so on. Perturbing or inactivating the NCC for any one specific conscious experience will affect the percept or cause it to disappear. If the NCC could be induced artificially, for instance by cortical microstimulation in a prosthetic device or during neurosurgery, the subject will experience the associated percept. This definition of the NCC stresses the word "minimal," because the question of interest is which subcomponents of the brain are actually needed. For instance, while neural activity in the cerebellum may ultimately affect some behaviors elicited by the presentation of a stimulus (such as eye movements), it is likely that such activity has little to do with the generation of the conscious percept of that stimulus, and thus is not part of the NCC.

Many questions can be asked: What characterizes the NCC for a specific experience? What do the NCC for different experiences have in common? Do the NCC involve just the thalamocortical system, or do they extend to structures such as the hippocampus, the claustrum, or the basal ganglia? Do they involve all pyramidal neurons in cortex at any given point in time? Or only a subset of cells in frontal lobes that project to the sensory cortices in the back? Only layer 5 cortical cells? Neurons that fire in a phasic, synchronous, or oscillatory manner? Or neurons that are included in reentrant loops? These are some of the proposals that have been advanced over the past years (Chalmers 2000).

Much of the contemporary work aimed at characterizing the NCC has concentrated on changes in specific visual contents of consciousness (or awareness, which is here used interchangeably), in part because visual experience is easy to manipulate experimentally, and in part because more is known about the anatomy and function of visual areas in primates than about any other brain regions. Visual psychologists have perfected a number of techniques—masking, binocular rivalry, continuous flash suppression, motion-induced blindness, change blindness, inattentional blindness—in which the seemingly simple and unambiguous relationship between a physical stimulus in the world, the resulting neural activity, and its associated percept is disrupted (Kim & Blake 2005). We first consider what such approaches have revealed about the brain areas that underlie the NCC, focusing specifically on the visual system. In the following sections we ask whether the NCC for visual percepts corresponds to some special kind of neural activity.

A Test Case: The NCC in Visual Cortex

Many experiments exploit perceptual illusions in which the physical stimulus remains fixed while the percept fluctuates. The best known example is the Necker cube, whose 12 lines can be perceived in one of two different ways in depth. Another perceptual illusion that is easy to vary parametrically is binocular rivalry (Blake & Logothetis 2002): a small image, for example a horizontal grating, is presented to the left eye and another image, for example a vertical grating, is shown to the corresponding location in the right eye. In spite of the constant visual stimulus, observers consciously see the horizontal grating alternate every few seconds with the vertical one. The brain does not allow for the simultaneous perception of both images.

Macaque monkeys can be trained to report whether they see the left or the right image. The distribution of the switching times and the way in which changing the contrast in one eye affects the reports leaves little doubt that monkeys and humans experience the same basic phenomenon. In a series of elegant experiments, Logothetis and colleagues (Leopold & Logothetis 1996; Logothetis 1998) recorded from a variety of visual cortical areas in the awake macaque monkey while the animal performed a binocular rivalry task. In primary visual cortex (V1), only a small fraction of cells weakly modulated their response as a function of the percept of the monkey. The majority of cells responded to one or the other retinal stimulus with little regard to what the animal perceived at the time. In contrast, in a high-level cortical area such as the inferior temporal (IT) cortex along the ventral pathway, almost all neurons responded only to the perceptual dominant stimulus, that is, to the stimulus that was being reported. For example, when a face and a more abstract design were presented, one of these to each eye, a "face" cell fired only when the animal indicated by its performance that it saw the face and not the design presented to the other eye. This result implies that the NCC involve activity in neurons in inferior temporal cortex (but not, of course, that the NCC are local to IT).

In a related perceptual phenomenon, flash suppression (Wolfe 1984), the percept associated with an image projected into one eye is suppressed by flashing another image into the other eye (while the original image remains). A methodological advantage over binocular rivalry is that the timing of the perceptual transition is determined by an external trigger rather than by an internal event. The majority of responsive cells in inferior temporal cortex and in the superior temporal sulcus follow the monkey's behavior—and therefore its percept. That is, when the animal perceives a cell's preferred stimulus, the neuron fires; when the stimulus is present on the retina but is perceptually suppressed, the cell falls silent, even though legions of V1 neurons fire vigorously to the same stimulus (Sheinberg & Logothetis 1997). Single neuron recordings in the medial temporal lobe of epileptic patients during flash suppression likewise demonstrate abolition of their responses when their preferred stimulus is present on the retina but not seen (Kreiman et al. 2002).

In a powerful combination of binocular rivalry and flash suppression, a stationary image in one eye can be suppressed for minutes on end by continuously flashing different images into the other eye (continuous flash suppression; Tsuchiya & Koch 2005). This paradigm lends itself naturally to further investigation of the relationship between neural activity—whether assayed at the single neuron or at the brain voxel level—and conscious perception. Imaging experiments with such perceptual illusions demonstrate quite conclusively that BOLD activity in the upper stages of the ventral pathway (e.g., the fusiform face area and the parahippocampal place area) follow the percept and not simply the retinal stimulus (Tong et al. 1998; Rees & Frith 2007).

There is a lively debate about the extent to which neurons in primary visual cortex simply encode the visual stimulus or are directly contributing to the subject's conscious percept (Tong 2003). That is, is V1 part of the NCC (Crick & Koch 1995)? It is clear that retinal neurons are not part of the NCC for visual experiences. While retinal neurons often correlate with visual experience, the spiking activity of retinal ganglion cells does not accord with visual experience (e.g., there are no photoreceptors at the blind spot; yet no hole in the field of view is apparent, in dreams vivid imagery occurs despite closed eyes, and so on). A number of compelling observations link perception with fMRI BOLD activity in human V1 and even in the lateral geniculate nucleus (LGN) (Tong et al. 1998; Lee et al. 2005). These data are at odds with single-neuron recordings from the monkey. This discrepancy is probably explained by the often tight relationship between consciousness and attention that was mentioned above (see section "Consciousness and Attention"). Unless attentional effects are carefully controlled for, their neural correlates cannot be untangled from those of consciousness (Huk et al. 2001; Tse et al. 2005). This has now been achieved in an elegant study of Lee, Blake, and Heeger (2007). Using a dual-task paradigm they found that hemodynamic BOLD activity in human V1 reflects attentional processes but does not directly correlate with the conscious percept of the subject. The experiment by Bahrami and colleagues (Bahrami et al. 2007) comes to a similar conclusion—they show that the fMRI signal in V1 associated with percep-

tually invisible line drawings can still be modulated by selective visual attention. Also, Haynes and Rees (2005) exploited multivariate decoding techniques to read out perceptually suppressed information (the orientation of a masked stimulus) from V1 BOLD activity, even though the stimulus orientation was so efficiently masked that subjects performed at chance levels when trying to guess the orientation. That is, although subjects did not give any behavioral indication that they saw the orientation of the stimulus, its slant could be predicted on a single-trial basis with better-than-chance odds from the V1 (but not from V2 or V3) BOLD signal.

In conclusion, information pertaining to visual stimulus can be registered in primary visual cortex that may or may not be accessible to the subject. It may be modulated by attention, but it does not appear to correlate directly with the subject's percept. In that sense much of the neural activity in V1 probably does not belong to the NCC. Moreover, as suggested by PET experiments in patients in a persistent vegetative state, in whom stimuli evoked strong but localized activity in primary auditory and primary somatosensory cortices (Laureys et al. 2000b; Laureys et al. 2002), it may well be that none of the primary sensory cortices contributes directly to sensory consciousness.

Consciousness and Neural Dynamics

The studies discussed above indicate that, even within the cerebral cortex, changes in neural activity do not necessarily correlate with changes in conscious experience. Also, we saw earlier that most of the cortex is active during early NREM sleep and anesthesia, not to mention during generalized seizures, but subjects have little conscious content to report. Thus, it is natural to suggest that some additional dynamic feature of neural activity must be present to generate conscious content. Here we consider the roles of i) sustained versus phasic activity, ii) reentrant versus feedforward activity, and iii) synchronous or oscillatory activity.

Sustained versus Phasic Activity

A plausible idea is that neural activity may contribute to consciousness only if it is sustained for a minimum period of time, perhaps around a few hundred ms. At the phenomenological level, there is no doubt that the "now" of experience unfolds at a time scale comprised between tens and several hundred ms (Bachmann 2000) and in some aspects may even stretch to one or two seconds (Poppel & Artin 1988). Other experiments have made use of the attentional blink phenomenon: when an observer detects a target in a rapid stream of visual stimuli, there is a brief period of time during which the detection of subsequent targets is impaired. Remarkably, targets that directly follow the first target are less impaired than those that follow after 200 to 400 ms (Raymond et al. 1992). By manipulating attention, identical visual stimuli can be made conscious or unconscious. In such studies, event-related potentials reflecting early sensory processing (the P1 and N1 components) were identical for seen and unseen stimuli but quickly diverged around 270 ms, suggesting that stimuli only become visible when a sustained wave of activation spreads through a distributed network of cortical association areas (Vogel et al. 1998; Sergent et al. 2005).

More generally, the requirement for sustained discharge might account for why fast, reflex responses of the kind mediated by, say, the spinal cord, do not seem to contribute to consciousness. Fast, reflex-like responses also take place in the cerebral cortex. For example, the action-oriented dorsal visual stream rapidly adjusts movements that remain outside of consciousness (Goodale & Milner 2005). Perhaps these reflex-like adjustments to fast-changing aspects of the environment that must be tracked online are incompatible with the development of sustained discharge patterns. By contrast, such sustained patterns may be necessary for the ventral stream to build a stable representation of a visual scene. By the same token, if the ventral stream could be forced to behave in a reflex-like manner, it should cease to be part of the NCC. Indeed, this can be achieved by pushing the ventral system to perform ultra-rapid categorizations such as deciding whether a natural image contains an animal or not (Thorpe et al. 1996; Bacon-Mace et al. 2005; Kirchner & Thorpe 2006). In such cases, a sweep of activity travels from the retina through several stages of feedforward connections along the hierarchy of ventral visual areas, until it elicits an appropriate categorization response. This process takes as little as 150 ms, which leaves only about 10 ms of processing per stage. Thus, only a few spikes can be fired before the next stage produces its output, yet they are sufficient to specify selective responses for orientation, motion, depth, color, shape, and even animals, faces, or places conveying most of the relevant information about the stimulus (Hung et al. 2005). While this fast feedforward sweep within the ventral system is sufficient for the near-automatic categorization of stimuli and a behavioral response, it seems insufficient to generate a conscious percept (VanRullen & Koch 2003). For example, if another image (the mask) is flashed soon after the target image, subjects are still able to categorize the target, though they may deny having seen it consciously. Thus, consciousness would seem to require that neural activity in appropriate brain structures lasts for a minimum amount of time, perhaps as much as is needed to guarantee interactions among multiple areas.

On the other hand, other data would seem to suggest that it may actually be the phasic, onset, or offset discharge of neurons that correlates with experience. The most stringent data come again from studies of visual masking (for a review see Macknik 2006). To be effective, masking stimuli must either precede (forward masking) or follow (backward masking) target stimuli at appropriate time intervals and usually need to be spatially contiguous. Macknik, Martinez-Conde, and collaborators showed, using a combination of psychophysics, unit recordings in animals, and neuroimaging in humans, that for simple, unattended target stimuli, masking stimuli suppress visibility if their "spatiotemporal edges" overlap with the spatiotemporal edges of the targets, that is, if they begin or end when target stimuli begin or end, in space and time. They confirmed that such spatiotemporal edges correspond to transient bursts of spikes in primary visual cortex. If these bursts are inhibited, for example if the offset discharge elicited by the target stimulus is obliterated by the onset of the mask, the target becomes invisible. Most likely, these spatiotemporal edges of increased firing are both generated (target stimuli) and suppressed (masking stimuli) by mechanisms of lateral inhibition, which are ubiquitous in sensory systems (Macknik 2006).

Additional evidence for the importance of phasic, transient activation of neurons in determining the visibility of stimuli comes from studies of microsaccades—the small, involuntary movements that our eyes make continually (Martinez-Conde et al. 2004). If microsaccades are counteracted by image stabilization on the retina, stationary objects fade and become completely invisible. In a recent study (Martinez-Conde et al. 2006), subjects were asked to fixate a central dot (which tends to reduce microsaccades) while attending to a surrounding circle. Soon, the circle fades and merges into the background (the Troxler illusion). It was found that before a fading period, the probability, rate, and magnitude of microsaccades decreased. Before transitions toward visibility, the probability, rate, and magnitude of microsaccades increased, compatible with the hypothesis that microsaccades are indeed necessary for visibility. Importantly, in macaque monkeys, when an optimally oriented line was centered over the receptive field of cells in V1, the cells' activity increased after microsaccades and tended to emit bursts

(Martinez-Conde et al. 2002), suggesting again that phasic activity may be crucial for visibility.

One should remember, however, that the importance of phasic discharges for stimulus awareness has only been demonstrated for early visual cortex; but, as we saw above, the NCC are more likely to lie elsewhere. Psychophysically, masking is similarly effective when masking stimuli are presented monoptically (through the same eye as the target) and dichoptically (through the other eye). The analysis of fMRI data in humans shows that a correlate of monoptic visual masking can be found in all retinotopic visual areas, whereas dichoptic masking is only seen in retinotopic areas downstream of V2 within the occipital lobe (Tse et al. 2005), suggesting an anatomical lower bound for the NCC. Thus, it could be that phasic onset and offset discharges are important not in and of themselves, but because they are particularly effective in activating downstream areas that directly support the NCC. In these downstream areas, perhaps, the NCC may actually require sustained firing. Indeed, the duration of the activation of face-selective neurons in IT is strongly correlated with the visibility of masked faces (Rolls et al. 1999).

Reentrant versus Feedforward Activity

Another possibility is that it is not so much sustained firing that triggers the awareness of a stimulus, but rather the occurrence of a "reentrant" wave of activity (also described as recurrent, recursive, or reverberant) from higher to lower cortical areas. In this view, when a stimulus evokes a feedforward sweep of activity, it is not seen consciously, but it becomes so when the feedforward sweep is joined by a reentrant sweep (Lamme & Roelfsema 2000). This logic could apply both to early sensory areas such as V1 and to higher areas such as IT. For example, when face neurons in the fusiform face area are first activated, we would not see a face consciously, although we could turn our eyes toward it or press a button to indicate our unconscious categorization as a face. However, when face-selective neurons receive a backward volley from some higher area, for example frontal cortex, the face would become visible.

This view is based on several considerations. An important one, though rarely confessed, is that a mere sequence of feedforward processing steps seems far too "straightforward" and mechanical to offer a substrate for subjective experience. Reentrant processes, by "closing the loop" between past and present activity, or between predicted and actual versions of the input, would seem to provide a more fertile substrate for giving rise to reverberations (Lorente de Nó 1938), generating emergent properties through cell assemblies (Hebb 1949), implementing hypothesis testing through resonances (Grossberg 1999), linking present with past (Edelman & Mountcastle 1978; Edelman 1989), and subject with object (Damasio 1999).

A more concrete reason why reentrant activity is an attractive candidate for the NCC is that it travels through back connections, of which the cerebral cortex is extraordinarily rich (Felleman & Van Essen 1991). In primates, feedforward connections originate mainly in supragranular layers and terminate in layer 4. Feedback connections instead originate in both superficial and deep layers and usually terminate outside of layer 4. The sheer abundance of back connections in sensory regions suggests that they ought to serve some important purpose, and giving rise to a conscious percept might just fit the bill. However, back connections and associated reentrant volleys are just as numerous between V1 and visual thalamus, which is usually denied any direct contribution to awareness. Also, there does not seem to be any lack of back connections within the dorsal stream. It should be emphasized that the strength and termination pattern of back connections seem more suited to a modulatory/synchronizing role than to driving their target neurons. For example, the focal inactivation of area 18 can slightly increase or decrease discharge rates of units in area 17, but it does not change their feature selectivity for location and orientation (Martinez-Conde et al. 1999). Also, the numerosity of backward connections is a natural consequence of the hierarchical organization of feedforward ones. For instance, cells in the LGN are not oriented, while cells in area 17 are. To be unbiased, feedback to any one LGN cell should come from area 17 cells of all orientations, which requires many connections; on the other hand, since at any given time only area 17 cells corresponding to a given orientation would be active, feedback effects would not be strong. If they were, properties of area 17 cells, such as orientation selectivity, would be transferred upon LGN cells, which they are not (to a first approximation). Backward signals certainly play a role in sensory function: for instance, they can mediate some extraclassical receptive field effects, provide a natural substrate for both attentional modulation and imagery, and can perhaps dynamically route feedforward processing according to prior expectations. But are backward signals really critical for consciousness?

The most intriguing data in support of a role for reentrant activity in conscious perception have come from neurophysiological experiments. In awake monkeys trained to signal whether or not they see a salient figure on a background, the early, feedforward response of V1 neurons was the same, no matter whether or not the monkey saw the figure (Super et al. 2001). However, a later response component was suppressed when the monkey did not see the figure. Light anesthesia also eliminated this later component without affecting the initial response. Late components are thought to reflect reentrant volleys from higher areas, although other studies have disputed this claim (Rossi et al. 2001). The late response component crucial for the visibility of stimuli under backward masking might also be due to a reentrant volley (Lamme & Roelfsema 2000). In this case the timing of maximal backward masking should be independent of target duration, since it would be determined exclusively by the time needed for the early component to travel to higher areas and return to primary visual cortex. Instead, the timing of maximal masking depends on the timing of target offset, suggesting that the component that is obliterated is a feedforward offset discharge, not a reentrant one (Macknik 2006). Moreover, the late component can be dissociated from a behavioral response simply by raising the decision criterion (Super et al. 2001), and it can occur in the absence of report during change and inattentional blindness (Scholte et al. 2006). Perhaps in such cases subjective experience is present but, due to an insufficient involvement of frontal areas, it cannot be reported (Block 2005; Tsuchiya & Koch 2005; Lamme 2006). But then, by the same token, why should we rule out subjective experience during the feedforward sweep?

Another main source of evidence for a role of reentrant volleys in consciousness comes from experiments using TMS. In an early experiment, Pascual-Leone and Walsh applied TMS to V5 to elicit large, moving phosphenes (Pascual-Leone & Walsh 2001). They then applied another, subthreshold TMS pulse to a corresponding location in V1. When TMS to V1 was delivered after TMS to V5 (+5 to +45 ms), subjects often did not see the V5 phosphene, and when they saw one, it was not moving. Their interpretation was that disruption of activity in V1 at the time of arrival of a reentrant volley from V5 interferes with the experience of attributes encoded by V5. In a subsequent study (Silvanto et al. 2005), it was shown that, when a subthreshold pulse was applied over V5, followed 10 − 40 ms later by a suprathreshold pulse over V1, subjects reported a V5-like phosphene (large and moving), rather than a V1 phosphene (small and stationary). Their interpretation was that activity in V5 that, on its own, is insufficient to induce a moving percept can produce such a percept if the level of induced activity in V1 is high enough.

In another study (Boyer et al. 2005), subjects where shown either an oriented bar or a colored patch— stimuli that are processed in visual cortex. If, around 100 ms later, a TMS pulse was applied to V1, the stimulus became perceptually invisible, although on forced choice subjects could still discriminate orientation or color. This result indicates that, without any overt participation of V1, stimuli can reach extrastriate areas without eliciting a conscious percept, just as in blindsight patients. It also suggests that, since the forward sweep reaches V1 after just 30 or 40 ms, the TMS pulse may abolish the awareness of the stimulus not so much by blocking feedforward transmission as by interfering with the backward volley (see also Ro et al. 2003). On the other hand, it cannot be ruled out that the TMS pulse may act instead by triggering a cortical–thalamo–cortical volley that interferes with the offset discharge triggered by the stimulus, as may indeed be the case in backward masking.

Yet another study, this time using fMRI, examined the neural correlates of brightness (perceptual lightness) using backward masking. The psychometric visibility function was not correlated with the stimulated portion of V1, but with downstream visual regions, including fusiform cortex, parietal–functional areas, and with the sectors of V1 responding to the unstimulated surround (Haynes et al. 2005). Remarkably, visibility was also correlated with the amount of coupling (effective connectivity) between fusiform cortex and the portion of V1 that responded to the surround. Once again, this result could be explained by the activation of reentrant connections, though fMRI cannot distinguish between forward and backward influences.

Synchronization and Oscillations

Another influential idea is that consciousness may require the synchronization, at a fine temporal scale, of large populations of neurons distributed over many cortical areas, in particular via rhythmic discharges in the gamma range (30–70 Hz and beyond) (Crick & Koch 1990). The emphasis on synchrony ties in well with the common assumption that consciousness requires the "binding" together of a multitude of attributes within a single experience, as when we see a rich visual scene containing multiple objects and attributes that is nevertheless perceived as a unified whole (Singer 1999). According to this view, the NCC of such an experience would include two aspects: first, the underlying activation pattern (groups of neurons that have increased their firing rates) would be widely distributed across different areas of the cerebral cortex, each specialized in signaling a different object or attribute within the scene; and second, the firing of these activated neurons would be synchronized on a fast time scale to signal their binding into a single percept. In this respect, synchrony seems ideally suited to signal relatedness: for example, in the presence of a red square, some neurons would respond to the presence of a square, while others would respond to the presence of the color red. If they synchronize at a fast time scale, they would indicate to other groups of neurons that there is a red square, "binding" the two features together (Tononi et al. 1992). By contrast, signaling relatedness by increased firing rates alone would be more cumbersome and probably slower (Singer 1999). Also, fine-temporal-scale synchrony has the welcome property of disambiguating among multiple objects—if a green cross were present simultaneously with the red square, cross and green neurons would also be active, but false conjunctions would be avoided by precise phase locking (Tononi et al. 1992). Moreover, computational models predict that, for the same level of firing, synchronous input is more effective on target neurons than asynchronous input (Abeles 1991; Tononi et al. 1992), and indeed synchrony makes a difference to the outputs to the rest of the brain (Brecht et al. 1999; Schoffelen et al. 2005). Finally, large-scale models predict that synchrony in the gamma range occurs due to the reciprocal connectivity and loops within the thalamocortical system (Lumer et al. 1997a, b), and indeed phase alignment between distant groups of neurons in the gamma range anticipates by a few ms an increase in gamma-band power (Womelsdorf et al. 2007). In this respect, oscillatory activity, even when subthreshold, could further facilitate synchronous interactions by biasing neurons to discharge within the same time frame (Engel et al. 2001).

Experimental evidence concerning the role of synchrony/synchronous oscillations in perceptual operations was initially obtained in primary visual areas of anesthetized animals (for a review see Singer & Gray 1995). For example, in primary visual cortex, neurons have been found that respond to a coherent object by synchronizing their firing in the gamma range. Stimulus-specific, gamma-range synchronization is greatly facilitated when the EEG is activated by stimulating the mesencephalic reticular formation (Munk et al. 1996; Herculano-Houzel et al. 1999). It is similarly facilitated by attention (Roelfsema et al. 1997) and by increases in a dominant stimulus under binocular rivalry even though firing rates may not change (Fries et al. 1997, 2001).

Other evidence has come from EEG studies of phase locking in humans. A recent study compared the neural correlates of words that were consciously perceived with those of masked words that had been processed and semantically decoded but had remained unconscious (Melloni et al. 2007). The results showed that consciously perceived words induced theta oscillations in multiple cortical regions until the test stimulus was presented and a decision reached, while a burst of gamma activity occurred over central and frontal leads just prior to and during the presentation of the test stimulus. Importantly, the earliest event distinguishing conscious and unconscious processing was not visible in the power changes of oscillations but in their phase locking. About 180 ms after presentation of stimuli that were consciously perceived, induced gamma oscillations recorded from a large number of regions exhibited precise phase locking both within and across hemispheres for around 100 ms. These results have been interpreted to indicate that a transient event of gamma synchrony resets multiple parallel processes to a common time frame. The global theta rhythm that follows after this trigger event could provide the time frame for allowing a global integration of information provided by sensory inputs and internal sources. Or perhaps beta–gamma synchrony could enable the integration of activity patterns within local cortical areas, while theta synchrony would permit the integration of more globally distributed patterns: the more global the representation, the longer the time scale for the integration of distributed information.

It would be premature to conclude, however, that synchrony in one or another frequency band is necessarily a marker of NCC. As revealed by an increasing number of EEG, MEG, electrocorticography, and multiunit recordings, cognitive tasks are associated with complex modes of synchronous coupling among populations of neurons that shift rapidly both within and across different frequency bands, within and between areas, and in relation to the timing of the task (Womelsdorf et al. 2007). It would rather seem that, given the brain's remarkable connectivity, synchrony is an inevitable accompaniment of neural activity, and that it is bound to change just as activity patterns change, depending on the precise experimental conditions. Whether a particular kind of synchrony, for example in the gamma range, is uniquely associated with consciousness is still unclear. For example, high beta and gamma synchrony can be found in virtually every brain region investigated, including some that are unlikely to contribute directly to consciousness. Also, it is not yet clear whether synchrony in the gamma range vanishes during early NREM sleep, during anesthesia, or even during seizures. Human studies are still inconsistent on this point, whereas animal studies show a paradoxical increase in gamma synchrony when rats lose the righting reflex (thought to correspond more or less to the loss of consciousness in humans; see Imas et al. 2005a, b). It would seem that there can be synchrony without consciousness, though perhaps not consciousness without synchrony, at least in mammalian brains.

Finally, there are some difficult conceptual problems in characterizing synchrony as an essential ingredient that unifies perceptual states and thereby makes them conscious. While many experiences do indeed involve several different elements and attributes that are "bound" together into a unified percept, there are many other experiences, equally conscious, that do not seem to require much binding at all: for instance, an experience of pure darkness or of pure blue, or a loud sound that briefly occupies consciousness and has no obvious internal structure, would merely seem to require the strong activation of the relevant neurons, with no need for signaling relatedness to other elements, and thus no need for synchrony. Also, the idea that the NCC of a given conscious experience are given by active neurons bound by synchrony discounts the importance of inactive ones: information specifying that particular unified experience must be conveyed both by which neurons are active and which are not, yet for inactive neurons there does not seem to be anything to bind. On the other hand, if most neurons in the cortex were to become active hypersynchronously, as is the case in generalized seizures, they should result in maximal "binding," but consciousness vanishes rather than become more vivid..

Consciousness from a Theoretical Perspective

Progress in the study of the NCC will hopefully lead to a better understanding of what distinguishes neural structures or processes that are associated with consciousness from those that are not. But even if we come closer to this goal, we still need to understand *why* certain structures and processes have a privileged relationship with subjective experience. For example, why is it that neurons in thalamocortical circuits are essential for conscious experience, whereas cerebellar neurons, despite their huge numbers, are not? And what is wrong with many cortical circuits, including those in V1, that makes them unsuitable to yield subjective experience? Or why is it that consciousness wanes during slow-wave sleep early in the night, despite levels of neural firing in the thalamocortical system that are comparable to those in quiet wakefulness? Other questions are even more difficult to address in the absence of a theory. For example, is consciousness present in animals that have a nervous system considerably different from ours? And what about computerized robots or other artifacts that behave intelligently but are organized in a radically different way from human brains?

Consciousness as Integrated Information

To address these questions, it would seem that we need a theoretical approach that tries to establish, at the fundamental level, what consciousness is, how it can be measured, and what requisites a physical system must satisfy in order to generate it. The *integrated information theory* of consciousness represents such an approach (Tononi 2004b).

According to the theory, the most important property of consciousness is that is extraordinarily *informative*. This is because, whenever you experience a particular conscious state, it rules out a huge number of alternative experiences. Classically, the reduction of uncertainty among a number of alternatives constitutes information. For example, you lie in bed with eyes open and experience pure darkness and silence. This is one of the simplest experiences you might have, one that may not be thought as conveying much information. One should realize, however, that the informativeness of what you just experienced lies not in how complicated it is to describe, but in how many alternatives were ruled out when you experienced it: you could have experienced any one frame from any of innumerable movies, or the smoke and flames of your room burning, or any other possible scene, but you did not—instead, you experienced darkness and silence. This means that when you experienced darkness and silence, whether you think or not of what was ruled out (and you typically don't), you actually gained access to a large amount of information. This point is so simple that its importance has been overlooked.

It is essential to realize, however, that the information associated with the occurrence of a conscious state is *integrated* information. When you experience a particular conscious state, that conscious state is an integrated whole—it cannot be subdivided into components that are experienced independently. For example, the conscious experience of the particular phrase you are reading now cannot be experienced as subdivided into, say, the conscious experience of how the words look independently of the conscious experience of how they sound in your mind. Similarly, you cannot experience visual shapes independently of their color, or perceive the left half of the visual field of view independently of the right half.

Based on these and other considerations, the theory claims that *the level of consciousness of a physical system is related to the repertoire of causal states (information) available to the system as a whole (integration)*. That is, whenever a system enters a particular state though causal interactions among its elements, it is conscious in proportion to how many system states it has thereby ruled out, provided these are states of the system as a whole, not decomposable into states of causally independent parts. More precisely, the theory introduces a measure of integrated information called Φ, quantifying the reduction of uncertainty (i.e., the information) that is generated when a system enters a particular state through causal interactions among its parts, above and beyond the information that is generated independently within the parts themselves (hence integrated information). The parts should be chosen in such a way that they can account for as much nonintegrated (independent) information as possible.

If a system has a positive value of Φ (and it is not included within a larger subset having higher Φ) it is called a *complex*. For a complex, and only for a complex, it is appropriate to say that when it enters a particular state, it generates an amount of integrated information corresponding to Φ. Since integrated information can only be generated *within* a complex and not outside its boundaries, consciousness is necessarily subjective, private, and related to a single point of view or perspective (Tononi & Edelman 1998). Some properties of complexes are worth pointing out. A given physical system, such as a brain, is likely to contain more than one complex, many small ones with low Φ values, and perhaps a few large ones. We suspect that in the brain there is at any given time a complex of comparatively much higher Φ, which we call the *main complex*. Also, a complex can be causally connected to elements that are not part of it through *ports-in* and *ports-out*. In that case, elements that are part of the complex contribute to its conscious experience, while elements that are not part of it do not, even though they may be connected to it and exchange information with it through ports-in and ports-out. One should also note that the Φ value of a complex is dependent on both spatial and temporal scales that determine what counts as a state of the underlying system. In general, the relevant spatial and temporal scales are those that jointly maximize Φ (Tononi 2004b). In the case of the brain, the spatial elements and time scales that maximize Φ may be local collections of neurons such as minicolumns and periods of time comprised between tens and hundreds of milliseconds, respectively, though at this stage it is difficult to adjudicate between minicolumns and individual neurons.

Accounting for Neurobiological Observations

Measuring Φ and finding complexes is not easy for realistic systems, but it can be done for simple networks that bear some structural resemblance to different parts of the brain (Tononi 2004b, 2005). For example, by using computer simulations, it is possible to show that high Φ requires networks that conjoin functional specialization (due to its specialized connectivity, each element has a unique functional role within the network) with functional integration (there are many pathways for interactions among the elements.). In very rough terms, this kind of architecture is characteristic of the mammalian thalamo-cortical system: different parts of the cerebral cortex are specialized for different functions, yet a vast network of connections allows these parts to interact profusely. Indeed, the thalamo-cortical system is precisely the part of the brain which cannot be severely impaired without loss of consciousness.

Conversely, Φ is low for systems that are made up of small, quasi-independent modules. This may be why the cerebellum, despite its large number of neurons, does not contribute much to consciousness: its synaptic organization is such that individual patches of cerebellar cortex tend to be activated independently of one another, with little interaction between distant patches (Cohen & Yarom 1998; Bower 2002).

Computer simulations also show that units along multiple, segregated incoming or outgoing pathways are not incorporated within the repertoire of the main complex. This may be why neural activity in afferent pathways (perhaps as far as V1), though crucial for triggering this or that conscious experience, does not contribute directly to conscious experience; nor does activity in efferent pathways (perhaps starting with primary motor cortex), though it is crucial for reporting each different experience.

The addition of many parallel cycles also generally does not change the composition of the main complex, although Φ values can be altered. Instead, cortical and subcortical cycles or loops implement specialized subroutines that are capable of influencing the states of the main thalamocortical complex without joining it. Such informationally insulated cortico-subcortical loops could constitute the neural substrates for many unconscious processes that can affect and be affected by conscious experience (Baars 1988; Tononi 2004a, b), such as those that enable object recognition, language parsing, or translating our vague intentions into the right words. At this stage, however, it is hard to say precisely which cortical circuits may be informationally insulated. Are primary sensory cortices organized like massive afferent pathways to a main complex "higher up" in the cortical hierarchy? Is much of prefrontal cortex organized like a massive efferent pathway? Do certain cortical areas, such as those belonging to the dorsal visual stream, remain partly segregated from the main complex? Do interactions *within* a cortico-thalamic minicolumn qualify as intrinsic miniloops that support the main complex without being part of it? Unfortunately, answering these questions and properly testing the predictions of the theory require a much better understanding of cortical neuroanatomy than is presently available (Ascoli 1999).

Other simulations show that the effects of cortical disconnections are readily captured in terms of integrated information (Tononi 2004b): a "callosal" cut produces, out of large complex corresponding to the connected thalamocortical system, two separate complexes, in line with many studies of split-brain patients (Gazzaniga 1995). However, because there is great redundancy between the two hemispheres, their Φ value is not greatly reduced compared to when they formed a single complex. Functional disconnections may also lead to a restriction of the neural substrate of consciousness, as is seen in neurological neglect phenomena, in psychiatric conversion and dissociative disorders, and possibly during dreaming and hypnosis. It is also likely that certain attentional phenomena may correspond to changes in the composition of the main complex underlying consciousness. Phenomena such as the attentional blink, where a fixed sensory input may at times make it to consciousness and at times not, may also be due to changes in functional connectivity: access to the main thalamocortical complex may be enabled or not based on dynamics intrinsic to the complex (Dehaene et al. 2003). Phenomena such as binocular rivalry may also be related, at least in part, to dynamic changes in the composition of the main thalamocortical complex caused by transient changes in functional connectivity (Lumer 1998). Computer simulations confirm that functional disconnection can reduce the size of a complex and reduce its capacity to integrate information (Tononi 2004b). While it is not easy to determine, at present, whether a particular group of neurons is excluded from the main complex because of hard-wired anatomical constraints, or is transiently disconnected due to functional changes, the set of elements underlying consciousness is not static, but form a *dynamic complex* or *dynamic core* (Tononi & Edelman 1998).

From the perspective of integrated information, a reduction of consciousness during early sleep would be consistent with the ensuing bistability of cortical circuits. As we have seen, studies using TMS in conjunction with high-density EEG show that early NREM sleep is associated either with a breakdown of the effective connectivity among cortical areas, and thereby with a loss of integration (Massimini et al. 2005, 2007), or with a stereotypical global response suggestive of a loss of repertoire and thus of information (Massimini et al. 2007). Computer simulations also indicate that the capacity to integrate information is reduced if neural activity is extremely high and near synchronous, due to a dramatic decrease in the available degrees of freedom (Balduzzi and Tononi, in preparation). This reduction in degrees of freedom could be the reason why consciousness is reduced or eliminated in absence seizure and other conditions characterized by hyper-synchronous neural activity.

Finally, we have seen that consciousness not only requires a neural substrate with appropriate anatomical structure and appropriate physiological parameters, it also needs time (Bachmann 2000). The theory predicts that the time requirement for the generation of conscious experience in the brain emerge directly from the time requirements for the build-up of an integrated repertoire among the elements of the thalamocortical main complex (Balduzzi and Tononi II, in preparation). To give an obvious example, if one were to perturb half of the elements of the main complex for less than a millisecond, no perturbations would produce any effect on the other half within this time window, and the repertoire measured by Φ would be equal to zero. After say 100 ms, however, there is enough time for differential effects to be manifested, and Φ should grow.

Some Implications

The examples discussed above show that the integrated information theory can begin to account, in a coherent manner, for several puzzling facts about consciousness and the brain. This goes beyond proposing a provisional list of candidate brain areas for the NCC and of seemingly important neural ingredients, such as synchronization, sustained or phasic firing, reentrant activity, or widespread "broadcasting," without a principled explanation of why they would be important or whether they would be always necessary. Naturally, the integrated information theory converges with other neurobiological frameworks (e.g., Crick & Koch 2003; Edelman 1989; Dehaene et al. 2006) and cognitive theories (Baars 1988) on certain key facts: that our own consciousness is generated by distributed thalamocortical networks, that reentrant interactions among multiple cortical regions are important, that the mechanisms of consciousness and attention overlap but are not the same, and that there are many "unconscious" neural systems.

The integrated information theory avoids the pitfalls associated with assigning conscious qualities to individual brain elements. For example, it is sometimes assumed loosely that the firing of specific thalamocortical elements (e.g., those for red) conveys some specific information (e.g., that there is something red) and that such information becomes conscious either as such, or perhaps if it is disseminated widely. However, a given thalamocortical element has no information about whether what made it fire was a particular color rather than a shape, a visual stimulus rather than a sound, a sensory stimulus rather than a thought. All it knows is whether it fired or not, just as each receiving element only knows whether it received an input or not. Thus, the information specifying "red" cannot possibly be in the message conveyed by the firing of any neural element, whether it is located in a high-order cortical area or whether it is broadcasting widely. According to the theory, that information resides instead in the reduction of uncertainty occurring when a whole complex enters one out of a large number of available states—the complex, and not its elements, is the locus of consciousness. Indeed, within a complex, both active and inactive neurons count, just as the sound of an orchestra is specified both by the instruments that are playing and by those that are silent. Though it would be too long to address the issue here, the theory proposes that, just as the quantity of consciousness is given by the amount of integrated information generated within a complex, the particular quality of consciousness—including the redness of red—is given by the specific informational relationships among the elements of the complex (Tononi 2004b).

The integrated information theory also predicts that consciousness depends exclusively on the ability of a system to integrate information, whether or not it has a strong sense of self, language, emotion, or is immersed in an environment, contrary to some common intuitions. Nevertheless, the theory recognizes that these same factors are important historically because they favor the development of neural circuits forming a main complex of high Φ. For example, integrated information grows as that system incorporates statistical regularities from its environment and learns (Tononi et al. 1996). In this sense, the emergence of consciousness in biological systems is predicated on a long evolutionary history, on individual development, and on experience-dependent change in neural connectivity.

Finally, the integrated information theory says that the presence and extent of consciousness can be determined, in principle, also in cases in which we have no verbal report, such as in infants or animals, or in neurological conditions such as minimally conscious states, akinetic mutism, psychomotor seizures, and sleepwalking. In practice, of course, measuring Φ accurately in such systems will not be easy, but approximations and informed guesses are certainly conceivable. The theory also implies that consciousness is not an all-or-none property but is graded: specifically, it increases in proportion to a system's repertoire of available states. In fact, any physical system with some capacity for integrated information would have some degree of experience, irrespective of the stuff of which it is made, and independent of its ability to report.

At present, the validity of this theoretical framework and the plausibility of its implications rest on its ability to account, in a coherent manner, for some basic phenomenological observations and for some elementary but puzzling facts about consciousness and the brain. Experimental developments, such as ways to concurrently stimulate and record the activity of broad regions of the brain, should permit stringent tests of some of the theory's predictions. Especially important will be paradigms to test the counterintuitive prediction that experience can change even though the underlying neural activity stays the same: if one inactivates neurons that are silent, the current firing pattern would not change, but the repertoire of available neural states would shrink and consciousness should be diminished.

Conclusions

As this chapter demonstrates, the study of consciousness has entered an intense experimental phase, a refreshing change from the previous millennia when the only approach available to students of the mind was philosophical speculation. The two dominant experimental paradigms are the study of brain differences between the awake, conscious state and various degrees of unconsciousness, such as deep sleep, anesthesia, or coma, and the study of the brain basis of the changing content of consciousness, as in when one visual stimulus is consciously perceived but then becomes invisible and vice versa.

In order to make progress, it will be imperative to record from a large number of neurons simultaneously at many locations throughout the cortico-thalamic system and related satellites in behaving subjects. Such experiments cannot, of course, be done in humans. Progress in understanding the circuitry of consciousness therefore demands a battery of behaviors (akin to but different from the well-known Turing test for intelligence) that the subject—a newborn infant, immobilized patient, or nonhuman animal—has to pass before considering him, her, or it to possess some measure of conscious experience. This is not an insurmountable step for mammals such as the monkey or the mouse that share many behaviors and brain structures with humans. For example, one particular mouse model of contingency awareness (Han et al. 2003) is based on the differential requirement for awareness of trace versus delay associative eyeblink conditioning in humans (Clark & Squire).

The growing ability of neuroscientists to manipulate in a reversible, transient, deliberate, and delicate manner identified populations of neurons using methods from molecular biology combined with optical stimulation (Aravanis et al. 2007; Han & Boyden 2007; Zhang et al. 2007) enables the intrepid neuroengineer to move from correlation—observing that a particular conscious state is associated with some neural or hemodynamic activity—to causation. For example, rather than just noting that motion perception is associated with an elevated firing rate in projection neurons in cortical area MT, we will be able to perturb the system by inactivating genetically distinct subpopulations of cells in a highly targeted manner. Exploiting these increasingly powerful tools depends on the simultaneous development of appropriate behavioral assays and model organisms amenable to large-scale genomic analysis and manipulation, in particularly in mice (Lein et al. 2007) and rats.

Finally, as we have argued here, it is imperative to complement experimental studies with the development of full-blown theories that try to capture the essential properties of consciousness; suggest ways to measure them; can be validated through counterintuitive experimental tests; permit the extrapolation to pathological conditions, animals, and even artifacts; and begin to offer a framework to understand how and why the different modalities of consciousness map onto different brain architectures and processes. Only the combination of fine-grained neuronal analysis in mice, rats, and monkeys; ever more sensitive psychophysical and brain imaging techniques in patients and healthy individuals; and the development of a robust theoretical framework can lend hope to the belief that human ingenuity can, ultimately, understand in a rational manner one of the central mysteries of life.

Conflict of Interest

The authors declare no conflicts of interest.

References

Abeles, M. (1991). *Corticonics Neural circuits of the cerebral cortex*. Cambridge, UK, New York: Cambridge University Press.

Alkire, M. T., & Miller, J. (2005). General anesthesia and the neural correlates of consciousness. *Prog. Brain Res., 150*, 229–244.

Alkire, M. T., Haier, R. J., & Fallon, J. H. (2000). Toward a unified theory of narcosis: Brain imaging evidence for a thalamocortical switch as the neurophysiologic basis of anesthetic-induced unconsciousness. *Conscious Cogn., 9*, 370–386.

Alkire, M. T., McReynolds, J. R., Hahn, E. L., & Trivedi, A. N. (2007). Thalamic microinjection of nicotine reverses sevoflurane-induced loss of righting reflex in the rat. *Anesthesiology, 107*, 264–272.

Amedi, A., Malach, R., & Pascual-Leone, A. (2005). Negative BOLD differentiates visual imagery and perception. *Neuron, 48*, 859–872.

Aravanis, A. M., Wang, L. P., Zhang, F., Meltzer, L. A., Mogri, M. Z., et al. (2007). An optical neural interface: In vivo control of rodent motor cortex with integrated fiberoptic and optogenetic technology. *J. Neural Eng., 4*, S143–156.

Ascoli, G. A. (1999). Progress and perspectives in computational neuroanatomy. *Anat. Rec., 257*, 195–207.

Baars, B. J. (1988). *A cognitive theory of consciousness*. New York: Cambridge University Press.

Baars, B. J. (2005). Global workspace theory of consciousness: Toward a cognitive neuroscience of human experience. *Prog. Brain Res., 150*, 45–53.

Bachmann, T. (2000). *Microgenetic approach to the conscious mind*. Amsterdam and Philadelphia: John Benjamins Pub. Co.

Bacon-Mace, N., Mace, M. J., Fabre-Thorpe, M., & Thorpe, S. J. (2005). The time course of visual processing: Backward masking and natural scene categorisation. *Vision Res., 45*, 1459–1469.

Bahrami, B., Lavie, N., & Rees, G. (2007). Attentional load modulates responses of human primary visual cortex to invisible stimuli. *Curr. Biol., 17*, 509–513.

Barcelo, F., Suwazono, S., & Knight, R. T. (2000). Prefrontal modulation of visual processing in humans. *Nat. Neurosci., 3*, 399–403.

Bauby, J. -D. (1997). *The diving-bell and the butterfly: A memoir of life in death*. New York: Alfred A. Knopf.

Blake, R., & Logothetis, N. K. (2002). Visual competition. *Nat. Rev. Neurosci., 3*, 13–21.

Block, N. (2005). Two neural correlates of consciousness. *Trends Cogn. Sci., 9*, 46–52.

Blumenfeld, H. (2005). Consciousness and epilepsy: Why are patients with absence seizures absent? *Prog. Brain Res., 150*, 271–286.

Blumenfeld, H., & Taylor, J. (2003). Why do seizures cause loss of consciousness? *Neuroscientist, 9*, 301–310.

Blumenfeld, H., McNally, K. A., Vanderhill, S. D., Paige, A. L., Chung, R., et al. (2004). Positive and negative network correlations in temporal lobe epilepsy. *Cereb. Cortex, 14*, 892–902.

Blumenfeld, H., Westerveld, M., Ostroff, R. B., Vanderhill, S. D., Freeman, J., et al. (2003). Selective frontal, parietal, and temporal networks in generalized seizures. *Neuroimage, 19*, 1556–1566.

Bower, J. M. (2002). The organization of cerebellar cortical circuitry revisited: implications for function. *Ann. N. Y. Acad. Sci., 978*, 135–155.

Boyer, J. L., Harrison, S., & Ro, T. (2005). Unconscious processing of orientation and color without primary visual cortex. *Proc. Natl. Acad. Sci. U.S.A., 102*, 16875–16879.

Braun, J., & Sagi, D. (1990). Vision outside the focus of attention. *Percept. Psychophys., 48*, 45–58.

Braun, J., & Julesz, B. (1998). Withdrawing attention at little or no cost: Detection and discrimination tasks. *Percept. Psychophys.*, *60*, 1–23.

Braun, J., Koch, C., & Davis, J. (Eds.). (2001). *Visual attention and cortical circuits*. Cambridge, MA: MIT Press.

Brecht, M., Singer, W., & Engel, A. K. (1999). Patterns of synchronization in the superior colliculus of anesthetized cats. *J. Neurosci.*, *19*, 3567–3579.

Buchel, C., Price, C., Frackowiak, R. S., & Friston, K. (1998). Different activation patterns in the visual cortex of late and congenitally blind subjects. *Brain*, *121*(Pt 3), 409–419.

Campagna, J. A., Miller, K. W., & Forman, S. A. (2003). Mechanisms of actions of inhaled anesthetics. *N. Engl. J. Med.*, *348*, 2110–2124.

Chalmers, D. (2000). What is a neural correlate of consciousness? In T. Metzinger (Ed.), *Neural correlates of consciousness: Empirical and conceptual questions* (pp. 17–40). Cambridge, MA: MIT Press.

Chun, M., & Wolfe, J. (2000). Visual attention. In E. B. Goldstein (Ed.), *Blackwell's handbook of perception* (pp. 272–310). Oxford, UK: Blackwell.

Clark, R. E., & Squire, L. R. (1998). Classical conditioning and brain systems: the role of awareness. *Science*, *280*, 77–81.

Cohen, D., & Yarom, Y. (1998). Patches of synchronized activity in the cerebellar cortex evoked by mossy-fiber stimulation: Questioning the role of parallel fibers. *Proc. Natl. Acad. Sci. U.S.A.*, *95*, 15032–15036.

Crick, F., & Koch, C. (1990). Some reflections on visual awareness. *Cold Spring Harbor Symposia on Quantitative Biology*, *55*, 953–962.

Crick, F., & Koch, C. (1995). Are we aware of neural activity in primary visual cortex? *Nature*, *375*, 121–123.

Crick, F., & Koch, C. (1998). Consciousness and neuroscience. *Cereb. Cortex*, *8*, 97–107.

Crick, F., & Koch, C. (2003). A framework for consciousness. *Nat. Neurosci.*, *6*, 119–126.

Damasio, A. R. (1999). *The feeling of what happens: Body and emotion in the making of consciousness* (1st ed.). New York: Harcourt Brace.

Dehaene, S., Sergent, C., & Changeux, J. P. (2003). A neuronal network model linking subjective reports and objective physiological data during conscious perception. *Proc. Natl. Acad. Sci. U.S.A.*, *100*, 8520–8525.

Dehaene, S., Changeux, J. P., Naccache, L., Sackur, J., & Sergent, C. (2006). Conscious, preconscious, and subliminal processing: A testable taxonomy. *Trends Cogn. Sci.*, *10*, 204–211.

Desimone, R., & Duncan, J. (1995). Neural mechanisms of selective visual attention. *Annual Review of Neuroscience*, *18*, 193–222.

Destexhe, A., Hughes, S. W., Rudolph, M., & Crunelli, V. (2007). Are corticothalamic "up" states fragments of wakefulness? *Trends Neurosci.*, *30*, 334–342.

Edelman, G. M. (1989). *The remembered present: A biological theory of consciousness*. New York: BasicBooks.

Edelman, G. M., & Mountcastle, V. B. (1978). *The mindful brain: Cortical organization and the group-selective theory of higher brain function*. Cambridge, MA: MIT Press.

Engel, A. K., Fries, P., & Singer, W. (2001). Dynamic predictions: oscillations and synchrony in top-down processing. *Nat. Rev. Neurosci.*, *2*, 704–716.

Felleman, D. J., & Van Essen, D. C. (1991). Distributed hierarchical processing in the primate cerebral cortex. *Cereb. Cortex*, *1*, 1–47.

Franks, N. P. (2006). Molecular targets underlying general anaesthesia. *Br. J. Pharmacol.*, *147*(Suppl 1), S72–81.

Fries, P., Roelfsema, P. R., Engel, A. K., Konig, P., & Singer, W. (1997). Synchronization of oscillatory responses in visual cortex correlates with perception in interocular rivalry. *Proc. Natl. Acad. Sci. U.S.A.*, *94*, 12699–12704.

Fries, P., Neuenschwander, S., Engel, A. K., Goebel, R., & Singer, W. (2001). Rapid feature selective neuronal synchronization through correlated latency shifting. *Nat. Neurosci.*, *4*, 194–200.

Gazzaniga, M. S. (1995). Principles of human brain organization derived from split-brain studies. *Neuron*, *14*, 217–228.

Goodale, M., & Milner, A. (2005). *Sight unseen: An exploration of conscious and unconscious vision*. Oxford, UK: Oxford University Press.

Grossberg, S. (1999). The link between brain learning, attention, and consciousness. *Conscious Cogn.*, *8*, 1–44.

Guilleminault, C. (1976). Cataplexy. In C. Guilleminault, W. Dennet, & P. Passouant, (Eds.), *Narcolepsy* (pp. 125–143). New York: Spectrum.

Han, C. J., O'Tuathaigh, C. M., van Trigt, L., Quinn, J. J., Fanselow, M. S., et al. (2003). Trace but not delay fear conditioning requires attention and the anterior cingulate cortex. *Proc. Natl. Acad. Sci. U.S.A.*, *100*, 13087–13092.

Han, X., & Boyden, E. S. (2007). Multiple-color optical activation, silencing, and desynchronization of neural activity, with single-spike temporal resolution. *PLoS ONE*, *2*, e299.

Hardcastle, V. (1997). Attention versus consciousness: A distinction with a difference. *Studies: Bulletin of the Japanese Cognitive Science Society*, *4*, 56–66.

Hasson, U., Nir, Y., Levy, I., Fuhrmann, G., & Malach, R. (2004). Intersubject synchronization of cortical activity during natural vision. *Science*, *303*, 1634–1640.

Haynes, J. D., Driver, J., & Rees, G. (2005). Visibility reflects dynamic changes of effective connectivity between V1 and fusiform cortex. *Neuron*, *46*, 811–821.

He, S., Cavanagh, P., & Intriligator, J. (1996). Attentional resolution and the locus of visual awareness. *Nature*, *383*, 334–337.

Hebb, D. O. (1949). *The organization of behavior: A neuropsychological theory*. New York: Wiley.

Herculano-Houzel, S., Munk, M. H., Neuenschwander, S., & Singer, W. (1999). Precisely synchronized oscillatory firing patterns require electroencephalographic activation. *J. Neurosci.*, *19*, 3992–4010.

Hobson, J. A., & Pace-Schott, E. F. (2002). The cognitive neuroscience of sleep: Neuronal systems, consciousness and learning. *Nat. Rev. Neurosci.*, *3*, 679–693.

Hobson, J. A., Pace-Schott, E. F., & Stickgold, R. (2000). Dreaming and the brain: toward a cognitive neuroscience of conscious states. *Behav. Brain Sci.*, *23*, 793–842; discussion 904–1121.

Hollins, M. (1985). Styles of mental imagery in blind adults. *Neuropsychologia, 23*, 561–566.

Huk, A. C., Ress, D., & Heeger, D. J. (2001). Neuronal basis of the motion aftereffect reconsidered. *Neuron, 32*, 161–172.

Hung, C. P., Kreiman, G., Poggio, T., & DiCarlo, J. J. (2005). Fast readout of object identity from macaque inferior temporal cortex. *Science, 310*, 863–866.

Imas, O. A., Ropella, K. M., Ward, B. D., Wood, J. D., & Hudetz, A. G. (2005a). Volatile anesthetics enhance flash-induced gamma oscillations in rat visual cortex. *Anesthesiology, 102*, 937–947.

Imas, O. A., Ropella, K. M., Ward, B. D., Wood, J. D., & Hudetz, A. G. (2005b). Volatile anesthetics disrupt frontal-posterior recurrent information transfer at gamma frequencies in rat. *Neurosci. Lett., 387*, 145–150.

Iwasaki, S. (1993). Spatial attention and two modes of visual consciousness. *Cognition, 49*, 211–233.

Jiang, Y., Costello, P., Fang, F., Huang, M., & He, S. (2006). A gender- and sexual orientation-dependent spatial attentional effect of invisible images. *Proc. Natl. Acad. Sci. U.S.A., 103*, 17048–17052.

Joliot, M., Ribary, U., & Llinas, R. (1994). Human oscillatory brain activity near 40 Hz coexists with cognitive temporal binding. *Proc. Natl. Acad. Sci. U.S.A., 91*, 11748–11751.

Jones, E. G. (1998). A new view of specific and nonspecific thalamocortical connections. *Adv. Neurol., 77*, 49–71; discussion 72–43.

Kim, C. Y., & Blake, R. (2005). Psychophysical magic: rendering the visible "invisible." *Trends Cogn. Sci., 9*, 381–388.

Kirchner, H., & Thorpe, S. J. (2006). Ultra-rapid object detection with saccadic eye movements: visual processing speed revisited. *Vision Res., 46*, 1762–1776.

Koch, C., & Tsuchiya, N. (2007). Attention and consciousness: Two distinct brain processes. *Trends Cog. Sci. 11*, 16–22.

Kosslyn, S. M., Ganis, G., & Thompson, W. L. (2001). Neural foundations of imagery. *Nat. Rev. Neurosci., 2*, 635–642.

Kreiman, G., Fried, I., & Koch, C. (2002). Single-neuron correlates of subjective vision in the human medial temporal lobe. *Proc. Natl. Acad. Sci. U.S.A., 99*, 8378–8383.

Lamme, V. A. (2003). Why visual attention and awareness are different. *Trends Cogn. Sci., 7*, 12–18.

Lamme, V. A. (2006). Towards a true neural stance on consciousness. *Trends Cogn. Sci., 10*, 494–501.

Lamme, V. A., & Roelfsema, P. R. (2000). The distinct modes of vision offered by feedforward and recurrent processing. *Trends Neurosci., 23*, 571–579.

Langston, J., & Palfreman, J. (1995). *The case of the frozen addicts.* New York: Vintage Books.

Laureys, S., Owen, A. M., & Schiff, N. D. (2004). Brain function in coma, vegetative state, and related disorders. *Lancet Neurol., 3*, 537–546.

Laureys, S., Faymonville, M. E., Luxen, A., Lamy, M., Franck, G., et al. (2000a). Restoration of thalamocortical connectivity after recovery from persistent vegetative state. *Lancet, 355*, 1790–1791.

Laureys, S., Faymonville, M. E., Degueldre, C., Fiore, G. D., Damas, P., et al. (2000b). Auditory processing in the vegetative state. *Brain, 123*(Pt 8), 1589–1601.

Laureys, S., Faymonville, M. E., Peigneux, P., Damas, P., Lambermont, B., et al. (2002). Cortical processing of noxious somatosensory stimuli in the persistent vegetative state. *Neuroimage, 17*, 732–741.

Laureys, S., Pellas, F., Van Eeckhout, P., Ghorbel, S., Schnakers, C., et al. (2005). The locked-in syndrome: What is it like to be conscious but paralyzed and voiceless? *Prog. Brain Res., 150*, 495–511.

Lee, S. H., Blake, R., & Heeger, D. J. (2005). Traveling waves of activity in primary visual cortex during binocular rivalry. *Nat. Neurosci., 8*, 22–23.

Lee, S. H., Blake, R., & Heeger, D. J. (2007). Hierarchy of cortical responses underlying binocular rivalry. *Nat. Neurosci., 10*, 1048–1054.

Lein, E. S., et al. (2007). Genome-wide atlas of gene expression in the adult mouse brain. *Nature, 445*, 168–176.

Leopold, D. A., & Logothetis, N. K. (1996). Activity changes in early visual cortex reflect monkeys' percepts during binocular rivalry. *Nature, 379*, 549–553.

Li, F. F., VanRullen, R., Koch, C., & Perona, P. (2002). Rapid natural scene categorization in the near absence of attention. *Proc. Natl. Acad. Sci. U.S.A., 99*, 9596–9601.

Logothetis, N. K. (1998). Single units and conscious vision. *Philos. Trans. R. Soc. Lond. B Biol. Sci., 353*, 1801–1818.

Lorente de Nó, R. (1938). The cerebral cortex: Architecture, intracortical connections and motor projections. In J. Fulton (Ed.), *Physiology of the nervous system* (pp. 291–339). London: Oxford University Press.

Lumer, E. D. (1998). A neural model of binocular integration and rivalry based on the coordination of action-potential timing in primary visual cortex. *Cereb. Cortex, 8*, 553–561.

Lumer, E. D., Edelman, G. M., & Tononi, G. (1997a). Neural dynamics in a model of the thalamocortical system. 2. The role of neural synchrony tested through perturbations of spike timing. *Cerebral Cortex, 7*, 228–236.

Lumer, E. D., Edelman, G. M., & Tononi, G. (1997b). Neural dynamics in a model of the thalamocortical system. 1. Layers, loops and the emergence of fast synchronous rhythms. *Cerebral Cortex, 7*, 207–227.

Mack, A., & Rock, I. (1998). *Inattentional blindness.* Cambridge, MA: MIT Press.

Macknik, S. L. (2006). Visual masking approaches to visual awareness. *Prog. Brain Res., 155*, 177–215.

Maquet, P., Péters, J., Aerts, J., Delfiore, G., Degueldre, C., et al. (1996). Functional neuroanatomy of human rapid-eye-movement sleep and dreaming. *Nature, 383*, 163–166.

Markowitsch, H. J., & Kessler, J. (2000). Massive impairment in executive functions with partial preservation of other cognitive functions: The case of a young patient with severe degeneration of the prefrontal cortex. *Exp. Brain Res., 133*, 94–102.

Markram, H. (2006). The blue brain project. *Nat. Rev. Neurosci., 7*, 153–160.

Martinez-Conde, S., Macknik, S. L., & Hubel, D. H. (2002). The function of bursts of spikes during visual fixation in the awake primate lateral geniculate nucleus and primary visual cortex. *Proc. Natl. Acad. Sci. U.S.A., 99*, 13920–13925.

Martinez-Conde, S., Macknik, S. L., & Hubel, D. H. (2004). The role of fixational eye movements in visual perception. *Nat. Rev. Neurosci., 5*, 229–240.

Martinez-Conde, S., Macknik, S. L., Troncoso, X. G., & Dyar, T. A. (2006). Microsaccades counteract visual fading during fixation. *Neuron, 49,* 297–305.

Martinez-Conde, S., Cudeiro, J., Grieve, K. L., Rodriguez, R., Rivadulla, C., et al. (1999). Effects of feedback projections from area 18 layers 2/3 to area 17 layers 2/3 in the cat visual cortex. *J. Neurophysiol., 82,* 2667–2675.

Mason, M. F., Norton, M. I., Van Horn, J. D., Wegner, D. M., Grafton, S. T., et al. (2007). Wandering minds: The default network and stimulus-independent thought. *Science, 315,* 393–395.

Massimini, M., Huber, R., Ferrarelli, F., Hill, S., et al. (2004). The sleep slow oscillation as a traveling wave. *J. Neurosci., 24,* 6862–6870.

Massimini, M., Ferrarelli, F., Huber, R., Esser, S. K., Singh, H., et al. (2005). Breakdown of cortical effective connectivity during sleep. *Science, 309,* 2228–2232.

Massimini, M., Ferrarelli, F., Esser, S. K., Riedner, B. A., Huber, R., et al. (2007). Triggering sleep slow waves by transcranial magnetic stimulation. *Proc. Natl. Acad. Sci. U.S.A., 104,* 8496–8501.

Mataro, M., Jurado, M. A., Garcia-Sanchez, C., Barraquer, L., Costa-Jussa, F. R., et al. (2001). Long-term effects of bilateral frontal brain lesion: 60 years after injury with an iron bar. *Arch. Neurol., 58,* 1139–1142.

Melloni, L., Molina, C., Pena, M., Torres, D., Singer, W., et al. (2007). Synchronization of neural activity across cortical areas correlates with conscious perception. *J. Neurosci., 27,* 2858–2865.

Merikle, P. M., & Joordens, S. (1997). Parallels between perception without attention and perception without awareness. *Conscious Cogn., 6,* 219–236.

Miller, J. W., & Ferrendelli, J. A. (1990). Characterization of GABAergic seizure regulation in the midline thalamus. *Neuropharmacology, 29,* 649–655.

Miller, J. W., Hall, C. M., Holland, K. D., & Ferrendelli, J. A. (1989). Identification of a median thalamic system regulating seizures and arousal. *Epilepsia, 30,* 493–500.

Montaser-Kouhsari, L., & Rajimehr, R. (2004). Attentional modulation of adaptation to illusory lines. *J. Vis., 4,* 434–444.

Munk, M. H., Roelfsema, P. R., Konig, P., Engel, A. K., & Singer, W. (1996). Role of reticular activation in the modulation of intracortical synchronization. *Science, 272,* 271–274.

Naccache, L., Blandin, E., & Dehaene, S. (2002). Unconscious masked priming depends on temporal attention. *Psychol. Sci., 13,* 416–424.

Nakakimura, K., Sakabe, T., Funatsu, N., Maekawa, T., & Takeshita, H. (1988). Metabolic activation of intercortical and corticothalamic pathways during enflurane anesthesia in rats. *Anesthesiology, 68,* 777–782.

O'Regan, J. K., & Noe, A. (2001). A sensorimotor account of vision and visual consciousness. *Behav. Brain Sci., 24,* 939–973; discussion 973–1031.

Ori, C., Dam, M., Pizzolato, G., Battistin, L., & Giron, G. (1986). Effects of isoflurane anesthesia on local cerebral glucose utilization in the rat. *Anesthesiology, 65,* 152–156.

Owen, A. M., Coleman, M. R., Boly, M., Davis, M. H., Laureys, S., et al. (2006). Detecting awareness in the vegetative state. *Science, 313,* 1402.

Pascual-Leone, A., & Walsh, V. (2001). Fast backprojections from the motion to the primary visual area necessary for visual awareness. *Science, 292,* 510–512.

Pashler, H. (1998). *The psychology of attention.* Cambridge, MA: MIT Press.

Poppel, E., & Artin, T. (1988). *Mindworks: Time and conscious experience.* Boston: Harcourt Brace Jovanovich.

Posner, M. I. (1994). Attention: The mechanisms of consciousness. *Proc. Nat. Acad. Sci. U.S.A., 91,* 7398–7403.

Raymond, J. E., Shapiro, K. L., & Arnell, K. M. (1992). Temporary suppression of visual processing in an RSVP task: An attentional blink? *J. Exp. Psychol. Hum. Percept. Perform., 18,* 849–860.

Reddy, L., & Koch, C. (2006). Face identification in the near-absence of focal attention. *Vision Res., 46,* 2336–2343.

Reddy, L., Wilken, P., & Koch, C. (2004). Face-gender discrimination is possible in the near-absence of attention. *J. Vis., 4,* 106–117.

Rees, G., & Frith, C. (2007). Methodologies for identifying the neural correlates of consciousness. In M. Velmans & S. Schneider (Eds.), *The Blackwell companion to consciousness* (pp. 553–566). Oxford, UK: Blackwell.

Ro, T., Breitmeyer, B., Burton, P., Singhal, N. S., & Lane, D. (2003). Feedback contributions to visual awareness in human occipital cortex. *Curr. Biol., 13,* 1038–1041.

Roelfsema, P. R., Engel, A. K., Konig, P., & Singer, W. (1997). Visuomotor integration is associated with zero time-lag synchronization among cortical areas. *Nature, 385,* 157–161.

Rolls, E. T., Tovee, M. J., & Panzeri, S. (1999). The neurophysiology of backward visual masking: information analysis. *J. Cogn. Neurosci., 11,* 300–311.

Rossi, A. F., Desimone, R., & Ungerleider, L. G. (2001). Contextual modulation in primary visual cortex of macaques. *J. Neurosci., 21,* 1698–1709.

Schiff, N. D. (2006a). Multimodal neuroimaging approaches to disorders of consciousness. *J. Head Trauma Rehabil., 21,* 388–397.

Schiff, N. D. (2006b). Measurements and models of cerebral function in the severely injured brain. *J. Neurotrauma, 23,* 1436–1449.

Schiff, N. D., Giacino, J. T., Kalmar, K., Victor, J. D., Baker, K., et al. (2007). Behavioural improvements with thalamic stimulation after severe traumatic brain injury. *Nature, 448,* 600–603.

Schoffelen, J. M., Oostenveld, R., & Fries, P. (2005). Neuronal coherence as a mechanism of effective corticospinal interaction. *Science, 308,* 111–113.

Scholte, H. S., Witteveen, S. C., Spekreijse, H., & Lamme, V. A. (2006). The influence of inattention on the neural correlates of scene segmentation. *Brain Res., 1076,* 106–115.

Sergent, C., Baillet, S., & Dehaene, S. (2005). Timing of the brain events underlying access to consciousness during the attentional blink. *Nat. Neurosci., 8,* 1391–1400.

Sheinberg, D. L., & Logothetis, N. K. (1997). The role of temporal cortical areas in perceptual organization. *Proc. Natl. Acad. Sci. U.S.A., 94,* 3408–3413.

Siegel, J. (2000). Narcolepsy. *Sci. Am., 282,* 76–81.

Silvanto, J., Cowey, A., Lavie, N., & Walsh, V. (2005). Striate cortex (V1) activity gates awareness of motion. *Nat. Neurosci.*, *8*, 143–144.

Singer, W. (1999). Neuronal synchrony: A versatile code for the definition of relations? *Neuron*, *24*, 49–65, 111–125.

Singer, W., & Gray, C. M. (1995). Visual feature integration and the temporal correlation hypothesis. *Ann. Rev. Neurosci.*, *18*, 555–586.

Sperling, G., & Dosher, B. (1986). Strategy and optimization in human information processing. In K. Boff, L. Kaufman, & J. Thomas (Eds.), *Handbook of perception and human performance* (pp. 1–65). New York: Wiley.

Steriade, M. (2003). The corticothalamic system in sleep. *Front. Biosci.*, *8*, D878–899.

Steriade, M., Timofeev, I., & Grenier, F. (2001). Natural waking and sleep states: a view from inside neocortical neurons. *J. Neurophysiol.*, *85*, 1969–1985.

Super, H., Spekreijse, H., & Lamme, V. A. (2001). Two distinct modes of sensory processing observed in monkey primary visual cortex (V1). *Natl. Neurosci.*, *4*, 304–310.

Thorpe, S., Fize, D., & Marlot, C. (1996). Speed of processing in the human visual system. *Nature*, *381*, 520–522.

Tong, F. (2003). Primary visual cortex and visual awareness. *Nat. Rev. Neurosci.*, *4*, 219–229.

Tong, F., Nakayama, K., Vaughan, J. T., & Kanwisher, N. (1998). Binocular rivalry and visual awareness in human extrastriate cortex. *Neuron*, *21*, 753–759.

Tononi, G. (2004a). Consciousness and the brain: Theoretical aspects. In G. Adelman & B. Smith (Eds.), *Encyclopedia of neuroscience* (3rd ed.). Elsevier.

Tononi, G. (2004b). An information integration theory of consciousness. *BMC Neurosci.*, *5*, 42.

Tononi, G. (2005). Consciousness, information integration, and the brain. *Prog. Brain Res.*, *150*, 109–126.

Tononi, G., & Edelman, G. M. (1998). Consciousness and complexity. *Science*, *282*, 1846–1851.

Tononi, G., Sporns, O., & Edelman, G. M. (1992). Reentry and the problem of integrating multiple cortical areas: Simulation of dynamic integration in the visual system. *Cereb. Cortex*, *2*, 310–335.

Tononi, G., Sporns, O., & Edelman, G. M. (1996). A complexity measure for selective matching of signals by the brain. *Proc. Natl. Acad. Sci. U.S.A.*, *93*, 3422–3427.

Tse, P. U., Martinez-Conde, S., Schlegel, A. A., & Macknik, S. L. (2005). Visibility, visual awareness, and visual masking of simple unattended targets are confined to areas in the occipital cortex beyond human V1/V2. *Proc. Natl. Acad. Sci. U.S.A.*, *102*, 17178–17183.

Tsuchiya, N., & Koch, C. (2005). Continuous flash suppression reduces negative afterimages. *Nat. Neurosci.*, *8*, 1096–1101.

Vahle-Hinz, C., Detsch, O., Siemers, M., & Kochs, E. (2007). Contributions of GABAergic and glutamatergic mechanisms to isoflurane-induced suppression of thalamic somatosensory information transfer. *Exp. Brain Res.*, *176*, 159–172.

VanRullen, R., & Koch, C. (2003). Visual selective behavior can be triggered by a feed-forward process. *J. Cogn. Neurosci.*, *15*, 209–217.

Velly, L. J., Rey, M. F., Bruder, N. J., Gouvitsos, F. A., Witjas, T., et al. (2007). Differential dynamic of action on cortical and subcortical structures of anesthetic agents during induction of anesthesia. *Anesthesiology*, *107*, 202–212.

Vogel, E. K., Luck, S. J., & Shapiro, K. L. (1998). Electrophysiological evidence for a postperceptual locus of suppression during the attentional blink. *J. Exp. Psychol. Hum. Percept. Perform.*, *24*, 1656–1674.

Voss, H. U., Uluc, A. M., Dyke, J. P., Watts, R., Kobylarz, E. J., et al. (2006). Possible axonal regrowth in late recovery from the minimally conscious state. *J. Clin. Invest.*, *116*, 2005–2011.

Wolfe, J. M. (1984). Reversing ocular dominance and suppression in a single flash. *Vision Res.*, *24*, 471–478.

Womelsdorf, T., Schoffelen, J. M., Oostenveld, R., Singer, W., Desimone, R., et al. (2007). Modulation of neuronal interactions through neuronal synchronization. *Science*, *316*, 1609–1612.

Zhang, F., Wang, L. P., Brauner, M., Liewald, J. F., Kay, K., et al. (2007). Multimodal fast optical interrogation of neural circuitry. *Nature*, *446*, 633–639.

Index of Contributors

Addis, D.R., 39–60
Aharoni, E., 145–160
Andrews-Hanna, J.R., 1–38

Buckner, R.L., 1–38, 39–60
Burgess, N., 77–97

Casey, B.J., 111–126

de Oliveira-Souza, R., 161–180

Funk, C., 145–160

Gazzaniga, M., 145–160
Grady, C.L., 127–144

Hare, T.A., 111–126

Jones, R.M., 111–126

Kingstone, A., ix
Koch, C., 239–261

Làdavas, E., 98–110
Lambon Ralph, M.A., 61–76

Miller, M.B., ix
Moll, J., 161–180

Owen, A.M., 225–238

Patterson, K., 61–76

Rushworth, M.F.S., 181–207

Schacter, D.L., 1–38, 39–60
Sinnott-Armstrong, W., 145–160

Todorov, A., 208–224
Tononi, G., 239–261

Zahn, R., 161–180